Burg · Dummer (Eds.)

Strategies for Immunointerventions in Dermatology

Springer
Berlin
Heidelberg
New York
Barcelona
Budapest
Hong Kong
London
Milan
Paris
Santa Clara
Singapore
Tokyo

Günter Burg Reinhard G. Dummer (Eds.)

Strategies for Immunointerventions in Dermatology

With 35 Figures und 22 Tables

Springer

Burg, Günter, Prof. Dr.
Chairman of the Department of
Dermatology
University Hospital Zurich
Gloriastrasse 31

CH-8091 Zurich, Switzerland

Dummer, Reinhard G., PD Dr.
Department of Dermatology
University Hospital Zurich
Gloriastrasse 31

CH-8091 Zurich, Switzerland

Sponsored by an educational grant from
Novartis Pharma Schweiz AG

Library of Congress Cataloging-in-Publication Data
Strategies for immunointerventions in dermatology / Günter Burg, Reinhard Dummer (eds.).
p. cm.
Includes bibliographical references and index.
ISBN-13: 978-3-642-64539-6 e-ISBN-13: 978-3-642-60752-3
DOI: 10.1007/978-3-642-60752-3
1. Skin-Diseases-Immunological aspects. 2. Dermatopharmacology. 3. Immunopharmacology. I. Burg, Günter. II. Dummer, Richard, 1960-
RL97.S77 1997
616.5'061-dc21

Production and Supervision: W. Bischoff, Heidelberg
Cover Design: Design & Production, Heidelberg
Typesetting and Reproduction of Figures: Renner Typografie & Satz, Wiesenbach

SPIN: 10554459 23/3134 – 5 4 3 2 1 0 – Printed on acid-free paper

Preface

The skin provides the structural and functional prerequisites for an array of cellular and humoral immune reactions assocoiated with a broad spectrum of dermatoses. Depend-ing on the type of disease, immunosuppresive or immunostimulatory therapeutic strategies may offer specific and well-tolerated treatment modalities. This book gives an updated overview – which is necessarily incomplete – of those substances and drugs currently in use which show immunostimulatory or immunosuppressive effects. The use of these substances is described from a clinician's point of view for various indications, such as autoimmune diseases, and neoplasias in particular malignant melanoma.

The constributors are all experts, most with long standing experience in treating patients, which makes this book a primary source of knowledge of the extremely exciting and clinically important issue of immunointervention. Clinicians are informed about recent developments and researchers about the clinical and immunologic aspects of skin diseases.

Günter Burg, M.D.
Reinhard Dummer, M.D.

Contents

1 Basic Aspects

A Rational Approach to Immune Intervention
T.M. Kündig 1

Skin as an Immunocompetent Organ in Health and Disease
T. Bieber and A. Wollenberg 21

2 Immunosuppressive and Antiinflammatory Compounds

Cyclosporin A
T. Wrone-Smith and B.J. Nickoloff 29

Rapamycin
F. O. Nestle 43

FK-506/Tacrolimus
A. Wollenberg and T. Bieber 53

Low-Dose Methotrexate: An Immunomodifying Therapeutic Strategy for Dermatologic Diseases
I. Boehm and R. Bauer 59

Leflunomide
R. Dummer, G. Hofbauer, G. Burg, and R. R. Bartlett 71

Fusion Toxins
F. M. Foss 79

Dermatological Phototherapy: A Prime Example of Ultraviolet Radiation-Induced Immunointervention
J. Krutmann 89

Cytokines with Immunosuppressive Capacities
T.A. Luger and M. Böhm 101

Extracorporeal Photochemotherapy
M. Girardi and P. Heald 119

Glucocorticosteroids
C. A. Akdis 131

High-Dose Intravenous Immunoglobulins
G. Messer and M. Meurer 147

3 Immunostimulatory Substances and Vaccination Therapies

Interferon-α Therapy in Dermatology
M. Micksche 161

Tumor Necrosis Factors
R.M. Trüeb 169

Cytokines and Cytokine Gene Transfer in Cancer Treatment
D. Schadendorf 181

Development of a DNA Vaccine Against Malignant Melanoma
K. Moelling, B. Strack, M. Nawrath, J. Heinrich, C. Döhring, S. N. Wagner, and J. Pavlovic 195

Low Molecular Weight Cytokine Inducers
P. Stütz and E. Liehl 207

4 Clinical Aspects of Immunosuppression and Immunostimulation

4.1 Dermatoses Treated with Immunosuppressives 217

Autoimmune Bullous Diseases
D. Zillikens and L.A. Diaz 217

Rheumatic Disease Group
R.M. Trüeb 227

Atopic Dermatitis
U. Reinhold 243

Psoriasis – Mediation of Skin Phenotype by Circulatory Pathogenic T Lymphocytes
B.J. Nickoloff 253

Vasculitis Allergica
B. Zelger 263

Contact Dermatitis
A.H. Enk and J. Knop 273

Pyoderma Gangrenosum
P. Schmid-Grendelmeier 283

4.2 Dermatoses Treated with Immunostimulatory Drugs and Vaccination Therapies 293

4.2.1 Infections 293

Viral Infections: Human Papillomavirus Infections Treated with Immunostimulatory Drugs and Vaccination Therapies
G. Gross 293

Immunostimulation and Vaccination Therapy of Human Immunodeficiency Virus Infection
N.S. Penneys 307

Cytokine Therapy and Vaccination in Tropical Diseases:
Leishmaniasis and Leprosy
G. Kolde and C. Sunderkötter 311

4.2.2 Neoplasms 321

Cutaneous Lymphomas
G. Burg, R. Dummer, and F. O. Nestle 321

Non-melanoma Skin Cancer
S.A. Buechner 337

Therapy of Kaposi's Sarcoma
W. Kempf 347

4.2.3 Strategies for Immunointervention in Malignant Melanoma 357

Adjuvant Melanoma Therapy
A. Hauschild and E. Stockfleth 357

Cytokine-Based Treatments for Advanced Melanoma
U. Keilholz and C. Scheibenbogen 365

Gene Therapy: A New Perspective for the Treatment of Malignant Melanoma
D. Schadendorf and R. Dummer 375

Topical Immunotherapy of Malignant Melanoma
K. Zepter and A. Häffner 387

Vaccination with Dendritic Cells — A Specific Immunomodulatory Approach
for the Treatment of Malignant Melanoma
D. Schadendorf, S. Grabbe, and F.O. Nestle 399

Subject Index 410

List of Contributors

Akdis, C.A., M.D.
Swiss Institute of Allergy and Asthma Research (SIAF),
Obere Str. 22,
CH-7270 Davos, Switzerland

Bartlett, R. R., M.D.
Biomedical Research, TA Rheumatology/ Immunology, Hoechst Marion Roussel,
Hoechst AG Werk Kalle-Albert,
65174 Wiesbaden, Germany

Bauer, R., M.D.
Rhein. Friedrich-Wilhelms-Universität
Klinik und Poliklinik für
Haut und Geschlechtskrankheiten
Sigmund-Freud-Str. 25
53105 Bonn, Germany

Bieber, T., Prof. Dr. Dr.
Dermatologische Klinik und Poliklinik der Ludwig-Maximilians-Universität München,
Frauenlobstr. 9–11,
80337 München, Germany

Boehm, I., M.D.
Department of Dermatoloy,
University of Bonn,
Sigmund-Freud-Str. 25,
53105 Bonn, Germany

Böhm, M., M.D..
Department of Dermatology,
University of Münster,
Von-Esmarch-Str. 56,
48149 Münster, Germany

Buechner, S. A., M.D.
Dermatologische Universitätspoliklinik,
Kantonsspital Basel,
Petersgraben 4,
CH-4031 Basel, Switzerland

Burg, G., M.D.
Chairman of the Department of Dermatology,
University Hospital Zurich,
Gloriastr. 31,
CH-8091 Zurich, Switzerland

Diaz, L. A., M.D.
Department of Dermatology,
Medical College of Wisconsin,
8701 Watertown Plank Road,
Milwaukee, WI 53226, USA

Döhring, C., M.D.
Basel Institute for Immunology,
Grenzacher Str. 487,
CH-4005 Basel, Switzerland

Dummer, R., M.D.
Department of Dermatology,
University Hospital Zurich,
Gloriastr. 31,
CH-8091 Zurich, Switzerland

Enk, A.H., M.D.
Klinikum,
Department of Dermatology,
Johannes Gutenberg-Universität Mainz,
Langenbeckstr. 1,
55131 Mainz, Germany

Foss, F. M., M.D.
Boston University Medical Center,
88 East Newton Street,
Boston, MA 02118, USA

Girardi, M., M.D.
Yale University School of Medicine,
Dermatology Department,
15 York Street,
New Haven, CT 06510, USA

Grabbe, S., M.D.
Department of Dermatology,
University of Münster,
Von-Esmarch-Str. 56,
48149 Münster, Germany

Gross, G., M.D.
Dermatologische Klinik und Poliklinik,
Medizinische Fakultät,
Universität Rostock,
Augustenstr. 80–85,
18055 Rostock, Germany

Häffner, A., M.D.
Department of Dermatology,
University of Zurich,
Gloriastr. 31,
CH-8091 Zurich, Switzerland

Hauschild, A., M.D.
Department of Dermatology,
University of Kiel,
Schittenhelmstr. 7,
24105 Kiel, Germany

Heald, P.W., M.D.
Yale University School of Medicine,
Dermatology Department,
15 York Street,
New Haven, CT 06510, USA

Hofbauer, G., M.D.
Department of Dermatology,
University Hospital Zurich,
Gloriastr. 31,
CH-8091 Zurich, Switzerland

Keilholz, U., M.D.
Department of Medicine V,
University of Heidelberg,
Hospitalstr. 3,
69115 Heidelberg, Germany

Kempf, W., M.D.
Department of Dermatology,
University Hospital Zurich,
Gloriastr. 31,
CH-8091 Zurich, Switzerland

Knop, J., M.D.
Klinikum, Department of Dermatology,
Johannes Gutenberg-Universität Mainz,
Langenbeckstr. 1,
55131 Mainz, Germany

Kolde, G., M.D.
Department of Dermatology,
Virchow-Klinikum,
Humboldt-University of Berlin,
Augustenburger Platz 1,
13353 Berlin, Germany

Krutmann, J., Univ.-Prof. Dr.
Clinical and Experimental
Photodermatology,
Department of Dermatology,
Heinrich-Heine-University,
Moorenstr. 5,
40225 Düsseldorf, Germany

Kündig, T., M.D.
Department of Dermatology,
University Hospital Zurich,
Gloriastr. 31,
CH-8091 Zurich, Switzerland

Liehl, Ekke, M.D.
Sandoz Forschungsinstitut GmbH,
Brunner Str. 59,
A-1235 Vienna, Austria

Luger, T.A., M.D.
Department of Dermatology,
University of Münster,
Von-Esmarch-Str. 56,
48149 Münster, Germany

Messer, G., M.D.
Department of Dermatology,
Ludwig-Maximilians-Universität
München,
Frauenlobstr. 9-11,
80337 München, Germany

Meurer, M., M.D.
Department of Dermatology,
Medizinische Fakultät Carl Gustav Carus,
Technische Universität Dresden,
Fetscherstr. 74,
01307 Dresden, Germany

Micksche, M., M.D.
Department of Applied & Experimental
Oncology, Institute for Tumor
Biology/Cancer Research,
Vienna University Medical School,
Borschkegasse 8a,
A-1090 Vienna, Austria

Moelling, K., M.D.
Institute of Medical Virology,
University of Zurich,
Gloriastr. 30,
CH-8028 Zurich, Switzerland

Nawrath, M., M.D.
Institute of Medical Virology,
University of Zurich,
Gloriastr. 30,
CH-8028 Zurich, Switzerland

Nestle, F. O., M.D.
Department of Dermatology,
University of Zurich Medical School,
Gloriastr. 31,
8091 Zurich, Switzerland

Nickoloff, B. J., M.D., Ph.D.
Department of Pathology,
Skin Disease Research Laboratories,
Loyola University Medical Center,
Oncology Institute-Room 301,
2160 South First Avenue,
Maywood, IL 60153-5385, USA

Pavlovic, J., M.D.
Institute of Medical Virology,
University of Zurich,
Gloriastr. 30,
CH-8028 Zurich, Switzerland

Penneys, N. S., M.D., Ph.D., M.B.A.
Department of Dermatology,
Saint Louis University
Medical Science Center,
1402 S.Grand Blvd,
St. Louis, 63104, USA

Reinhold, U., M.D.
Universitäts-Hautklinik,
Sigmund-Freud-Str. 25,
53105 Bonn, Germany

Schadendorf, M.D.
Klinische Kooperationseinheit
für Dermatoonkologie (DKFZ),
Hautklinik des Klinikum Mannheim
Theodor-Kutzer-Ufer 1
68135 Mannheim, Germany

Scheibenbogen, C., M.D.
Department of Medicine V,
University of Heidelberg,
Hospitalstr. 3,
69115 Heidelberg, Germany

Schmid-Grendelmeier, P., M.D.
Dermatologisches Ambulatorium des
Stadtspitals Triemli,
Herman Greulich-Str. 70,
CH-8004 Zürich, Switzerland

Stockfleth, E., M.D.
Department of Dermatology,
University of Kiel,
Schittenhelmstr. 7,
24105 Kiel, Germany

Strack, B., M.D.
Institute of Medical Virology,
University of Zurich,
Gloriastr. 30,
CH-8028 Zurich, Switzerland

Stütz, P., PhD
Sandoz Forschungsinstitut GmbH,
Brunner Str. 59,
A-1235 Vienna, Austria

Sunderkötter, C., M.D.
Department of Dermatology and
Institute of Experimental Dermatology,
University of Münster,
Von-Esmarch-Str. 56,
48149 Münster, Germany

Trüeb, R.M., M.D.
Department of Dermatolotgy,
University Hospital of Zürich,
Gloriastr. 31,
CH-8091 Zürich, Switzerland

Wagner, S.N., M.D.
Klinik und Poliklinik für Dermatologie,
Venerologie und Allergologie,
Universitätsklinikum Essen,
Hufelandstr. 55,
45147 Essen, Germany

Wollenberg, A., M.D.
Dermatologische Klinik und Poliklinik
der Ludwig-Maximilians-Universität
München,
Frauenlobstr. 9–11,
80337 München, Germany

Wrone-Smith, T., M.D.
Loyola University Medical Center,
Oncology Institute-Room 30,
2160 South First Avenue,
Maywood, IL 60153-5385, USA

Zelger, B., M.D.
Department of Dermatology,
University of Innsbruck,
Anichstr. 35,
A-6020 Innsbruck, Austria

Zepter, K., M.D.
Klinikum Aachen,
Department of Dermatology, RWTH
Pauwelsstr. 20
52074 Aachen, Germany

Zillikens, D., M.D.
Department of Dermatology,
Medical College of Wisconsin,
8701 Watertown Plank Road,
Milwaukee, WI 53226, USA

1 Basic Aspects

A Rational Approach to Immune Intervention

T. M. Kündig

Introduction

How the Immune System Recognizes Invaders but Tolerates the Body

Change of Concepts

Not too long ago, it was still a mystery how the immune system was able to recognize the infinite number of viruses, bacteria, and other parasites and foreign elements. It was thought that antigens served as a template around which antibodies molded themselves to gain a complementary form. In 1955, Niels K. Jerne was the first to suggest that the immune response was selective rather than instructive, i.e., that the immune system has the capacity to synthesize billions of different antibodies and that encountering antigen only increases production of the antibody that makes the best fit. Soon afterwards, Macfarlane Burnet and David Talmage suggested that each lymphocyte bears only one particular antibody as a receptor and that, after encounter with antigen, it divides to start mass production of the relevant antibody. Later, Susumu Tonegawa elucidated the molecular mechanism that generates the enormous diversity of antibodies, and discovery of the genes coding for the T cell receptor (TCR) by Tak W. Mak revealed that TCR diversity is generated in a similar way.

After it had become clear that the immune system can recognize millions of antigens by random generation of diverse TCR and antibodies, the next question was how reactivity against self-antigens was prevented. Joshua Lederberg therefore suggested that immature lymphocytes, in contrast to mature lymphocytes, die instead of becoming activated when encountering specific antigen, a theory later called the clonal deletion theory. Clonal deletion of immature T cells in the thymus is still regarded as the most important mechanism of self tolerance.

Current Concept of Self – Nonself Discrimination

T cell maturation and the random rearrangement of the TCR takes place in the thymus. Immature T cells recognizing antigens present in the thymus are deleted. However, not all self-antigens are present in the thymus. Many self-proteins are expressed exclusively in highly differentiated organ tissue, such as the pancreas or the kidney. It is now clear that T cells specific for such exclusively extrathymic antigens mature normally and recirculate in the periphery. Potentially self-reactive lymphocyte receptors may also arise in the periphery from somatic mutations during proliferation of mature lympho-

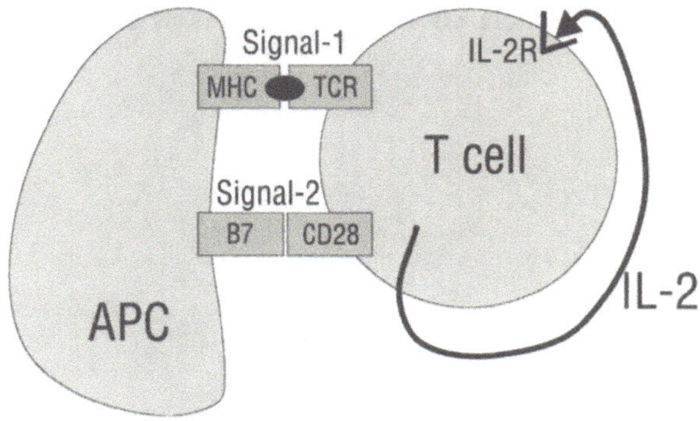

Fig. 1. Two-signal model of T cell activation. The T cell receives signal 1 through T cell receptor (*TCR*) binding to an antigenic peptide presented on major histocompatibility complex (*MHC*) molecules. Signal 2 is mediated via CD28 binding to B7 molecules on the professional antigen-presenting cell (*APC*). Signal 2 significantly enhances interleukin (*IL*)-2 production by the T cell, which stimulates T cell proliferation in an autocrine fashion. *IL-2R*, IL-2 receptor

cytes (formerly called "forbidden clones"). Thus there must be an additional, peripheral tolerance mechanism which prevents these potentially self-reactive T cells from causing disease.

The two-signal model of lymphocyte activation is considered the most important mechanism of peripheral tolerance (Fig. 1). The induction of naive, resting T lymphocytes to produce effector cells requires two sets of signaling events. The first signal (signal 1) is antigen specific and is received through the TCR after engaging antigenic peptide on major histocompatibility complex (MHC) molecules. The first signal alone is insufficient for the induction of T cell responses. Secondary, costimulatory signals (signal 2) are required for T cells to proliferate and differentiate into effector cells. Originally proposed by Bretscher and Cohen for B cells [12], this two-signal model of lymphocyte activation has been expanded to all lymphocyte subpopulations [63, 96].

Cells involved in the processing of exogenous foreign antigens, such as macrophages, dendritic cells, Langerhans cells, and B cells, are the only cells which can provide costimulatory signals and thus induce immune responses. They are therefore called professional antigen-presenting cells (APC). Since no other cells of the body can provide T cells with costimulation, tissue-specific self-antigens do not result in the induction of T cell responses, and autoimmunity is avoided. Furthermore, if T cells receive signal 1 via the TCR in the absence of signal 2, this is not merely a neutral event for the cell; such encounters with antigen induce a state of T cell unresponsiveness to further antigenic stimulation, a state called T cell anergy [96]. Thus the immunogenicity of an antigen is determined by the cell that presents the antigen to the immune system.

At the molecular level, the second signal is most importantly mediated by B7 molecules, which are present on the surface of professional APC [51]. The interaction of this B7 molecule with the CD28 receptor on the T cell markedly increases the production of interleukin (IL)-2, the major growth hormone of the immune system. In an autocrine fashion, IL-2 then promotes T cell proliferation, which is a prerequisite for an efficient T cell response. In the absence of the second signal, the insufficient production of IL-2 allows only for some abortive T cell proliferation before cells become anergic. Importantly, anergy can be prevented or even reversed when exogenous IL-2 is provided [96, 97].

Goals of Immune Intervention

The goals of immune intervention comprise augmentation of the immune response against tumors and pathogens, suppression of the immune response causing autoimmune disease and graft rejection, and deviation of misled immune responses causing allergies. This review focuses on tumor vaccination, immune suppression in autoimmune disease, and immune deviation in allergies, as these three topics are of primary interest in dermatology.

Augmentation of the Immune Response

The Problem in Tumor Immunology

The current concept of central and peripheral T cell tolerance discussed above is good and bad news as far as developing vaccines against cancer is concerned. The upside is that the central tolerance mechanism is incomplete and not all T cells reactive to self-antigens, such as tumor-specific antigens, are deleted in the thymus, so that T cells with potential reactivity to tumor-specific antigens mature and recirculate in the periphery. The downside is the existence of a peripheral tolerance mechanism which prevents activation of T cells potentially reactive to tissue-specific self-antigens and which may even anergize these T cells. However, this mechanism does not only efficiently protect normal organ tissue from autoimmune disease. Since tumors derived from such organs do not express costimulatory molecules either, this mechanism also protects tumor-specific antigens from being recognized by T cells and may even anergize tumor-specific T cells.

Tumor-Specific Antigens

The ideal target for immunotherapy of tumors are antigens which are exclusive to the tumor. Against such "truly" tumor-specific antigens no clonal deletion of T cells in the thymus occurs, and thus specific T cells can be expected to be present. In addition, immune destruction of cells bearing such antigens would have no side effects on normal tissues.

As long as the search for tumor-associated proteins was done using monoclonal antibodies, it seemed as if these proteins would usually also be expressed in the normal tissue counterpart or, in the case of oncofetal antigens, during certain stages of tissue development, such as carcinoembryonic antigen (CEA [7]).

However, since the search for tumor-specific antigens has focused on MHC class I presented peptides, the range of tumor-specific antigens has dramatically increased. The identification of antigens recognized by CD8+ T cells on tumor cells is now progressing at a tremendous pace as new techniques are being developed, including genetic [13] and peptide elution approaches [21].

Indeed, reactions of autologous T cells have now been demonstrated against several antigens which are exclusive to tumors. Such antigens include oncogene products activated by mutation or rearrangment, such as position 12 mutation in p21 *ras* [52], the p120 product of *bcr/abl* rearrangement in chronic myeloid leukemia (CML), and mutated tumor suppressor gene products, such as p53 [43]. Viral gene products expressed in virus-associated tumors form another group of "truly" tumor-specific antigens, and the presence of T cells specific for gene products of human T cell leukemia virus (HTLV) [74], Epstein-Barr virus (EBV)-associated B cell lymphoma [37], and human papillomavirus (HPV)-associated anogenital tumors have been demonstrated [11, 18, 20, 71]. In addition, idiotypic epitopes on T and B cell receptors of lymphomas, which due to random rearrangement are always unique to one specific T or B cell clone, represent "truly" tumor-specific antigens [26, 62]. Further, certain reactivated embryonic gene products may be expressed "almost exclusively" in tumors. Several such antigens have been described for malignant melanoma, e.g., MAGE-1 (melanoma-associated antigen) is expressed only in malignant melanoma and in testis [113]. Furthermore, differentiation antigens, which are expressed on cells that are not necessary for the survival of the host, may also be a target for vaccination, e.g., antigens that are specific to normal melanocytes and melanomas, such as tyrosinase, Melan-A/MART-1 (melanoma antigen recognized by T cells), gp100, and gp75 [114].

CD8$^+$ T Cells Are Antitumor Effector Cells of First Choice

In the last decade it became clear that the majority of tumor-specific antigens are mutated or rearranged oncogenes or mutated tumor suppresser genes, which are characteristic of virtually all malignancies. Most cellular proteins are intracellular in location, and these tumor-specific antigens are no exception. Therefore, most tumor-specific antigens are not accessible to antibody therapy. However, since peptides of all intracellular proteins are presented on MHC molecules, it is now emerging that T cells must be the primary effectors in antitumor vaccination strategies [10, 85, 86, 114]. Among the T cells, the CD8$^+$ subpopulation constitutes the logical primary effectors. There are two reasons for this: (1) Tumor cells usually express class I MHC molecules, and only few cell types express class II molecules (expression of class II MHC molecules is typical of professional APC, which need no help in inducing an immune response) and (2) CD8$^+$ T cells are the most effective "killer cells" of the immune system.

How To Induce a Tumor-Specific T Cell Response

Since T cells are induced most efficiently by professional APC, two strategies are possible. Either tumor cells are manipulated such that T cells mistake them for professional APC, or professional APC are made to express tumor-specific antigens.

Strategy I: Manipulation of Tumor Cells To Resemble Professional Antigen-Presenting Cells

One key parameter defining the immunogenicity of a professional APC is to provide a second signal stimulating CD28 on the T cell, which will then start producing the IL-2 it needs as an autocrine growth factor. Thus, tumor cells can be manipulated to stimulate

CD28 on the T cell by transfection with B7 [6, 19, 110]. Alternatively, bispecific antibodies binding to a tumor-specific antigen and to CD28 have been successfully used to stimulate CD28 on the T cell [91, 92]. Transfection of tumor cells with IL-2 or other costimulatory cytokines may be regarded as a "short cut," circumventing the need for stimulation of CD28 [28, 36, 68]. An alternative way to enhance CD28 stimulation is to block CTLA-4 (cytotoxic T lymphocyte-associated antigen) by the use of antibodies [3, 66]. CTLA-4 is the counterregulatory receptor for CD28 [118]. It is upregulated on activated T cells, binds to B7 with a 20-fold higher affinity than CD28, and downregulates the T cell response. This vaccination strategy may therefore be regarded as "releasing the brakes" on the T cell response which is naturally going on against the tumor [84].

Another key parameter defining the immunogenicity of professional APC is the capacity to migrate and present the antigen in a lymphoid environment. Immune responses are usually generated in the regional lymph nodes, and experimental blocking of lymphoid vessels draining a skin flap abrogates induction of T cell responses against antigens on the flap [5, 35]. We have recently shown that tumor cells may become highly immunogenic if given this migratory capacity by injection directly into lymphoid organs [60]. We further demonstrated that, in these organs, prolonged antigen presentation seems to render T cell responses independent of costimulatory signals [59, 61, 100].

Strategy II: Making Professional Antigen-Presenting Cells Present Tumor-Specific Antigens

Cells from all growing tumors eventually die and are phagocytosed by professional APC such as macrophages. However, such phagocytosed tumor-specific antigens do not usually leave the endosomal pathway and therefore enter the class I MHC pathway of antigen presentation inefficiently [38, 123], although there is recent evidence that some class I presentation may take place, at least during late tumor stages [16, 46]. This insufficient presentation of tumor-specific antigens can be dramatically enhanced by infusion of professional APC pulsed with tumor-specific antigens in vitro [124]. Dendritic cells are the first choice among professional APC, since they most potently induce CD8+ T cell responses [106], and it is now possible to obtain sufficient numbers of dendritic cells by in vitro culture of precursor cells from blood samples [49, 93]. In vitro, tumor-specific antigens can be loaded onto class I MHC molecules externally by incubation with high concentrations of the relevant class I binding peptide [17, 127]. If the class I presented peptide is not known, soluble antigen can be forced into the class I pathway in the presence of granulocyte-macrophage colony-stimulating factor (GM-CSF) [83], which is regarded as a "pro-presentation" cytokine for dendritic cells [94].

The capacity of GM-CSF to promote the differentiation of hemotogenic precursors to dendritic cells and then to enhance their capacity to present soluble antigen on class I MHC molecules [94] may also explain why tumor cells transfected with GM-CSF were found to be highly efficient vaccines [24].

Another way to make professional APC present tumor-specific antigens is immunization of the host with recombinant viruses expressing tumor-specific antigens [11].

Finally, peptides in liposomes containing lipid A can efficiently induce $CD8^+$ T cells by delivering the peptide to professional APC [4].

Naked DNA Vaccination

One way of inducing tumor-specific T cell responses which does not fit into the above-mentioned concept is naked DNA vaccination. Expression of vaccine antigens after injection of DNA plasmids into muscle cells has been found to efficiently induce long-lasting T cell responses [111, 122], although muscle cells do not express costimulatory molecules. It may, however, be speculated that it is the prolonged expression of the antigen that makes the T cell response independent of costimulation [61].

Mechanisms of Evading the Immune System Used by Tumors

Despite all the enthusiasm for vaccination protocols against cancer, it must be remembered that tumors are usually clinically diagnosed at a late stage. One gram of tumor already contains approximately 10^9 cells, and even the best vaccination protocol in mice is not able to completely clear this tumor burden.

At these late stages, it must be assumed that an immune response has already taken place. However, either the immune response was inefficient or the tumor was able to escape the immune response [31]. In fact, both probably happened, otherwise the tumor would not have reached the "diagnostic stage."

There is good evidence that "spontaneous" immune responses against tumors occur, at least during the late stages, as demonstrated by the phenomenon of concomitant immunity, i.e., mice carrying large established tumors are often protected against rechallenge with the same tumor [39]. In some tumors activated tumor-specific T cells have been demonstrated [108, 114], and in several tumors tumor-infiltrating lymphocytes (TIL) carry clonally expanded TCR sequences, suggesting antigen-specific proliferation [99]. In addition, selective pressure on tumor cells to downregulate molecules involved in immune recognition seems to exist, further suggesting that an immune response has taken place. Tumor escape mechanisms include downregulation or loss of MHC molecules [30], loss of tumor-specific antigens [112], increased expression of regulators of complement activation, such as CD46, CD55, and CD59 [31], production of T cell suppressive cytokines such as transforming growth factor (TGF)-β [107], and probably induction of T cell anergy. The latter is suggested by the finding of abnormal T cell signaling patterns in TIL [75], which can be normalized after transfection of tumor cells with IL-2 [125]. Further evidence for spontaneously occurring immune responses against tumors is the frequent observation of spontaneous tumor regression, especially in renal cell carcinoma and malignant melanoma [81].

Strategies To Prevent Immune Evasion

The fact that the tumor has already escaped the immune system is no reason to give up on tumor vaccination. Similar to bacteria, which can often escape one antibiotic monotherapy, but which can hardly escape an antibiotic combination therapy, the chances that several immune escape mutations will occur in a tumor cell at the same time are improbable. Thus the tumor has probably only escaped the predominant and first immune effector mechanism. In further analogy to antibiotic therapy, it may be important to vaccinate against several epitopes at the same time, in order to hinder escape mutants. In mice, it has been shown that a virus can readily escape a monoclonal T cell response, but not a polyclonal T cell response [88].

Suppression of the Immune Response

Autoimmune Disease

It was realized early in the study of the immune system, by Paul Ehrlich, that the powerful effector mechanisms used to defend the host against infection could turn against the host and cause severe tissue damage. In humans, autoimmune disease usually arises spontaneously. However, there is a correlation between the onset of autoimmune disease and infection. In animal models, too, the usual way of inducing experimental autoimmune disease is to mix the target tissues with adjuvants containing bacterial components. The susceptibility to autoimmune disease shows a significant genetic component. The most clear-cut and consistent susceptibility marker is the MHC genotype, and with more accurate HLA genotyping these associations become stronger. All effector mechanisms except for IgE have been shown to cause autoimmune disease, and autoimmune diseases may be classified by the mechanisms of immunological tissue damage suggested by Coombs and Gell: examples of type II antibody-mediated diseases are autoimmune hemolytic anemia, autoimmune thrombocytopenia, rheumatic fever, and pemphigus vulgaris. Glomerulonephritis, vasculitis, and arthritis seen in patients with systemic lupus erythematosus are caused by type III immune complex disease, whereas diabetes mellitus, rheumatoid arthritis, and multiple sclerosis are prototypes of type IV T cell-mediated disease.

Ways of Suppressing Immune Responses

As discussed above, several effector mechanisms may cause autoimmune disease. However, all these effector mechanisms have one thing in common, namely that the immune response begins with antigen presentation and activation of specific T cells, which then either provide help for B cells to produce antibodies or which cause the damage directly. Therapeutic attempts to target APC are dangerous, as APC such as macrophages are part of the nonspecific, nonadaptive immune system, which is indispensable for our daily survival. In contrast, T cells are the optimal target. The fact that part of the immune system still functions without them gives us a wider therapeutic range. In addition, T cell responses are sophisticatedly regulated, which in future will allow similarly sophisticated therapeutic modulation.

The induction of a T cell response requires the presence of three things (see Fig. 1): specific T cells, signal 1, and signal 2, thus providing three checkpoints for interference: (1) deletion of T cells, (2) interference with signal 1, or (3) interference with signal 2. Elimination of specific T cells and antigen-specific interference with T cell induction are the mechanisms to be preferred, as all nonspecific approaches cause considerable side effects.

Immunosuppressive Drugs

T cells involved in unwanted immune responses proliferate rapidly and may therefore be efficiently depleted by the use of cytotoxic drugs such as cyclophosphamide and azathioprin. Signal 1 can be intercepted by the use of cyclosporin A, which specifically blocks IL-2 synthesis at a late stage of the TCR signaling. Signal 2 is intercepted by rapamycin and by leflunomide, which inhibit the signaling pathway used by the IL-2 receptor. Therefore, the use of rapamycin together with cyclosporin A, blocking signaling via the IL-2 receptor as well as IL-2 production, is a highly effective combination. Corticosteroids regulate an estimated 1% of all human genes, which makes the list of anti-inflammatory and immunosuppressive effects a very long one. Not surprisingly, these highly potent inhibitors of the immune response have as many unwanted side effects. The above-mentioned drugs are reviewed by Nickoloff, Nestle, Boehm and Bauer, Dummer et al. and Akdis (this volume). However, drugs fail to take advantage of the most important feature of the immune response, i.e., antigen specificity and clonal specificity.

Antibodies

Antibodies can be used to either deplete or inhibit lymphocytes. Anti-lymphocyte globulin, a polyclonal antiserum from animals immunized with human T lymphocytes, and more recently monoclonal antibodies against the TCR, CD4 or CD8, or against integrins mediating T cell binding to APC, have all been successfully used to inhibit immune responses. However, all the above antibody therapies have the common disadvantage that they suppress both the harmful and the normal T cells, thus leading to nonspecific immune suppression.

Antigen specificity may be obtained by an approach in which nondepleting anti-CD4 antibodies are administered together with primary exposure of the antigen, thereby inducing a long-lasting state of T cell tolerance [117].

The fact that some murine autoimmune disease models show a predominant use of certain variable regions of the TCR, such as Vβ elements, raised the hope that antibody therapy against these TCR could be used [1, 2, 44]. However, in human autoimmune disease, no consistent Vβ usage has been found so far, so that high hopes in this therapeutic approach are not justified. Vaccination against T and B cell receptor idiotypes is equally difficult, since the pathogenic T and B cell responses are polyclonal.

A major drawback of antibody therapy is the fact that antibodies against human proteins can only be produced in another species, such as mice, and humans rapidly develop an anti-antibody response inhibiting their activity and producing immune complex-mediated side effects. This problem is currently being solved by the use of three approaches [121]:

1. Cloning human V regions into phage display libraries and selecting for binding to human antigens, so that entirely human antibodies are obtained.
2. Alternatively, mice lacking endogenous immunoglobulin genes can be made transgenic for human immunoglobulin loci. Since mice are not tolerant to human antigens they can readily be immunized, and hybridomas producing human antibodies specific for human antigens can be derived.

3. A third approach is the "humanization" of antibodies, i.e., construction of antibodies with antigen binding regions of the mouse grafted onto the framework of human immunoglobulins.

Fusion Proteins and Toxin Immunoconjugates

A fusion protein made from CTLA-4, a high-affinity ligand of B7, and the Fc portion of a human immunoglobulin (CTLA-4Ig) has been successfully used to block the costimulatory pathway, e.g., to prolong graft survival [67].

The cytotoxicity of monoclonal antibodies can be enhanced by conjugation of a variety of cytotoxic agents to the antibody [116]. Immunotoxins are reviewed in detail by Foss (this volume).

Altered Peptide Ligands

Until recently, signaling through the TCR has been thought of as a binary event, i.e., the TCR either does or does not deliver a signal to the T cell. In recent years, this concept has dramatically changed. The analysis of peptide analogues revealed that the TCR is able to selectively trigger T cell effector functions [23, 27, 101]. Similar to many other receptors, not only agonists, but also partial agonists and antagonists exist.

The TCR binds to a bimolecular ligand composed of the MHC molecule presenting an antigenic peptide of 8–15 amino acids in length. The crystal structures of peptide-MHC complexes revealed that only three to four amino acid side chains of the peptide are accessible to the TCR, while other amino acid side chains are involved in binding to the MHC molecule [9, 22, 34, 69]. By manipulating exclusively TCR contact residues of immunogenic peptides, while leaving the MHC binding residues unchanged, so-called altered peptide ligands can be derived, which still bind to the MHC molecule. While first described for $CD4^+$ T cells [23, 27, 101], the phenomenon of selectively triggering T cell functions or even antagonizing T cell function has also been extended to $CD8^+$ T cells [50, 82, 90].

Only peptides which provide an optimal fit for the TCR activate all functions of the T cell; such peptides are referred to as agonists. Peptides which produce a suboptimal fit of the TCR, however, induce only partial T cell activation. Such peptides may act as partial agonists by inducing only some T cell functions, but they may also act as antagonists by inhibiting the effects of wild-type peptide (Fig. 2). A third class of ligands, although binding to the MHC, induce no measurable response of the T cell and are therefore called null ligands.

How the TCR can perceive different ligands is presently a matter of debate [55]. It appears that, in contrast to wild-type peptides, partial agonist peptides not only deliver a quantitatively different, but also a qualitatively different signal, resulting in unique phosphorylation patterns of molecules involved in TCR signaling, such as the TCR-ζ chain, and failure to activate the ZAP-70-kinase [70, 103]. This signaling pattern is unique in that it cannot be reproduced simply by titrating down the agonist peptide.

The demonstration of such altered peptide ligands has offered the intriguing possibility of exclusively manipulating T cells specific for one antigenic peptide. In this respect it is particularly interesting that altered peptide ligands are able to induce T cell anergy in vitro [101, 102], i.e., T cells specific for an antigen can be selectively tolerized.

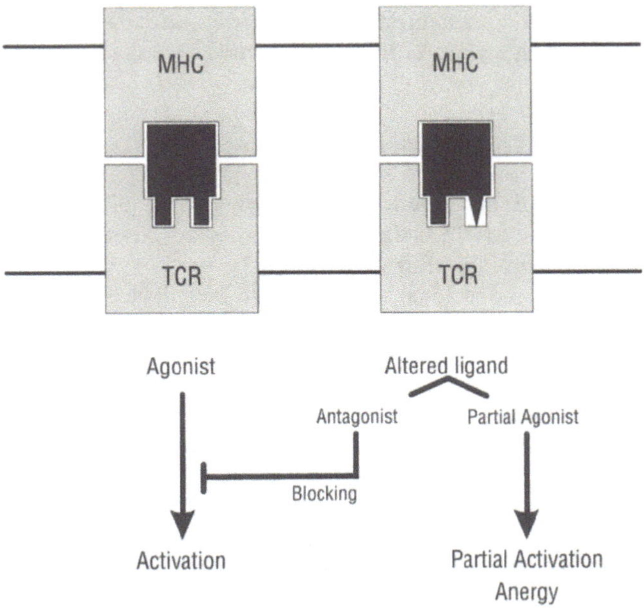

Fig. 2. Altered peptide ligands. Peptides providing an optimal fit for the T cell receptor (*TCR*) act as agonists and activate all functions of the T cell. Altered peptide ligands producing a suboptimal fit for the TCR may act as antagonists by inhibiting the effects of wild-type peptide ("blocking"), or they may act as partial agonists by inducing only some T cell functions, including induction of T cell anergy. *MHC*, major histocompatibility complex

In recent years, several studies have successfully used peptide therapy to treat autoimmune disease, such as experimental allergic encephalomyelitis (EAE) [32, 57, 104, 119]. In this model, immunization of animals with myelin basic protein (MBP) induces a $CD4^+$ T cell response causing demyelinating disease. Pretreatment of mice by injection of a MBP-peptide analogue with only one single amino acid change rendered mice resistant to induction of MBP-induced EAE [104]; the resistance lasted for up to 2 weeks [119]. Similar experiments in an adjuvant arthritis model demonstrated that inhibition of the arthritogenic T cells was antigen specific [119]. In contrast, administration of a MHC-blocker peptide, i.e., of a totally unrelated peptide with high affinity for the involved MHC molecule, induces only short-lasting inhibition of MBP-induced EAE [64, 65]. MHC-blocking peptides must be given chronically to prevent disease [47]. Thus injection of peptide analogues does not simply compete for MHC binding with the wild-type peptide, but induces a prolonged and specific inhibition of pathogenic T cells.

The finding that altered peptide ligands can trigger certain T cell functions selectively also offers the intriguing possibility not only of inhibiting an immune response, but also modulating it. Further studies in the EAE model demonstrated that injection of the altered peptide ligand changed the immune response from the pathogenic Th1 phenotype to the Th2 phenotype [78, 120].

Interestingly, viruses which have a vital interest in studying our immune system found ways to interfere and to antagonize a T cell response long before immunologists did. It has recently been found that peptides of naturally selected human immunodeficiency virus (HIV) and hepatitis B virus variants may act as antagonist peptides [8, 56], inhibiting the ability of cytotoxic T cells to lyse infected cells [73]. These viruses demonstrate that inhibition of T cell responses by suboptimal ligands may in fact be the "Achilles heel of T cells" [55]. Thus, the recent finding of altered peptide ligand-induced T cell inhibition may represent a breakthrough on our way to antigen-specific immune suppression, i.e., immune suppression without side effects.

Deviation of the Immune Response

Allergies

There is now clear evidence that alterations of T cell function cause atopic allergic disease. This concept was originally suggested by the observation that patients with primary T cell immunodeficiency disorders tend to have elevated serum IgE antibody levels and skin lesions identical to atopic dermatitis [15]. Furthermore, in Wiskott-Aldrich syndrome, normalization of immune responsiveness after bone marrow transplantation is paralleled by disappearance of skin lesions [87]. It now emerges that atopic disorders are caused by an imbalance in the T-helper (Th) cell response.

Increasing Variety of T Cell Subsets

Studies in recent years have identified two functional subsets of Th cells, Th1 and Th2 cells, which are characterized by their cytokine profiles. Mouse Th1 cells produce IL-2, interferon (IFN)-γ, and lymphotoxin, whereas Th2 cells produce IL-4, IL-5, IL-6, IL-9, IL-10, and IL-13. Human Th1 and Th2 cells produce similar patterns, but IL-6, IL-10, and IL-13 production is not as tightly restricted to Th2 cells. Other cytokines, such as IL-3, tumor necrosis factor-α, and GM-CSF are produced by both Th1 and Th2 cells. Further analysis revealed the existence of Th cells producing cytokines of both patterns, now called Th0 cells, and cells producing large amounts of TGF-β, called Th3 cells; the longer Th cell clones are held in culture, the more cytokine secretion patterns were found. In vivo and in short-term culture, however, the Th1–Th2 dichotomy remains the important functional division. Functionally, Th1 cytokines drive the immune response towards cell-mediated cytotoxic and inflammatory reactions, whereas Th2 cytokines "push" the immune response towards antibody production. In particular, IgE production and the eosinophilic response are strongly dependent on Th2 cytokines. Th1 and Th2 responses mutually inhibit each other. Th1 cytokines such as IFN-γ inhibit Th2 responses, and IL-10 and IL-4 inhibit Th1 responses. Thus, once the Th cell response has chosen its direction, it will perpetuate itself and inhibit the other type of response.

Who Decides Which Way To Go?

Th1 and Th2 cells originate from a common IL-2-secreting precursor cell. The central question is, therefore, what pushes the precursor cell in one or the other direction. Experimental evidence shows that, quite similar to the already committed Th1 or Th2 cell, the uncommitted precursor cell goes toward Th1 responses when stimulated with IFN-γ, IL-12, and TGF-β, whereas IL-4 promotes differentiation towards Th2 responses

[76]. However, during the initiation phase of the response, antigen-specific T cells have a very low frequency, so that the source of cytokines promoting either Th1 or Th2 differentiation cannot be the T cells themselves, but must be other cell types. T cells bearing γδ TCR have recently been invoked as the regulators of the Th1–Th2 balance [29]. T cells bearing γδ receptors are strategically positioned at ports of antigen entry, such as mucosal surfaces. Due to their limited specificity for certain antigens and their relatively high numbers, they can even participate in the very early phase of the immune response. Depending on the pathogen, γδ T cells were found to produce different cytokine patterns [29]. They may therefore play an important role in Th cell differentiation. Other cells which participate early in the immune response and produce characteristic cytokine patterns are natural killer (NK) cells producing IFN-γ, NK1.1-positive T cells producing IL-4, macrophages producing IL-12, and mast cells producing IL-4 and IL-10 [89].

Antigen and Immunogenetics Decide on the Type of T-Helper Cell Response

Some antigens, such as parasitic worms, cause a Th2 type response in nearly all individuals of a population. In this case, IL-4 and IL-5 production and the consecutive eosinophilic response are an important effector mechanism of host defense, as eosinophils – via their high-affinity Fc receptor for IgE – attack parasites opsonized with IgE [40]. Other antigens, such as bacterial antigens, seem to almost invariably elicit a Th1-type response. Both the proinflammatory Th cell response and the cytotoxic T cell response are crucial for host survival during bacterial and many viral infections, respectively [54, 126]. While the atopic or nonatopic disposition of an individual may enhance or decrease one or the other response, it cannot affect the vital capacity of an individual to react with either a Th1 or a Th2 response.

While potentially beneficial against parasitic worms, however, the atopic disposition is a nuisance when the individual is confronted with innocuous substances, such as pollen. It is possibly because these substances are presented to the immune system in extremely low doses that only atopic individuals which efficiently mount Th2 responses produce IgE (Fig. 3).

The hereditary component of atopic disease is well known. In the search for atopy genes, two have been localized, one in the chromosomal region of the b-chain of the high-affinity Fc receptor for IgE on chromosome 11q [95], another in a region of chromosome 5q which also codes for Th2 cytokines such as IL-4 and IL-5 [72].

Application Dose and Route of Antigen Influence Type of T-Helper Cell Response

Most allergens are proteins inhaled in desiccated particles such as pollen or mite feces. Allergens are usually highly soluble and have a low molecular weight, so that they are readily eluted from the particle and can diffuse into the mucosa. However, only minimal doses of antigen pass via this transmucosal way and are presented to the immune system. It is thought that low antigen doses favor the induction of Th2 cells over the induction of inflammatory Th1 cells. In fact, the antigen dose can influence the Th1–Th2 balance. Lowering the antigen dose can switch the immune response from the Th1 to

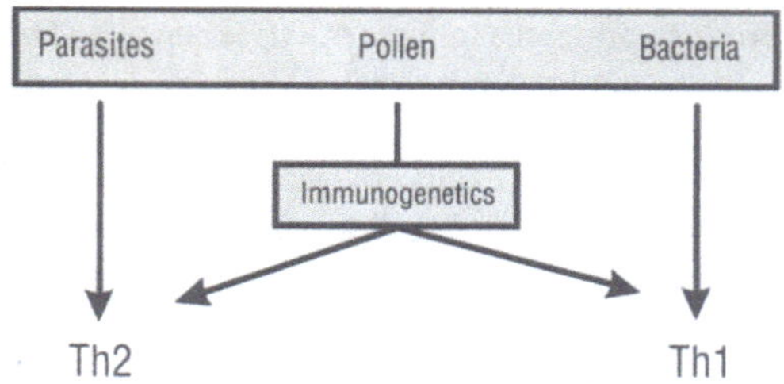

Fig. 3. Determination of T-helper cell (*Th*) differentiation. The type of antigen and immunogenetics (e.g., atopic disposition) determine the type of Th cell response. Certain antigens, such as parasites, induce a Th2 response in all individuals, whereas bacterial antigens almost invariably induce a Th1 response in all individuals. For a third group of antigens, however, the immunogenetics of the individual are decisive

the Th2 type [76]. As specific B cells carrying the highest-affinity antigen receptors in the form of surface immunoglubulins most efficiently pick up and present low-dose antigens, it is tempting to speculate that B cells preferentially induce Th2 responses, whereas antigen presentation by macrophages, which pick up the antigen left over by the B cells after administration of high antigen doses (e.g., desensitization), would preferentially induce Th1 responses. In fact, macrophages produce Th1-promoting cytokines such as IL-12 and IFN-α [45]. However, these mechanisms are not well understood and are still a matter of debate, since the influence of the antigen dose on the Th1–Th2 balance cannot be generalized. When a wide range of antigen doses are studied, biphasic curves are also observed, with low and high antigen doses inducing delayed-type hypersensitivity (DTH) and intermediate doses inducing Th2-mediated antibody responses [76]. In addition, consistent experimental evidence that the type of professional APC determines Th cell differentiation has yet not beenobtained, since macrophages, B cells, and dendritic cells are all able to induce both Th1 and Th2 responses, depending on the cytokines present [76]. A final objection is that primary T cell responses are in any case elicited by dendritic cells. Personally, I do not believe in such an exclusive role for dendritic cells [60,61], but even if it were exclusively dendritic cells priming the T cell response, later repeated exposures to allergens and presentation on other APC could drive the response in the Th1 or Th2 direction.

In contrast to typical allergens, antigens eliciting Th1-type responses, such as bacterial or viral antigens, are present in abundance and systemically, as they cause systemic infection.

Clinical Implications

New immunological therapies for the treatment of allergies and atopic dermatitis must focus on the modulation of the Th2–Th1 imbalance. While modern basic sciences struggle to define parameters determining Th cell differentiation, clinicians introduced specific immunotherapy as a treatment for pollinosis as early as 1911 [33,79]. Immunotherapy by repeated subcutaneous injections of increasing doses of allergen extracts leads to an initial increase of specific serum IgE levels, followed by a long-term increase of allergen-specific IgG, which belongs predominantly to the IgG4 subclass [25,77,105]. The IgG is thought to block antigen-stimulated mediator release by mast cells and basophils sensitized by IgE antibody [80]. In fact, the shift from IgE towards IgG production seems to be the consequence of Th1 cells gaining the upper hand over Th2 cells, as can be demonstrated during late-phase reactions in successfully desensitized individuals [53, 80, 98, 115]. In vitro and in vivo evidence suggests that immunotherapy may anergize Th2 cells [14, 41, 48].

Clinical trials using Th1 cytokine treatment such as injections with IFN-γ or IFN-α did indeed show some beneficial effects on the course of atopic skin disease, but could not lower IgE antibody levels [42, 109]. Perhaps future combinations using desensitization procedures and Th1 cytokine therapy simultaneously will increase the efficiency of such treatments.

As discussed for the treatment of autoimmune disease, altered peptide ligands may be a new hope for the future. Alteration of the relevant allergen peptides might be used either to antagonize a Th2-type response or, even more elegantly, to shift a Th2-type towards a Th1-type response [78, 120].

Summary

The immune system has to be able to protect us against countless pathogens, yet it has to tolerate every tissue cell and protein in the body. Thus the immune response must be tightly regulated, since both failure to attack a pathogen as well as an accidental attack against the body can have catastrophic results. Increasing knowledge of how the immune system is regulated may allow us to use it as a powerful therapeutic tool. The goals are to augment the immune response against cancer and pathogens, to encourage tolerance of transplanted tissue, to reprogram inappropriate responses such as allergies, and to control autoimmune disease. This chapter reviews some of the current immunological concepts behind the above-mentioned therapeutic approaches.

References

1. Acha-Orbea H, Mitchell DJ, Timmermann L, Wraith DC, Tausch GS, Waldor MK, Zamvil SS, McDevitt HO, Steinman L (1988) Limited heterogeneity of T cell receptors from lymphocytes mediating autoimmune encephalomyelitis allows specific immune intervention. Cell 54:263–273
2. Acha-Orbea H, Steinman L, McDevitt HO (1989) T cell receptors in murine autoimmune disease. Annu Rev Immunol 7:371–405
3. Allison JP, Krummel MF (1995) The yin and yang of T cell costimulation. Science 270:932–934
4. Alving CR, Koulchin V, Glenn GM, Rao M (1995) Liposomes as carriers of peptide antigens: induction of antibodies and cytotoxic T lymphocytes to conjugated and unconjugated peptides. Immunol Rev 145:1–30
5. Barker CF, Billingham RE (1967) The role of regional lymphatics in the skin homograft response. Transplantation 5:962–974
6. Baskar S, Ostrand-Rosenberg S, Nabavi N, Nadler LM, Freeman GJ, Glimcher LH (1994) Constitutive expression of B7 restores immunogenicity of tumor cells expressing truncated MHC class II molecules. Proc Natl Acad Sci USA 90:5687–5693
7. Benchimol S, Fuks A, Jothy S, Beauchemin N, Shirota K, Stanners CP (1989) Carcinoembryonic antigen, a human tumor marker, functions as intracellular adhesion molecule. Cell 57:327–333
8. Bertoletti A, Sette A, Chisari FV, Penna A, Levrero M, De Carli M, Fiaccadori F, Ferrari C (1994) Natural variants of cytotoxic epitopes are T-cell receptor antagonists for antiviral cytotoxic T cells. Nature 369:407–410
9. Bjorkman PJ, Saper MA, Samraoui B, Bennett WS, Strominger JL, Wiley DC (1987) Structure of the human class I histocompatibility antigen, HLA-A2. Nature 329:506–511

10. Boon T, van der Bruggen P (1996) Human tumor antigens recognized by T lymphocytes. J Exp Med 183:725–729
11. Borysiewicz LK, Fiander A, Nimako M, Man S, Wilkinson GWG, Westmoreland D, Evans AS, Adams M, Stacey SN, Boursnell MEG, Rutherford E, Hickling JK, Inglis SC (1996) A recombinant viaccina virus encoding human papillomavirus types 16 and 18, E6 and E7 proteins as immunotherapy for cervical cancer. Lancet 347:1523
12. Bretscher P, Cohn M (1970) A theory of self-nonself discrimination. Science 169:1042
13. Brichard V, Van Pel A, Wölfel T, Wölfel C, De Plaen E, Lethe B, Coulie P, Boon T (1993) The tyrosinase gene codes for an antigen recognized by autologous cytolytic T lymphocytes on HLA-A2 melanomas. J Exp Med 178:489–495
14. Briner TJ, Kuo MC, Keating KM, Rogers BL (1993) Peripheral T cell tolerance induced in naive and primed mice by subcutaneous injection of peptides from the major cat allergen Fel d I. Proc Natl Acad Sci USA 90:7608–7612
15. Buckley RH, Fiscus SA (1975) Serum IgD and IgE concentrations in immunodeficiency diseases. J Clin Invest 55:157–165
16. Carbone FR, Bevan MJ (1990) Class I-restricted processing and presentation of exogenous cell-associated antigen in vivo. J Exp Med 171:377–387
17. Celluzzi CM, Mayordomo JI, Storkus WJ, Lotze MT, Falo LD Jr (1996) Peptide pulsed dendritic cells induce antigen-specific CTL-mediated protective tumor immunity. J Exp Med 183:283–287
18. Chen L, Thomas EK, Hu S, Hellstrom I, Hellstrom KE (1991) Human papillomavirus type 16 nucleoprotein E7 is a tumor rejection antigen. Proc Natl Acad Sci USA 88:110–114
19. Chen L, Asche S, Brady WA, Hellström I, Hellström EK, Ledbetter JA, McGowan P, Linsley PS (1992a) Costimulation of antitumor immunity by the B7 counterreceptor for the T lymphocyte molecules CD28 and CTLA-4. Cell 71:1093–1102
20. Chen L, Mizuno MT, Singhal MC, Shiu-Lok H, Galloway DA, Hellström I, Hellström KE (1992b) Induction of cytotoxic T lymphocytes specific for a syngeneic tumor expressing the E6 oncoprotein of huma papilloma virus type 16. J Immunol 148:2617–2621
21. Cox AL, Skipper J, Chen Y, Henderson RA, Darrow TL, Shabanowitz J, Engelhard VH, HUnt DF, Slingluff CL Jr (1994) Identification of a peptide recognized by five melanoma-specific human cytotoxic T cell lines. Science 264:716–719
22. Davis MM, Bjorkman PJ (1988) T-cell antigen receptor genes and T-cell recognition. Nature 334:395–402
23. De Magistris MT, Alexander J, Coggeshall M, Altman A, Gaeta FCA, Grey HM, Sette A (1992) Antigen analog-major histocompatibility complex acts as antagonist of the T cell receptor. Cell 68:625–634
24. Dranoff G, Jaffee E, Lazenby A, Golumbek P, Levitsky H, Brose K, Jackson V, Hamada H, Pardoll D, Mulligan R (1993) Vaccination with irradiated tumor cells engeniered to secrete murine granulocyte-macrophage colony-stimulating factor stimulates potent, specific, and long-lasting anti-tumor immunity. Proc Natl Acad Sci USA 90:3539–3543
25. Einarsson R, Dreborg S, Hammarström L, Löfkvist T, Smith CIE, Svensson G (1992) Monitoring of mite dermatophagoides farinae allergen-specific IgG and IgG subclass distribution in patients on immunotherapy. Allergy 47:76–82
26. Eisen HN, Sakato N, Hall SJ (1975) Myeloma proteins as tumor specific antigens. Transplant Proc 7:209–229
27. Evavold BD, Allen PM (1991) Separation of IL-4 production from Th cell proliferation by an altered T cell receptor ligand. Science 252:1308–1310
28. Fearon ER, Pardoll DM, Itaya T, Golumbek P, Levitsky HI, Simons JW, Karasuyama H, Vogelstein B, Frost P (1990) Interleukin-2 production by tumor cells bypasses T helper function in the generation of an antitumor response. Cell 60:397–403
29. Ferrick DA, Schrenzel MD, Mulvania T, Hsieh B, Ferlin WG, Lepper H (1995) Gamma-delta T cells differentially produce interferon-gamma and interleukin-4 to Th1- and Th2-stimulating pathogens in vivo. Nature 373:255–257
30. Ferrone S, Marincola FM (1995) Loss of HLA class I antigens by melanoma cells: molecular mechanisms, functional significance and clinical relevance. Immunol Today 16:487–494

31. Fleurin GJ, Gorter A, Kuppen PJK, Litvinov S, Warnaar SO (1995) Tumor heterogeneity and immunotherapy of cancer. Immunol Rev 145:91–122
32. Franco A, Southwood S, Arrhenius T, Kuchroo VK, Grey HM, Sette A, Ishioka GY (1994) T cell receptor antagonist peptides are highly effective inhibitors of experimental allergic encephalomyelitis. Eur J Immunol 24:940–946
33. Freeman J (1911) Further observations on the treatment of hay fever by hypodermic inoculation of pollen vaccine. Lancet 2:814–817
34. Fremont DH, Matsumura M, Stura EA, Peterson PA, Wilson IA (1992) Crystal structure of two viral peptides in complex with murine MHC class I H-2kb. Science 257:919–927
35. Frey JR, Wenk P (1957) Experimantal studies on the pathogenesis on contact eczema in the guinea pig. Int Arch Allergy Appl Immunol 11:81–94
36. Gansbacher B, Zier K, Danials B, Cronin K, Bannerji R, Gilboa E (1990) Interleukin-2 gene transfer into tumor cells abrogates tumorigenicity and induces protective immunity. J Exp Med 172:1217–1224
37. Gavioli R, De Campos-Lima PO, Kurilla MG, Kieff E, Klein G, Masucci MG (1992) Recognition of the EBV encoded nuclear antigens EBNA-1 and EBNA-6 by HLA-A11 restricted cytotoxic T lymphocytes. Implications for down-regulation of HLA-A11 in Burkitt's lymphoma. Proc Natl Acad Sci USA 89:5862–5967
38. Germain RN (1986) The ins and outs of antigen processing and presentation. Nature 322: 687–689
39. Gorelik E (1983) Concomitant immunity and the resistance to a second tumor challenge. Adv Cancer Res 39:71–120
40. Gounni AS, Lamkhioued B, Ochiai K, Tanaka Y, Delaporte E, Capron A, Kinet JP, Capron M (1994) High affinity IgE receptor on eosinophils is involved in defense against parasites. Nature 367:183–186
41. Greenstein JL, Morgenstern JP, LaRaia J, Counsell CM, Goodwin WH, Lussier A, Creticos PS, Norman PS, Barman RD (1992) Ragweed immunotherapy decreases T cell reactivity to recombinant Amb a I. J Allergy Clin Immunol 89:322–328
42. Hanifin J, Schneider LC, Leung DYM, Ellis CN, Jaffe HS, Izu AE, Bucalo LR, Hirabayashi SE, Tofte SJ, Cantu GC (1993) Recombinant interferon-gamma therapy for atopic dermatitis. J Am Acad Dermatol 28:189–197
43. Houbiers JG, Nijman HW, Van der Burg SH, Drijhout JW, Kenemans P, Van de Velde CHJ, Brand A, Momburg F, Kast WM, Melief CJM (1993) In vitro induction of human cytotoxic T lymphocyte responses against peptides of mutant and wild-type p53. Eur J Immunol 23: 2072–2077
44. Howell MD, Winters ST, Olee T, Powell HC, Carlo DJ, Brostoff SW (1989) Vaccination against experimental allergic encephalomyelitis with T cell receptor peptides. Science 246:668–670
45. Hsieh CS, Macatonia SE, Tripp CS, Wolf CS, O'Garra A, Murphy KM (1993) Development of Th1 CD4 cells through IL-12 produced by listeria-induced macrophages. Science 260:547–549
46. Huang AYC, Golumbek P, Ahmadzadeh M, Jaffee E, Pardoll D, Levitsky H (1994) Role of bone marrow derived cells in presenting MHC class I-restricted tumor antigens. Science 164: 961–965
47. Hurtenbach U, Lier E, Adorini L, Nagy ZA (1993) Prevention of autoimmune diabetes in nonobese diabetic mice by treatment with a class II major histocompatibility complex binding peptide. J Exp Med 177:1499–1504
48. Iliopoulos O, Proud D, Adkinson NF, Creticos PS, Norman PS, Kagey-Sobotka A, Lichtenstein LM, Naclerio RM (1991) Effects of immunotherapy in the early, late and rechallenge nasal reaction to provocation with allergen: changes in inflammatory mediators and cells. J Allergy Clin Immunol 87:855–866
49. Inaba K, Steinman RM, Pack MW, Aya H, Inaba M, Sudo T, Wolpe S, Schuler G (1992) Identification of proliferating dendritic cell precursors in mouse blood. J Exp Med 175: 1157–1167
50. Jameson SC, Carbone FR, Bevan MJ (1993) Clone-specific T cell receptor antagonists of major histocompatibility complex class I-restricted cytotoxic T cells. J Exp Med 177:1541–1550

51. June CH, Bluestone JA, Nadler LM, Thompson CB (1994) The B7 and CD28 receptor families. Immunol Today 15:321–332
52. Jung S, Schluesener HJ (1991) Human T lymphocytes recognize a peptide of single point mutated oncogenic ras proteins. J Exp Med 173:273–279
53. Jutel M, Skribic D, Urwyler A, Pichler WJ, Müller U (1995) Ultra rush bee venom immunotherapy results in decrease of IL4 and IL5 secretion and increase of IFN-gamma in specific allergen stimulated cultures. J Immunol 154:4187–4194
54. Kaufmann SHE (1993) Immunity to intracellular bacteria. In: Paul WE (ed) Fundamental immunology. Raven, New York, pp 1251–1286
55. Kersh GJ, Allen PM (1996) Essential flexibility in the T-cell recognition of antigen. Nature 380:495–498
56. Klenerman P, Rowland-Jones S, McAdam S, Edwards J, Daenke S, Lalloo D, Köppe B, Rosenberg W, Boyd D, Edwards A, Giangrande P, Phillips RE, McMichael AJ (1994) Cytotoxic T-cell activity antagonized by naturally occurring HIV-1 Gag variants. Nature 369:403–407
57. Kuchroo VK, Greer JM, Kaul D, Ishioka G, Franco A, Sette A, Sobel RA, Lees MB (1994) A single TCR antagonist peptide inhibits experimental allergic encephalomyelitis mediated by a diverse T cell repertoire. J Immunol 153:3326–3332
58. Kündig TM, Bachmann MF, Lefrancois L, Puddington L, Hengartner H, Zinkernagel RM (1993a) Nonimmunogenic tumor cells may efficiently restimulate tumor antigen-specific cytotoxic T cells. J Immunol 150:4450–4456
59. Kündig TM, Schorle H, Bachmann MF, Hengartner H, Zinkernagel RM, Horak I (1993b) Immune responses in IL-2 deficient mice. Science 262:1059–1061
60. Kündig TM, Bachmann MF, DiPaolo C, Simard JL, Battegay M, Lother H, Gessner A, Kühlke K, Ohashi PS, Hengartner H, Zinkernagel RM (1995) Fibroblasts as efficient antigen-presenting cells in lymphoid organs. Science 268:1343–1347
61. Kündig TM, Shahinian A, Kawai K, Mittrücker HW, Sebzda E, Mak TW, Ohashi P (1996) Duration of T cell receptor stimulation determines costimulatory requirements of T cells. Immunity (in press)
62. Kwak LW, Campbell MJ, Czerwinski DK, Hart S, Miller RA, Levy R (1993) Induction of immune responses in patients with B-cell lymphoma against the surface immunoglobulin idiotype expressed by their tumors. N Engl J Med 327:1209–1215
63. Lafferty K, Woolnough J (1977) The origin and mechanism of allograft reaction. Immunol Rev 35:231–262
64. Lamont AG, Powell MF, Colon SM, Miles C, Grey HM, Sette A (1990a) The use of peptide analogs with improved stability and MHC binding capacity to inhibit antigen presentation in vitro and in vivo. J Immunol 144:2493–2498
65. Lamont AG, Sette A, Fujinami R, Colon SM, Miles C, Grey HM (1990b) Inhibition of experimental autoimmune encephalomyelitis induction in SJL/J mice by using a peptide with high affinity for IAs molecules. J Immunol 145:1687–1693
66. Leach DR, Krummel MF, Allison JP (1996) Science 271:1734–1738
67. Lenschow DJ, Zeng Y, Thistlethwaite R, Montag A, Brady W, Gibson MG, Linsley PS, Bluestone JA (1993) Long-term survival of xenogeneic pancreatic islet grafts induced by CTLA4Ig. Science 257:789–793
68. Ley V, Langlade-Demoyen P, Kourilsky P, Larsson-Sciard EL (1991) Interleukin-2 dependent activation of tumor specific cytotoxic T lymphocytes in vivo. Eur J Immunol 21:851–854
69. Madden DR, Gorga JC, Strominger JL, Wiley DC (1991) The structure of HLA-B27 reveals nonamer self-peptides bound in an extended conformation. Nature 353:321–325
70. Madrenas J, Wange RL, Wang JL, Isakov N, Samelson LE, Germain RN (1995) Zeta-phosphorylation without ZAP-70 activation induced by TCR antagonists or partial agonists. Science 267:515–518
71. Mandelboim O, Berke G, Fridkin M, Feldman M, Eisenstein M, Eisenbach L (1994) CTL induction by a tumor-associated antigen octapeptide derived from a murine lung carcinoma. Nature 369:67–71

72. Marsh DG, Neely JD, Breazeale TM, Ghosh TM, Freidhoff LR, Ehrlich-Kautzky E, Schou C, Krishnaswamy G, Beaty TH (1994) Linkage analysis of IL4 and other chromosome 5q31.1 markers and total serum IgE concentrations. Science 264:1152–1156
73. Meier UC, Klenerman P, Griffin P, James W, Köppe B, Larder B, McMichael A, Phillips R (1995) Cytotoxic T lymphocyte lysis inhibited by viable HIV mutants. Science 270:1360–1364
74. Mitsuza H, Matis LA, Megson M, Bunn PA, Murray C, Mann DL, Gallo RC, Broder S (1983) Generation of an HLA-restricted cytotoxic T cell line reactive against cultured tumor cells from a patient infected with human T cell leukemia/lymphoma virus. J Exp Med 158:994–1000
75. Mizoguchi H, O'Shea JJ, Longo DL, Loeffler CM, McVicar DW, Ochoa AC (1992) Alterations in signal transduction molecules in T lymphocytes from tumor bearing mice. Science 258:1795–1798
76. Mosmann TR, Sad S (1996) The expanding universe of T cell subsets. Immunol Today 17:138–145
77. Nakagawa T (1991) The role of IgG subclass antibodies in the clinical response to immunotherapy in allergic disease. Clin Exp Allergy 21:289–296
78. Nicholson LB, Greer JM, Sobel RA, Lees MB, Kuchroo VK (1995) An altered peptide ligand mediates immune deviation and prevents autoimmune encephalomyelitis. Immunity 3:397–405
79. Noon L (1911) Prophylactic inoculation for hay fever. Lancet 1:1572–1573
80. Norman PS (1993) Modern concepts of immunotherapy. Curr Opin Immunol 5:968–973
81. Oliver RTD, Nouri AME (1991) T cell immune response to cancer in humans and its relevance for immunodiagnosis and therapy. Cancer Surv 13:173–193
82. Ostrov D, Krieger J, Sidney J, Sette A, Concannon P (1993) T cell receptor antagonism mediated by interaction between T cell receptor junctional residues and peptide antigen-analogues. J Immunol 150:4277–4283
83. Paglia P, Chiodoni C, Rodolfo M, Colombo MP (1996) Murine dentritic cells loaded in vitro with soluble protein prime cytotoxic T lymphocytes against tumor specific antigens in vivo. J Exp Med 183:317–322
84. Pardoll D (1996) Releasing the brakes on antitumor immune response. Science 271:1691
85. Pardoll DM (1993) Cancer vaccines. Immunol Today 14:310–316
86. Pardoll DM (1994) A new look for the 1990s. Nature 369:357–358
87. Parkman R (1985) Complete correction of the Wiskott-Aldrich syndrome by allogeneic bone marrow transplantation. N Engl J Med 298:921–925
88. Pircher HP, Moskophidis D, Rohrer U, Bürki K, Hengartner H, Zinkernagel RM (1990) Viral escape by selection of cytotoxic T cell-resistant virus variants in vivo. Nature 346:629–633
89. Plaut M, Pierce JH, Watson CJ, Hanley-Hyde J, Nordan RP, Paul WE (1989) Mast cell lines produce lymphokines in response to cross-linkage of Fc RI or to calcium ionophores. Nature 339:64–67
90. Racioppi L, Ronchese F, Matis LA, Germain RN (1993) Peptide-major histocompatibility complex class II complexes with mixed agonist/antagonist properties provide evidence for ligand-related differences in T cell receptor-dependent intracellular signaling. J Exp Med 177:1047–1060
91. Renner C, Pfreundschuh M (1995) Tumor therapy by immune recruitment with bispecific antibodies. Immunol Rev 145:199–220
92. Renner C, Jung W, Sahin U, Denfeld R, Pohl C, Trümper L, Hartmann F, Diehl V, van Lier R, Pfreundschuh M (1994) Cure of xenografted human tumors by bispecific monoclonal antibodies and human T cells. Science 264:833–835
93. Romani N, Gruner S, Brand D, Kampgen E, Lenz A, Trockenbacher B, Konwalinka G, Fritsch PO, Steinman RM (1994) Proliferating dendritic cell progenitors in human blood. J Exp Med 180:83–93
94. Sallusto F, Lanzavecchia A (1994) Efficient presentation of soluble antigen by cultured human dendritic cells is maintained by granulocyte/macrophage colony-stimulating factor plus interleukin-4 and downregulated by tumor necrosis factor. J Exp Med 179:1109–1118

95. Sandford AJ, Shirakawa T, Moffat MF, Daniels SE, Ra C, Faux JA, Young RP, Nakamura Y, Lathrop GM, Cookson WOCM, Hopkin JM (1993) Localisation of atopy and β subunit of high-affinity IgE receptor (Fc RI) on chromosome 11q. Lancet 341:332–334
96. Schwartz RH (1990) A cell culture model for T lymphocyte clonal anergy. Science 248:1349–1356
97. Schwartz RH (1996) Models of T cell anergy: is there a common molecular mechanism. J Exp Med 184:1–8
98. Secrist H, Chelen CJ, Wen Y, Marshall JD, Umetsu DI (1993) Allergen immunotherapy decreases interleukin-4 production in $CD4^+$ T cells from allergic individuals. J Exp Med 178:2132–2130
99. Sensi M, Parmiani G (1995) Analysis of TCR usage in human tumors: a new tool for assessing tumor-specific immune responses. Immunol Today 16:588–595
100. Shahinian A, Pfeffer K, Lee KP, Kündig TM, Kishihara K, Wakeham A, Kawai K, Ohashi PS, Thompson CB, Mak TW (1993) Differential costimulatory requirements in CD28-deficient mice. Science 261:609–612
101. Sloan-Lancaster J, Evavold BD, Allen PM (1993) Induction of T cell anergy by altered T-cell-receptor ligand on live antigen-presenting cells. Nature 363:156–159
102. Sloan-Lancaster J, Evavold BD, Allen PM (1994a) Th2 cell clonal anergy as a consequence of partial activation. J Exp Med 180:1195–1205
103. Sloan-Lancaster J, Shaw AS, Rothbard JB, Allen PM (1994b) Partial T cell signaling: altered phosho-zeta and lack of ZAP-70 recruitment in APL induced T cell anergy. Cell 79:913–922
104. Smilek DE, Wraith DC, Hodkinson S, Dwivedy S, Steinman L, McDevitt HO (1991) A single amino acid change in a myelin basic protein peptide confers the capacity to prevent rather than induce experimental autoimmune encephalomyelitis. Proc Natl Acad Sci USA 88: 9633–9637
105. Sondergaard I, Poulsen LK, Osterballe O, Weeke B (1992) Evidence for a common regulation of IgE and IgG-subclass antibodies in humans during immunotherapy. Allergy 47:467–470
106. Steinman RM (1991) The dendritic cell system and its role in immunogenicity. Annu Rev Immunol 9:271–296
107. Sulitzeanu D (1993) Immunosuppressive factors in human cancer. Adv Cancer Res 60:147–167
108. Topalian SL, Solomon D, Rosenberg SA (1989) Tumor specific cytolysis by lymphocytes infiltrating human melanomas. J Immunol 142:3714–3725
109. Torrelo A, Harto A, Sendagorta E, Czarnetzki B, Ledo A (1992) Interferon-γ therapy in atopic dermatitis. Acta Derm Venereol (Stockh) 72:370–372
110. Townsend SE, Allison JP (1993) Tumor rejection after direct costimulation of $CD8^+$ T cells by B7-transfected melanoma cells. Science 259:368–372
111. Ulmer JB, Donnelly JJ, Parker SE, Rhodes GH, Felgner PL, Dwarki VJ, Gromkowski SH, Deck RR, DeWitt CM, Friedman A, Hawe LA, Leander KR, Martinez D, Perry HC, Shiver JW, Montgomery DL, Liu MA (1993) Heterologous protection against influenza by injection of DNA encoding a viral protein. Science 259:1745–1749
112. Uyttenhove C, Maryanski J, Boon T (1983) Escape of mouse mastocytoma P815 after nearly complete rejection is due to antigen loss variants rather than immunosuppression. J Exp Med 157:1040–1052
113. van der Bruggen P, Traversari C, Chomez P, Lurquin C, De Plaen E, Van den Eynde B, Knuth A, Boon T (1991) A gene encoding an antigen recognized by cytolytic T lymphocytes on a human melanoma. Science 254:1643–1648
114. Van Pel A, van der Bruggen P, Coulie P, Brichard VG, Lethe B, Van den Eynde B, Uyttenhove C, Renauld JC, Boon T (1995) Genes coding for tumor antigens recognized by cytolytic T lymphocytes. Immunol Rev 145:229–250
115. Varney V, Hamid QA, Gaga M, Ying S, Jacobson M, Frew AJ, Kay AB, Durham SR (1993) Influence of grass pollen immunotherapy on cellular infiltration and cytokine mRNA expression during allergen-induced late phase cutaneous responses. J Clin Invest 92:644–651
116. Vitetta ES, Thorpe PE, Uhr JW (1993) Immunotoxins: magic bullets of misguided missiles? Immunol Today 14:252–259

117. Waldmann H, Cobbold S (1993) The use of monoclonal antibodies to achieve immunological tolerance. Immunol Today 14:247–251
118. Waterhouse P, Penninger JM, Timms E, Wakeham A, Shahinian A, Lee KP, Thompson CB, Griesser H, Mak TW (1995) Lymphoprolifertaive disorders with early lethality in mice deficient in CTLA-4. Science 270:985–989
119. Wauben MHM, Boog CJP, Van der Zee R, Joosten I, Schlief A, van Eden W (1992) Disease inhibition by major histocompatibility complex binding peptide analogues of disease-associated epitopes: more than just blocking alone. J Exp Med 176:667–677
120. Windhagen A, Scholz C, Höllsberg P, Fukaura H, Sette A, Hafler DA (1995) Modulation of cytokine patterns of human autoreactive T cell clones by a single amino acid substitution of their peptide ligand. Immunity 2:373–380
121. Winter G, Harris WJ (1993) Humanized antibodies. Immunol Today 14:243–246
122. Wolff JA, Malone RW, Williams P, Chong W, Acsadi G, Jani A, Felgner PL (1990) Direct gene transfer into mouse muscle in vitro. Science 247:1465–1468
123. Yewdell JW, Bennink JR (1990) The binary logic of antigen processing and presentation to T cells. Cell 62:203–206
124. Young JW, Inaba K (1996) Dendritic cells as adjuvants for class I major histocompatibility complex-restricted anti-tumor immunity. J Exp Med 183:7–11
125. Zier K, Gansbacher B, Salvadori S (1996) Preventing abnormalities in signal transduction of T cells in cancer: the promise of cytokine gene therapy. Immunol Today 17:39–45
126. Zinkernagel RM (1994) Immunity to viruses. In: Paul WE (ed) Fundamental immunology. Raven, New York, pp 1211–1250
127. Zitvogel L, Mayordomo JI, Storkus WJ, Tjandrawan T, DeLeo AB, Clarke MR, Lotze MT (1996) Therapy of murine tumors with tumor peptide pulsed dendritic cells: dependence on T cells, B7 costimulation, and Th1-associated cytokines. J Exp Med 183:87–79

Skin as an Immunocompetent Organ in Health and Disease

T. Bieber and A. Wollenberg

Introduction

Covering the human body, the skin represents the main interface organ directly in contact with the environment. The skin divides wet and dry, warm and cold, own and foreign, thus enabling us to keep all of our body systems in working order. Here, at the very border of our entire organism, the immunologic properties of the skin, our largest organ, are of vital importance. In addition to its well-known physical protective properties, human skin is a target for a series of agents, e.g., of microbiologic or physical nature, and an amazing source of various mediators that either initiate or accompany defense responses, e.g., inflammation (Fig. 1). Impaired barrier function, ultraviolet (UV) radiation, cell death, and encounter with bacteria, viruses, fungi, and protozoa belong to the broad spectrum of signals that are capable of initiating this inflammatory response, thus activating the cutaneous immune system. The aim of this chapter is not to go into experimental details, which may be read in excellent reviews on this topic [1, 2], but rather to provide the reader with an overview of simple and basic concepts that have been developed in almost two decades of progress in immunodermatologic research for a better understanding of the rationale of the strategies discussed in this book.

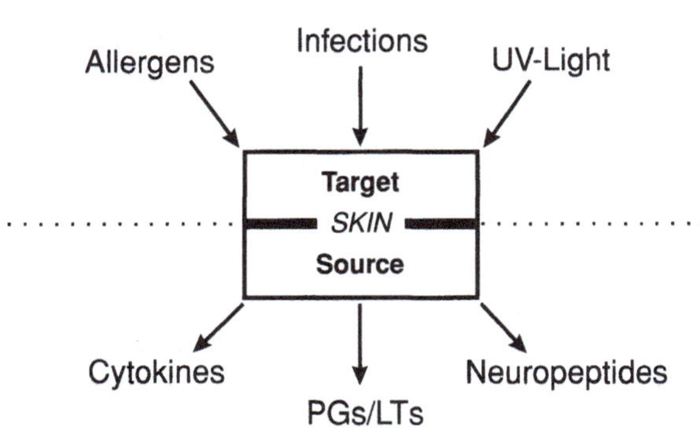

Fig. 1. The skin as a target for various agents and in response to this as the source of an extending array of mediators. *PGs*, prostaglandins; *LTs*, leukotrienes; *UV*, ultraviolet

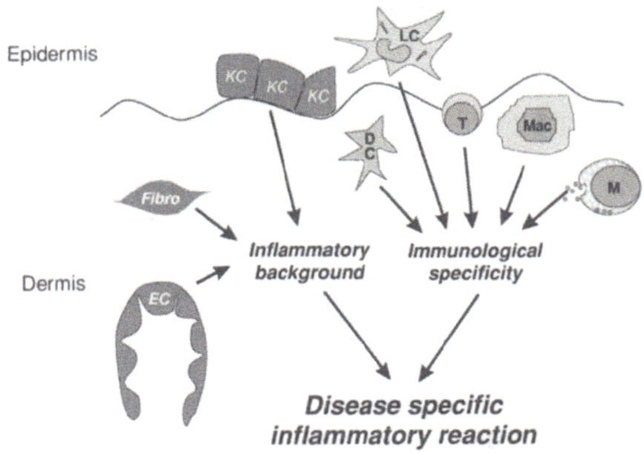

Fig. 2. The two components of the skin immune system (SIS). The static component provides the "bed of the inflammatory reaction" (*KC*, keratinocytes; *EC*, endothelial cells; *Fibro*, fibroblasts); the dynamic component provides its specificity (*LC*, Langerhans cells; *T*, T lymphocytes; *DC*, dermal dendritic cells; *M*, mast cells; *Mac*, macrophages)

Components of the Skin Immune System

The immune system faces several challenges: (1) the repertoire of recognition must be sufficiently diverse to recognize all the molecules which are encountered; (2) it has to eliminate cells with self-recognition; (3) it must be able to develop a diverse set of cellular and humoral effectors; and (4) it has to fashion effectors that do not destroy the system. The so-called skin immune system (SIS), a concept proposed by Bos et al. [1], is an organ-related unit of this complex network which has to fulfill a variety of protective and effector functions due to the interface status of the skin.

In addition to the clear anatomic architecture composed of epidermis and dermis, from an immunologic point of view two main components may be distinguished in the SIS, a static one and a more dynamic one (Fig. 2). Cellular elements of the more static components are those cells which on the one hand anatomically contribute to the classical architecture, e.g., keratinocytes, fibroblasts, and endothelial cells, and on the other hand provide the "bed of the immune reaction" by producing proinflammatory cytokines [2]. In contrast, the dynamic component is composed of leukocytes, i.e., T lymphocytes, macrophages, Langerhans cells, and other dendritic cells which are committed to spending a limited time in the skin. Schematically, these cells equipped with immune recognition receptors, i.e., T cell receptors (TCR) and Fc receptors (FcR), provide the specificity of the immune reaction. As an example, a recirculating pool of skin-homing T cells, identified by the CLA antigen [3], represents the cellular basis of the immunologic memory of the skin and, at the same time, the cellular basis of many skin diseases, such as allergic contact dermatitis. Thus the great variations in the clinical appearance of skin diseases are the product of complex and subtle interactions between the static and the dynamic components, and the characteristic lesions of a defined condition, e.g., psoriasis, most probably reflect a distinct and unique pattern of the immunologic microenvironment.

Skin Immune System in Health – Waiting for Antigens

Epidermal Langerhans cells and lymphocytes, both part of the dynamic component, may together be regarded as the "minimal organ of immunology." In a normal, noninflammatory environment, Langerhans cells and related dendritic cells [4] continuously filter their extracellular fluid, degrade intact protein allergens to immunogenic peptides, load them into major histocompatibility complex (MHC) molecules, and present these peptides on their cell surface [5]. Distinct signals probably provided by the static components, e.g., keratinocytes, initiate Langerhans cell migration to the regional lymph node. Simultaneously, profound phenotypic and functional changes convert the migrating Langerhans cell from a good antigen-processing, but weakly antigen-presenting cell into a poorly processing, extraordinary effective stimulator of naive T cells [6]. This stimulation takes place in the paracortical region of the lymph node.

For an effective immune response, HLA molecules, costimulatory molecules, and adhesion molecules are required on antigen-presenting cells, whereas T cell receptors and adhesion molecules are involved on the T cell surface. In the next step, T cells may activate B lymphocytes to secrete antigen-specific immunoglobulins of the G, A, M, D, and E subtype. These immunoglobulins may be measured in the peripheral blood, thus providing the physician with useful information, e.g., on the state of immunization in vaccination therapy or sensitization in atopic diseases. Cellular and humoral defense are closely linked. Surface-bound IgE molecules, for example, enable the immune system to induce immunoglobulin-mediated and -facilitated antigen presentation by FcεRI- or FcεRII/CD23-expressing, antigen-presenting cells, e.g. dendritic cells/monocytes or B cells [7, 8].

Such mechanisms may lead to an amplification and diversification of the IgE response. As opposed to the elicitation phase, this crucial sensitization phase or primary immune response, which involves the entire skin-associated lymphoid tissue (SALT) [2, 9], remains imperceptible. Consequently, strategies for intervention at this level cannot be guided by any clinical signs.

Skin Immune System in Disease – Cutaneous Inflammation

Under inflammation, the entire epidermodermal cell pool shifts from homeostasis towards an active battlefield. High numbers of cells from the dynamic component of the skin immune system invade the skin. In the epidermis, keratinocytes shorten their epidermal transit time from 1 month to a few days and may, depending on the actual microenvironment, express MHC class II molecules as well as their constitutive MHC class I structures. Langerhans cells upregulate costimulatory molecules and FcR. Novel cell types such as inflammatory dendritic epidermal cells (IDEC) with abundant MHC class II expression and disease-specific surface receptor expression profiles migrate to the epidermal compartment [10]. In the dermis, lymphocytes, histiocytes, macrophages, and dermal dendritic cells are present and fulfil their defense tasks against the pathogen. Lymphocytes equipped with skin-homing receptors such as the CLA antigen assemble in the inflamed skin. Distinctive changes in the inflammatory microenvironment are the basis of the different dermatologic diagnoses, initially established decades ago on a morphologic and histopathologic basis. The perivascular area of the postcapillary venules of the papillary dermis thereby contains the highest concentration of immune response-related cells. This area, referred to as the "dermal perivascular unit" [1], represents a histopathologic correlate to the clinical reaction pattern of follicular eczema. Since, in contrast to almost all other human organs and tissue, the static and dynamic components of the skin immune system are an easily accessible target for organ-specific immunomodulation, much effort has been undertaken in development of these strategies.

Skin Tumors and Tumor Escape Mechanisms

In contrast to bacteria, helminths, and other pathogenic organisms, most of a tumor cell's proteins are present in the source tissue of the tumor and are therefore well known to the immune system. In its effort to successfully defend the human body against growing tumor cells, the immune system needs to identify tumor-specific antigens. To maintain the immune response, these tumor antigens have to be presented repeatedly from an antigen-presenting cell, coexpressing some kind of costimulatory molecules. Malignant tumors frequently have acquired mechanisms to escape the immune system. Downregulation of costimulatory molecules, leading to tolerance induction, and inhibition of dendritic cell migration out of tumor tissue, are some of these escape mechanisms.

Benign and malignant melanocytic tumors are generally surrounded by a more or less pronounced inflammatory infiltrate, mainly consisting of lymphocytes. Recently, much effort has been made in establishing procedures for modulation of the immune response against malignant tumors, especially melanoma. Transfection of tumor cells with costimulatory molecules followed by reimplantation or ex vivo generation and growing of large numbers of tumor-specific T lymphocytes by various antigen presentation techniques are some of the approaches that are currently under investigation.

Functional Concepts of the Skin Immune System

Many theories have been developed to better describe the immune system and thereby help us to understand this fascinating part of the human body. The classical concept of immunology is that of an immune system which predominantly differentiates between "self" and "non-self" by secondary immune responses. Modifications in the inborn "self/non-self" classification are performed by primary immune responses and tolerance induction, both involving professional antigen-presenting cells, i.e., dendritic cells. Describing the same phenomena, but following a different concept, the immune system senses "danger" instead of "non-self," and the fate of every single T cell is functionally determined by its contact with the relevant antigen in the presence or absence of danger signals [11]. Candidates for the deliverance of this presently ill-defined "danger" information include costimulatory molecules detectable on many cell systems, such as B7-1 and B7-2. Although there are some exceptions to this classical rule, intracellular (e.g., viral) antigens are generally presented to $CD8^+$ T cells via MHC class I molecules, whereas extracellular antigens (e.g., allergens) are presented by antigen-presenting cells, via MHC class II molecules, to $CD4^+$ T cells.

Subsequent identification of functional T helper cell subpopulations in mice and men gave rise to the so-called Th1/Th2 concept based on their cytokine profile. Although some markers such as CD27 and CD30 have been proposed as specific for some Th classes, no reliable immunophenotypes are currently available to distinguish between these subpopulations. Th1 cells typically secrete, among other things, the cytokines interleukin (IL)-2 and interferon (IFN)-γ. A Th1-dominated response leads to a cure of skin diseases such as cutaneous leishmaniosis and verruca vulgaris. In contrast, Th2 cells typically secrete, among other things, the cytokines IL-4 and IL-5. A Th2-dominated response leads to a cure of helminthic infections. Most cytokines which contribute to IgE production can be regarded as Th2 associated, and aeroallergen-specific CD4+ and CD8+ T cell clones with a Th2, but also with Th1 and Th0 profiles have been isolated from atopic dermatitis skin [12, 13]. Clinical aspects of this Th1/Th2 dichotomy have recently been reviewed in detail [14].

Activation of the Immune System

The skin immune system may be fully activated by various signals, by no means all of which are well understood at present. Impaired skin barrier function, as frequently induced by improper skin care or occupationally enforced washing procedures, leads to exsiccation eczema. UV radiation induces a cutaneous inflammatory response in addition to its downregulatory effects. Necrotic cell death, as caused by trauma, tumor, or infection, is a strong inductor of polymorphic cellular infiltrates. Fungal infection, e.g., tinea corporis, leads to an inflammatory reaction pattern involving granulocyte extravasation into the epidermal compartment. Skin infection with *Borrelia* and *Treponema* species results in a cutaneous inflammation usually dominated by plasma cells. Viral skin infections are dominated by lymphocytic infiltrates. Infection of the skin with helminths induces Th2 responses. Most benign and malignant skin tumors also possess an immunoactivating capacity. All nevocytic nevi, as well as malignant melanoma, have a more or less pronounced lymphocytic infiltrate resulting from an encounter of the tumor cells with the immune system. The Sutton nevus, a benign nevocytic tumor successfully removed by the immune system, is probably the best example of an ongoing antitumor response in humans.

In clinical dermatology, the question of ongoing inflammation is generally addressed on a yes-or-no basis. Following a more investigative approach of inflammation, it seems more reasonable to describe cutaneous inflammation as a quantitative process that becomes clinically manifest once an individual threshold is exceeded in loco. In fact, there is evidence that in some individuals, namely atopic dermatitis patients, there is a phenomenon of ongoing minimal disease and subclinical inflammation. Taken together, cutaneous inflammation may be regarded as an initially uniform, later differential response to danger. Minimal danger signals are reduced by negative feedback mechanisms and remain clinically undetectable. Stronger danger signals are augmented and lead to clinically present inflammation. Current research has shed some light on particular segments of the complex inflammation initiation cascade. However, very little is known about the mechanisms leading to the termination of an ongoing inflammation. Apoptosis of many cell types from the dynamic component of the skin immune system has been attributed and, in part, shown to be the basis of the powerful immunosuppressive treatment available for inflammatory skin diseases. In the absence of this artificial immunomodulation, dermal macrophages have been suggested to play a key role in the physiologic downregulation of ongoing cutaneous inflammation and/or the induction of tolerance [15, 16]. However, more functional studies are urgently needed to support this suggestion.

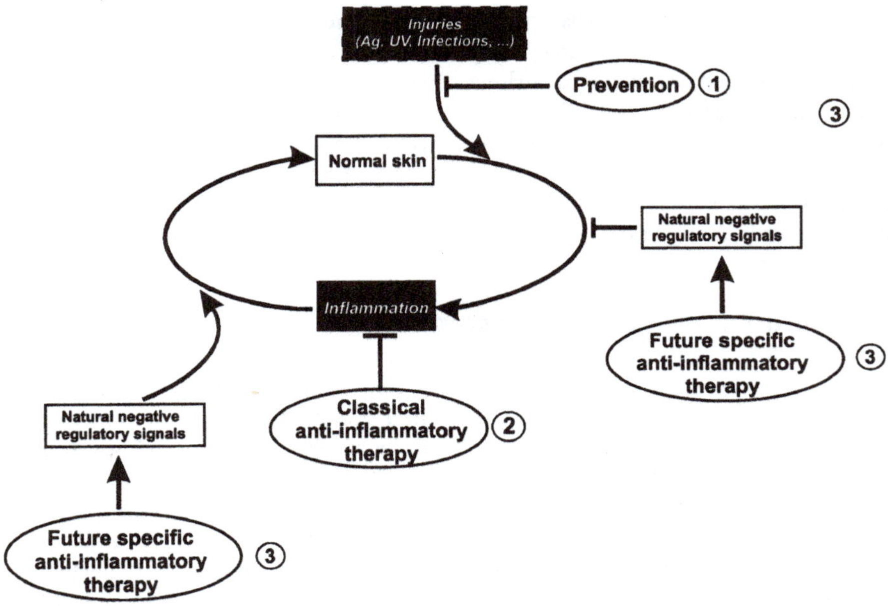

Fig. 3. Evolution of an inflammatory reaction offers three putative possibilities for immunointervention: *1*, desensitization for prophylaxis; *2*, immunosuppression of ongoing reactions; *3*, support for negative regulating mechanisms leading to clearance of the reaction. *Ag*, antigen; *UV*, ultraviolet

Therapeutic compounds and procedures modulating an underlying immunologic response and directing it in a biologic and clinically helpful direction are therefore an invaluable tool for the dermatologist.

Skin as a Target for New Immunointervention Strategies

Clinical experience and basic research have broadened the spectrum of immunomodulatory tools and substances for the dermatologist in the clinic and in research. From a theoretical viewpoint, one has to distinguish two phases in the evolution of an inflammatory reaction on which present and future strategies should focus (Fig. 3). In addition to prophylactic measures, which are aimed at avoiding the initiation of a given inflammatory reaction, current classical therapies are aimed at suppressing the ongoing inflammatory reaction. On the other hand, a better undestanding of the natural negative regulatory mechanisms leading to clearing of the inflammation should provide targets for future strategies designed to initiate and support such mechanisms.

Many immunosuppressive and anti-inflammatory strategies are important. Glucocorticosteroids have multiple effects on the immune system, e.g., inhibition of leukocyte migration, induction of apoptosis in lymphocytes and dendritic cells, and inhibition of T cell activation. For short treatment periods, oral and topical drugs are generally well tolerated and may be regarded as safe. Long-term application is limited because of undesirable side effects, in particular skin atrophy. Cyclosporin A and the two immunophilins FK-506 and ascomycin inhibit various immunologic cell functions, at least in part by calcineurine-mediated blocking of nuclear factor (NF)-AT-dependent cytokine production. The lipophilic molecule structure of FK-506 has led to the development of topical drugs. Methotrexate is mainly given for the inhibition of antibody production. Fundamental and clinical aspects of these and other immunosuppressive substances are discussed in detail in the respective chapters of this book.

UVB light is a highly effective immunosuppressive therapy for many superficial dermatoses, but favors the induction of skin cancer. UVA light penetrates deeper into the skin, but induces skin aging. The combination of photosensitizing drugs such as 8-methoxypsoralene and UVA (PUVA) is even more effective in the treatment of inflammatory skin diseases, such as psoriasis. Topical sensitization using the PUVA bath regimen has overcome both the unwanted prolonged sensitization period and gastro-intestinal side effects of oral PUVA. In extracorporal photophoresis, peripheral blood cells are subjected to PUVA treatment ex vivo and reinfused afterwards. This relatively expensive procedure leads to improvement in some patients with scleroderma, but has classically been used in mycosis fungoides and more recently with success in severe atopic dermatitis.

In dermatology, all immunostimulatory strategies are used at present more on an investigational than a clinically routine basis. Systemic INF therapy, which has been proved effective for human papillomavirus infection in multiple trials, is of benefit in patients with various infectious diseases cured by Th1 responses, e.g., cutaneous leishmaniosis. The high costs of recombinant INF limit their routine use in dermatology, and this also applies to many other cytokines as well. Further aspects of these and other immunostimulatory regimens are discussed in detail in the respective chapters of this book.

At present, only a few skin diseases may causally or symptomatically be cured with immunotherapy. In alopecia areata, induction of mild contact dermatitis by obligate contact sensitizers, e.g., DCP, often leads to regrowth induction and subsequent restitutio ad integrum. Two hundred years after Jenner's first virus inoculation, an effective vaccination therapy is available for many pediatric diseases predominantly affecting the skin. Highly standardized allergen preparations have revolutionized the field of desensitizing immunotherapy, with the highest curative rate in allergy to venoms of hymenoptera.

Conclusion

In spite of all the past and present research activities undertaken, many immunologic aspects of skin biology are still not well understood. Some of the open questions include the connection between emotional distress and flare-up of atopic dermatitis, the cause of psoriasis, why drug reactions follow distinct morphologic patterns, the relevant escape mechanisms of melanoma cells, and the basis of fixed drug eruptions. Intensive laboratory and clinical investigation needs to be continued in the hope that some of these fascinating questions will be solved in the near future and will substantially contribute to developing new and more disease-specific therapeutic strategies.

Summary

Haemopoetic as well as epithelial and mesenchymal cells contribute to building up the finely tuned defense mechanisms provided by the skin immune system. This system plays a pivotal role in the defense against foreign structures such as infectious agents, chemicals or allergens, but also neoantigens from tumors. Recent progress in the understanding of the skin immune system will hopefully inaugurate a new era in dermatological therapy where more specific strategies can be developed to alter ongoing inflammatory reactions or to reestablish successful tumor elimination.

References

1. Bos JD, Kapsenberg ML (1993) The skin immune system: progress in cutaneous biology. Immunol Today 14:75–78
2. Luger T, Schwarz T (eds) (1994) Epidermal growth factors and cytokines. Dekker, New York
3. Babi LFS, Picker LJ, Soler MTP, Drzimalla K, Flohr P, Blaser K, Hauser C (1995) Circulating allergen-reactive T cells from patients with atopic dermatitis and allergic contact dermatitis express the skin-selective homing receptor, the cutaneous lymphocyte-associated antigen. J Exp Med 181:1935–1940
4. Steinman RM (1991) The dendritic cell system and its role in immunogenicity. Annu Rev Immunol 9:271–296
5. Lanzavecchia A (1996) Mechanisms of antigen uptake for presentation. Curr Opin Immunol 8:348–354
6. Schuler G, Steinman RM (1985) Murine epidermal Langerhans cells mature into potent immunostimulatory dendritic cells in vitro. J Exp Med 161:526–546
7. Bieber T (1996) Fc epsilon R1 on human antigen presenting cells. Curr Opin Immunol 8:773–777
8. Mudde GC, Bheekha R, Bruijnzeelkoomen CAFM (1995) Consequences of IgE/CD23-mediated antigen presentation in allergy. Immunol Today 16:380–383
9. Streilein JW (1983) Skin-associated lymphoid tissues (SALT): origin and functions. J Invest Dermatol [Suppl] 80:12s–16s
10. Wollenberg A, Kraft S, Hanau D, Bieber T (1996) Immunomorphological and ultrastructural characterization of Langerhans cells and a novel, inflammatory dendritic epidermal cell (IDEC) population in lesional skin of atopic eczema. J Invest Dermatol 106:446–453
11. Matzinger P (1994) Tolerance, danger, and the extended family. Annu Rev Immunol 12:991–1045
12. Van Reijsen FC, Bruijnzeel-Koomen CAFM, Kalthoff FS, Maggi E, Romagnani S, Westland JKT, Mudde GC (1992) Skin derived aeroallergen-specific T cell clones of Th2 phenotype in patients with atopic dermatitis. J Allergy Clin Immunol 90: 184–193
13. Sager N, Feldmann A, Schilling G, Kreitsch P, Neumann C (1992) House dust mite-specific T cells in the skin of subjects with atopic dermatitis: frequency and lymphokine profile in the allergen patch test. J Allergy Clin Immunol 89:801–810
14. Mosmann TR, Sad S (1996) The expanding universe of T-cell subsets: Th1, Th2 and more. Immunol Today 17:138–146
15. Hammerberg C, Duraiswamy N, Cooper KD (1994) Active induction of unresponsiveness (tolerance) to DNFB by in vivo ultraviolet-exposed epidermal cells is dependent upon infiltrating class II MHC(+) CD11b(bright) monocytic/macrophagic cells. J Immunol 153:4915–4924
16. Lonati A, Mommaas M, Pasolini G, Lavazza A, Rowden G, De Panfilis G (1996) Macrophages, but not Langerhans cell-like cells of dendritic lineage, express the CD36 molecule in normal human dermis: relevance to downregulatory cutaneous immune responses? J Invest Dermatol 106:96–101

2 Immunosuppressive and Antiinflammatory Compounds

Cyclosporin A

T. Wrone-Smith and B.J. Nickoloff

Introduction

CsA (ciclosporin, cyclosporine, Sandimmune, SIM) is derived from the fungus *Tolypocladium inflatum* and is a neutral, lipophilic, cyclic undecapeptide that has a molecular weight of 1203. Borel and colleagues [4] showed CsA to be a powerful inhibitor of T cell activation induced by mitogen or mixed lymphocyte reaction (MLR). They also observed the concentration of CsA needed to inhibit T cell activation was noncytotoxic, reversible, and did not block the proliferation of other cell types at low concentrations, suggesting it might make a useful immunosuppressant. This prediction was accurate, as CsA is today the first-line drug for preventing allograft rejection in organ and bone marrow transplant recipients. Additionally, CsA has been used in treating autoimmune diseases such as systemic lupus erythematosus (SLE), myasthenia gravis, adult-onset and juvenile diabetes, and rheumatoid arthritis.

The effect of CsA in skin was first demonstrated in animal studies [5] in which CsA treatment prevented delayed-type hypersensitivity (DTH) to the tuberculin test in guinea pigs and contact hypersensitivity to dinitrochlorobenzene (DNCB) and oxazolone in mice. The clinical relevance of CsA in dermatology was initially demonstrated by Mueller and Hermann [54], who serendipitously observed that patients treated for psoriatic arthritis also had significant improvement of their skin disease. This study led to further clinical trials of CsA in treating psoriasis and other dermatoses and subsequently established CsA as a method of treatment in various skin diseases.

The cellular and molecular components in the cell affected by CsA have been extensively studied in order to improve its efficacy and reduce toxic side effects. The molecular mechanism of action of CsA has been best characterized in the T cell, but CsA also has direct effects on other immunocytes as well as nonimmune cells such as Keratinocytes (KC), endothelial cells, and vascular smooth muscle cells [25, 29, 57]. Furthermore, other immune processes in addition to T cell activation and lymphokine secretion are affected by CsA that are relevant in understanding its efficacy in the clinical setting. This chapter will review and discuss the following: (a) immunomodulation and mechanism of action of CsA, (b) the pharmacology of CsA, (c) and the effect of CsA on skin and its clinical efficacy in dermatologic diseases.

Immunomodulation and Mechanism of Action

T Cell Activation

The T cell is central in many dermatoses, including psoriasis, atopic dermatitis, contact sensitivity, graft-versus-host disease in the skin, and the autoimmune disease, SLE. Activated T cells in skin secrete lymphokines, which can stimulate growth of KC, recruit and activate other immune cells in the skin, or alternatively prime other T cells to destroy the tissue. T cells require two signals for activation and subsequent proliferation and acquisition of function, one through the T cell antigen receptor (TCR) - CD3 complex and a second signal from lymphokines or through costimulatory molecules, i.e., CD28 on the T cell surface. Once activated, a sequence of biochemical signals (phosphatidylinositol hydrolysis, increased intracellular calcium, translocation of protein kinase C, and increased cytoplasmic cAMP) occurs in the T cell with gene activation leading to transcription of intermediate-early (c-*fos*, c-*jun*), early (c-*myc*; interleukin-2, (IL-2); interleukin-3, (IL-3), and late genes that encode, among others, lymphokine receptors (IL-2 receptor, (IL-2R). Lymphokines binding to lymphokine receptors promote autocrine and paracrine stimulation of T cell proliferation.

CsA acts within several hours of the activation stimulus: if the drug is given within 4–8 h after the stimulus, T cell proliferation is inhibited; if it is given after 8 h following the stimulus, no effect is observed on T cell proliferation induced in naive, resting T cells. However, the inhibition of T cell proliferation can be partially reversed with addition of exogenous IL-2 to the cultures, suggesting the block in T cell function due to CsA is proximal to this step. Indeed, *in vitro* studies [64] confirmed CsA inhibits early T cell signal transduction pathways leading to the activation of lymphokine genes; addition of this immunosuppressive agent prevents transcription of mRNA encoding IL-2, IL-3, IL-4, interferon (IFN)-γ, tumor necrosis factor (TNF)-α, and others without inhibiting lymphokine receptor, i.e., IL-2R activation.

T cell responses requiring signaling through the TCR–CD3 complex, as in primary and secondary mixed lymphocyte response, MLR and autologous MLR, are sensitive to CsA. CsA also inhibits T cell proliferation induced by mitogenic lectins, superantigens, cross-linking CD2 on the T cell surface, or by the combination of phorbol 12-myristate 13-acetate (PMA), an activator of protein kinase C, and the calcium ionophore, ionomycin. Interestingly, each of these CsA-sensitive pathways is associated with an initial rise in intracellular calcium, suggesting that a common intermediate may be the molecular target of this drug. Other T cell activation pathways such as IL-2-dependent growth without mitogen or antigen stimulation by T cell clones are resistant to CsA. Furthermore, the combination of anti-CD28 monoclonal antibody (mAb) and PMA, which can induce vigorous proliferation of T cells in the absence of accessory cells, is also resistant to CsA [44]. Thus not all modes of T cell activation, especially those not associated with an increase in intracellular calcium, are susceptible to the suppressive actions of CsA.

Molecular Mechanism of Action in T Cells

The molecular mechanism of action of CsA in T cells was of great interest to immunologists and transplantation biologists alike to not only improve the efficacy of this drug, but also to have a means of dissecting the complex machinery involved in T cell activation. A summary of these works will be presented below, and the reader is referred to these excellent reviews for further reading [3, 50, 59, 61].

CsA is cell permeable and binds to a family of receptors, termed cyclophilins, which are a tye of immunophilin. Cyclophilins are ubiquitous and phylogenetically conserved and have been described in bacteria, fungi, rodents, and humans [6]. Studies using both biochemical and molecular approaches have shown these CsA-binding proteins to be present as cytosolic, membrane-associated and secreted forms [75]. In T cells, the predominant receptor for CsA is CyPA, a 17-Da protein located in the cytoplasm. Cyclophilins were later shown to be identical to *cis-trans* peptidyl-prolyl isomerases (also called rotamases) [26, 66]. Rotamases accelerate protein folding in proline-containing protein substrates in cells, and CsA can inhibit this activity. However, the inhibition of rotamase activity by CsA was found to be unrelated to its immunosuppressive abilities because (a) the concentration of CsA needed to inhibit T cell activation was far less than that needed to inhibit the rotamase activity of cyclophilins, and (b) non-immunosuppressive analogues of CsA could inhibit rotamase activity.

Later studies showed that the target of CsA is the protein calcineurin (Cn), a serine/threonine phosphatase, also known as phosphatase 2B, that is ubiquitous and highly conserved from mammals to yeast. It is expressed in T cells and is critical for transducing membrane-associated signals to the nucleus during T cell activation [12]. Cn is a heterodimer composed of two subunits: a 59-kDa catalytic A subunit with a binding site for calmodulin and a 19-kDa calcium-binding regulatory B subunit that is required for enzymatic activity. In the presence of calcium, calmodulin binds to and activates Cn, explaining the calcium requirements for CsA-sensitive intracellular pathways. An important observation by Liu et al. [51] was that only the complex of CsA and cyclophilin inhibited the phosphatase activity of Cn, and neither CsA nor cyclophilin alone would bind to or inhibit the activity of Cn.

The next focus was on the identification of phosphoprotein substrates for Cn in T cells. One potential substrate was the transcription factor NFAT (nuclear factor of activated T cells), the activity of which is required for optimal transcription of IL-2. The NFAT complex consists of a ubiquitously expressed nuclear component and a preexisting cytoplasmic component, NFATp/c. The murine NFATp and human NFATc are homologous phosphoproteins and have similar binding characteristics. Upon T cell activation, increases in intracellular calcium induce the translocation of NFATp/c from the cytoplasm to the nucleus, where it interacts with the AP1 elements Fos and Jun and binds to its cognate DNA-binding site within the IL-2 promoter. *In vitro* studies [53] demonstrated that NFATp/c is a substrate of Cn and that its dephosphorylation by Cn was inhibited by CsA. In short, the complex of cyclophilin/CsA directly binds Cn and prevents it from dephosphorylating NFATp/c, subsequently preventing the translocation of NFATp/c to the nucleus to initiate transcription of IL-2. However, it should be noted that CsA-regulatory sites other than NFAT (i.e., NF-κB) exist within the IL-2 promoter and therefore calcium inducibility and CsA sensitivity of T cell cytokines may be mediated by a combination of NFAT sites and non-NFAT sites.

CsA also inhibits the transcription of other cytokines secreted by activated T cells, including IL-3, IL-4, granulocyte-macrophage colony-stimulating factor (GM-CSF), IFN-γ, and TNF-α. NFAT and NFAT-like sites that are sensitive to CsA have been identified in the promoter regions of these cytokine genes in T cells [9, 13, 31]. Furthermore, CsA treatment inhibits the calcium-dependent production of TNF-α in surface immunoglobulin (Ig) cross-linked B cells, inhibits IL-3, IL-4, and GM-CSF in PMA- and ionomycin-treated mast cells, and inhibits IL-6 production in activated monocytes. Wang and colleagues [71] identified NFATp in B cells, natural killer (NK) cells, mast cells, monocytes, macrophages, and endothelial cells, but not in fibroblasts or neutrophils. Thus, from these experimental data, one can conclude that CsA can directly inhibit calcium-dependent cytokine gene transcription not only in T cells, but also in other classes of immunocytes during the immune response.

Effect on Immunocytes

CsA also affects other calcium-dependent functions of immunocytes in addition to inhibition of lymphokine production (for a review, see [64]). CsA is anti-inflammatory, as *in vitro* studies in mouse and human [11] demonstrate that CsA can block degranulation of mast cells, cytotoxic T lymphocytes (CTL), and basophils and inhibit leukotriene synthesis in mast cells. CsA treatment of human skin-derived mast cells *in vitro* [65] can also inhibit their histamine and prostaglandin synthesis, which may be relevant in the pathogenesis of atopic dermatitis and psoriasis.

The generation of CTL is inhibited by CsA, but that of suppressor T cells is not; immunosuppressive activity in some experimental systems may even be enhanced by CsA treatment [39]. The ability of CsA to suppress functional T cell-dependent B cell differentiation and antibody production is primarily through the inhibition of T-helper lymphokine secretion. CsA can however, directly inhibit B cell proliferation induced by anti-Ig antibodies or PMA and ionomycin treatment at the same concentrations used to inhibit T cell activation [72].

Numerous studies do not indicate a significant direct effect of CsA on antigen uptake and processing in murine and human monocytes, macrophages, dendritic cells, epidermal antigen-presenting cells (APC), and Langerhans cells. Rather, the sensitivity of APC to CsA is more indirect, i.e., block of lymphokine secretion, which may have profound effects on major histocompatibility complex (MHC) expression and maturation of these cells [34]. In summary, despite these additional effects of CsA on the immune system, it appears that the drug acts primarily by suppressing lymphokine production and reducing the activation of T-helper cells and CTL.

Pharmacology

CsA is insoluble in water and must be dissolved in ethanol or olive oil to remain in solution at room temperature. It is stabilized with castor oil for intravenous administration or with olive oil for oral administration. After oral administration, CsA is slowly and erratically absorbed. Peak blood levels are reached 2–4 h after ingestion, and the serum half-life is 8–24 h, with an average of 18 h [45].

CsA is widely distributed in the body, with the highest concentrations in adipose tissues, epidermis, lymphoid tissues, kidneys, and liver. In the blood, CsA has a high affinity for erythrocytes and lipoproteins; only 5%–10% of the drug remains free. Therefore, whole blood is the preferred matrix to measure CsA levels by radioimmunoassay (RIA) or high-performance liquid chromatography (HPLC). However, on an individual basis, blood CsA levels correlate poorly with efficacy and toxicity. Recently, a microemulsion-based formulation, Neoral (Sandoz, Vienna, Austria), demonstrated

CsA absorption which was significantly faster, more extensive, and more predictable than the standard oral formulation, However, pronounced changes in long-term side effects are not expected, since Neoral is composed with the same active ingredient as the old formulation (for a review, see [58]).

Cyclosporin is metabolized primarily in the liver via cytochrome P-450 IIIA microsomal enzymes. Elimination is by hepatic metabolism and biliary secretion. Caution is warranted with concomitant administration of drugs that interact with the P-450 system, as they may affect cyclosporine metabolism. Drugs that induce cytochrome P-450 enzymes (ketoconazole, erythromycin) decrease the blood concentration of CsA; conversely, drugs that inhibit P-450 enzymes (rifamycin, phenobarbital) increase CsA levels.

Hypertension and nephrotoxicity are the most common side effects of CsA treatment. Other side effects include hepatotoxicity, electrolyte imbalance, gingival hypertrophy, hypertrichosis, and neurologic symptoms such as tremors and paresthesia. Most of these side effects are reversible upon dosage reduction or cessation of therapy. Compared to other immunosuppressive agents, CsA has a lower incidence of infection and oncogenic potential. However, transplant recipients receiving CsA therapy are at a greater risk of developing infections with herpes zoster, herpes simplex, cytomegalovirus, and *Pneumocystis carinii* [33]. Malignancies that appear to be at an increased frequency with CsA therapy in transplant and dermatologic patients include non-Hodgkins B cell lymphomas, squamous cell carcinomas, and basal cell carcinomas. An important point is that the adverse side effects are much less frequent and the increased risk of infection and malignancy much lower in dermatologic patients; this is reflective of dosage (starting doses of 15 mg/kg per day in transplant patient vs. 3–5 mg/kg per day in dermatologic patients) and the fact that transplant patients are generally in poorer health and are frequently on a variety of other treatments [48].

Effect on Skin and Clinical Efficacy in Dermatologic Diseases

In Vitro Studies

The basis for the use of CsA in dermatology began from a series of serendipitous observations, without a thorough understanding of its mechanism of action. It is clear from the literature that CsA is immunosuppressive and anti-inflammatory, and it is not surprising that CsA has been successful to date in treating certain skin diseases, including psoriasis, atopic dermatitis, and others with inflammatory and immunological components. However, the question arises as to what effect CsA has directly on the nonimmunologic components of the skin, i.e., the KC. KC can become hyperproliferative and secrete chemotactic and immunostimulatory cytokines that are increased and even dysregulated in certain skin diseases such as psoriasis. Since CsA has been shown to inhibit proliferation and cytokine secretion in immunocytes, the question remains whether its clinical success in dermatology is due in part to its ability to directly inhibit these activities in KC.

As previously mentioned, the receptor for CsA, cyclophilin, is ubiquitous and expressed in all cells and tissues studied to date. Griffiths and colleagues [35] demonstrated by western blot analysis and [^{3}H]CsA-binding assays that cyclophilin is indeed present and can bind CsA in human KC and epidermis. They detected no difference in cyclophilin levels between normal, psoriatic-involved, and psoriatic-uninvolved skin samples or cultured cells, suggesting the therapeutic effect of CsA in psoriasis is independent of cyclophilin content. Using polyacrylamide gel electrophoresis (PAGE) and isoelectric focusing (IEF) radiobinding assays, Chatellard-Gruaz and colleagues [10] detected different isoforms of cyclophilin in KC that differed upon differentiation of KC in culture and between normal and psoriatic skin samples. What the different isoforms represent in KC and what role they may play in CsA treatment remains to be determined. In conclusion, these studies demonstrate that cyclophilin is present in the epidermis, binds to CsA, and also explains the high epidermal accumulation of CsA – ten times serum trough levels – reported in psoriatic patients treated with oral CsA [27].

Numerous studies have been conducted in cell culture and animal models to determine whether CsA can directly inhibit KC proliferation. In general, in most cell culture systems utilizing serum-free media, CsA at 1–10 μg/ml is cytostatic to KC, and CsA concentrations greater than 10 mg/ml are cytotoxic with vacuole formation in the KC [57, 62, 67]. In addition, inhibition of CsA proliferation *in vitro* is dose and time dependent in serum-free media and reversible at cytostatic concentrations, i.e., 5 μg/ml, upon removal of CsA from the media. In contrast, studies in which serum was included in the media showed CsA did not inhibit KC proliferation [46] or inhibited it almost equally compared to CsA administered in serum-free media [17]. Furthermore, a direct *in vivo* antiproliferative effect of CsA was demonstrated in human skin grafted onto nude mice. High-dose subcutaneous injections of CsA (50 mg/kg per day) revealed a significant decrease in bromodeoxyuridine (BrdU)-positive KC in the human grafts [69].

The significance of these findings is unclear when translating to the clinical setting. Determinations of the skin levels of CsA in psoriasis patients have shown that tissue concentrations of 1.0–2.9 μg/ml are reached using therapeutic doses of 3–5 mg/kg per day [22]. Furthermore, serum is obviously present in patients, and it has been demonstrated that lack of serum in culture almost doubles the intracellular accumulation of CsA in KC compared to KC treated in serum-containing media [27]. In conclusion, the intracellular concentration of CsA demonstrated to inhibit the proliferation of KC *in vitro* may not be achievable in patients, and thus it is unlikely that the primary clinical efficacy of CsA treatment is due to direct inhibition of KC growth. Further support for this conclusion was provided by Ho and colleagues [41], who demonstrated that lamellar ichthyosis, a hyperproliferative skin disease, is not affected by CsA treatment.

The effect of CsA on cytokine secretion by KC has also been studied, since activated KC may play an important role in initiating or maintaining cutaneous inflammation in certain dermatoses. KC exposed to immune system-derived cytokines IL-1, IFN-γ, and TNF-α *in vitro* secrete IL-1β, IL-6, and IL-8, among others, which are known to be chemotactic and proinflammatory to immunocytes and which also serve as autocrine factors for KC. Furthermore, it is thought that the secretion and response to cytokines in psoriasis may be dysregulated [56]. Therefore, it becomes important to determine whether the effects on CsA on KC cytokine production *in vivo* is a direct result of CsA or indirect, i.e., blockade of immune system activation.

Elder and colleagues [20] demonstrated by northern blot analysis that IL-1β and IL-8 RNA were elevated in lesional skin from psoriasis patients and significantly lowered after 1 week of low-dose CsA therapy. However, they could not demonstrate CsA inhibited the induction of IL-8 mRNA in response to IL-1β or TNF-α and IFN-γ stimulation in cultured normal human KC with doses up to 12 mg/ml. In contrast, Won et al. [73] demonstrated by northern analysis the ability of CsA to decrease IL-1α, IL-1β, and IL-8 in human and murine KC cell lines, albeit at higher doses and longer incubation times (2–5 days). However, the cell lines used were transformed, and their similarity to KC in a diseased patient's skin is unclear. In conclusion, cytokines secreted by KC may be elevated and significantly decreased by CsA treatment *in vivo*, but it appears unlikely that this is due to direct inhibition by CsA on the KC, but probably to the reduction of KC-stimulatory cytokines secreted by activated immunocytes. In support of these conclusions, CsA concentrations required to inhibit activation, proliferation, and secretion of cytokines (10–1000 ng/ml) by various immunocytes are demonstrable in patient's skin undergoing CsA therapy.

Clinical Applications

CsA has been used in the treatment of a variety dermatologic diseases. The most responsive and well-studied diseases will be briefly reviewed below and include the following:

- Psoriasis
- Atopic dermatitis
- Lichen planus
- Immunobullous diseases
- Alopecia areata
- Pyoderma gangrenosum
- Connective tissue diseases

The reader is also referred to reviews by Ho and Zloty [40] and Kauver and Stiller [47] for further reading.

Psoriasis. Psoriasis is a complex disease characterized by hyperplastic KC and increased numbers of immunocytes within the epidermis and dermis, including lymphokine-secreting activated T cells, activated APC (Langerhans cells, macrophages, and dendritic cells), and polymorphonuclear leukocytes (PMN). The efficacy of systemic CsA treatment of psoriasis has been well established by a number of studies [21, 22]. CsA is successful in treating plaque-type, erythrodermic, and pustular forms of psoriasis as well as psoriatic arthritis.

Although higher doses of CsA have been used, the recommended systemic dosage to treat psoriasis is 3–5 mg/kg per day in order to minimize side effects. Intralesional injections of psoriasis are efficacious [7]; however, to date topical preparations of CsA have proven ineffective [18]. The combination of low-dose CsA with other immunosuppressants, i.e., psoralens and ultraviolet A therapy (PUVA), methotrexate, ultraviolet B (UVB), to reduce toxicity have not proven to be as or more effective than CsA treatment alone. A gradual recurrence of psoriasis occurs within weeks or months after discontinuation of therapy. In general, due to side effects, CsA is not recommended as monotherapy for psoriasis. Rather, short-term therapy with CsA is recommended to control acute psoriatic flares and/or induce remission followed by less toxic immunosuppressants, i.e., PUVA, for maintenance therapy.

Experimental data support the efficacy of CsA treatment in psoriasis is due to diminution of T cell activation in plaques with decreased subsequent lymphokine production. A decrease in total numbers of T cells (both $CD4^+$ and $CD8^+$) as well as activated, i.e., IL-$2R^+$ HLA-DR^+, T cells is noted in lesions following CsA treatment. In addition, expression of the activation markers HLA-DR and intercellular adhesion molecule (ICAM)-1 on KC and endothelial cells, and the secretion of the chemokine IP-10 by KC, all induced by *in vivo* exposure to lymphokines such as IFN-γ, are decreased following CsA treatment [74]. However, continual expression of hyperproliferative keratin K16 and overexpression of epidermal growth factor receptors (EGF-R) and transforming growth factor (TGF)-α by KC within psoriatic plaques during CsA therapy reinforces the idea that immunocytes, and not KC, are the direct target of CsA [32].

Atopic Dermatitis. Oral CsA at 5 mg/kg per day is efficacious in treating the T cell-mediated inflammatory disease atopic dermatitis, even severe forms that are resistant to conventional therapy with corticosteroids [8,70]. By contrast, topical CsA does not seem to be particularly effective in treating atopic dermatitis. Relapses occur when cyclosporine is withdrawn, and continued treatment is required to maintain long-term remission. CsA does not appear to affect the allergic reaction in atopic dermatitis, as treatment does not interfere with patch tests to dust mite antigens or intracutaneous skin tests [55]. Rather, CsA therapy results in inhibition of hyperstimulatory Langerhans cells present in lesional atopic dermatitis skin and in reduction of activated T cells and the cytokines they secrete (IL-5), Langerhans cells bearing IgE, and macrophages [14].

Lichen Planus. Systemic CsA treatment (6 mg/kg per day) is efficacious in the treatment of cutaneous lichen planus [42], a disease characterized histologically by lymphocytic infiltrate at the dermoepidermal junction and KC damage by CTL. Treatment of oral lichen planus with topical forms of CsA by either the "swish and spit" method or digital application of an oily solution has varied from beneficial to ineffective [19, 28, 63]. Systemic absorption of CsA by topical application is undetectable or detected at low levels in the blood, with no correlation of blood levels to clinical efficacy demonstrated. Clinical improvement with CsA treatment is associated with a decrease in expression of KC ICAM-1 and HLA-DR expression and a reduction in numbers of infiltrating activated i.e., HLA-DR^+ T cells.

Immunobullous Diseases. Oral CsA (6–12 mg/kg per day) has been effective in treating the autoimmune blistering diseases pemphigus and bullous pemphigoid, primarily as a steroid-sparing agent or in combination with corticosteroids [1, 68]. A significant reduction in blister formation is seen within several weeks of therapy, and relapse of disease is common upon cessation of treatment. Epidermolysis bullosa acquisita (EBA), a disease resistant to other immunosuppressive agents, is responsive to CsA treatment [49]. The response to CsA in patients with pemphigus and bullous pemphigoid is associated with a decrease in serum titers of autoantibodies and a decrease in immune deposits in the skin. A similar decrease in serum autoantibodies was not noted in EBA [16], and the precise mechanism by which CsA ameliorates EBA is unknown.

Alopecia Areata. Hypertrichosis is a common side effect of CsA therapy and thus became of interest in the treatment of alopecia. Cosmetically acceptable hair growth has been reported in patients receiving oral CsA therapy (6 mg/kg per day) for alopecia areata (AA) [30, 37]. However, hair loss occurs within months of discontinuing CsA therapy. To date, topical CsA treatment has not been shown to have a significant effect on AA. Hair growth with oral CsA treatment was associated with a decrease in expression of HLA-DR and ICAM-1 on follicular KC and a reduction in T cells (CD4+ and $CD8^+$) and Langerhans cells surrounding the follicles [38].

Pyoderma Gangrenosum. This skin disease has been characterized as an immune-mediated lymphocytic vasculitis with infiltration by activated T cells and neutrophil accumulation within the lesions. There have been numerous case reports [24, 52, 60] demonstrating the efficacy of oral CsA in treating this disease, especially those lesions that are resistant to other forms of immunosuppressive therapy. Dosages of 5–10 mg CsA/kg per day are reported to result in a significant improvement in weeks and complete clearing within months without relapse.

Connective Tissue Diseases. Oral CsA (5–10 mg/kg per day) has been demonstrated to benefit some patients with either the cutaneous or systemic forms of lupus erythematous or systemic sclerosis, and dermatomyositis [15, 23, 43]. Overall, the treatment response is variable, and CsA is more therapeutic when combined with corticosteroid treatment. CsA must be used with caution in patients with SLE and systemic sclerosis, who may have disease associated with renal dysfunction.

Conclusions

CsA is an immunosuppressive and anti-inflammatory drug that primarily exerts its effect by preventing activation and lymphokine gene transcription in T cells as well as B cells, monocytes/macrophages, and mast cells. By preventing transcription of IL-2 in T cells, activation and acquisition of T-helper or CTL function is prevented, thus crippling an effective immune response.

CsA has been used successfully in treating a variety of dermatoses, the best response being achieved in those with immunological and/or inflammatory components, i.e., psoriasis, atopic dermatitis, and lichen planus. CsA accumulates in the skin via its intracellular receptor, cyclophilin, which is expressed in KC. The levels of CsA that accumulate in the skin after systemic administration are high enough to inhibit lymphokine secretion and activation of immunocytes, but probably not high enough to directly inhibit proliferation or cytokine secretion by KC. Therefore, the efficacy of CsA treatment in skin diseases mentioned above primarily results from its direct effects on the immune system and not the KC.

At present, CsA is not recommended as the first-choice treatment for patients requiring systemic therapy due to the serious side effects it has, namely nephrotoxicity. Rather, CsA is indicated in patients for whom conventional therapies have failed or are inappropriate. Grossman and colleagues [36] found that the incidence of side effects even with low-dose CsA treatment increase with time and age of the patient and recommend that CsA not be used as a long-term monotherapy for diseases such as psoriasis. Other negating factors to consider with CsA use is that it is expensive to use because of the need to monitor liver and kidney function in the patients and that its effect is reversible. *In vivo* and *in vitro* studies [2] indicate the activation and secretion of cytokines by T cells is rapidly reversible upon cessation of CsA treatment or its removal from the culture medium. This probably explains in part the relapse seen in many patients once CsA therapy is discontinued.

Future areas of investigation for CsA use in dermatology lie in developing successful topical applications to minimize systemic absorption and side effects. To date, there is no convincing data that topical preparations of CsA are efficacious in dermatoses such as psoriasis and atopic dermatitis. Other areas include developing less toxic CsA analogues, perhaps with less affinity for kidney epithelial cells. In conclusion, CsA has proven to be highly efficacious in treating intractable skin diseases, and with careful administration to the patient it will continue to be a drug that has a role in the treatment of several diseases of the skin.

Summary

Cyclosporin A (CsA), a fungal metabolite, is a powerful immunosuppressant of humoral and cell-mediated immunity that has been effectively used to prevent allograft rejection in solid organ and bone marrow transplantation. CsA inhibits signal transduction pathways that are characterized by an initial rise in intracellular calcium concentration, which includes the transcription of lymphokine genes in T cells and other immune cells. The cytosolic receptors for CsA, cyclophilins, are found in nearly every cell and tissue examined and therefore CsA can affect the function of other cells present within the skin, including Langerhans cells, mast cells, endothelial cells, and keratinocytes. Since the 1980s, CsA has been used to treat a variety of dermatoses, with those primarily involving inflammatory or immune-mediated mechanisms, i.e., psoriasis and atopic dermatitis, having the best response. The study of CsA in culture, animal models, and in the clinic will further our understanding of the pathologic mechanisms underlying certain dermatologic diseases.

References

1. Barthelemy H, Fraapaz A, Cambazard F, Mauduit G, Rouchouse B, Kanitakis J, Souteyrand P, Claudy AL, Thivolet J (1988) Treatment of nine cases of pemphigus vulgaris with cyclosporine. J Am Acad Dermatol 18:1262–1266
2. Batiuk TD, Pazderka F, Enns J, DeCastro L, Halloran PF (1995) Cyclosporine inhibition of calcineurin activity in human leukocytes in vivo is rapidly reversible. J Clin Invest 96:1254–1260
3. Bierer BE, Hollander G, Fruman D, Burakoff SJ (1993) Cyclosporin A and FK506: molecular mechanisms of immunosuppression and probes for transplantation biology. Curr Opin Immunol 5:763–773
4. Borel JF, Feurer C, Gubler HU, Stahelin H (1976) Biological effects of cyclosporin A: a new antilymphocytic agent. Agents Actions 6:468–475
5. Borel JF, Feurer C, Magnee C, Stahelin H (1977) Effects of the new antilymphocytic peptide cyclosporin A in animals. Immunology 32:1017–1025
6. Braun W, Kallen J, Mikol V, Walkinshaw MD, Wuthrich K (1995) Three-dimensional structure and actions of immunosuppressants and their immunophilins. FASEB J 9:63–72
7. Burns MK, Ellis, CN, Eisen D, Duell E, Griffiths CEM, Annesley TM, Hamilton TA, Birnbaum JE, Voorhees JJ (1992) Intralesional cyclosporine for psoriasis. Arch Dermatol 128:786–790
8. Camp RDR, Reitamo S, Friedman PS, Ho V, Heule F (1993) Cyclosporin A in severe, therapy-resistant atopic dermatitis: report of an international workshop, April 1993. Br J Dermatol 129:217–220

9. Campbell PM, Pimm, J, Ramassar V, Halloran PF (1996) Identification of a calcium-inducible, cyclosporine-sensitive element in the IFNγ promoter that is a potential NFAT binding site. Transplantation 61:933–939
10. Chatellard-Gruaz D, Saurat J-H, Siegenthaler G (1994) Differential expression of cyclophilin isoforms during keratinocyte differentiation. Biochem J 303:863–867
11. Cirillo R, Triggiana M, Siri L, Ciccarelli A, Pettit GR, Condorelli M, Marone G (1990) Cyclosporin A rapidly inhibits mediator release from human basophils presumably by interacting with cyclophilin. J Immunol 150:2591–2598
12. Clipstone NA, Crabtree GR (1992) Identification of calcineurin as a key signalling enzyme in T-lymphocyte activation. Nature 357:695–697
13. Cockerill PN, Shannon MF, Bert AG, Ryan GR, Vadas MA, (1993) The granulocyte-macrophage colony-stimulating factor/interleukin 3 locus is regulated by an inducible cyclosporin A-sensitive enhancer. Proc Natl Acad Sci USA 90:2466–2470
14. Cooper KD (1994) Atopic dermatitis: recent trends in pathogenesis and therapy. J Invest Dermatol 102:128–137
15. Correia O, Polonia J, Nunes JP, Resende C, Delgado L (1992) Severe acute form of adult dermatomyositis treated with cyclosporine. Int J Dermatol 31:517–519
16. Crow LL, Finkle JP, Gammon WR, Woodley DT (1988) Clearing of epidermolysis bullosa acquisita with cyclosporine. J Am Acad Dermatol 19:937–942
17. Duncan JI (1994) Differential inhibition of cutaneous T-cell-mediated reactions and epidermal cell proliferation by cyclosporin A, FK-506, and rapamycin. J Invest Dermatol 102:84–88
18. Duncan JI, Wakeel RA, Winfield AJ, Ormerod AD, Thomson AW (1993) Immunomodulation of psoriasis with a topical cyclosporin A formulation. Acta Derm Venereol (Stockh) 73:84–87
19. Eisen D, Griffiths CEM, Ellis CN, Nickoloff BJ, Voorhees JJ (1990) Cyclosporin wash for oral lichen planus. Lancet 335:535–536
20. Elder JT, Hammerberg C, Cooper KD, Kojima T, Nair RP, Ellis CN, Voorhees JJ (1993) Cyclosporin A rapidly inhibits epidermal cytokine expression in psoriasis lesions, but not in cytokine-stimulated cultured keratinocytes. J Invest Dermatol 101:761–766
21. Ellis CN, Gorsulowsky DC, Hamilton TA, Billings JK, Brown MD, Headington JT, Cooper KD, Baadsgaard O, Duell EA, Annesley TM, Turcotte JG, Voorhees JJ (1986) Cyclosporine improves psoriasis in a double-blind study. JAMA 256:3110–3116
22. Ellis CN, Fradin MS, Messana JM, Brown MD, Siegel MT, Hartley AH, Rocher LL, Wheeler S, Hamilton TA, Parrish TG, Ellis-Madu M, Duell E, Annesley TM, Cooper KD, Voorhees JJ (1991) Cyclosporine for plaque-type psoriasis. Results of a multidose, double-blind trial. N Engl J Med 324:277–284
23. Favre H, Miescher PA, Lemoine R (1994) Use of cyclosporine in the treatment of autoimmune disorders. Transplant Proc 26:3194–3196
24. Fedi MC, Quercetani R, Lotti T (1993) Recalcitrant pyoderma gangrenosum responsive to cyclosporine. Int J Dermatol 32:119
25. Ferns G, Reidy M, Ross R (1990) Vascular effects of cyclosporin A in vivo and in vitro. Am J Pathol 137:403–413
26. Fischer G, Wittman-Liebold B, Lang K, Kiefhaber T, Schmid FX (1989) Cyclophilin and peptidyl-prolyl cis-trans isomerase are probably identical proteins. Nature 337:476–478
27. Fisher GJ, Duell EA, Nickoloff BJ, Annesley TM, Kowalke JK, Ellis CN, Voorhees JJ (1988) Levels of cyclosporine in epidermis of treated psoriasis patients differentially inhibit growth of keratinocytes cultured in serum free versus serum-containing media. J Invest Dermatol 91:142–146
28. Frances C, Boisnic S, Etienne S, Szpirglas H (1988) Effect of the local application of cyclosporin A on chronic erosive lichen planus of the oral cavity. Dermatologica 177:194–195
29. Furue M, Gaspari AA, Katz SI (1988) The effect of cyclosporin A on epidermal cells. II. Cyclosporin A inhibits proliferation of normal and transformed keratinocytes. J Invest Dermatol 90:796–800
30. Gebhart W, Schmidt JB, Schemper M, Spona J, Kopsa H, Zazgornik S (1986) Cyclosporin-A-induced hair growth in human renal allograft recipients and alopecia areata. Arch Dermatol Res 278:238–240

31. Goldfeld A McCaffrey PG, Strominger J, Rao A (1993) Identification of a novel cyclosporin-sensitive element in the human tumour necrosis factor-α gene promoter. J Exp Med 178: 1365–1379
32. Gottlieb AB, Grossman RM, Khandke L, Carter DM, Sehgal PB, Fu SM, Granelli-Piperno A, Rivas M, Barazani L, Krueger JG (1992) Studies of the effect of cyclosporine in psoriasis in vivo: combined effects on activated T lymphocytes and epidermal regenerative maturation. J Invest Dermatol 98:302–309
33. Graham R (1994) Cyclosporine: mechanisms of action and toxicity. Cleve Clin J Med 61:308–313
34. Granelli-Piperno A, Keane M, Steinman RM (1988) Evidence that cyclosporin inhibits cell-mediated immunity at the level of the T lymphocyte rather than the accessory cell. Transplantation 46:53S–60S
35. Griffiths CEM, Fisher GJ, Harding MW, Elder JT, Voorhees JJ (1990) Cyclophilin content of normal and psoriatic epidermis. J Invest Dermatol 94:436–440
36. Grossman RM, Chevret S, Abi-Rachad J, Blanchet F, Dubertret L (1996) Long-term safety of cyclosporine in the treatment of psoriasis. Arch Dermatol 132:623–629
37. Gupta AK Ellis CN, Tellner DC, Voorhees JJ (1988) Cyclosporine A in the treatment of severe alopecia areata. Transplant Proc 20:105–108
38. Gupta AK, Ellis CN, Cooper KD, Nickoloff BJ, Ho VC, Chan LS, Hamilton TA, Tellner DC, Griffiths CEM, Voorhees JJ (1990) Oral cyclosporine for the treatment of alopecia areata: a clinical and immunohistochemical analysis. J Am Acad Dermatol 22:242–250
39. Hess AD, Tutschka PJ (1981) Effect of cyclosporin A on human lymphocyte responses in vitro. I. CsA allows for the expression of alloantigen-activated suppressor cells while preferentially inhibiting the induction of cytolytic effector lymphocytes in the MLR. J Immunol 124:2601–2608
40. Ho VC, Zloty DM (1993) Immunosuppressive agents in dermatology. Dermatol Clin 11:73–85
41. Ho VC, Gupta AK, Ellis CN, Cooper KD, Nickoloff BJ, Voorhees JJ (1989) Cyclosporine in lamellar ichthyosis. Arch Dermatol 125:511–514
42. Ho VC, Gupta AK, Ellis CN, Nickoloff BJ, Voorhees JJ (1990) Treatment of severe lichen planus with cyclosporine. J Am Acad Dermatol 22:64–68
43. Ippoliti G, Miori L, Negri M, Rovati B, Lorenzutti F, Zerbinati N, Rabbiosi G (1994) Cyclosporine in treatment of progressive systemic sclerosis: clinical and immunologic findings. Transplant Proc 26:3117–3118
44. June CH, Ledbetter JA, Gillespie MM, Lindstein T, Thompson CB (1987) T-cell proliferation involving the CD28 pathway is associated with cyclosporine-resistant interleukin 2 gene expression. Mol Cell Biol 7:4472–4481
45. Kahan BD, VanBuren CT, Nierberger W (1983) Cyclosporine: pharmokinetics, metabolism and drug interaction. Transplant Proc 15:2409–2412
46. Kato N, Halprin KM, Taylor JR (1987) Cyclosporin A does not inhibit epidermal cell growth at therapeutic levels. J Invest Dermatol 88:52–54
47. Kauver AB, Stiller MJ (1994) Cyclosporine in dermatology: pharmacology and clinical use. Int J Dermatol 33:86–96
48. Krupp P, Monka C (1990) Side-effect profile of cyclosporin A in patients treated for psoriasis. Br J Dermatol 122 [Suppl 36]:47–56
49. Layton AM, Cunliffe WJ (1990) Clearing of epidermolysis bullosa acquisita with cyclosporine. J Am Acad Dermatol 22:535–536
50. Liu J (1993) FK506 and cyclosporin, molecular probes for studying intracellular signal transduction. Immunol Today 14:290–295
51. Liu J, Farmer JDJ, Lane WS, Friedman J, Weissman I, Schreiber SL (1991) Calcineurin is a common target of cyclophilin-cyclosporin A and FKBP-FK506 complexes. Cell 66:807–815
52. Matis WL, Ellis CN, Griffiths CEM, Lazarus GS (1992) Treatment of pyoderma gangrenosum with cyclosporine. Arch Dermatol 128:1519–1529
53. McCaffrey PG, Perrino BA, Soderling TR, Rao A (1993) NF-ATp, a T lymphocyte DNA-binding protein that is a target for calcineurin and immunosuppressive drugs. J Biol Chem 268:3747–3752

54. Mueller W, Herrmann B (1979) Cyclosporin A for psoriasis. N Engl J Med 301:555
55. Munro CS, Higgins EM, Marks JM, Daly BM, Friedman PS, Shuster S (1991) Cyclosporin A in atopic dermatitis: therapeutic response is dissociated from affects on allergic reactions. Br J Dermatol 124:43–48
56. Nickoloff B (1991) The cytokine network in psoriasis. Arch Dermatol 127:871–884
57. Nickoloff BJ, Fisher GJ, Mitra RS, Voorhess JJ (1988) Additive and synergistic antiproliferative effect of cyclosporin A and gamma interferon on cultured human keratinocytes. Am J Pathol 131:12–18
58. Noble S, Markham A (1995) Cyclosporin. A review of the pharmokinetic properties, clinical efficacy and tolerability of a microemulsion-based formulation (Neoral). Drugs 50:924–41
59. Rao A (1995) NFATp, a cyclosporin-sensitive transcription factor implicated in cytokine gene induction. J Leukoc Biol 57:536–542
60. Schmitt EC, Pigatto PD, Boneschi V, Bubola D, Finzi AF (1993) Pyoderma gangrenosum treated with low-dose cyclosporin. Br J Dermatol 128:230–231
61. Schrieber SL, Crabtree GR (1992) The mechanism of action of cyclosporin A and FK506. Immunol Today 13:136–142
62. Sharpe GR Fisher C (1990) Time-dependent inhibition of growth of human keratinocytes and fibroblasts by cyclosporin A: effect on keratinocytes at therapeutic blood levels. Br J Dermatol 123:207–213
63. Sieg P, Von Domarus H, Von Zitzewitz V, Iven H, Farber L (1995) Topical cyclosporin in oral lichen planus: a controlled, randomized, prospective trial. Br J Dermatol 132:790–794
64. Sigal NH, Dumont FJ (1992) Cyclosporin A, FK-506, and rapamycin: pharmacological probes of lymphocyte signal transduction. Annu Rev Immunol 10:519–560
65. Stellato C, de Paulis A, Ciccarelli A, Cirillo R, Patella V, Casolaro V, Marone G (1992) Anti-inflammatory effect of cyclosporin A on human skin mast cells. J Invest Dermatol 800–804
66. Takahashi N, Hayano T, Suzuki M (1989) Peptidyl-prolyl cis-trans isomerase is the cyclosporin A-binding protein cyclophilin. Nature 337:473–475
67. Taniguchi S, Kono T, Ishii M, Hamada T (1995) Effects of cyclosporin and ultraviolet radiation on growth and ornithine decarboxylase activity in cultured human epidermal keratinocytes. Br J Dermatol 132:703–709
68. Thivolet J, Barthelemy H, Rigot-Muller G, Bendelac A (1985) Effects of cyclosporin on bullous pemphigoid and pemphigus. Lancet 1:334–335
69. Urabe A, Kaniakis J, Viac J, Thivolet J (1989) Cyclosporin A inhibits directly in vivo keratinocyte proliferation of living human skin. J Invest Dermatol 92:755–757
70. Van Joost T, Heule F, Korstanje M, Van Den Broek MJTB, Stenveld HJ, Van Vloten WA (1994) Cyclosporin in atopic dermatitis: a multicentre placebo-controlled study. Br J Dermatol 130:634–640
71. Wang DZ, McCaffrey, PG, Rao A (1995) The cyclosporin-sensitive transcription factor NFATp is expressed in several classes of cells in the immune system. Ann N Y Acad Sci 766:182–194
72. Wicker LS, Boltz RC, Matt V Nichols EA, Peterson LB, Sigal NH (1990) Suppression of B-cell activation by cyclosporin-A, FK506, and rapamycin. Eur J Immunol 20:2277–2283
73. Won Y-H, Sauder DN, Mckenzie RC (1994) Cyclosporin A inhibits keratinocyte cytokine gene expression. Br J Dermatol 130:312–319
74. Wong RL, Winslow CM, Cooper KD (1993) The mechanisms of action of cyclosporin A in the treatment of psoriasis. Immunol Today 14:69–74
75. Zav'yalov VP, Denesyuk AI, Lundell J, Korpela T (1995) Some new aspects of molecular mechanisms of cyclosporin A effect on immune response. APMIS 103:401–415

Rapamycin

F. O. Nestle

Introduction

Rapamycin (sirolimus, rapamune), a macrolide antibiotic, was initially identified more than 20 years ago as an antifungal agent during antibiotic screening at Ayerst Research Laboratories. It is produced by *Streptomyces hygroscopicus* isolated from a soil sample obtained from the Vai Atore region of Easter Island (Rapa Nui) [56]. Although lacking antibacterial activity, rapamycin is a potent inhibitor of yeast growth [50]. In addition to its fungicidal activity, rapamycin exerts tumoricidal effects through its growth-inhibiting effect [17]. The structural organisation of rapamycin ($C_{51}H_{79}NO_{13}$; see Fig. 1) demonstrated the molecule to be a mixture of two conformational isomers of the 31-membered macrolide ring [18], and the proposed chemical structure was later confirmed by the total organic synthesis [42].

The first demonstration of its immunosuppressive activity was obtained from studies showing its inhibitory effect in two animal models of human autoimmune disease, experimental autoimmune encephalitis and adjuvant arthritis [31]. Ironically, rapamycin was not developed as an immunosuppressant at that time. Nearly a decade later, FK506, another macrolide antibiotic produced by *Streptomyces tsubakensis*, was discovered during a screen for natural products that inhibit interleukin (IL)-2 production [27]. The structural similarities between FK506 and rapamycin (see Fig. 1) and the fact that FK506 was an immunosuppressant 100-fold more potent than cyclosporin A

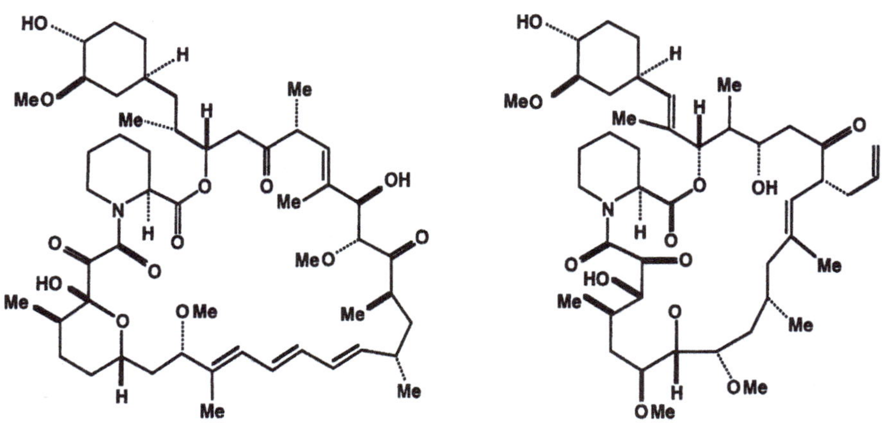

Fig. 1. Structure of rapamycin (*left*) and FK506 (*right*)

(CsA) [28] provoked a resurgence of interest in rapamycin as a candidate immunosuppressive drug. Subsequent studies demonstrated potent immunosuppressive activity in mouse as well as rat heart transplant recipients [40] and in larger animal models [5]. Soon it became also evident that rapamycin and FK506 have different mechanisms of action [14, 15], and the search for the intracellular binding partners as well as molecular and biochemical mechanisms of this drug began.

Molecular Mechanisms

Similar to FK506 and CsA, rapamycin binds to a family of proteins called immunophilins [52]. This protein family interfaces with a wide range of signal transduction systems inside the cell, especially those relating to calcium and phosphorylation [52]. The major cytosolic receptor for CsA is cyclophilin A (CyPA), while the major FK506- and rapamycin-binding protein (FKBP) is FKBP12 [30, 55]. CyPA–CsA and FKBP12–FK506 complexes bind to and inhibit the same target protein, the Ca^{2+}-dependent serine-threonine phosphatase calcineurin, a critical component of T cell receptor (TCR)-linked signal transduction which leads to cytokine gene transcription [12]. In contrast, formation of the FKBP–rapamycin complex in T cells interferes with the ability of T cell growth factors to drive the progression of these cells from G1 to the S phase of the cell cycle [36]. Five groups, working independently, have recently identified the intracellular target proteins for the immunophilin–rapamycin complexes, so-called mammalian targets of rapamycin (mTOR; also called sirolimus effector protein SEP or RAP target RAPT; for an excellent review, see [2]). These mTOR are highly conserved in eukaryotes and contain a kinase-like domain in the C-terminal 400 amino acids which exhibits 25% protein identity with the kinase domain of phosphatidylinositol (PI) 3-kinase. This family of kinases is believed to be involved in a broad range of physiologic processes linked to control of the cell cycle. The most recent addition to this expanding family of signal transducers is the product of the human AT gene, which is mutated in the autosomal recessive disorder ataxia teleangiectatica [47], resulting in immunologic and cell cycle abnormalities as well as a predisposition to cancer.

Further biochemical activities of rapamycin include the interference with a Ras-independent signal transduction pathway required for the activation of the 70-kDa S6 protein kinase ($p70^{sk6}$) [29, 45]. The inhibition of p70sk6 might explain the growth-suppressive effect of rapamycin on lymphoid cells.

Another cellular effect of rapamycin is interference with cyclin-associated protein kinases (cyclin-cdk), which orchestrate the progression of mammalian cells from G1 to M phase. Rapamycin is thought to tip the balance between activation and inhibition of cyclin-cdks toward the inhibitory side by blocking the downregulation of Kip1 protein, which is part of a novel family of negative regulators of the cell cycle [43].

The above-mentioned and other studies of the mechanism of action of rapamycin are beginning to uncover a previously unrecognized signal transduction pathway that may play a general role in the control of growth of normal and transformed mammalian cells.

Effect of Rapamycin on Tumor Growth

Similar to other antiproliferative and immunosuppressive compounds such as azathioprin and cyclophosphamide, rapamycin also has antitumor activities in mice. Initially, rapamycin was found to be active against certain mouse mammary and intestinal tumors [13], but it has also been found to be active against certain brain tumors xenografted in nude mice [21]. The antitumor efficacy of rapamycin is route dependant [17]. Intraperitoneal or intramuscular injections are superior to subcutaneous or oral routes. Interestingly, unlike other more general antiproliferative immunosuppressants, rapamycin seems to allow bone marrow and intestinal cells to proliferate normally [38]. Unfortunately, the antineoplastic activity in preclinical models seems to be less potent than its antifungal and immunosuppressive activity. Therefore, increase of antitumor efficacy by optimization of its dose and route or by combination with other compounds has to be obtained before application of rapamycin to clinical studies in humans.

Effect of Rapamycin on the Immune System

For rapamycin to suppress allograft rejection or autoimmune diseases (see below), it must alter the normal functions of the immune system. The immunosuppressive effects of rapamycin result from its suppression of T and B cell activity. It blocks T cell proliferation induced by antigen, mitogenic lectins, alloantigen, cross-linking of T cell surface markers (e.g., CD28), and phorbol ester [14, 23, 25] in the mid- to late G_1 phase of the cell cycle, employing either calcium-dependent or -independent pathways [15, 37, 53]. In contrast to the effects of CsA or FK506 signaling through CD28, the major costimulatory ligand of a T cell, but not the TCR itself is sensitive to rapamycin [3]. Rapamycin blocks the clonal expansion of helper and cytotoxic T cells induced by alloantigen [14, 24, 26], but does not inhibit the effector function of cytotoxic T cells [36]. Rapamycin also inhibits proliferation of B cells induced by both calcium-dependent or -independent pathways in the mid- to late G_1 phase [1]. In vivo, rapamycin treatment can suppress antibody production to alloantigen, but has little effect on subsequent challenge and production of secondary antibodies [46, 54]. Taken together, these results suggest that rapamycin can directly affect the function of T and B cells.

An important mechanism of interference with the amplification of an immune response is the inhibition of responses to cytokines. Rapamycin can readily inhibit proliferation induced by cytokines such as IL-1 [60], IL-2 [10], IL-6 [23], colony-stimulating factors [11], and many others (for a review, see [35]). In long-term cardiac allograft recipients, rapamycin has also been demonstrated to reduce the expression of T-helper (Th)1 cytokines (IL-2, IL-12) and preservation of Th2 cytokines (IL-4, IL-10) [58].

It is important to mention that many studies have demonstrated synergistic effects of rapamycin and CsA in the in vitro and in vivo inhibition of T cell and B cell proliferation [14, 23]. The above-mentioned in vitro and in vivo results indicate that rapamycin could be highly effective in diseases in which a suppression of T cell- or B cell-mediated (auto)immune responses would be desirable.

Animal Models

Studies of the effectiveness of rapamycin in models of allogeneic organ transplantation [5, 40] have awakened interest in its use in organ transplantation.

In animal models of cardiac transplantation, it has been shown that rapamycin is not only an effective prophylaxis against acute rejection, but it can also reverse ongoing rejection [41]. Recent work also suggests that rapamycin may be very effective in preventing antibody-mediated accelerated rejection and in prolonging allograft survival in previously sensitized recipients [8, 48]. Furthermore, low doses of rapamycin in combination with CsA prevented monkey allograft heart rejection more effectively than either drug alone [38]. These initial studies suggest that the combined use of rapamycin and CsA may afford the benefits of increased immunosuppressive efficacy without the risk of decreased safety. Rapamycin is not only effective in heart transplantation, it is also effective in other animal models of organ transplantation, such as small-bowel transplantation in the mouse [9], skin transplant rejection [19], and renal transplant rejection [49].

The discovery of rapamycin to control allograft rejection in experimental animal models has also renewed the interest in the use of rapamycin to treat autoimmune diseases. Prolonged treatment with rapamycin increases the survival of MRL/lpr mice, an animal model of systemic lupus erythematosus, and prevents the typical rise of anti-double-stranded DNA antibody levels [57]. Reports on the effectivity of rapamycin to interfere with experimentally induced arthritides have been published [6, 7]. Rapamycin significantly reduced both periarticular inflammation and bony erosions compared to controls and was at least as effective as CsA. Furthermore, rapamycin inhibits the growth of synovial fibroblasts from patients with rheumatoid arthritis [34]. In some of these rodent models of autoimmunity, rapamycin appeared to be more potent than CsA.

Human Studies

Application of rapamycin in human trials has just begun. Several studies to determine the effectiveness of rapamycin are currently underway, such as an acute renal rejection pilot study, an acute cardiac rejection study, a renal prophylaxis study, and studies in recalcitrant psoriasis. Results from a multicenter phase II trial (149 patients) in renal transplantation were presented at a recent meeting in Barcelona (Sirolimus Meeting, 28 August 1996, Barcelona). The six-arm, randomized, placebo-controlled single-blinded study examined the impact of sirolimus (rapamycin) in combination with tapering doses of corticosteroids on the prevention of acute rejection episodes and dose reduction of CsA. There was a reduction from 40% acute rejection episodes to 11% among full-dose CsA and to 26% among reduced-dose CsA (B.D. Kahan et al. 1996, oral presentation). Therefore, during the first 6 post-transplant months, addition of rapamycin to a CsA/corticosteroid regimen markedly reduced acute rejection incidences in renal transplant patients. Although the combination of CsA and rapamycin had an enhanced immunosuppressive effect, the overall risk of infectious complications did not appear to significantly increase (Y. Vanrenterghem et al. 1996, oral presentation).

A phase I study showed that a single dose of sirolimus (rapamycin) up to 15 mg/m^2 was tolerated and safe in stable renal transplant recipients [4]. The drug was rapidly absorbed, with peak values being reached within 3 h after administration of the dose. No serious side effects occurred. Preliminary clinical studies with rapamycin involved the use of an oral vehicle that contained dimethylacetamide (DMA), with more recent studies using a new vehicle without DMA. The bioavailibility is approximately 15%. The absorption is rapid, reaching peak concentrations within 1 h (for a review, see [59]).

Toxicity in animal models includes weight loss, lethargy, and testicular atrophy; no nephrotoxicity of this agent has been demonstrated in the doses used for the prevention of transplant rejection in animals [33]. Extensive experiences in humans are currently missing. The most frequent side effect in one phase I study was headache (in six of 24 patients [22]). No toxicity was observed at any of the dose levels. In the above-mentioned phase II study, a cluster of infections with *Pneumocystis carinii* was experienced at one center. Addition of rapamycin increased serum lactate dehydrogenase (LDH), cholesterol, and triglycerides and decreased platelets (B. D. Kahan et al. 1996, oral presenation). The absence of renal side effects would make rapamycin a valuable addition to already existing immunosuppressive drugs, such as CsA. An explanation for the more restricted side effects may be that rapamycin's antiproliferative action is less generalized than that of other immunosuppressive drugs such as CsA and FK506. Its actions may be more targeted and its toxicity limited [39]. Several studies have demonstrated the synergistic or additive effects of combining rapamycin with either CsA or FK506 [14, 23, 24, 51]. CsA levels and clearance in humans do not change after rapamycin administration [22]. The possibility of using the combined effects of rapamycin and CsA or FK506 is intriguing and will hopefully increase immunosuppressive activity, while decreasing overall toxicity in future human studies. This has been recently shown in one phase II study on acute rejection episodes in renal transplantation (B. D. Kahan et al. 1996, oral presentation).

Apart from application in human organ transplantation, rapamycin may be useful in autoimmune diseases such as rheumatoid arthritis. Animal models of arthritis demonstrated effectiveness of rapamycin in preventing the onset of the disease (see above). Since toxicity in phase I studies seems acceptable, investigation of rapamycin with or without combination with CsA in humans for both prevention of transplant rejection and treatment of autoimmune diseases such as inflammatory arthritis seems warranted.

Applications in Skin Diseases

Inflammatory T cell-mediated skin diseases such as psoriasis were always rewarding applications to study the effectiveness of new immunosuppressive drugs. Treatment with CsA has been proven to be very effective in psoriasis and other T cell-mediated skin diseases [44]. Phase II studies investigating the effect of rapamycin alone or in combination with CsA in psoriasis are currently underway. No definitive results have been published yet (M. Gioud-Paquet, personal communication).

Effects of rapamycin on delayed-type hypersensitivity reactions (DTH) of the skin have been shown in animal models. Rapamycin inhibits the bovine serum-induced DTH reaction in mice more potently than CsA [6]. In contrast, rapamycin had no inhibitory effect in a guinea pig model of DTH to dinitrofluorbenzene (DNFB) when given systemically or topically [16]. Rapamycin did not significantly inhibit T cell infiltration or skin reddening, while exerting a strong inhibitory effect on keratinocyte growth in vitro. In another animal model of acute skin inflammation, rapamycin significantly inhibited carrageenan paw edema at higher doses in rats [7]. In this model, doses approximately ten to 20 times greater than active doses in T cell-mediated models were required. Rapamycin also inhibits passive cutaneous anaphylaxis caused by IgE-like antibodies stimulated by immunization with egg albumin [31]. In this study, it was concluded that rapamycin rather suppresses the formation of antibodies causing passive anaphylaxis than suppressing mediators of response.

Another interesting issue is site-specific immune suppression using topical formulations of immunosuppressive drugs. FK506 has been shown to be very potent in this regard [16, 32]. Data about the effectiveness of rapamycin are inconsistent. While rapamycin has been shown to be ineffective in concentrations of up to 1.2% in a pig skin model of allergic contact dermatitis [32] and in concentrations of up to 2% in a guinea pig model of allergic contact dermatitis [16], rapamycin (0.01%) was effective in combination with CsA (0.1%) in a dual skin allograft model or a mouse contact dermatitis model using oxazolone as allergen [20]. Rapamycin was particularly efficacious during the late-local inflammatory-immune phase.

All these animal models indicate that rapamycin could be effective in T cell- or antibody-mediated skin diseases and justify further investigation of the effect in inflammatory diseases of the skin.

Summary

The search for immunosuppressant drugs to increase success in organ transplantation has led to the discovery of macrolide fermentation products such as rapamycin and FK506. Rapamycin displays a distinct inhibitory effect on the immune system by interfering with the T cell activation program. Rapamycin forms active complexes with a new family of intracellular receptors, FKBP, and acts through recently defined target proteins to block progression of T cells from the G_1 to the S phase of the cell cycle.

Rapamycin has been shown to be promising in several animal models of organ transplantation and autoimmunity. The synergistic effects of rapamycin and CsA or FK506 open new ways in immunosuppression by hopefully increasing the immunosuppressive activity, while decreasing the associated side effects. Currently, several phase II/III studies on the effectiveness of rapamycin in organ transplantation and T cell- mediated skin diseases such as psoriasis are underway. The future will show whether rapamycin will be an effective, well-tolerated addition to our arsenal of immunosuppressive drugs in dermatology.

Acknowledgements. I thank Dr. M. Gioud-Paquet (Immunology Department, Wyeth-Lederle, Paris) for providing some of the information regarding clinical studies with rapamycin. This work was supported by grants from the Cancer League Zurich and the Swiss Cancer League.

References

1. Aagaard-Tillery KM, Jelinek DF (1994) Inhibition of human B lymphocyte cell cycle progression and differentiation by rapamycin. Cell Immunol 156:493–507
2. Abraham RT, Wiederrecht GJ (1996) Immunopharmacology of rapamycin. Annu Rev Immunol 14:483–510
3. Bierer BE, Schreiber SL, Burakoff SJ (1991) The effect of the immunosuppressant FK-506 on alternate pathways of T cell activation. Eur J Immunol 21:439–445
4. Brattstrom C, Tyden G, Sawe J, Herlenius G, Claesson K, Groth CG (1996) A randomized, double-blind, placebo-controlled study to determine safety, tolerance, and preliminary pharmacokinetics of ascending single doses of orally administered sirolimus (rapamycin) in stable renal transplant recipients. Transplant Proc 28:985–986
5. Calne RY, Collier DS, Lim S, Pollard SG, Samaan A, White DJ, Thiru S (1989) Rapamycin for immunosuppression in organ allografting. Lancet 2:227
6. Carlson RP, Baeder WL, Caccese RG, Warner LM, Sehgal SN (1993a) Effects of orally administered rapamycin in animal models of arthritis and other autoimmune diseases. Ann N Y Acad Sci 685:86–113
7. Carlson RP, Hartman DA, Tomchek LA, Walter TL, Lugay JR, Calhoun W, Sehgal SN, Chang JY (1993b) Rapamycin, a potential disease-modifying antiarthritic drug. J Pharmacol Exp Th34Ser 266:1125–1138
8. Chen H, Luo H, Daloze P, Xu D, Shan X, St-Louis G, Wu J (1993) Long-term in vivo effects of rapamycin on humoral and cellular immune responses in the rat. Immunobiology 188: 303–315
9. Chen H, Qi S, Xu D, Wu J, Daloze P (1996) The immunosuppressive effect of rapamycin on mouse small bowel transplantation. Transplantation 61:523–526
10. Chung J, Kuo CJ, Crabtree GR, Blenis J (1992) Rapamycin-FKBP specifically blocks growth-dependent activation of and signaling by the 70 kd S6 protein kinases. Cell 69:1227–1236
11. Cooper MH, Gregory SH, Starzl TE, Wing EJ (1994) Rapamycin but not FK506 inhibits the proliferation of mononuclear phagocytes induced by colony-stimulating factors. Transplantation 57:433–439
12. Crabtree GR, Clipstone NA (1994) Signal transmission between the plasma membrane and the nucleus in T lymphocytes. Annu Rev Biochem 63:1045–1083
13. Douros J, Suffness M (1981) New antitumor substances of natural origin. Cancer Treat Rev 8:63
14. Dumont FJ, Melino MR, Staruch MJ, Koprak SL, Fischer PA, Sigal NH (1990a) The immunosuppressive macrolides FK-506 and rapamycin act as reciprocal antagonists in murine T cells. J Immunol 144:1418–1424
15. Dumont FJ, Staruch MJ, Koprak SL, Melino MR, Sigal NH (1990b) Distinct mechanisms of suppression of murine T cell activation by the related macrolides FK-506 and rapamycin. J Immunol 144:251–258
16. Duncan JI (1994) Differential inhibition of cutaneous T-cell-mediated reactions and epidermal cell proliferation by cyclosporin A, FK-506, and rapamycin. J Invest Dermatol 102:84–88
17. Eng CP, Sehgal SN, Vezina C (1984) Activity of rapamycin (AY-22,989) against transplanted tumors. J Antibiot (Tokyo) 37:1231–1237
18. Findlay JA, Radics L (1980) On the chemistry and high field nuclear magnetic resonance spectroscopy of rapamycin. Can J Chem 58:579–590
19. Gardner CR (1995) The pharmacology of immunosuppressant drugs in skin transplant rejection in mice and other rodents. Gen Pharmacol 26:245–271
20. Hewitt CW, Black KS (1996) Overview of a 10-year experience on methods and compositions for inducing site-specific immunosuppression with topical immunosuppressants. Transplant Proc 28:922–923
21. Houchens DP, Ovejera AA, Riblet SM, Slagel DE (1983) Human brain tumor xenografts in nude mice as a chemotherapy model. Eur J Cancer Clin Oncol 19:799–805

22. Johnson EM, Zimmerman J, Duderstadt K, Chambers J, Sorenson AL, Granger DK, Almond PS, Fryer J, Leventhal JR, Scarola J, Matas AJ, Canafax DM (1996) A randomized, double-blind, placebo-controlled study of the safety, tolerance, and preliminary pharmacokinetics of ascending single doses of orally administered sirolimus (rapamycin) in stable renal transplant recipients. Transplant Proc 28:987
23. Kahan BD, Gibbons S, Tejpal N, Chou TC, Stepkowski S (1991a) Synergistic effect of the rapamycin-cyclosporine combination: median effect analysis of in vitro immune performances by human T lymphocytes in PHA, CD3, and MLR proliferative and cytotoxicity assays. Transplant Proc 23:1090–1091
24. Kahan BD, Gibbons S, Tejpal N, Stepkowski SM, Chou TC (1991b) Synergistic interactions of cyclosporine and rapamycin to inhibit immune performances of normal human peripheral blood lymphocytes in vitro. Transplantation 51:232–239
25. Kay JE, Kromwel L, Doe SE, Denyer M (1991) Inhibition of T and B lymphocyte proliferation by rapamycin. Immunology 72:544–549
26. Kimball PM, Kerman RH, Kahan BD (1991) Production of synergistic but nonidentical mechanisms of immunosuppression by rapamycin and cyclosporine. Transplantation 51: 86–490
27. Kino R, Hatanaka H, Hashimoto M, Nishiyama M, Goto T, Okuhara M, Kohsaka M, Aoki H, Imanaka H (1987a) FK-506, a novel immunosuppressant isolated from Streptomyces. I. Fermentation, isolation and physico-chemical and biological characteristics. J Antibiot (Tokyo) 40:1249–1255
28. Kino T, Hatanake H, Miyata S, Inamura N, Nishiyama M, Yajima T, Goto T, Okuhara M, Kohsaka M, Aoki H, Ochai T (1987b) FK-506, a novel immunosuppressant, isolated from Streptomyces. II. Immunosuppressive effect of FK-506 in vitro. J Antibiot (Tokyo) 40:1256–1265
29. Kuo CJ, Chung J, Fiorentino DF, Flanagan WM, Blenis J, Crabtree GR (1992) Rapamycin selectively inhibits interleukin-2 activation of p70 S6 kinase. Nature 358:70–73
30. Liu J, Farmer JD Jr, Lane WS, Friedman J, Weissman I, Schreiber SL (1991) Calcineurin is a common target of cyclophilin-cyclosporin A and FKBP-FK506 complexes. Cell 66:807–815
31. Martel RR, Klicius J, Galet S (1977) Inhibition of the immune response by rapamycin, a new antifungal antibiotic. Can J Physiol Pharmacol 55:48–51
32. Meingassner JG, Stutz A (1992) Immunosuppressive macrolides of the type FK 506: a novel class of topical agents for treatment of skin diseases? J Invest Dermatol 98:851–855
33. Merkel PA, Letourneau EN, Polisson RP (1995) Investigational agents for rheumatoid arthritis. Rheum Dis Clin North Am 21:779–796
34. Migita K, Eguchi K, aoyagi T, Tsukada T, Tsuboi M, Kawabe Y, Nagataki S (1996) The effects of the immunosuppressant rapamycin on the growth of rheumatoid arthritis (RA) synovial fibroblast. Clin Exp Immunol 104:86–91
35. Molnar-Kimber KL (1996) Mechanism of action of rapamycin (Sirolimus, Rapamune). Transplant Proc 28:964–969
36. Morice WG, Brunn GJ, Wiederrecht G, Siekierka JJ, Abraham RT (1993a) Rapamycin-induced inhibition of p34cdc2 kinase activation is associated with G1/S-phase growth arrest in T lymphocytes. J Biol Chem 268:3734–3738
37. Morice WG, Wiederrecht G, Brunn GJ, Siekierka JJ, Abraham RT (1993b) Rapamycin inhibition of interleukin-2-dependent p33cdk2 and p34cdc2 kinase activation in T lymphocytes. J Biol Chem 268:22737–22745
38. Morris RE (1992) Rapamycin: antifungal, antitumor, antiproliferative, and immunosuppressive macrolides. Transplant Rev 6:39–87
39. Morris RE (1993) New small molecule immunosuppressants for transplantation: review of essential concepts. J Heart Lung Transplant 12:S275–286
40. Morris RE, Meiser BM (1989) Identification of a new pharmacologic function for an old compound. Med Sci Res 17:609–610
41. Nair RV, Morris RE (1995) Immunosuppression in cardiac transplantation: a new era in immunopharmacology. Curr Opin Cardiol 10:207–217
42. Nicolau KC, Chakraborty TK, Piscopio AD, Minowa N, Bertinato P (1993) Total synthesis of rapamycin. J Am Chem Soc 115:4419–4420

43. Nourse J, Firpo E, Flanagan WM, Coats S, Polyak K, Lee MH, Massague J, Crabtree GR, Roberts JM (1994) Interleukin-2-mediated elimination of the p27Kip1 cyclin-dependent kinase inhibitor prevented by rapamycin. Nature 372:570–573
44. Powles AV, Baker BS, Fry L (1989) Cyclosporin A and skin diseases. In: Thomson AW (ed) Cylosporin: mode of action and clinical application. Kluwer, Dordrecht, pp 191–212
45. Price DJ, Grove JR, Calvo V, Avruch J, Bierer BE (1992) Rapamycin-induced inhibition of the 70-kilodalton S6 protein kinase. Science 257:973–977
46. Propper DJ, Woo J, Macleod AM, Catto GR, Thomson AW (1992) The effects of rapamycin on humoral immunity in vivo. Suppression of primary responses but not of ongoing alloantibody synthesis or memory responses. Transplantation 54:1058–1063
47. Savitsky K, Bar-Shira A, Gilad S, Rotman G, Ziv Y, Vanagaite L, Tagle DA, Smith S, Uziel T, Sfez S, Askenazi M, Pecker I, Frydman M, Harnik R, Patanjali SR, Simmons A, Clines GA, Sartiel A, Gatti RA, Chessa L, Sanal O, Lavin MF, Jaspers NGJ, Taylor AMR, Arlett CF, Miki T, Weissmann SM, Lovett M, Collins FS, Shiloh Y (1995) A single ataxia teleangiectatica gene with a product similar to PI-3 kinase. Science 268:1749–1753
48. Schmidbauer G, Hancock WW, Wasowska B, Badger AM, Kupiec-Weglinski JW (1994) Abrogation by rapamycin of accelerated rejection in sensitized rats by inhibition of alloantibody responses and selective suppression of intragraft mononuclear and endothelial cell activation, cytokine production, and cell adhesion. Transplantation 57:933–941
49. Sehgal SN (1995) Rapamune (sirolimus, rapamycin): an overview and mechanism of action. Ther Drug Monit 17:660–665
50. Sehgal SN, Baker H, Vezina C (1975) Rapamycin (AY-22,989), a new antifungal antibiotic. II. Fermentation, isolation and characterization. J Antibiot (Tokyo) 28:727–732
51. Sigal NH, Lin CS, Siekierka JJ (1991) Inhibition of human T-cell activation by FK 506, rapamycin, and cyclosporine A. Transplant Proc 23:1–5
52. Snyder SH, Sabatini DM (1995) Immunophilins and the nervous system. Nat Med 1:32–37
53. Terada N, Lucas JJ, Szepesi A, Franklin RA, Domenico J, Gelfand EW (1993) Rapamycin blocks cell cycle progression of activated T cells prior to events characteristic of the middle to late G1 phase of the cycle. J Cell Physiol 154:7–15
54. Thomson AW, Propper DJ, Woo J, Whiting PH, Milton JI, Macleod AM (1993) Comparative effects of rapamycin, FK 506 and cyclosporine on antibody production, lymphocyte populations and immunoglobulin isotype switching in the rat. Immunopharmacol Immunotoxicol 15:355–369
55. Van Duyne GD, Standaert RF, Karplus PA, Schreiber SL, Clardy J (1993) Atomic structures of the human immunophilin FKBP-12 complexes with FK506 and rapamycin. J Mol Biol 229:105–124
56. Vezina C, Kudelski A, Sehgal SN (1975) Rapamycin (AY-22,989), a new antifungal antibiotic. I. Taxonomy of the producing streptomycete and isolation of the active principle. J Antibiot (Tokyo) 28:721–726
57. Warner LM, Adams LM, Sehgal SN (1994) Rapamycin prolongs survival and arrests pathophysiologic changes in murine systemic lupus erythematosus. Arthritis Rheum 37:289–297
58. Wasowska B, Wieder KJ, Hancock WW, Zheng XX, Berse B, Binder J, Strom TB, Kupiec-Weglinski JW (1996) Cytokine and alloantibody networks in long term cardiac allografts in rat recipients treated with rapamycin. J Immunol 156:395–404
59. Yatscoff RW (1996) Pharmacokinetics of rapamycin. Transplant Proc 28:970–973
60. Yoshimura N, Ohmoto Y, Yasui H, Ohsaka Y, Bong JM, Kobayashi Y, Oka T (1994) The direct effect of FK506 and rapamycin on interleukin (beta) and immunoglobulin production in vitro. Transplantation 57:1815–1818

FK-506/Tacrolimus

A. Wollenberg and T. Bieber

History

Tacrolimus (FK-506) was first isolated in May 1984 from the culture broth of a soil microorganism found in Tsukuba, Japan. In contrast to Flemming's penicillin, it was no accidental finding but the result of a thoroughly undertaken screening project for new immunomodulatory substances by researchers of an industrial company. Following 3 years of extensive research, the first report on this new drug was published by Kino et al. [1]. The newly identified drug-producing fungus was named after its origin as *Streptomyces tsukubaensis* and is characterized by a grey mycelium color, rectiflexible spore chains with smooth spore surfaces, nonchromogenicity, and a limited carbohydrate usage [2].

Biochemical Properties

Although it has similar biological properties to cyclosporin A, FK-506 has no structural relationship to it. FK-506 is a macrolide lactone with a hemiketal masked a,b-diketoamide incorporated in a 23-member ring [2] (Fig. 1). In its natural form, FK-506 is a white powder with an atomic weight of 822.05 Da, a melting point of 127°–129 °C, and the molecular formula $C_{44}H_{69}NO_{12}$ H_2O [3]. Due to its hydrophobicity, FK-506 is freely soluble in methanol, chloroform, acetone, and ethanol, but virtually insoluble in water. The resulting poor intestinal absorption has successfully been overcome by a solid dispersible formulation on hydroxypropyl methylcellulose [4]. In contrast to cyclosporin A, topically applied FK-506 penetrates the skin in variable amounts, depending on the drug concentration and integrity of the treated skin. Therefore, topical FK-506 treatment of skin diseases is possible.

Molecular Mode of Action

On the molecular level, tacrolimus inhibits T cell receptor-mediated Ca^{2+}-associated signal transduction pathways and the transcriptional activation of several lymphokine genes. Similar to cyclosporin A, the activation and maturation of various cell types, including those involved in cell-mediated immunity, is inhibited. FK-506 exerts its biological effects after binding to cytosolic proteins (immunophillins or FK-506-binding proteins, FK-BP). The resulting complex functionally blocks the calcium-dependent serine/threonine phosphatase calcineurin, one of the effects being inhibition of the dephosphorylation of the transcription factor NF-ATp and thereby inhibition of its translocation to the nucleus [5]. Since NF-ATp is an essential transcription-activating

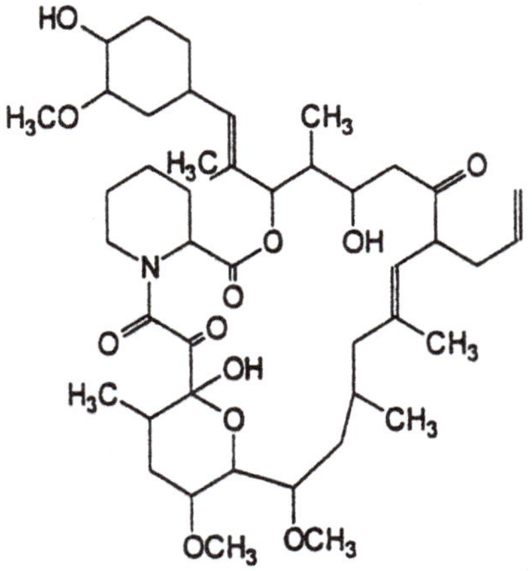

Fig. 1. Molecule structure of FK-506

factor of the interleukin (IL)-2 gene, FK-506 in the end blocks the T cell response by IL-2 transcription inhibition [6]. Other targets involving the NF-AT pathway, such as the IL-5 gene [7] and IL-4 gene [8], have been reported. Furthermore, anti-CD40-induced murine B cell proliferation, in the presence or absence of IL-4 is, like the response to anti-immunoglobulin, abrogated by 1–5 ng FK-506/ml [9]. Another immunomodulatory substance, rapamycin, competes with FK-506 for the FK-BP. Since rapamycin exerts biological effects that are different from and often contrary to FK-506, the entire FK-506/rapamycin/FK-BP system has gained much interest in basic research. The effects of rapamycin are discussed in "Rapamycin" (this volume).

Effects on Skin Cells In Vitro

In normal human skin cell systems, among other biological effects, FK-506 affects the maturation of Langerhans cells and modulates the appearance/increase of distinct, functionally relevant molecules such as the IL-2 receptor (CD25), B7.1 (CD80), and B7.2 (CD86) [10]. This may explain the observed decrease in their allostimulatory activity in the skin mixed lymphocyte reaction [10]. In vitro studies with cultured human foreskin keratinocytes showed 70% reduction of IL-8 receptor RNA expression 1 h after FK-506 incubation, leading to reduced protein binding of IL-8 to its receptor after 24 h [11]. Mast cells and basophils are targets for FK-506 as well. Histamine release from skin mast cells and basophils, activated by anti-IgE, was inhibited by incubation with FK-506 [12]. In contrast, degranulation resulting from the activation of protein kinase C by phorbol ester was not inhibited [13].

Effects on Skin Cells Ex Vivo/In Vivo

In inflammatory skin conditions, keratinocytes, Langerhans cells, fibroblasts, lymphocytes, mast cells, and inflammatory dendritic epidermal cells (IDEC) [14] may, among other cell types, be simultaneously altered in their biological function. Keratinocytes in psoriasis have been shown to respond dose dependently to FK-506 by downregulation of the IL-8 receptor [15]. In atopic eczema, FK-506 treatment leads to downregulation of the high-affinity IgE receptor (FceRI) [16]. Furthermore, the cell numbers of IDEC subsequently fall below the detection limit [16]. Finally, the antigen-presenting capacity of lesional epidermal cell suspensions towards their autologous lymphocytes is lowered under topical FK-506 treatment [16]. As compared to cyclosporin A, approximately 100 times lower FK-506 concentrations may be considered therapeutic in vitro and in vivo [2].

Clinical Application in Dermatology

For treatment in dermatology, the physician has the choice of oral and systemic FK-506 formulations. This therapeutic choice is made on the basis of the respective effects and side effects in the given skin disease. If there is sufficient drug delivery to the disease location by topical administration, e.g., atopic eczema, this will be the method of choice.

The oral formulation of FK-506 [4] is a most powerful regimen, which might be used on an experimental basis for many dermatologic disorders known to respond to steroids or cyclosporin A. In clinical dermatology, interest has focused on oral FK-506 administration since 1992, when Jegasothy et al. [17] reported the clearing of disease in four psoriasis patients under oral FK-506 treatment. The clinical effectivity of oral FK-506 in psoriasis has been confirmed in a controlled clinical trial by the European FK-506 Multicenter Psoriasis Study Group [18]. Similar beneficial effects have been reported for atopic eczema. However, keeping in mind the susceptibility of atopic patients to cutaneous and extracutaneous infections, systemic FK-506 has been and will be used with caution. Side effects may limit the usage of oral FK-506; arterial hypertension, electrolyte disturbance, neurotoxicity, nephrotoxicity, and disturbances of glucose metabolism are among the reported side effects in transplantation medicine. However, the most important unwanted effect is the obligatory general immunosuppression, potentially leading to cutaneous and extracutaneous systemic infections.

Topical FK-506 formulations have been developed as a means of delivering therapeutic concentrations to the disease area while minimizing the risk of systemic toxicity. In fact, these topical FK-506 formulations have been used in a few atopic eczema patients, where they have been shown to be an effective drug [19, 20]. A large, placebo-controlled, double-blinded clinical multicenter trial involving over 200 atopic eczema patients proved the safety and efficacy of topical FK-506 in this disease. Allergic contact dermatitis is responsive to topical FK-506 as well. The efficacy in this condition was reported in humans [21] and further investigated in guinea pig [22]. Whether topical FK-506 is also effective in psoriasis vulgaris remains to be verified.

Clinical Prospects

At present (in 1996), the main indication for oral FK-506 is the prevention of allograft rejection in transplantation medicine. Severe psoriasis vulgaris, atopic eczema, and some other skin diseases that respond to cyclosporin A may additionally be considered rare indications for the oral dosage form. Topical FK-506 must be regarded a highly promising drug for atopic eczema. Since topical FK-506 treatment does not lead to most of the topical steroid side effects, e.g., epidermal atrophy or striae distensae, it should broaden the therapeutic options for many patients with chronic inflammatory skin disease. In the future, topical FK-506 could be a therapeutic option for alopecia areata, lupus erythematodes, lichen planus, and various other inflammatory skin diseases that are currently treated with topical steroids alone.

Summary

FK-506/Tacrolimus is an immunomodulatory macrolide first isolated from the fungus *Streptomyces tsukubaenis* in 1984. FK-506 functionally resembles Cyclosporine A, but is effective at 100-fold lower concentrations. Biological activities include functional blocking of calcineurin and inhibition of NF-ATp-dependent cytokines. The hydrophobicity of FK-506 allows an effective drug delivery following topical application to eczematous skin lesions. Since topical FK-506 therapy circumvents most of the unwanted topical steroid side effects (e.g. epidermal and dermal atrophy, striae distensae), it is regarded as a highly promising drug for inflammatory skin diseases.

References

1. Kino T, Hatanaka H, Hashimoto M et al (1987) FK-506, a novel immunosuppressant isolated from a Streptomyces. I. Fermentation, isolation, and physico-chemical and biological characteristics. J Antibiot Tokyo 40(9):1249–1255
2. Goto T, Kino T, Hatanaka H et al (1991) FK 506: historical perspectives. Transplant Proc 23:2713–2717
3. Tanaka H, Kuroda A, Marusawa H et al (1987) Physicochemical properties of FK-506, a novel immunosuppressant isolated from Streptomyces tsukubaensis. Transplant Proc 19 [5; Suppl 6]:11–16
4. Honbo T, Kobayashi M, Hane K, Hata T, Ueda Y (1987) The oral dosage form of FK-506. Transplant Proc 19 [5; Suppl 6]:17–22
5. Wesselborg S, Fruman DA, Sagoo JK, Bierer BE, Burakoff SJ (1996) Identification of a physical interaction between calcineurin and nuclear factor of activated T cells (NFATp). J Biol Chem 271:1274–1277
6. Schreiber SL, Crabtree GR (1992) The mechanism of action of cyclosporin A and FK506. Immunol Today 13:136–142
7. Mori A, Suko M, Nishizaki Y et al (1995) IL-5 production by CD4+ T cells of asthmatic patients is suppressed by glucocorticoids and the immunosuppressants FK506 and cyclosporin A. Int Immunol 7:449–457
8. Schneider G, Heinfling A, Klein HS, Schomberg C, Chuvpilo S, Serfling E (1995) The inducible transcription factor NF-AT plays an important role in the activation of the murine interleukin-4 promoter. Immunobiology 193:268–272
9. Klaus GG, Choi MS, Holman M (1994) Properties of mouse CD40. Ligation of CD40 activates B cells via a Ca(++)-dependent, FK506-sensitive pathway. Eur J Immunol 24:3229–3232
10. Panhans A, Bieber T (1996) FK506 (tacrolimus) impairs the phenotypic and functional differentiation of human epidermal Langerhans cells. J Invest Dermatol 107:485
11. Michel G, Ried C, Beetz A (1993) FK-506 blocks expression of interleukin-8 receptor in normal human keratinocytes. J Invest Dermatol 100:449
12. de Paulis A, Stellato C, Cirillo R, Ciccarelli A, Oriente A, Marone G (1992) Anti-inflammatory effect of FK-506 on human skin mast cells. J Invest Dermatol 99:723–728
13. Nakajima K, Koichi H, Takaishi T (1992) Antiallergic action of a new immunosuppressive agent, FK 506. Yamanashi Kenritsu Chuo Byoin Nenpo 19:27–30
14. Wollenberg A, Kraft S, Hanau D, Bieber T (1996) Immunomorphological and ultrastructural characterization of Langerhans cells and a novel, inflammatory dendritic epidermal cell (IDEC) population in lesional skin of atopic eczema. J Invest Dermatol 106:446–453
15. Schulz BS, Michel G, Wagner S et al (1993) Increased expression of epidermal IL-8 receptor in psoriasis. Down-regulation by FK-506 in vitro. J Immunol 151:4399-4406

16. Wollenberg A, Regele D, Sharma S, Haberstok J, Panhans A, Bieber T (1996) Topical tacrolimus treatment leads to profound alterations of the antigen presenting cells in lesional atopic dermatitis skin. J Invest Dermatol 107:468
17. Jegasothy BV, Ackerman CD, Todo S, Fung JJ, Abu EK, Starzl TE (1992) Tacrolimus (FK 506) a new therapeutic agent for severe recalcitrant psoriasis. Arch Dermatol 128:781–785
18. The European FK 506 Multicentre Psoriasis Study Group (1996) Systemic tacrolimus (FK 506) is effective for the treatment of psoriasis in a double-blind, placebo-controlled study. Arch Dermatol 132:419–423
19. Nakagawa H, Etoh T, Ishibashi Y et al (1994) Tacrolimus ointment for atopic dermatitis. Lancet 344:8926
20. Aoyama H, Tabata N, Tanaka M, Uesugi Y, Tagami H (1995) Successful treatment of resistant facial lesions of atopic dermatitis with 0.1% FK506 ointment. Br J Dermatol 133:494–496
21. Lauerma AI, Maibach HI, Granlund H, Erkko P, Kartamaa M, Stubb S (1992) Inhibition of contact allergy reactions by topical FK506 (letter). Lancet 340:8818
22. Lauerma AI, Stein BD, Homey B, Lee CH, Bloom E, Maibach HI (1994) Topical FK506: suppression of allergic and irritant contact dermatitis in the guinea pig. Arch Dermatol Res 286:337–340

Low-Dose Methotrexate: An Immunomodifying Therapeutic Strategy for Dermatologic Diseases

I. Boehm and R. Bauer

Introduction

Methotrexate (4-amino-N^{10}-methylpteroyl-glutamate, MTX), a folic acid antagonist that binds to the active catalytic site of dihydrofolate reductase, inhibits the synthesis of C1 units, which are important metabolites for the production of purine nucleotides, thymidylate, and the amino acids serine and methionine. Consequently, RNA, DNA, and protein synthesis are altered in a dose-dependent manner, so that MTX works as a cytostatic compound.

As far as cytostatic agents are concerned, folic acid antagonists have been used by dermatologists for psoriasis since the early 1950s to control increased epidermal cell proliferation. Early studies already suggested that low-dose MTX has an immunomodifying ability. Due to intense use by rheumatologists for rheumatoid arthritis (RA) in the past 10 years and to immunologic research, it became evident that low-dose MTX has anti-inflammatory and immunomodulating effects.

Indications

MTX is an established therapeutic agent for psoriasis. Despite the introduction of new antipsoriatic drugs, low-dose MTX is still one of the most effective and safest agents for the treatment of severe psoriasis if the suggested guidelines are closely adhered to. Unlike other antipsoriatics, MTX also improves psoriatic arthritis and nail psoriasis. Initially, in the therapeutic use of MTX, dermatologists focused almost exclusively on psoriatic patients. Later, it became evident that this drug is beneficial for dermatomyositis, sarcoidosis, lupus erythematosus (LE), and Wegener's granulomatosis. Although prospective, randomized, double-blind, placebo-controlled multicenter studies are lacking, preliminary results of clinical trials indicate efficacy of low-dose MTX in a growing number of noninfectious inflammatory skin diseases, including the following:

- Severe psoriasis (psoriatic erythroderma, psoriatic arthritis, pustular psoriasis)
- Nail psoriasis
- Reiter's disease
- Pityriasis rubra pilaris
- Pityriasis lichenoides et varioliformis acuta (Mucha-Habermann disease)
- Vasculitis
- Polyarteritis nodosa
- Giant cell (temporal) arteritis
- Takayasu's arteritis

- Urticaria vasculitis
- Wegener's granulomatosis
- LE
- Cardiolipin antibody syndrome
- Scleroderma
- Eosinophilia-myalgia syndrome
- Dermatomyositis
- Bullous pemphigoid
- Pemphigus vulgaris
- Benign familial chronic pemphigus
- Behcet's disease
- Melkersson-Rosenthal syndrome
- Sarcoidosis
- Drug-induced pustulosis
- Job's syndrome
- Atopic dermatitis
- Steroid-resistant urticaria
- Lymphomatoid papulosis
- Cutaneous T cell lymphoma (Sézary syndrome)
- Multiple keratoacanthomata
- Keloids

For long-term treatment of chronic dermatoses such as bullous pemphigoid, low-dose MTX has a steroid-sparing effect; Paul and colleagues stated that MTX is a first-line agent for this indication [34]. Different forms of vasculitis respond with a favorable efficacy to risk ratio to low-dose MTX, including severe recalcitrant polyarteritis nodosa [7]. MTX has even been suggested for the treatment of patients with atopic dermatitis [11]. Moreover, low-dose MTX has been demonstrated in an animal model to ameliorate interleukin (IL)-2-induced pulmonary vascular leak syndrome [15] and might be helpful in IL-2-treated oncologic patients in future.

Dose, Application, and Dose Adjustment

MTX is usually given as an oral or intravenous weekly bolus in doses ranging from 5 to 25 mg. Depending on disease severity and individual MTX toxicity risk factors, it is initially administered in doses up to 25 mg per week. If long-term treatment is necessary, it is recommended that the minimal disease-controlling dose be administered. When the maximum of clinical benefit has been achieved, an attempt can be made to withdraw MTX. If this is not possible, one can try to reduce the single administered dose and/or increase the administration intervals up to 2 weeks. In order to minimize the total cumulative dose, van Dooren-Greebe and colleagues [49] suggest an interruption of MTX administration in long-term treatment, and Weinstein and White [53] propose a rotational therapy for psoriasis with successive change of treatment modalities.

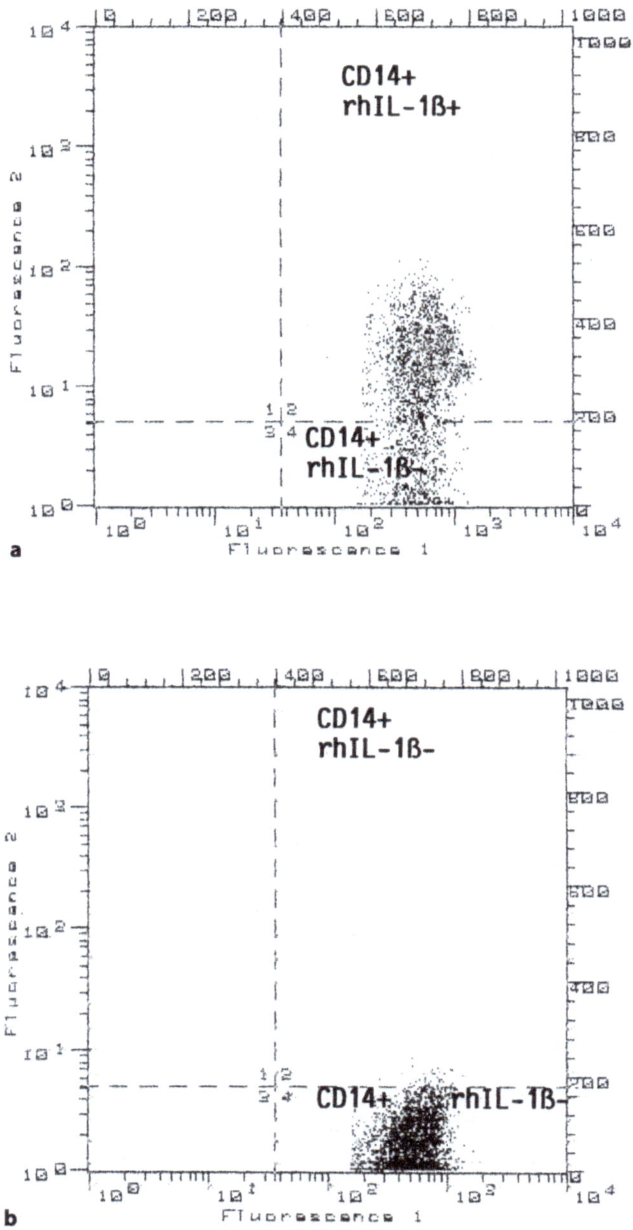

Fig. 1a,b. Flow cytometric dot plot analysis of CD^{14+} (fluorescence 1) monocytes. **a** Without methotrexate (MTX), binding of phycoerythrin (PE)-labeled recombinant human interleukin (*rhIL*)-1β (fluorescence 2). **b** With MTX, lack of binding to rhIL-1β

Mode of Action

MTX is a cytostatic agent whose mechanism of action in a low-dose weekly regimen is not completely understood; however, several lines of evidence indicate that it has anti-inflammatory rather than immunosuppressive effects. The onset of action is rapid. When used in pustular psoriasis, early treatment effects were visible 48 h after the first MTX injection [6], and even erythrodermic patients improved significantly more quickly when receiving MTX [21]. Recently, it has been shown that low-dose MTX improved the condition of a patient with subacute cutaneous LE (SCLE) within 2 weeks [4]. Moreover, usually neither leukocytes nor lymphocytes decrease under low-dose MTX treatment [32, 46]. This prompted several researchers to investigate cytokines, mediators, and other functional immunocellular mechanisms in association with MTX. Segal and colleagues [41] were the first to investigate the influence of MTX on IL-1. They did not find any reduction of IL-1 production or secretion, but their data indicated an inhibition of IL-1 activity. This has been confirmed by other investigators. Analyzing the ability of MTX on cytokine release, they revealed that MTX inhibited neither cell-associated nor secreted IL-1β levels [36, 40], but without affecting IL-1 production MTX inhibited IL-1 activity [9]. In an in vitro assay, we demonstrated that MTX interferes with IL-1 and inhibits binding to its cell surface receptor [5] (Fig. 1). Based on these data, MTX seems to be the first discovered low molecular weight anticytokine for IL-1.

In vitro, MTX has no effect on lipopolysaccharide (LPS)-induced IL-1 synthesis by macrophages [24]. In vivo, however, several investigators have found that macrophages or peripheral blood mononuclear cells (PBMC) from MTX-treated individuals produce less IL-1 upon stimulation than those from untreated and pretreated subjects, respectively [3, 10, 24, 26, 42]. As the IL-1 receptor antagonist (IL-1ra) has been shown to inhibit IL-1-induced IL-1 production in PBMC [18], it is tempting to speculate that a similar mechanism might be responsible for the decreased IL-1 synthesis in MTX-treated patients or animals. This speculation is based on the fact that a significantly lower IL-1ra to IL-1β ratio before treatment and an increase of this ratio due to MTX treatment has been detected in association with clinical response [42]. In addition to inhibition of IL-1 activity, these results suggest that MTX induces the production of IL-1ra, the naturally occurring antagonist of IL-1 activity.

IL-1, an important proinflammatory cytokine, plays a central pathogenetic role in cutaneous inflammatory events, e.g., by activating chemotaxis of neutrophils, activating endothelial cells, inducing adhesion molecules and chemokines, activating nuclear factor (NF)-kB, and stimulating the production of nitric oxide. Consequently, IL-1 has been detected as a pivotal mediator of various dermatoses such as psoriasis [13], sarcoidosis [17], scleroderma [27], and LE [39]. Therefore, the clinical benefit of low-dose MTX in these dermatoses appears to depend particularly on MTX-mediated blocking of IL-1 activity. Recent in vitro investigations indicate that proliferating lymphoid cells rather than epithelial cells are a major cellular target of MTX in psoriasis [25].

Invasion of leukocytes from the circulating blood into the skin is a crucial step in inflammatory skin diseases. Therefore, the pharmacological blocking of this event may offer an attractive therapeutic tool. Reduced numbers of skin-infiltrating polymorphonuclear leukocytes (PMN) in MTX-treated patients with psoriasis [29] as well as

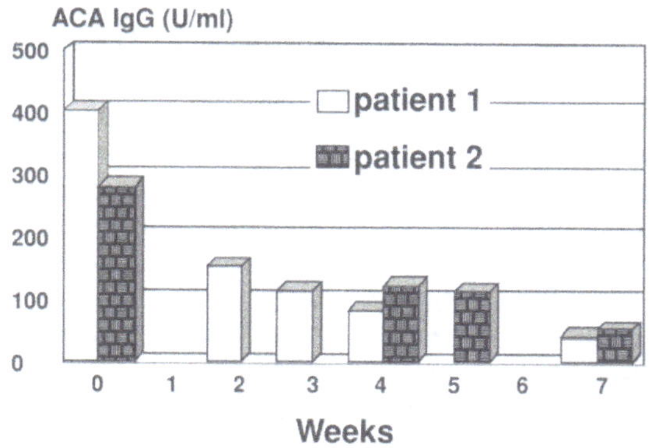

Fig. 2. Follow-up of the levels of anticardiolipin antibodies (ACA) in two patients with phospholipid syndrome under low-dose methotrexate (MTX) treatment

reduced numbers of leukocytes and neutrophils in the synovial fluid and decreased influx of macrophages into synovial tissue in MTX-treated patients with RA have been registered [26, 46]. This suggests that MTX acts particularly by reducing the migration of leukocytes into inflamed tissue. This effect may be due to attenuation of platelet-activating factor (PAF)-induced leukocyte-endothelial cell adhesion in postcapillary venules via activation of A2 receptors on the leukocyte by MTX [2]. Furthermore, MTX inhibits leukotriene B_4 (LTB_4) and/or C5a-induced neutrophil and macrophage chemotaxis [45, 51]. Inhibition of PMN accumulation in the skin may contribute to its action on inflammatory dermatoses, especially those with prominent extravasation of neutrophils, e.g., pustular psoriasis [6]. Nevertheless, controlled trials are warranted to prove the efficacy in larger patient groups under clinical conditions.

In most instances, neither leukocytes nor lymphocyte subsets decrease under low-dose MTX [32, 46]. However, treatment with low-dose MTX in systemic LE [22] and SCLE (I. Boehm and R. Rauer, manuscript submitted) appears to be associated with an increase in diminished T cell subsets such as $CD3^+$ $CD4^+$ cells. The amelioration of the T cell counts was accompanied by clinical improvement of LE. Nevertheless, the mechanism by which MTX increases $CD4^+$ cells is unknown, but it may be speculated that anti-$CD4^+$ T cell autoantibodies responsible for low T cell counts in LE might be downregulated by MTX. This seems likely, because MTX is able to suppress Ig production. O'Meara and coworkers [33] found that MTX at a concentration of 5×10^{-9} *M* markedly decreased all classes of Ig synthesis; Alarcon and associates [1] showed that MTX downregulated rheumatoid factor production; and we revealed in two patients with antiphospholipid syndrome a decrease in elevated anti-cardiolipin antibodies (ACA) in association with low-dose MTX (Fig. 2). Rosenthal and colleagues [37] suggested that inhibition of purine biosynthesis might be responsible for suppression of B cell function. Furthermore, several cytokines, such as IL-1, IL-6, and tumor necrosis factor (TNF)-α, have been implicated in the spontaneous Ig production in SLE. Blocking of these mediators by specific antibodies has been shown to decrease Ig production [30]. Therefore, it seems likely that, by interacting with IL-1, MTX might have similar effects on B cell function and could thus downregulate Ig synthesis. The clinical improvement of a variety of autoimmune diseases may be attributable to this effect of MTX, but further investigations are necessary to obtain closer insight into the therapeutic action of MTX.

A variety of other cytokines and mediators have been investigated to elucidate the therapeutic influence of low-dose MTX. MTX was completely inactive in inhibiting the release of IL-2, IL-4, IL-5, and IL-8 from monocytes and T cell subsets [40]. Interactions between IL-8 and endothelial cells play an important role in the emigration of mononuclear cells from the blood into areas of inflammation. MTX did not disturb the production of either IL-8 or monocyte chemoattractant protein (MCP)-1 by rheumatoid synoviocytes [31]. Furthermore, MTX had no effect on IL-8 secretion by endothelial cells [14]. In RA patients, MTX significantly reduces IL-6 and soluble IL-2 receptor (sIL-2R) in the circulating blood [12]. In contrast, Wascher and coworkers [52] demonstrated that, in patients with a successful clinical outcome, MTX treatment did not affect elevated levels of IL-6 and TNF-α. This leads to the assumption that MTX might inhibit the actions of IL-6 and TNF-α.

Furthermore, MTX slightly but significantly decreased the production of IL-10 at a concentration of 10 μM, and it thus seems likely that MTX is able to influence the Th1–Th2 misbalance [47] and possibly to improve atopic dermatitis [11].

Divergent results have been obtained when analyzing the effect of MTX on the production of 5-lipoxygenase (5-LO) metabolites. Whereas Sperling and coworkers [44] revealed significant reduction of neutrophil 5-LO pathway metabolites, Hawkes and associates [22] found an increase in the production of all measured 5-LO metabolites. These data may indicate that the influence on 5-LO metabolites is not a hallmark of MTX.

At concentrations of 10^{-3} to 10^{-7} M, MTX neither altered antibody-dependent cell-mediated cytotoxicity (ADCC) nor O_2^- and H_2O_2 secretion by phorbol myristate acetate (PMA)-stimulated macrophages [20]. Even at high doses, MTX did not disturb macrophage functional activity as asssessed by analysis of phagocytosis and ADCC [55]. On the other hand, MTX potentiates the release of hydrogen peroxide by stimulated polymorphonuclear neutrophils in a dose-dependent manner [19]. With respect to these results, nonspecific toxic effects of low-dose MTX on cell function seem to be rather unlikely.

A variety of other immunomodifying events of MTX have been discovered; these are summarized in Fig. 3.

Side Effects and Risk Factors

Controlled clinical trials and numerous case reports have shown low-dose MTX to be a second-line agent of high efficacy with an acceptable profile of safety and tolerability. A variety of possible side effects are associated with MTX treatment:

- Gastrointestinal intolerance (nausea, vomiting, diarrhea, transient noncirrhotic ascites, stomatitis, oral ulceration)
- Hepatotoxicity (hepatic enzyme elevation, liver fibrosis/cirrhosis, liver failure)
- Pulmonary complications (pulmonary fibrosis, pneumonitis, pulmonary edema, acute pleuritis, pleural effusion, respiratory failure)
- Pericardial tamponade
- Opportunistic infections (disseminated histoplasmosis, Mycobacterium avium intracellulare pneumonia, Pneumocystitis carinii pneumonia, nocardiosis, herpes simplex hepatitis, herpes zoster, systemic fungal infection)

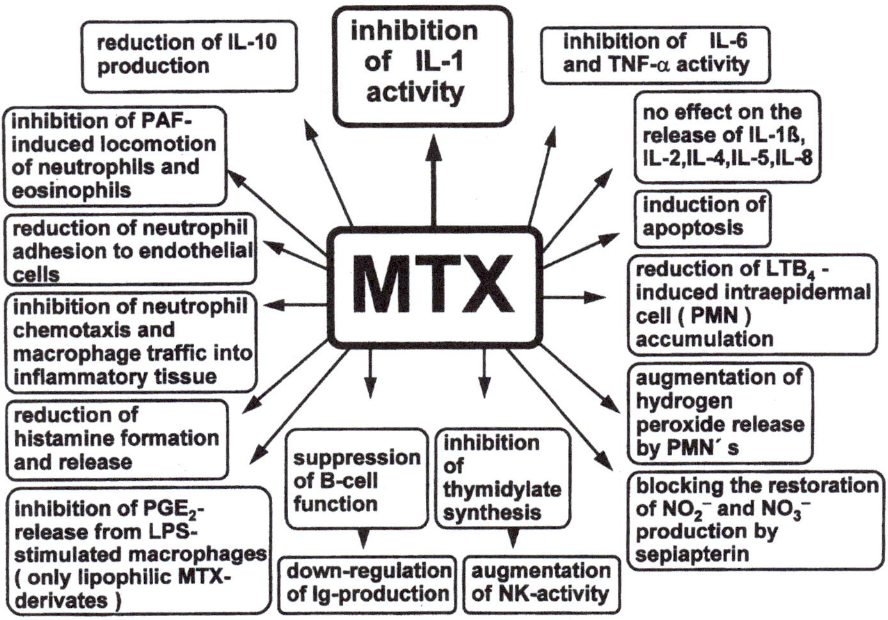

Fig. 3. Synopsis of the recent standpoint of scientific research concerning the mode of action of low-dose methotrexate (MTX)

- Hematotoxicity (leukopenia/pancytopenia, megaloblastic anemia, bone marrow failure)
- Anaphylaxis
- Neurotoxicity (headache, visual field defects, dementing illness with leukoencephalopathy)
- Accelerated nodulosis
- Skin disorders (reversible alopecia, erythema multiforme, toxic epidermal necrolysis, cutaneous pseudolymphoma, reactivation of sunburn)
- Teratogenesis
- Oligospermia
- Lymphoma
- Malignant neoplasm

However, the toxicity of MTX appears to be comparable to that of antimalarials [38]. During a 22-year period, van Dooren-Greebe and coauthors [48] did not observe any deaths or life-threatening side effects due to MTX treatment in psoriasis patients.

Nevertheless, mild and moderate side effects are common, but they rarely necessitate withdrawal of the drug. Psoriatic patients treated with MTX frequently develop gastrointestinal symptoms, which can be controlled with folate substitution [16]. Mucositis responds to folate administration less frequently. Elevations of transaminases are also common; in most cases, they are reversible after reducing the dose or increasing the administration intervals.

In short-term treatment, the risk for toxicity is low, but long-term toxicity has been analyzed in detail only for psoriatic patients. For other indications, long-term toxicity is uncertain. Serious side effects of MTX include hepatic, hematologic, and pulmonary toxicity. Most side effects of MTX – with the exception of anaphylaxis and other hypersensitivity reactions – are dose dependent and tend to increase in patients with preexisting risk factors, such as the following:

- Preexisting liver disorder
- Alcohol abuse
- Hepatotoxic co-medication
- Previous arsenic treatment
- Low serum albumin
- Elevated serum creatinine
- Total cumulative dose of MTX
- Low folate level
- Co-medication with other folic acid antagonists
- Co-medication with nonsteroidal anti-inflammatory drugs (NSAID; penicillin, cephalotine, colchicine, barbiturate, dipyridamole)
- Diabetes mellitus and obesity
- Preexisting lung disease
- Age (?)

The main serious side effect in psoriatic patients receiving low-dose MTX is hepatotoxicity. In a cohort of 183 MTX-treated psoriatic patients, biopsy-proven liver cirrhosis occurred in 19 (10.3 %) [54]. The authors also showed that the frequency of cirrhosis increased parallel to the duration of MTX treatment (13.5 % in patients treated for longer than 2 years, 25.6 % in patients treated for longer than 5 years). The cumulative MTX dose since liver cirrhosis was detected ranged from 590 to 8105 mg (mean, 2200 mg). Other investigators found hepatic fibrosis in 13 % of MTX-treated psoriatic patients, and cirrhosis in 4 % [48]. They did not reveal any correlation between liver histology and cumulative dose of MTX, nor between liver morphology and increase in transaminases. Serious liver disease is an uncommon complication of low-dose MTX therapy in RA. Liver fibrosis [43] and liver cirrhosis [8], as detected by liver biopsy, occur in less than 3 %. The accumulation of MTX polyglutamates within hepatocytes has been attributed to the hepatotoxicity of MTX. In additional, preexisting risk factors may support the development of liver fibrosis/cirrhosis.

Low-dose MTX therapy-related hematotoxic effects, pulmonary complications, and opportunistic infections seem to be more frequent in RA than in psoriatic or other dermatologic patients.

Monitoring and Managing Patients

Careful selection of patients for MTX therapy and close clinical and laboratory monitoring during treatment are essential in order to minimize or even prevent serious side effects. Intact renal, hepatic, and bone marrow function are important prerequisites for low-dose MTX treatment. Patients with (potential) risk factors (see above) should be excluded or, if no acceptable alternative exists, should be monitored at short intervals. Moreover, careful consideration of indications and combination with other medication are necessary. Hepatotoxic co-medication should be avoided if not absolutely necessary. As NSAID have been suspected to increase the toxicity of MTX, these should not be combined.

The total cumulative dose should be exactly documented. Reducing the total cumulative dose may reduce long-term side effects.

Dynamic hepatic scintigraphy is considered an appropriate diagnostic method for MTX-induced hepatic damage, but grading of the hepatic damage is not possible. Therefore, although dynamic hepatic scintigraphy may be useful for liver diagnostics in the future, liver biopsy is currently still superior to other noninvasive diagnostic methods [50].

Taken together, the suggested guidelines for treatment with MTX should be closely followed [28, 35].

Conclusions

Pharmacological manipulation of pathogenetic relevant cytokines with low molecular weight agents, as has been shown for MTX, provides a new therapeutic tool for immunomodifying strategies. Recent research discovered several other immunomodifying actions of MTX which might be responsible for the favorable clinical outcome of different inflammatory dermatoses. The synthesis of new MTX derivates is currently underway. The creation of a compound with anti-inflammatory activity without or much less toxic effects would be desirable.

MTX is not yet in general use in dermatology, but it could provide an interesting pharmacological approach and an effective alternative to other immunosuppressive regimens and should undergo further evaluation.

Summary

The efficacy of low-dose MTX in the treatment of severe psoriasis and a wide spectrum of inflammatory dermatoses has been documented. The mechanism of action of low-dose weekly MTX in inflammatory disorders remains unclear, but it appears to act as an anti-inflammatory agent, as supported by the rapid clinical response. Moreover, recent data suggest that low-dose MTX therapy attenuates the inflammatory status at the cellular level. Blocking of IL-1 activity and other proinflammatory mediators and cells may be the basis of the anti-inflammatory effect of MTX. Side effects such as hepatic, hematologic, and pulmonary toxicity are particularly associated with the total cumulative dose and individual risk factors. Careful baseline and follow-up monitoring is recommended to avoid or diminish adverse reactions.

References

1. Alarcon GS, Schrohenloher RE, Bartlucci AA, Ward JR, Williams HJ, Koopman WJ (1990) Suppression of rheumatoid factor production by methotrexate in patients with rheumatoid arthritis. Evidence for differential influences of therapy and clinical status on IgM and IgA rheumatoid factor expression. Arthritis Rheum 33:1156–1161
2. Asako H, Wolf RE, Granger DN (1993) Leukocyte adherence in rat mesenteric venules: effects of adenosine and methotrexate. Gastroenterology 104:31–37

3. Barrera P, Boerbooms AM, Demacker PN, van de Putte LB, Gallati H, van der Meer JW (1994) Circulating concentrations and production of cytokines and soluble receptors in rheumatoid arthritis patients: effects of a single dose of methotrexate. Br J Rheumatol 33:1017–1024
4. Boehm I, Uerlich M, Bauer R (1997) Dermatology (in press)
5. Brody M, Böhm I, Bauer R (1993) Mechanism of action of methotrexate: experimental evidence that methotrexate blocks the binding of interleukin 1b to the interleukin 1 receptor on target cells. Eur J Clin Chem Clin Biochem 31:667–674
6. Brody M, Niedecken HW, Biwer E, Boehm I, Bauer R (1994) Successful treatment of impetigo herpetiformis with low-dose methotrexate. Implications for the pathogenesis of psoriasis. Eur J Dermatol 4:437–439
7. Brody M, Böhm I, Biwer E, Bauer R (1994) Erfolgreiche Behandlung einer Panarteriitis nodosa mit Methotrexat Low-dose-Therapie. Hautarzt 45:476–479
8. Chandran G, Ahern MJ, Hall PD, Geddes R, Smith MD, Hill W, Harley JH (1994) Cirrhosis in patients with rheumatoid arthritis receiving low dose methotrexate. Br J Rheumatol 33:981–984
9. Chang DM, Baptiste P, Schur PH (1990) The effect of antirheumatic drugs on interleukin 1 (IL-1) activity and IL-1 inhibitor production by human monocytes. J Rheumatol 17:1148–1157
10. Chang DM, Weinblatt ME, Schur PH (1992) The effects of methotrexate on interleukin 1 in patients with rheumatoid arthritis. J Rheumatol 19:1678–1682
11. Cooper KD (1993) New therapeutic approaches in atopic dermatitis. Clin Rev Allergy 11:543–559
12. Crilly A, McInness IB, McDonald AG, Watson J, Capell HA, Madhok R (1995) Interleukin 6 (IL-6) and soluble receptor levels in patients with rheumatoid arthritis treated with low dose oral methotrexate. J Rheumatol 22:224–226
13. Debets R, Hegmans JP, Troost RJ, Benner R, Prens EP (1995) Enhanced production of biologically active interleukin-1 α and interleukin-1 β by psoriatic epidermal cells ex vivo: evidence of increased cytosolic interleukin-1 b levels and facilitated interleukin-1 release. Eur J Immunol 25:1624–1630
14. Deleuran B, Kristensen M, Paludan K, Zachariae C, Larsen CG, Zachariae E, Thestrup-Pedersen K (1992) The effect of second-line antirheumatic drugs on interleukin-8 mRNA synthesis and protein secretion in human endothelial cells. Cytokine 4:403–409
15. DeJoy SQ, Jeyaseelan R Sr, Torley LW, Schow SR, Wick MM, Kerwar SS (1995) Attenuation of interleukin-2-induced pulmonary vascular leak syndrome by low doses of oral methotrexate. Cancer Res 55:4929–4935
16. Duhra P (1993) Treatment of gastrointestinal symptoms associated with methotrexate therapy for psoriasis. J Am Acad Dermatol 28.466–469
17. Fink SD, Kremer JM (1994) Cutaneous and musculoskeletal features, diagnostic modalities, and immunopathology in sarcoidosis. Curr Opin Rheumatol 6:78–81
18. Granowitz EV, Clark BD, Vannier E, Callahan MV, Dinarello CA (1992) Effect of interleukin-1 (IL-1) blockade on cytokine synthesis: I. IL-1 receptor antagonist inhibits IL-1-induced cytokine synthesis and blocks the binding of IL-1 to its type II receptor on human monocytes. Blood 79:2356–2363
19. Gressier B, Lebegue S, Brunet C, Luyckx M, Dine T, Cazin M, Cazin JC (1994) Pro-oxidant properties of methotrexate: evaluation and prevention by an anti-oxidant drug. Pharmazie 49:679–681
20. Gudewicz PW (1988) Effect of anticancer drugs on macrophage-mediated antibody-dependent cytotoxicity and secretion of reactive oxygen intermediates. Cancer Lett 42:67–72
21. Harrison PV, Orrell DH, James R, Peat M, Stones RN (1989) Short-term methotrexate administration by low-dose infusion – does it influence clearance of psoriasis? Clin Exp Dermatol 14:291–294
22. Hashimoto M, Nonaka S, Furuta E, Wada T, Suenaga Y, Yasuda M, Shingu M, Nobunaga M (1994) Methotrexate for steroid-resistant systemic lupus erythematosus. Clin Rheumatol 13:280–283
23. Hawkes JS, Cleland LG, Proudman SM, James MJ (1994) The effect of methotrexate on ex vivo lipoxygenase metabolism in neutrophils from patients with rheumatoid arthritis. J Rheumatol 21:55–58

24. Hu SK, Mitcho YL, Oronsky AL, Kerwar SS (1988) Studies on the effect of methotrexate on macrophage function. J Rheumatol 15:206–209
25. Jeffes EWB, McCullough JL, Pittelkow MR, McCormick A, Almanzor J, Liu G, Dang M, Voss K, Voss J, Schlotzhauer A, Weinstein G (1995) Methotrexate therapy of psoriasis: differential sensitivity of proliferating lymphoid and epithelial cells to the cytotoxic and growth-inhibitory effects of methotrexate. J Invest Dermatol 104:183–188
26. Johnson WJ, DiMartino MJ, Meunier P, Muirhead KA, Hanna N (1988) Methotrexate inhibits macrophage activation as well as vascular and cellular inflammatory events in rat adjuvant induced arthritis. J Rheumatol 15:745–749
27. Kahaleh B (1993) Immunologic aspects of scleroderma. Curr Opin Rheumatol 5:760–765
28. Kremer JM, Alarcon GS, Lightfoot RW Jr, Willkens RF, Furst DE, Williams HJ, Dent PB, Weinblatt ME (1994) Methotrexate for rheumatoid arthritis. Suggested guidelines for monitoring liver toxicity. American College of Rheumatology. Arthritis Rheum 37:316–328
29. Lammers AM, van de Kerkhof PC, Mier PD (1987) Reduction of leukotriene B4-induced intraepidermal accumulation of polymorphonuclear leukocytes by methotrexate in psoriasis. Br J Dermatol 116:667–671
30. Linker-Israeli M, Deans RJ, Wallace DJ, Prehn J, Ozeri-Chen T, Klinenberg JR (1991) Elevated levels of endogenous IL-6 in systemic lupus erythematosus. J Immunol 147:117–123
31. Loetscher P, Dewald B, Baggiolini M, Seitz M (1994) Monocyte chemoattractant protein 1 and interleukin 8 production by rheumatoid synoviocytes. Effect of anti-rheumatic drugs. Cytokine 6:162–170
32. Martinez-Osuna P, Zwolinska JB, Sikes DH, Cory JG, Silveira LH, Jara LJ, Espinoza LR (1993) Lack of immunosuppressive effect of low-dose oral methotrexate on lymphocytes in rheumatoid arthritis. Clin Exp Rheumatol 11:249–253
33. O´Meara AMW, Brazil J, Reen DJ (1985) The effect of methotrexate on in vitro immunoglobulin production. J Immunopharmacol 7:235–245
34. Paul MA, Hyg MS, Jorizzo JL, Fleischer AB, White LW (1994) Low-dose methotrexate treatment in elderly patients with bullous pemphigoid. J Am Acad Dermatol 31:620–625
35. Roenigk HH Jr, Auerbach R, Maibach HI, Weinstein GD (1988) Methotrexate in psoriasis: revisted guidelines. J Am Acad Dermatol 19:145–156
36. Rordorf-Adam C, Lazdins J, Woods-Cook K, Alteri E, Henn R, Geiger T, Feige U, Towbin H, Erard F (1989) An assay for the detection of interleukin-1 synthesis inhibitors: effects of antirheumatic drugs. Drugs Exp Clin Res 15:355–362
37. Rosenthal GJ, Weigand GW, Germolec DR, Blank JA, Luster MI (1988) Suppression of B cell function by methotrexate and trimethrexate. Evidence of inhibition of purine biosynthesis as well as a major mechanism of action. J Immunol 141:410–416
38. Sandoval DM, Alarcon GS, Morgan SL (1995) Adverse events in methotrexate-treated rheumatoid arthritis patients. Br J Rheumatol 34 [Suppl 2]:49–56
39. Sauder DN, Wong D, Laskin C (1993) Epidermal cytokines in murine lupus. J Invest Dermatol 100:42S–46S
40. Schmidt J, Fleissner S, Heimann-Weitschat I, Lindstaedt R, Pomberg B, Werner U, Szelenyi I (1994) Effect of corticosteroids, cyclosporin A, and methotrexate on cytokine release from monocytes and T-cell subsets. Immunopharmacology 27:173–179
41. Segal R, Mozes E, Yaron M, Tartakovsky B (1989) The effects of methotrexate on the production and activity of interleukin 1. Arthritis Rheum 32:370–377
42. Seitz M, Loetscher P, Dewald B, Towbin H, Rordorf C, Gallati H, Baggiolini M, Gerber NJ (1995) Methotrexate action in rheumatoid arthritis: stimulation of cytokine inhibitor and inhibition of chemokine production by peripheral blood mononuclear cells. Br J Rheumatol 34:602–609
43. Shergy WJ, Polisson RP, Caldwell DS, Riece JR, Pisetsky DA, Allen NB (1988) Methotrexate-associated hepatotoxicity: retrospective analysis of 210 patients with rheumatoid arthritis. Am J Med 85:771–774
44. Sperling RI, Benincaso AI, Anderson RJ, Coblyn JS, Austen KF, Weinblatt ME (1992) Acute and chronic suppression of leukotriene B4 synthesis ex vivo in neutrophils from patients with rheumatoid arthritis beginning treatment with methotrexate. Arthritis Rheum 35:376–384

45. Suarez CR, Pickett WC, Bell DH, McClintock DK, Armsky AL, Kerwar SS (1987) Effect of low dose methotrexate on neutrophil chemotaxis induced by leukotriene B4 and complement C5a. J Rheumatol 14:9–11
46. Thomas R, Carroll GJ (1993) Reduction of leukocyte and interleukin-1 b concentration in the synovial fluid of rheumatoid arthritis patients treated with methotrexate. Arthritis Rheum 36:1244–1252
47. Tomkins PT, Cooper KL, Appleby P, Webber DG (1995) Effect of pharmacological agents on the productions of interleukin-10 by murine D10.G4.1 Th2 cell line in vitro. Int J Immunopharmacol 17:619–625
48. van Dooren-Greebe RJ, Kuipers ALA, Mulder J, de Boo T, van de Kerkhof PCM (1994) Methotrexate revisited: effects of long-term treatment in psoriasis. Br J Dermatol 130:204–210
49. van Dooren-Greebe RJ, Kuijpers ALA, Termorshuizen F, van de Kerkhof PCM (1995) Interruption of long-term methotrexate treatment in psoriasis. Acta Derm Venereol (Stockh) 75: 393–396
50. van Dooren-Greebe RJ, Kuijpers ALA, Buijs WCAM, Kniest PHM, Corstens FHM, Nagengast FM, de Boo T, Willems JL, Duller P, van de Kerkhof PCM (1996) The value of dynamic hepatic scintigraphy and serum aminoterminal propeptide of type III procollagen for early detection of methotrexate-induced hepatic damage in psoriasis patients. Br J Dermatol 134:481–487
51. Walsdorfer U, Christophers E, Schröder JM (1983) Methotrexate inhibits polymorphonuclear leukocyte chemotaxis in psoriasis. Br J Dermatol 108:451–454
52. Wascher TC, Hermann J, Brezinschek R, Brezinschek HP, Wilders-Trusching M, Rainer F, Krejs GJ (1994) Serum levels of interleukin-6 and tumor-necrosis-factor-alpha are not correlated to disease activity in patients with rheumatoid arthritis after treatment with low-dose methotrexate. Eur J Clin Invest 24:73–75
53. Weinstein GD, White GM (1993) An approach to the treatment of moderate to severe psoriasis with rotational therapy. J Am Acad Dermatol 28.454–459
54. Zachariae H, Kragballe K, Sogaard H (1980) Methotrexate induced liver cirrhosis. Br J Dermatol 102.407–412
55. Zeller JM, Gudewicz PW (1984) Functional resistance of inflammatory macrophages to methotrexate in vitro. J Leukoc Biol 35:475–487

Leflunomide

R. Dummer, G. Hofbauer, G. Burg, and R.R. Bartlett

Introduction

Leflunomide is a novel isoxazole derivative with immunomodulating and anti-inflammatory characteristics [3]. Following oral administration, leflunomide is rapidly absorbed and converted, by opening the isoxazole ring, to the active metabolite A77 1726 (Fig. 1). This new drug has shown efficacy in an array of animal models of autoimmune disease [1–4, 11, 22, 25, 27, 30] and organ graft rejection [4, 14, 17, 24, 29, 32]. It has also demonstrated efficacy and good tolerability in clinical phase II trials in patients with rheumatoid arthritis (RA) [19]. Leflunomide suppresses autoantibody formation, inhibits cell adhesion of leukocytes to endothelial cells [39], and acts as an antiproliferative agent. Leflunomide seems to be a rather specific immunomodulating drug which may inhibit crucial steps in the pathophysiology of psoriasis.

State of the Art

Preclinical Experience

The first publication dealing with leflunomide appeared in 1985, reporting results concerning the effects of this drug on the adjuvant disease of rats [1]. Classical nonsteroidal anti-inflammatory drugs (NSAID) inhibit the development of adjuvant arthritis once it has been initiated by injection of complete Freund's adjuvant, particularly affecting the systematic manifestations of the disease (swelling, joint damage) in the limbs, which start to appear after about 10 days. It was found that leflunomide not only inhibited the development of the adjuvant disorder, it also prevented the onset of the disease when administered on days 1–12 before systemic symptoms appeared, an action not seen with classical NSAID. This suggested that leflunomide acts like an immunosuppressive drug, such as cyclophosphamide. Lymphocytes taken from untreated adju-

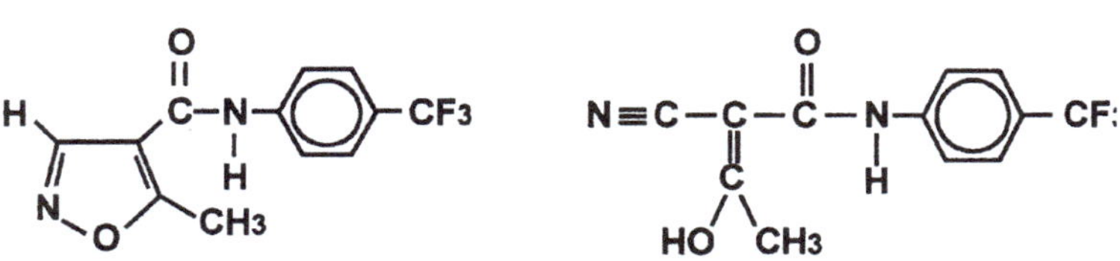

Fig. 1. Chemical structure of leflunomide (HWA 486; *left*) and its active metabolite A771726 (*right*)

vant arthritic rats already show a reduced response to stimulation with natural immunostimulants such as bacterial endotoxin, which is further reduced by cyclophosphamide. In contrast to the known immunosuppressants, however, it was found that leflunomide normalized the response to stimulation of these lymphocytes. Here, then, was a compound which was clearly not just anti-inflammatory, but also had an unusual action on the immune system.

In addition to adjuvant arthritis in rats, leflunomide has displayed efficacy in several other experimental autoimmune animal models, such as proteoglycan-induced arthritis in mice [1, 11], glomerulonephritis induced by antibasement membrane antibody in rats [22], autoimmune uveitis in rats [25], experimental autoimmune tubulointerstitial nephritis in rats [27], experimentally induced myasthenia gravis in rats [30], and autoimmunity in MRL/lpr mice [2]. In all of these models, leflunomide restored the immunopathological parameters of these animals to normal values.

Not only has leflunomide proven to be effective in autoimmunity, but also in reactions leading to organ graft rejection [12–17, 19, 20, 21, 23, 24, 26, 29, 31, 32, 34–36]. Schorlemmer et al. [24] were able to provide data demonstrating leflunomide's ability to induce specific allograft tolerance in two skin graft models. The authors also reported that this tolerance was adoptively transferable, an activity which could not be observed using cyclosporin A.

Many human diseases are caused by a loss of self-tolerance with the development of autoimmune responses to specific tissue components. The ultimate goal of any autoimmune therapy is not only to stop reactivity to autoantigens, but for the individual to regain his or her tolerance to self-antigens. As mentioned above, leflunomide was able to induce specific tolerance to alloantigens in a transplantation model; thus the question arised as to the ability of this drug to restore self-tolerance to autoimmune-diseased animals. This was shown to be the case in MRL/lpr-mice, a model of spontaneous systemic lupus erythematosis (SLE) [5]. Splenocytes from animals treated with leflunomide and displaying a long-term nondiseased state after therapy discontinuation were injected IV into 8-week-old MRL/lpr mice. In contrast to mice injected with spleen cells from diseased animals or animals not injected (normal disease control), none of the rodents developed symptoms of the SLE-like disorder. This indicates that leflunomide has immunorestoring activity.

It has been clearly shown that leflunomide is able to inhibit the growth of nonstimulated T cells and T cells stimulated with a variety of mitogens [3, 9]. Its antiproliferative activity was reversed by the addition of uridine to the cell culture, indicating that it acts at the level of the de novo pyrimidine biosynthesis pathway [6, 33, 40]. Binding studies using radiolabeled ligand demonstrate that the active metabolite binds to the human enzyme dihydroorotate dehydrogenase. It was shown that it inhibited the activity of the enzyme in concentrations lower than those which exert antiproliferative effects upon rapidly dividing cells. The production of lymphokines is not inhibited by leflunomide or its active metabolite at concentrations which block cell proliferation. However, expression of early activation markers such as interleukin (IL)-2 and transferin cell surface receptors were decreased after resting cells were stimulated and incubated with A77 1726 [38]. However, these concentrations were somewhat higher than those required to block cell proliferation. Interestingly, the metabolite of leflunomide inhibits epidermal growth factor (EGF)-stimulated proliferation of human foreskin fibroblasts and EGF-induced autophosphorylation of the EGF receptor. It also inhibits the T cell receptor (TCR)-CD3-mediated tyrosine phosphorylation of T cell leukemia cells as well as subsequent PLCgl (phospholipase) phosphorylation. The substance inhibits IL-2-stimulated proliferation of human T cells as well as the in vitro kinase activities of p56 and p59, two tyrosine kinases of the src family. These data indicate that the substance is a tyrosine kinase inhibitor [37] and that this may be, at least in part, a mechanism by which leflunomide inhibits T cell activation [7, 8, 10]. On the other hand, leflunomide did not inhibit the synthesis of leukotrienes after calcium ionophore stimulation of human peripheral blood mononuclear cells (PBMC). Leflunomide should thus not be associated with adverse effects typical of NSAID. In therapeutic doses in humans, leflunomide should act mainly on T cell proliferation without inhibiting the production of lymphokines and on the proliferation of other cells such as fibroblasts or keratinocytes by interfering with tyrosine kinases [18]. In addition, there is evidence that it has an effect upon the maturation to macrophages of adherent monocytes isolated from human PBMC (R.R. Bartlett et al., unpublished data). The constellation of these biological properties makes leflunomide a promising candidate for a successful and well-tolerated therapy of several inflammatory skin disorders such as psoriasis, lichen planus, and cutaneous lupus erythematosus.

Clinical Experience

In clinical phase II studies, leflunomide has been administered to over 500 patients with active RA. Of these, 270 patients have received the drug for over 18 months. The central study was a 6-month, multicenter, randomized, double-blind comparison of leflunomide at three dosage levels (5, 10, and 25 mg per day) with placebo [19]. A total of 402 patients with long-standing RA and a mean of 1.1 failed disease-modifying drugs (DMARD) were enrolled. Apart from a large placebo response, a statistically significant response was observed in the 10- and 25-mg/day dosage groups for primary variables such as the number of swollen joints, patient and physician overall assessment, or responder analysis according to the Paulus or ACR/WHO/ILAR criteria. After 1 month, onset of effect was evident and increased thereafter, stabilizing by 4–6 months. The 5-mg/day group showed no significant advantage over placebo, whereas the 10-mg/day group demonstrated significantly greater efficacy than placebo for all the above parameters except tender joint count; the 25-mg/day group had statistically significant improvement over placebo in all parameters. Statistical analysis indicated a dose–response relationship.

Twenty-three patients were withdrawn from the study because of adverse events. Ten of these were serious (septic arthritis, episcleritis, pleuritis, aseptic necrosis, and SLE; these were attributed to the underlying disease. In addition, one case each of anaphylaxis, skin rash, cholecystitis, and breast carcinoma and one death by suicide occurred. In total, 387 adverse events were reported in 195 patients. Adverse events judged to be related to study drug administration were rash/allergic reactions (5% under placebo, 6% at 5 mg/day, 4% at 10 mg/day, and 8% at 25 mg/day), gastrointestinal symptoms (3%, 16%, 10%, and 12%, respectively), weight loss (2%, 2%, 4%, and 4%, respectively), and reversible hair loss (1%, 1%, 1%, and 7%, respectively).

Mean plasma concentrations of A77 1726, the active metabolite into which leflunomide is rapidly and completely converted in vivo, were proportional to daily maintenance doses at 6 months. The pharmacokinetics of A77 1726 appeared to be linear over the dosage range of 5–25 mg per day. Mean plasma concentrations were proportional at 9 mg/ml, 19 mg/ml, and 52 ml/ml for the 5-mg, 10-mg, and 25-mg/day dosage groups, respectively. Mean plasma half-life was 15–18 days, with a total plasma clearance of 0.30 ml/kg per h. The active metabolite was extensively protein bound (> 99 %) and was cleared via several metabolic pathways, including biliary and urinary excretion. Administration of cholestyramine or activated charcoal rapidly decreases plasma levels of the active metabolite by 40–50 % within 24 h.

Clinical phase III studies in RA are underway. In addition, a double-blind multicenter study in patients with psoriasis has been initiated, comparing leflunomide at dosages of 5 mg, 10 mg, and 25 mg daily with placebo. The aim of the study is to determine the efficacy and tolerability of several doses of leflunomide in the treatment of severe disabling stationary chronic plaque-type psoriasis vulgaris. Efficacy is determined by clinical rating of signs and symptoms and area measurement (psoriasis area and severity index, PASI). In addition, an expanded program is included to determine the safety of the treatment. The patients are carefully monitored for changes in hematology, blood chemistry, urine analysis, stool, and serum drug levels. A weekly clinical examination checks for clinical variables, especially weight, skin condition, signs of infection, blood pressure measurements, and subjective tolerability. The treatment period is 4 weeks. After the end of treatment, patients undergo a post-treatment evaluation phase of 3 months. The trial is still ongoing. Our center has included 16 patients so far. Although we do not know the exact treatment of these 16 patients, we can nevertheless state that leflunomide is generally well tolerated. We did not observe any severe subjective or objective side effects. However, two patients had to be hospitalized because of progression of disease. We suspect that these patients were treated with placebo. Up to 30 % of the patients experienced a significant decrease in PASI score.

Discussion

A perfect immunosuppressive drug for cutaneous inflammatory disorders such as psoriasis, lichen planus, or discoid lupus erythematodes must be well-tolerated by the patient, without any subjective intolerability such as nausea, vomiting, or headaches [20, 28]. There should certainly not be any systemic toxicity, such as disturbances in hematology, liver, or renal functions. High tolerability is particularly necessary, since the mentioned inflammatory skin disorders have a benign clinical outcome. They usually do not affect extracutaneous organs and are thus never life-threatening. On the other hand, these skin conditions may dramatically affect the personal lifestyle of the patients by limiting their activities because of the impact on physical appearance or by itching. Leflunomide seems to be a rather specific immunomodulating drug. It inhibits crucial steps in the pathophysiology of psoriasis such as T cell proliferation and activation or proliferation of fibroblasts and keratinocytes. In addition, it inhibits the adherence of lymphocytes to endothelial cells and suppresses auto-antibody formation. It may also be important that it supports the maturation of monocytes to macrophages. The profile of the side effects during short-term and long-term application seems to be acceptable. However, it has not yet been clarified whether the drug has an influence on the development of epithelial or vascular skin neoplasms or lymphomas, as known for cyclosporin A. Patients that receive leflunomide for a longer period have to be carefully monitored for these events. There is reasonable hope that this drug might have a better therapeutic profile than other immunosuppressive drugs such as cyclosporin A, rapamycin, or FK506.

If diseases only affect the skin, topical application can be an elegant alternative in using immunomodulating drugs. Promising developments are under way to find formulations that contain leflunomide in a cream or lotion. By this approach, systemic side effects can be avoided.

In summary, leflunomide is certainly one of the most interesting immunomodulating drugs that can be expected to find a place in the therapeutic repertoire for inflammatory skin disorders.

Summary

Leflunomide is an isoxazole derivative with immunomodulating activities which has shown efficacy in an array of animal models of autoimmunity and organ graft rejection. Further, tolerance induction to transplanted organs as well as the restoration of self-tolerance in autoimmune animals has been observed after therapy with this drug. Leflunomide has biological effects on antibody formation, cell adhesion, intercellular signal transduction, and cell proliferation. Two molecular targets have been identified, tyrosine kinases and de novo pyrimidine biosynthesis, specifically dehydroorotate dehydrogenase (DHODH). This drug has demonstrated clinical efficacy and tolerability in international trials for RA. An ongoing clinical trial on the therapy of psoriasis is also showing promise. Leflunomide is an interesting candidate for a successful and well-tolerated therapy of psoriasis and other inflammatory skin disorders, especially if topical application is possible.

References

1. Bartlett RR, Schleyerbach R (1985) Immunopharmacological profile of a novel isoxazol derivative, HWA 486, with potential antirheumatic activity. Int J Immunopharmacol 7:7–18
2. Bartlett RR, Popovic S, Raiss RX (1988) Development of autoimmunity in MRL/lpr mice and the effects of drugs on this murine disease. Scand J Rheumatol [Suppl] 75:290–299
3. Bartlett RR, Anagnostopulos H, Zielinski T, Mattar T, Schleyerbach R (1993) Effects of leflunomide on immune responses and models of inflammation. Springer Semin Immunopathol 14:381–394
4. Bartlett RR, Zielinski T, Campion G, Musikic P, Schleyerbach R, Schorlemmer H-U (1994) Chapter 20: leflunomide: a novel immunomodulating drug. Nonsteroidal anti-inflammatory drugs. Decker, New York
5. Brendel S, Zielinski T, Bartlett RR (1996) Leflunomide induces transferable self-tolerance in autoimmune MRL/lpr-mice. In: 8th APLAR congress of rheumatology, Melbourne, abstract 4, p 1
6. Cherwinski HM, Byars N, Ballaron SJ, Nakano GM, Young JM, Ransom JT (1995) Leflunomide interferes with pyrimidine nucleotide biosynthesis. Inflamm Res 44:317–322
7. Cherwinski HM, Cohn RG, Cheung P, Webster DJ, Xu YZ, Caulfield JP, Young JM, Nakano G, Ransom JT (1995) The immunosuppressant leflunomide inhibits lymphocyte proliferation by inhibiting pyrimidine biosynthesis. J Pharmacol Exp Ther 275:1043–1049
8. Chong AS, Gebel H, Finnegan A, Petraitis EE, Jiang XL, Sankary HN, Foster P, Williams JW (1993) Leflunomide, a novel immunomodulatory agent: in vitro analyses of the mechanism of immunosuppression. Transplant Proc 25:747–749
9. Chong AS, Xiao F, Xu X, Williams JW (1994) In vivo and in vitro immunosuppression with leflunomide, vol 1. Recent developments in transplantation medicine. Physicians' and Scientists' Publishing, Glenview

10. Chong AS, Rezai K, Gebel HM, Finnegan A, Foster P, Xu X, Williams JW (1996) Effects of leflunomide and other immunosuppressive agents on T cell proliferation in vitro. Transplantation 61:140–145
11. Glant TT, Mikecz K, Bartlett RR, Deak F, Thonar EJ, Williams JM, Mattar T, Kuettner KE, Schleyerbach R (1992) Immunomodulation of proteoglycan-induced progressive polyarthritis by leflunomide. Immunopharmacology 23:105–116
12. Kemp E (1996) Xenotransplantation. J Intern Med 239:287–297
13. Kemp E, Dieperink H, Jensen J, Kemp G, Kuhlmann IL, Larsen S, Lillevang ST, Nielsen B, Salomon S, Steinbruchel D, Nielsen Thomsen F (1994) Newer immunosuppressive drugs in concordant xenografting – transplantation of hamster heart to rat. Xenotransplantation 1:102–108
14. Kuchle CC, Thoenes GH, Langer KH, Schorlemmer HU, Bartlett RR, Schleyerbach R (1991) Prevention of kidney and skin graft rejection in rats by leflunomide, a new immunomodulating agent. Transplant Proc 23:1083–1086
15. Lin Y, Sobis H, Vandeputte M, Waer M (1994) Induction therapy of leflunomide and cyclosporine allows for long-term xenograft survival under cyclosporine alone. Transplant Proc 26:3052
16. Lin Y, Sobis H, Vandeputte M, Waer M (1994) Long-term xenograft survival and suppression of xenoantibody formation in the hamster-to-rat heart transplant model using a combination therapy of leflunomide and cyclosporine. Transplant Proc 26:3202
17. Lin Y, Sobis H, Vandeputte M, Waer M (1995) Mechanism of leflunomide-induced prevention of xenoantibody formation and xenograft rejection in the hamster to rat heart transplantation model. Transplant Proc 27:305–306
18. Mattar T, Kochhar K, Bartlett R, Bremer EG, Finnegan A (1993) Inhibition of the epidermal growth factor receptor tyrosine kinase activity by leflunomide. FEBS Lett 334:161–164
19. Mladenovic V, Domljan Z, Rozman B, Jajic I, Mihajlovic D, Dordevic J, Popovic M, Dimitrijevic M, Zivkovic M, Campion G et al (1995) Safety and effectiveness of leflunomide in the treatment of patients with active rheumatoid arthritis. Results of a randomized, placebo-controlled, phase II study. Arthritis Rheum 38:1595–1603
20. Morris RE (1995) Mechanisms of action of new immunosuppressive drugs. Ther Drug Monit 17:564–569
21. Morris RE, Huang X, Cao W, Zheng B. & Shorthouse, R.A.: Leflunomide (HWA 486) and its analog suppress T- and B-cell proliferation in vitro, acute rejection, ongoing rejection, and antidonor antibody synthesis in mouse, rat, and cynomolgus monkey transplant recipients as well as arterial intimal thickening after balloon catheter injury. Transplant Proc 27:445–447
22. Ogawa T, Inazu M, Gotoh K, Hayashi S (1990) Effects of leflunomide on glomerulonephritis induced by antibasement membrane antibody in rats. Agents Actions 31:321–328
23. Popovic S, Bartlett RR (1987) The use of murine chronic graft versus host (CGVH) disease, a model for systemic lupus erythematosus (SLE), for drug discovery. Agents Actions 21:284–286
24. Schorlemmer HU, Seiler FR, Bartlett RR (1993) Prolongation of allogeneic transplanted skin grafts and induction of tolerance by leflunomide, a new immunosuppressive isoxazol derivative. Transplant Proc 25:763–767
25. Smith-Lang L, Glaser B, Weimer LK, Miller ST, Robertson SM, Aoki KR, Yanni JM (1992) Efficacy of novel immunomodulators leflunomide and rapamycin in autoimmune uveitis. FASEB J 6:A1048
26. Swan SK, Crary GS, Guijarro C, O'Donnell MP, Keane WF, Kasiske BL (1995) Immunosuppressive effects of leflunomide in experimental chronic vascular rejection. Transplantation 60: 887–890
27. Thoenes GH, Sitter T, Langer KH, Bartlett RR, Schleyerbach R (1989) Leflunomide (HWA 486) inhibits experimental autoimmune tubulointerstitial nephritis in rats. Int J Immunopharmacol 11:921–929
28. Thomson AW, Starzl TE (1993) New immunosuppressive drugs: mechanistic insights and potential therapeutic advances. Immunol Rev 136:71–98
29. Ulrichs K, Kaitschick J, Bartlett R, Muller-Ruchholtz W (1992) Suppression of natural xenophile antibodies with the novel immunomodulating drug leflunomide. Transplant Proc 24: 718–719

30. Vidic-Dankovic B, Kosec D, Damjanovic M, Apostolski S, Isakovic K, Bartlett RR (1995) Leflunomide prevents the development of experimentally induced myasthenia gravis. Int J Immunopharmacol 17:273–281
31. Wennberg L, Wallgren AC, Sundberg B, Rafael E, Zhu S, Liu J, Tibell A, Karlsson-Parra A, Groth CG, Korsgren O (1996) Immunosuppression with cyclosporin A in combination with leflunomide and mycophenolate mofetil prevents rejection of pig-islets transplanted into rats. Transplant Proc 28:819
32. Williams JW, Xiao F, Foster P, Clardy C, McChesney L, Sankary H, Chong AS (1994) Leflunomide in experimental transplantation. Control of rejection and alloantibody production, reversal of acute rejection, and interaction with cyclosporine. Transplantation 57:1223–1231
33. Williamson RA, Yea CM, Robson PA, Curnock AP, Gadher S, Hambleton AP, Woodward K, Bruneau J-M, Hambleton P, Moss D, Thomson TA, Spinella-Jaegle S, Morand P, Courtin O, Sautes C, Westwood R, Hercend T, Kou EA, Ruuth E (1995) Dihydroorotate dehydrogenase is a high affinity binding protein for A77 1726 and mediator of a range of biological effects of the immunomodulating compound. J Biol Chem 270:22467–22472
34. Wright JR Jr, Kearns H, McDonald AS (1994) Leflunomide and cyclosporin-A prolong fish-to-mouse islet xenograft survival in BALB/C mice. Transplant Proc 26:1310
35. Xiao F, Chong AS, Foster P, Sankary H, McChesney L, Koukoulis G, Yang J, Frieders D, Williams JW (1994) Leflunomide controls rejection in hamster to rat cardiac xenografts. Transplantation 58:828–834
36. Xiao F, Chong A, Shen J, Yang J, Short J, Foster P, Sankary H, Jensik S, Mital D, McChesney L et al (1995) Pharmacologically induced regression of chronic transplant rejection. Transplantation 60:1065–1072
37. Xu X, Williams JW, Bremer EG, Finnegan A, Chong AS (1995) Inhibition of protein tyrosine phosphorylation in T cells by a novel immunosuppressive agent, leflunomide. J Biol Chem 270:12398–12403
38. Zielinski T, Muller HJ, Bartlett RR (1993) Effects of leflunomide (HWA 486) on expression of lymphocyte activation markers. Agents Actions 38:C80–82
39. Zielinski T, Muller HJ, Schleyerbach R, Bartlett RR (1994) Differential effects of leflunomide on leukocytes: inhibition of rat in vivo adhesion and human in vitro oxidative burst without affecting surface marker modulation. Agents Actions 41:C276–C278
40. Zielinski T, Zeitter D, Muller S, Bartlett RR (1995) Leflunomide, a reversible inhibitor of pyrimidine biosynthesis? Inflamm Res 44:S207–208

Fusion Toxins

F. M. Foss

Introduction

Two different approaches have been undertaken to develop chimeric targeted biomolecules for therapeutics. The first was the construction of immunotoxins consisting of murine monoclonal antibodies chemically linked through a disulfide bond linker to a toxin or radionuclide. The plant toxin ricin and the bacterial exotoxins of *Pseudomonas aeruginosa* (*Pseudomonas* exotoxin A) and *Corynebacterium diphtheriae* (diphtheria toxin) have been used in the construction of the first immunotoxins. These enzymes inhibit protein synthesis by scission of the large ribosomal subunit in the case of ricin or by modification – adenosine diphosphate (ADP)-ribosylation – of elongation factor 2 in the case of the bacterial toxins. A detailed knowledge of the structure–function organization of these toxins separate domains which function in cell binding, membrane translocating, and catalytic activity has allowed for genetic manipulation of the toxin molecules to replace the native receptor-binding domains with the targeting antibody, preserving the necessary membrane-translocating sequences and active catalytic domain. While immunotoxins have demonstrated promising clinical activity in early studies, nonspecific binding and toxicities have been attributed to the instability of the chemical conjugation of the toxin moiety to the antibody, and therapeutic index has been compromised by the generation of neutralizing antibodies to the murine antibody component of the immunotoxin. Newer generations of immunotoxins have utilized murine complementarity-determining regions on human antibody frameworks to prevent immunogenicity of the immunotoxin; they have improved the chemical linkages to prevent dissociation of the toxin from the antibody and modified the toxin moieties to reduce nonspecific toxicities, such as deglycosylation in the case of the ricin A chain immunotoxins. Clinical studies are underway with these newer immunotoxins.

Recently, genetic engineering has led to the construction of fusion toxins in which the gene encoding the membrane-translocating and catalytic domains of a toxin is combined with a gene encoding a targeting ligand to produce a recombinant protein. Subsequent expression of these fusion genes in *Escherichia coli* results in the synthesis of a single biochemically stable gene product. This is in contrast to the production of immunotoxins, where chemical linkage reactions often give rise to mixtures of isomeric forms of the immunotoxin, thereby producing a heterogeneous product. In addition, since the fusion toxins are genetically constructed, the fusion junction, or point at which the targeting ligand is linked to the toxin fragment, can be precisely determined based on sequence data, thereby allowing for design of the optimal biologically active molecule by the generation of families of molecules containing different numbers of amino acids derived from the translocating and active domains of the toxin gene.

The first genetically constructed family of fusion toxins used diphtheria toxin as the toxophore for receptor-binding domain substitution. It was known quite early that native diphtheria toxin was a three-domain protein consisting of the enzymatically active domain (fragment A), the hydrophobic domain (N-terminal portion of fragment B), and the receptor-binding domain (C-terminal portion of fragment B) [8, 22]. The process by which native diphtheria toxin intoxicates sensitive eukaryotic cells involves the following steps: (a) binding of the toxin to its cell surface receptor, (b) activation of the catalytic domain by a proteolytic cleavage ("nicking") of the toxin in a sensitive, exposed 14-amino acid loop that is subtended by Cys-186 and Cys-201, (c) internalization of the bound toxin into endosomes by receptor-mediated endocytosis and subsequent acidification of the endocytic vesicle, and (d) facilitated delivery of the catalytic domain across the endocytic vesicle membrane and into the cytosol [4, 6, 10, 11, 18, 19]. Once delivered to the cytosol, fragment A rapidly catalyzes the ADP-ribosylation of elongation factor 2, which results in the inhibition of protein synthesis and subsequent death of the cell.

The first fusion toxin constructed was DAB_{486} α-melanocyte-stimulating hormone (α-MSH), in which the native diphtheria toxin receptor-binding domain was replaced with a-MSH [20]. This construct employed a unique *Sph*I restriction endonuclease site in the diphtheria toxin structural gene such that amino acid 486 served as the fusion junction between diphtheria toxin-related sequences and a-MSH. The α-MSH gene was selected because it was a small protein (13 amino acids) which could be easily synthesized in vitro and because it had previously been demonstrated that the receptor-binding region was located at the C-terminal end of the peptide, thereby allowing for N-terminal fusion with diphtheria toxin sequences. Despite the fact that DAB_{486} α-MSH was subject to marked proteolytic degradation in *E. coli*, sufficient amounts of the fusion toxin were purified to demonstrate specific toxicity for α-MSH receptor-bearing cells.

DAB_{486} α-MSH was subject to marked proteolytic degradation due to the small size of the peptide and the protease-sensitive sites appeared to be close to the fusion junction between diphtheria toxin and α-MSH; therefore, the next fusion toxins were constructed with a growth factor of larger mass to provide stearic hindrance and thereby minimize degradation. In 1987, Williams et al. [33] described the genetic construction, expression, and purification of the DAB_{486} interleukin (IL)-2 fusion toxin, in which the native receptor-binding domain of diphtheria toxin was replaced with IL-2 [1, 32–34]. The purified DAB_{486} IL-2 was biologically active and selectively inhibited protein synthesis with an IC_{50} of 10^{-10} *M* in cell lines bearing the high-affinity IL-2 receptor. Cells lacking the full component of the high-affinity IL-2 receptor were resistant to the fusion toxin, with an IC_{50} of 10^{-8} *M* for cells lacking IL-2 receptor expression. Bacha et al. [1] confirmed that receptor binding was required for fusion toxin-mediated cytotoxicity.

It has further been shown that only cells bearing the high-affinity isoform of the IL-2 receptor (p55, p75, p64) are preferentially more sensitive to intoxication by the IL-2 fusion toxins [32]. The early events following binding of DAB_{486} IL-2 to the high-affinity receptor have been shown to mimic those of IL-2, with increase in mRNA for IL-2, IL-2 receptor, c-*myc*, and interferon (IFN)-γ. This initial stimulation is rapidly followed by inhibition of protein synthesis such that, by 12 h, the mRNA profiles resemble those of a cell treated with cycloheximide [31]. Since the high-affinity form of the receptor is found only on activated proliferating T cells , recently activated B cells, and activated monocytes [29, 30], the natural killer (NK) cells which constitutively express the

Table 1. Diphtheria toxin-based cell receptor-targeted fusion proteins

Fusion toxin	Ligand
DAB_{486} α-MSH	α-MSH
DAB_{389} α-MSH	α-MSH
DAB_{486} IL-2	IL-2
DAB_{389} IL-2	IL-2
DAB_{389} mIL-4	IL-4
DAB_{389} IL-6	IL-6
DAB_{389} IL-7	IL-7
DAB_{389} EGF	EGF
DAB_{389} CD4	HIV gp120

MSH, melanocyte-stimulating hormone, IL, interleukin; EGF, epithial growth factor; HIV, human immunodeficiency virus; gp, glycoprotein

intermediate form of the receptor (p75, p64) and selected tumor cells expressing only Tac (p55) are much less sensitive to the action of the fusion toxin.

While DAB_{486} IL-2 demonstrated high specific activity in vitro, its half-life in vivo was less than 5 min. Efforts to reengineer the molecule were undertaken by Williams et al. [34], who demonstrated that the internal in-frame deletion of 97 amino acids from the diphtheria toxin fragment B resulted in a truncated form of the fusion toxin called DAB_{389} IL-2, which had a two- to threefold higher K_d than DAB_{486} IL-2 and a longer half-life, with a resulting tenfold increase in potency. Based on these results, it was determined that amino acid 389 of diphtheria toxin is the optimal site for the genetic fusion of cell receptor-binding ligands. DAB_{389} IL-2, like its progenitor, binds to and is selectively cytotoxic for high-affinity IL-2 receptor-bearing cells. As shown in Table 1, other cytokines and ligands have been substituted for IL-2, resulting in the generation of a family of fusion toxins built on the DAB_{389} skeleton. Of these, only the IL-2 and epithelial growth factor (EGF) fusion toxins have entered clinical trials thus far.

Pastan et al. [21] have created a family of fusion toxins using *Pseudomonas* exotoxin A. Like diphtheria toxin, *Pseudomonas* exotoxin is composed of three domains, but unlike diphtheria toxin., the protein synthesis-inhibiting domain is localized to the carboxy-terminal region of the molecule and the receptor-binding domain to the N-terminal region. Deletion of the first 252 amino acids of *Pseudomonas* exotoxin produces a 40-kDa protein (PE40), which cannot bind to cellular receptors but which, when conjugated to antibodies, is capable of inhibiting protein synthesis. A series of chimeric fusion toxins have been produced by fusing the PE40 gene with different targeting ligands, as shown in Table 2. Recently, Pastan and colleagues have designed fusion toxins consisting of single-chain variable heavy and light domains of monoclonal antibodies with PE40. The first of these agents to enter clinical trials will be the anti-Tac (Fv)–PE38, directed against the IL-2 receptor [12,13,24]. This ligand requires expression of only the Tac or p55 component of the IL-2 receptor on the target cells for internalization and cytotoxicity, compared to the cytokine ligand fusion toxins IL-2 PE or DAB_{389} IL2 fusion toxins, which require the presence of the high-affinity IL-2R complex (p55, p75, p64) for internalization [12]. Clinical trials with these single-chain antibody fusion toxins are underway.

Table 2. Pseudomonas exotoxin A fusion toxins

fusion toxin	Target
IL-2–PE40	IL-2 receptor neoplasms
IL-4–PE40	IL-4 receptor
IL-6–PE40	Il-6 receptor; myelomas, heptomas
Acidic FGF–PE40	FGF receptor
IGF-1–PE40	IGF-1 receptor
CD4(178)–PE40	HIV-infected cells
Anti-Tac (Fv)–PE38	IL-2 receptor
B3(Fv)–PE38KDEL	Many carcinomas

IL, interleukin; FGF, fibroplast growth factor; IGF, insulin-like growth factor; HIV, human immunodeficiency virus

State of the Art: Clinical Trials

DAB486 Interleukin-2 in Cancer

IL-2 receptor expression has been reported on subsets of hematopoietic malignancies, including Hodgkin's disease, low- and intermediate-grade non-Hodgkin's lymphoma, cutaneous T cell lymphoma, human T lymphotropic virus (HTLV)-1-associated adult T cell leukemia/lymphoma, and chronic lymphocytic leukemia [2, 3, 14, 23, 26–28].

A series of phase I/II clinical studies were developed to determine the safety, tolerability, and pharmacokinetics of the first-generation IL-2 fusion toxin DAB486 IL-2 in patients with refractory hematologic malignancies [5, 9, 15, 16, 25]. While IL-2 receptor expression was assayed on available tumor tissue of enrolled patients, expression was not required for eligibility. The initial clinical trials were designed as a three-patient cohort dose escalation in which single and multiple doses of the fusion toxin were administered by intravenous injection, either as a bolus or 90-min infusion. The initial dose was 700 ng/kg per day and was escalated to 400 μg/kg per day. Adverse effects were generally mild and included nausea/vomiting, hypersensitivity, fever/malaise/chills, and elevations in serum hepatic transaminases. The maximal tolerated dose for DAB486 IL-2 was 400 μg/kg per day, above which renal insufficiency occurred. All of the adverse effects observed in these studies were transient, not cumulative, and did not preclude repeated administration of the fusion toxin to patients who responded to therapy. In addition, there were no changes in circulating normal lymphocyte subsets during or following therapy, and no increased incidence of opportunistic infection was observed.

The time course of analysis of DAB486 IL-2 concentrations in serum, using a nonlinear mathematical model, showed that the clearance of the fusion toxin followed a one-component model with a $t_{1/2}$ of approximately 11 min at dose levels of 200–400 mg/kg [16]. Moreover, the pharmacokinetics of the fusion toxin did not change following multiple courses of administration.

In many patients, increased serum levels of soluble IL-2 receptor (sIL-2R) were detected; however, there was no correlation between the clearance rates of the fusion toxin from circulation and the level of sIL-2R. Bacha (personal communication) had previously found that the presence of 50|000 units sIL-2R per ml failed to inhibit the cytotoxic action of DAB486 IL-2 in vitro. Following administration of DAB486 IL-2,

Table 3. Clinical response to diphteria toxin fusion toxins

Diagnosis	DAB486 IL-2 (total CR+PR) (*n*)	(*n*)	(%)	DAB389 IL-2 (Total CR+PR (*n*)	(*n*)	(%)
NHL	51	4	8	17	3	18
HD	14	1	7	21	0	0
CTCL	26	6	17	35	13	37

NHL, non-Hodgkin's lymphoma; HD, Hodgkin's disease; CTL, cutaneous T cell lymphoma; IL, interleukin; CR, complete remission; PR, partial remission

approximately 60 % of the patients had an anamnestic response to the diphtheria toxin component of the fusion protein. Few patients, however, had anti-IL-2 titers prior to study entry. After one or more courses of fusion toxin administration, approximately half of the patients developed low titers of anti-IL-2 antibodies. As was seen with sIL-2R, the presence of either anti-diphtheria toxin-related or anti-IL-2 antibodies did not appear to prevent an antitumor response.

Clinical responses were seen in these phase I studies in patients with low- and intermediate-grade non-Hodgkin's lymphoma, Hodgkin's disease, and cutaneous T cell lymphoma, as shown in Table 3. All of these patients had refractory disease and had failed at least two prior chemotherapy regimens. While IL-2 receptor expression on the patient's tumor tissue was not a requirement for entry into this study, immunohistochemical studies were performed in patients in whom tissue was readily accessible for biopsy. All of the responders had demonstrable IL-2 receptor expression, as measured by immunoreactivity with the CD25 (anti-Tac) antibody. The most impressive responses in these studies occurred in patients with cutaneous T cell lymphoma. One patient with tumor-stage cutaneous T cell lymphoma had a complete remission with disappearance of all of his tumors, and he has remained disease free without further therapy for at least 5 years [9]. Another patient with diffuse plaque-stage disease had significant clearing of his lesions, and two patients with the Sézary syndrome experienced marked improvement in skin exfoliation and pruritis without a significant change in the numbers of circulating Sézary cells [5].

DAB389 Interleukin-2 in Neoplastic Disease

Because of the encouraging results demonstrated with DAB486 IL-2, further clinical studies were performed with the redesigned fusion toxin DAB389 IL-2. This molecule lacked 97 amino acids from the membrane- translocating region of DAB486 IL-2, thus conferring a tenfold increase in potency in vitro and a longer half-life of 60 min as compared to 5 min for DAB486 IL-2 [34]. A phase I/II study of DAB389 IL-2 was initiated in patients with non-Hodgkin's lymphoma, Hodgkin's disease, and cutaneous T cell lymphoma whose tumors expressed the IL-2 receptor, as determined by immunohistochemical staining using the anti-CD25 antibody and antibodies directed against the p75 component of the IL-2 receptor [17, M. Saleh, personal communication]. Immunostaining of more than 25 % of the patient's tumor cells was required for enrollment. Patients with human immunodeficiency virus (HIV)-associated T cell malignancy and HTLV-1-associated acute T cell leukemia/lymphoma were excluded. The study followed a cohort dose-escalation format, and the treatment schedule was five intravenous bolus infusions to be repeated every 21 days if toxicity permitted.

Of 230 patients screened for inclusion in to this study, IL-2 receptor was detected on tumor specimens from 109 patients (47 %), including 41% with non-Hodgkin's lymphoma, 62 % with cutaneous T cell lymphoma, and 83 % with Hodgkin's disease. Seventy-three patients were enrolled in this study. The median number of prior therapies was five, and 25 patients had undergone prior bone marrow transplantation.

Toxicities included treatment-associated fever and chills in 74 % and nausea/vomiting, asthenia, and hypotension in 50 %. The severity of these adverse events diminished with subsequent courses. Hypoalbuminemia (80 %) and reversible elevation of hepatic transaminases (62 %) were the most commonly observed laboratory abnormalities and were reversible in all patients. Of interest, hypoalbuminemia, hypotension, and edema was observed in eight patients with cutaneous T cell lymphoma and was felt to potentially represent mild vascular leak-type syndrome, similar to that observed with ricin A chain or *Pseudomonas* exotoxin A immunotoxin molecules. The dose-limiting toxicity was observed at the 31 mg/kg per day dosage and consisted of severe fatigue and asthenia. Overall, treatment was discontinued in 53 % of patients because of disease progression, while 16 % were taken off the study because of toxicity.

The kinetics of DAB389 IL-2 best fit a one-compartment model with an overall half-life of 72 min. The AUC increased with administered dose. Approximately 38 % of the patients demonstrated preexisting antibodies to DAB389 IL-2, and antibodies were detected in 92 % of the study population following two cycles of treatment. As was observed with DAB486 IL-2, preexisting antibody titers or antibody generation during therapy did not correlate with clinical response or toxicity.

Clinical responses were observed in 16 of the seventy-73 patients (22 %), as shown in Table 3. Thirteen of thirty-35 cutaneous T cell lymphoma patients (37 %) and three of 17 non-Hodgkin's lymphoma patients (18 %) demonstrated an objective clinical response. There were no responders among the Hodgkin's disease patients. The median time to response was 2 months (two cycles of treatment), and the median duration of response was 10 months. The most dramatic responses, including five of six complete responses, were observed in patients with cutaneous T cell lymphoma. Four of the five complete responders had failed prior photophoresis. An impressive complete response was achieved in a patient with extensive erythroderma (T4) and palpable adenopathy (stage III). The patient had debilitating plaque disease involving both hands and arms, resulting in palmar contractures bilaterally. He had previously failed photophoresis and psoralens ultraviolet A (PUVA) therapy. He was treated with a dosage of 15 μg/kg per day; objective response was documented following four cycles and biopsy-proven complete response following six cycles of DAB389 IL-2. A second patient who had previously failed topical therapy, phototherapy, chemotherapy, IFN, and local radiotherapy had dramatic shrinkage of cutaneous tumors following one cycle of treatment and complete regression of all visible lesions by the end of the second cycle. The patient had a=complete response of 12 months' duration. One patient with primary refractory non-Hodgkin's lymphoma, who had failed bone marrow transplantation, achieved a complete response which has been ongoing for more than 39 months. Clinical responses were seen at all dose levels.

The results of this study demonstrate that DAB389 IL-2 has enhanced antitumor activity compared to DAB486 IL-2, perhaps due to the increased half-life of the agent.

The achievement of objective antitumor responses in patients with refractory cutaneous T cell lymphoma is particularly impressive, especially since these responses in preliminary studies have been durable without other maintenance therapy. Based on these observations, two phase III clinical trials are currently ongoing using DAB_{389} IL-2 in the treatment of cutaneous T cell lymphoma patients whose tumors demonstrate expression of the IL-2 receptor. The first study is a double-blind analysis of two dose levels of DAB_{389} IL-2 in patients with refractory CTCL, and the other is a double-blind, randomized, placebo-controlled study in earlier-stage CTCL patients who have not received prior systemic therapy.

DAB_{389} Interleukin-2 in Benign Cutaneous Disease

DAB_{389} IL-2 has demonstrated preliminary activity in patients with psoriasis [7]. It was hypothesized that this agent may be efficacious in psoriasis due to the presence of activated antigen-presenting cells in skin lesions, high numbers of T lymphocytes infiltrating affected skin regions, and activation markers such as the IL-2 receptor (CD25) on the infiltrating lymphocytes. T cell activation in psoriasis is thought to be driven by an as yet unidentified cutaneous antigen which is presented to T cells by the activated dendritic cells in psoriatic lesions. As pathogenic T lymphocyte clones would control their proliferation through upregulated "normal" IL-2 receptors, disease-mediating T cell clones should be highly sensitive to DAB_{389} IL-2.

Of the few psoriatic patients treated with DAB_{389} IL-2, remarkable skin clearing or disease improvement has been noted in many [7]. Clinical improvement was coupled with reduction in the number of T lymphocytes infiltrating skin lesions and with marked improvement or elimination of keratinocyte hyperproliferation and other cellular aberrations that define the histopathology of psoriasis. While larger series are needed, the initial results suggest the potential of DAB_{389} IL-2 as an effective therapeutic agent for inflammatory or autoimmune skin disorders. The clinical responsiveness of atopic eczema, alopecia areata, lichen planus, and graft-versus-host disease (GVHD) to cyclosporine and other immunosuppressive agents suggests that these diseases are also logical candidates for DAB_{389} IL-2 therapy.

Discussion

Over the last decade, the design and genetic construction of targeted toxin-based therapies has been realized, based on a detailed understanding of the strucure–function relationships of both diphtheria toxin and *Pseudomonas* exotoxin A. A variety of fusion proteins have been constructed in which the native receptor-binding domain of either toxin has been replaced with either a polypeptide hormone, growth factor, or antibody determinant to produce chimeric proteins which selectively intoxicate receptor-bearing target cells in vitro. Moreover, cells that are devoid of the target receptor proteins are resistant to the action of these fusion toxins. The leading candidate fusion toxins which have reached clinical trials include DAB_{486} IL-2, DAB_{389} IL-2, DAB_{389} EGF, and the *Pseudomonas* exotoxin-based fusion toxins anti-Tac–PE40 and anti-Tac (Fv)–PE38. Clinical studies with the diphtheria toxin fusion toxins have now matured and have demonstrated promising activity of these agents in IL-2 receptor-bearing hematopoietic neoplasms as well as in psoriasis. These results suggest that IL-2-directed fusion toxins may be applicable to other diseases in which proliferating activated T cells play a major role in pathogenesis, including other benign dermatologic disorders, graft rejection, and other autoimmune disorders.

Future studies will be directed toward improvement of the activity profile of the existing agents as well as synthesis of molecules with new targeting ligands. One key issue to be addressed is that the response rates in the clincial studies with diphtheria toxin fusion toxin have been lower that what would be expected based on the level of detectable IL-2 receptor expression in patients' neoplastic cells. One reason for this may be inefficient delivery of fusion toxin to the tumor tissue. Further studies with different schedules of infusion would be useful in this regard. Another reason might involve insensitivity of the existing immunohistochemical tools in identifying the high-affinity IL-2 receptor isoform (p55, p75, p64) on tumor cells. It is known that expression of the p64 chain of the receptor is crucial for internalization and that internalization events depend on receptor clustering on the cell surface as well as possibly a signaling event. While these components of fusion toxin internalization have been identified in candidate cell lines, there is little data addressing the efficiency of internalization in fresh human tumor cells. Alternatively, a block in the postinternalization events involving the acidification of the internalized protein complex in the endosome and subsequent processing leading to liberation of active fragment A into the cytosol could lead to insensitivity of tumor cells. These events depend on furins which induce nicking of the fusion toxin and induction of pore formation in the endosome. Once the free fragment A is liberated and passes through the endosomal pore, it must be refolded accurately in the cytosol in order to bind to elongation factor 2. Studies are underway to evaluate these events in neoplastic cells. Recently, Murphy and colleagues have constructed mutants of diphtheria toxin fusion toxins which do not refold properly and are thus metabolically inactive. Information gathered from these and other studies will hopefully lead to development of genetically improved fusion toxins with enhanced biological activity. Clinical studies with the anti-Tac (Fv)–PE38 fusion toxin are early in development, and it remains to be seen whether this agent will, in fact , be more efficiently internalized by a larger number of neoplastic cells than a cytokine-based fusion toxin.

Summary

A variety of strategies have been undertaken to specifically direct therapeutic modalities toward populations of cells implicated in a disease while sparing the surrounding cells and tissues. Monoclonal antibodies were the first targeted effector molecules which, when used alone or conjugated with other agents such as toxins or radionuclides, could selectively kill cells or stimulate immune system destruction of tumors. The clinical utility of antibody-based therapies has been limited by large molecular weight, poor tissue penetration, nonspecific cross-reactivity, and generation of neutralizing antibodies directed against the murine epitopes. Recently, genetic engineering has led to the development of fusion toxins, "designer" targeted effector molecules which combine a targeting ligand, such as a growth factor, with a cytocidal moiety, such as a plant or bacterial toxin. The evolution of this technology and its implementation in the clinical therapy of disease is discussed.

References

1. Bacha P, Waters C, Williams J, Murphy JR, Strom TB (1988) Interleukin-2 targeted cytotoxicity: selective action of a diphtheria toxin-related interleukin-2 fusion protein. J Exp Med 167: 612–622
2. Barnett D, Wilson G, Lawrence A, Buckley G (1988) The interleukin-2 receptor and its expression in the acute leukemias and lymphoproliferative disorders. Dis Mark 6:133–139
3. Craig F, Banks P (1992) Detection of the alpha and beta components of the interleukin-2 receptor using immunologic techniques. Mod Pathol 5:118a
4. Donovan JJ, Simon MI, Draper RK, Montal M (1981) Diphtheria toxin forms transmembrane channels in planar lipid bilayers. Proc Natl Acad Sci USA 78:172–176
5. Foss F, Borkowski T, Gilliom M, Stetler-Stevenson M, Jaffe E, Tomkins A, Bastian A, Nylen P, Woodworth T, Udey M, Sausville E (1994) Chimeric fusion protein toxin DAB(486)IL2 in refractory mycosis fungoides and the Sezary syndrome: correlation of activity and IL2 receptor expression in a phase II study. Blood 84(6):1765–1774
6. Fuchs R, Schmid S, Mellman I (1989) A possible role for Na^+, K^+-ATPase in regulating ATP-dependent endosome acidification. Proc Natl Acad Sci USA 86:539–543
7. Gottlieb SL, Gilleaudeau P, Johnson R, Estis L, Woodworth T, Gottlieb AB, Krueger JG (1995) Response of psoriasis to a lymphocyte-selective toxin (DAB_{389} IL-2) suggests a primary immune, but not keratinocyte, pathogenic basis. Nature Med 1:442–447
8. Greenfield L, Johnson VG, Youle RJ (1987) Mutations in diphtheria toxin separate binding from entry and amplify immunotoxin selectivity. Science 238:536–539
9. Hesketh P, Caguioa P, Koh H, Dewey H, Facada A, McCaffrey R, Parker K, Nylen P, Woodworth T (1993) Clinical activity of a cytotoxic fusion protein in the treatment of cutaneous T cell lymphoma. J Clin Oncol 11:1628–1690
10. Hoch DH, Romero-Mira M, Ehrich BE, Finkelstein A, DasGupta BR, Simpson LL (1985) Channels formed by botulinum, tetanus, and diphtheria toxins in planar lipid bilayers: relevance to translocation of proteins across membranes. Proc Natl Acad Sci USA 82:336–343
11. Kagan BL, Finkelstein A, Colombini M (1981) Diphtheria toxin fragment forms large pores in phospholipid bilayer membranes. Proc Natl Acad Sci USA 78:4950–4954
12. Kreitman R, Chang C, Hudson D, Queen C, Bailon P, Pastan I (1994a) Anti-TAC (Fab)-PE40, a recombinant double chain immunotoxin which kills interleukin-2 receptor bearing cells and induces complete remission in an in vivo tumor model. Int J Cancer 57(56):856–864
13. Kreitman R, Bailon P, Chaudhary V, Fitzgerald D, Pastan I (1994b) Recombinant immunotoxins containing anti-Tac (Fv) and derivatives of Pseudomonas exotoxin produce complete regression in mice of an interleukin-2 receptor bearing carcinoma. Blood 83(2):426–434
14. Kung E, Meissner K, Loning T (1988) Cutaneous T-cell lymphoma: immunocytochemical study on activation/proliferation and differentiation associated antigens in lymph nodes, skin, and peripheral blood. Virchows Arch [A] Pathol Anat 413:539–549
15. LeMaistre CF, Meneghetti C, Rosenblum M, Reuben J, Parker K, Shaw J, Woodworth T, Parkinson D (1992) Phase I trial of an interleukin-2 receptor (IL-2R) fusion toxin (DAB486 IL-2) in hematologic malignancies expressing the IL-2 receptor. Blood 79:2547–2554
16. LeMaistre CF, Craig FE, Meneghetti C, McMullin B, Parker K, Reuben J, Boldt DH, Rosenblum M, Woodworth T (1993) Phase I trail of a 90-minute infusion of the fusion toxin DAB_{486} IL-2 in hematologic cancers. Cancer Res 53:3930–3934
17. LeMaistre F, Saleh M, Kuzel T, Foss F, Planaias L, Schwartz G, Ratain M, Rook A, Freytes C, Craig F, Revidin J, Nichols J (1997) Phase I trial of a ligand fusion toxin (DAB_{389} IL-2) in lymphomas expresssing the receptor for interleukin-2. (submitted)
18. Morris RE, Gerstein AS, Bonventre PF, Saelinger CB (1985) Receptor-mediated entry of diphtheria toxin into monkey kidney (Vero) cells: electron microscopic evaluation. Infect Immun 50:721–727
19. Moya M, Dautry-Versat A, Goud B, Louvard D, Boquet P (1985) Inhibition of coated pit formation in Hep cells blocks the cytotoxicity of diphtheria toxin but not that of ricin toxin. J Cell Biol 101:548–559

20. Murphy JR, Bishai W, Borowski M, Miyanohara A, Boyd J, Nagle S (1986) Genetic construction, expression, and melanoma-selective cytotoxicity of a diphtheria toxin a-melanocyte stimulating hormone fusion protein. Proc Natl Acad Sci USA 83:8258–8262
21. Pastan I, Chaudhary V, Fitzgerald D (1992) Recombinant toxins as novel therapeutic agents. Annu Rev Biochem 61:331–354
22. Rolf JM, Eidels L (1993) Structure-function analyses of diphtheria toxin by use of monoclonal antibodies. Infect Immun 61:944–1003
23. Rosolen A, Nakanishi M, Poplack D, Cole D, Quinines R, Reaman G, Cotelingam J, Trepel J, Sausville E, Marti G, Neckers L, Colamonici O (1992). Expression of interleukin-2 receptor beta subunit in hematopoietic malignancies. Blood 73:1968–1972
24. Saito T, Krietman R, Hanada S, Makino T, Utsunomiya A, Sumizawa T, Arima T, Chang C, Hudson D, Pastan I (1994) Cyutotoxicity of recombinant Fab and Fv immunotoxins on adult T-cell leukemia node and blood cells in the presence of soluble interleukin-2 receptor. Cancer Res 54(4):1059–1064
25. Schwartz G, Tepler I, Charette J, Kadin L, Parker K, Woodworth T, Schnipper L (1992) Complete response of a Hodgkin's lymphoma in a phase I trail of DAB_{486} IL-2. Blood 79:175a
26. Sheibani K, Winberg C, van de Velde S, Blayney D, Rappaport H (1987) Distributionof lymphocytes with interleukin-2 receptors (TAC antigens) in reactive lymphoproliferative processes, Hodgkins disease, and non-Hodgkins lymphomas. An immunohistochemical study of 300 cases. Am J Pathol 127:27–37
27. Strauchen J, Breakstone B (1987) IL-2 receptor expression in human lymphoid lesions. Am J Pathol 126:506–512
28. Uchiyama T, Hori T, Tsudo M, Wano Y, Umadome H, Tamori S, Yodoi J, Maeda M, Sawami H, Uchino H (1985) Interleukin-2 receptor (Tac antigen) expressed on adult T-cell leukemia cells. Clin Invest 76:446
29. Waldmann TA (1986) The structure, function, and expression of interleukin-2 receptors on normal and malignant T cells. Science 232:727–732
30. Waldmann TA (1990) The multichain interleukin-2 receptor. A target for immunotherapy in lymphoma, autoimmune disorders, and organ allografts. J Am Med Assoc 263:272–274
31. Walz G, Zanker B, Brand K, Swanlund D, Genbauffe F, Zeldis J, Murphy J, Strom T (1989) Sequential effects of interleukin-2/diphtheria toxin fusion protein on T-cell activation. Proc Natl Acad Sci USA 86:9485–9488
32. Waters CA, Schimke P, Snider CE, Itoh K, Smith KA, Nichols JC, Strom TB, Murphy JR (1990) Interleukin-2 receptor targeted cytotoxicity: receptor binding requirements for entry of IL-2-toxin into cells. Eur J Immunol 20:785–791
33. Williams D, Parker K, Bishai W, Borowski M, Genbauffe F, Strom TB, Murphy JR (1987) Diphtheria-toxin receptor binding domain substitution with interleukin-2: genetic construction and properties of a diphtheria toxin-related interleukin-2 fusion protein. Protein Eng 1:493–498
34. Williams D, Snider CE, Strom TB, Murphy JR (1990) Structure function analysis of IL-2 toxin (DAB IL-2): fragment B sequences required for the delivery of fragment A to the cytosol of target cells. J Biol Chem 265:11885–11889

Dermatological Phototherapy: A Prime Example of Ultraviolet Radiation-Induced Immunointervention

J. Krutmann

Introduction

Photoimmunology is a relatively new discipline of biomedical research which studies the effects of nonionizing electromagnetic radiation, in particular of ultraviolet (UV) radiation, on the immune system. Interest in photoimmunology originated from observations made in three different research fields: (1) photocarcinogenesis, (2) studies on the function of epidermal Langerhans cells, and (3) the increasing use of UV radiation for the treatment of skin diseases [13, 20, 37]. For dermatologic phototherapy, irradiation devices emitting either shortwave UV (UVB, 280–320 nm) or longwave UV (UVA, 320–400 nm) radiation are employed. Patients were originally treated with broadband UVB, broadband UVA, or combination regimens (UVA/UVB), but in recent years there has been a strong tendency towards the use of irradiation devices which allow exposure of human skin to selected emission spectra, e.g., 311-nm UVB (which uses long-wave UVB radiation 300 nm) [32] or high-dose UVA1 therapy (which selectively employs long-wave UVA radiation > 340 nm) [18]. In addition to phototherapy, photochemotherapy is widely used for the treatment of skin diseases [26]. The most popular photochemotherapeutic modality combines the oral or topical application of psoralens with subsequent UVA irradiation (PUVA therapy).

Phototherapy and photochemotherapy are of great benefit in the treatment of psoriasis, an inflammatory skin disease characterized by keratinocyte hyperproliferation. Both UV radiation and PUVA, by the induction of DNA photoproducts, transiently inhibit cell proliferation, and it has therefore been thought that the therapeutic effectiveness of phototherapeutic and photochemotherapeutic modalities mainly relates to their antiproliferative properties [1, 2]. Since the introduction of UVB radiation and PUVA in dermatological therapy, however, the number of skin diseases showing a favorable response to phototherapy or photochemotherapy has substantially grown [37]. The vast majority of these diseases are not characterized by hyperproliferative processes, but are immunologic in nature. In addition, studies on the role of UV radiation-induced immunosuppression in photocarcinogenesis and on the effects of UV radiation on the function of antigen-presenting Langerhans cells have provided increasing evidence that exposure to UVB, UVA, or PUVA exerts profound effects on the skin immune system [20]. These observations have stimulated studies in which the role of immunomodulation in phototherapy and photochemotherapy of skin diseases has been analyzed. The present chapter reviews current knowledge about immunointerventive principles associated with UVB, UVA, and PUVA therapy.

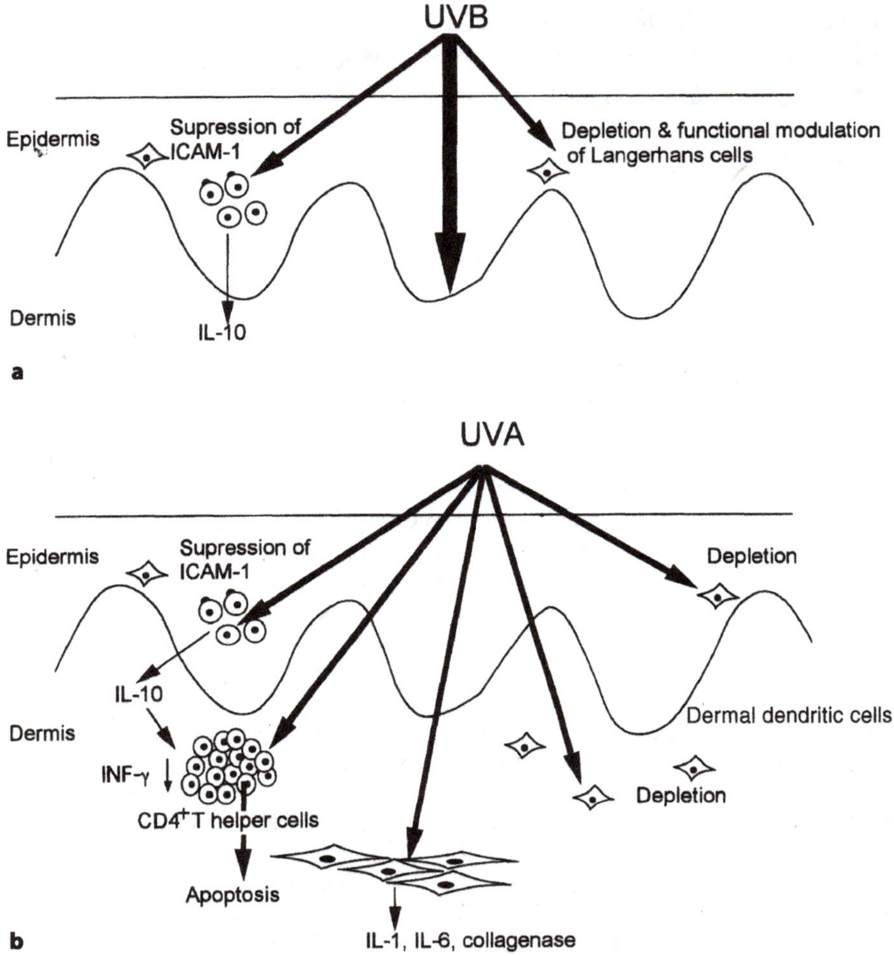

Fig. 1a,b. Immunomodulatory effects induced by **a** ultraviolet B (UVB)-induced or **b** *UVA*(1)-induced phototherapy. *ICAM*-1, intercellular adhesion molecule-1; *IFN*, interferon; *IL*, interleukin

Phototherapy- and Photochemotherapy-Induced Immunomodulation

Most of the immunomodulatory effects that are discussed in this chapter are not specific for a single modality, but may be observed in vitro after UVB, UVA, or PUVA treatment. It should be noted, however, that the in vivo relevance of these immunomodulatory effects for a given phototherapeutic regimen critically depends on the physical properties of the type of UV radiation employed [3]. For example, UVB phototherapy primarily affects the function of epidermal keratinocytes and Langerhans cells, whereas UVA radiation, which in contrast to UVB radiation is able to penetrate the dermal layers at significant doses, additionally affects dermal fibroblasts, dermal dendritic cells, endothelial cells, and also skin-infiltrating inflammatory cells such as T lymphocytes, mast cells, and granulocytes (Fig. 1). Moreover, UVB, UVA, and PUVA therapy, despite exhibiting similar or even identical immunomodulatory effects, differ greatly when their underlying photobiological mechanisms are compared.

Immunomodulatory effects associated with UVB, UVA, or PUVA have been studied in depth during the last 25 years, primarily by employing animal models and in vitro assay systems. A detailed summary of photoimmunological research is beyond the scope of this review, but can be found in a recent monograph [20]. The present chapter focuses mainly on studies in the field of human photoimmunology, with special emphasis on their relevance for dermatological phototherapy and photochemotherapy. Photoimmunological effects of therapeutic relevance fall into three major categories: (1) effects on soluble mediators, (2) modulation of the expression of cell surface associated molecules (e.g., adhesion molecules, cytokine receptors), and (3) the induction of apoptosis in pathogenetically relevant cells.

Effects on Soluble Mediators

Beneficial effects induced by phototherapeutic or photochemotherapeutic modalities may result either from the induction of mediators with anti-inflammatory and/or immunosuppressive properties or from suppression of the production of proinflammatory factors. In addition, recent studies indicate that some of the beneficial effects observed after UVA radiation therapy of scleroderma patients may be due to the induction of cytokines, which affect the expression of genes relevant for collagen metabolism. The capacity to affect the production of soluble, immunomodulatory mediators has been demonstrated extensively for UVB radiation and to some extent for UVA and UVA1 radiation [28]. In contrast, little is currently known about the effects of PUVA on the release of cytokines, neuropeptides, and prostanoids.

Induction of Anti-inflammatory/Immunosuppressive Factors

Epidermal keratinocytes and Langerhans cells, dermal fibroblasts, and endothelial cells, but also skin-infiltrating mast cells and T cells produce and secrete a variety of soluble mediators with both pro- and anti-inflammatory properties. Because of its physical properties, UVB radiation does not directly affect dermal cells, and studies on the effects of UVB radiation on the production of soluble mediators have therefore almost exclusively focused on epidermal keratinocytes. From these studies, it is now well established that UVB radiation is a potent inducer of the production of keratinocyte-derived cytokines, neuropeptides, and prostanoids [24].

UVB radiation-inducible cytokines include interleukin (IL)-1 and IL-6, which primarily exert proinflammatory effects and are held responsible, at least in part, for local and systemic symptoms associated with a sunburn reaction. Of much greater phototherapeutic interest is the recent observation that UV radiation may also induce the production of the anti-inflammatory/immunosuppressive cytokine IL-10. IL-10 is functionally defined by its capacity to suppress the production of interferon (IFN)-γ by T lymphocytes of the T-helper (Th)1-like subtype and by affecting the costimulatory repertoire of antigen-presenting cells such as dendritic cells and monocytes (for details, please see "Cytokines with Immunosuppressive Capacities," this volume). Recent in vitro studies have provided clear evidence that both UVB and UVA1 radiation have the capacity to significantly increase IL-10 mRNA and protein expression [8]. This mechanism may at least partially explain the observation that successful treatment of atopic dermatitis with UVA1 or UVA/UVB therapy leads to a significant downregulation of the in situ expression of the proinflammatory, T cell-derived cytokine IFN-γ [7]. In line with this assumption is the demonstration of increased IL-10 protein synthesis by epidermal keratinocytes following in vivo UV irradiation [9].

Recent studies indicate that human keratinocytes are capable of expressing mRNA specific for proopiomelanocortin (POMC) and of synthesizing biologically active POMC-derived peptides. In vitro exposure of human keratinocytes to either UVB or UVA1 radiation significantly induces the expression of POMC mRNA and increases the synthesis of POMC-derived peptides such as α-melanocyte-stimulating hormone (α-MSH) [24] (J. Krutmann and T.A. Luger, unpublished observation). α-MSH exhibits a variety of anti-inflammatory effects, e.g., inhibition of IL-1 or tumor necrosis factor (TNF)-α-mediated proinflammatory effects, and immunosuppressive effects, e.g., inhibition of the induction of contact hypersensitivity reactions, and UV radiation-induced increased production of keratinocyte-derived neuropeptides is therefore thought to represent an important UV radiation-inducible, anti-inflammatory principle [24].

Suppression of Proinflammatory Cytokines

In contrast to UVB radiation, UVA and in particular UVA1 radiation additionally affect cytokine production by dermal cells. For example, UVA1 radiation exerts direct effects on Th1-like cells by suppressing the production of IFN-γ, and this effect may contribute to the therapeutic effectiveness of high-dose UVA1 therapy in the treatment of atopic eczema, which was found to be associated with decreased in situ expression of this particular T cell cytokine [7, 27].

In a similar manner, UVB radiation-induced synthesis of prostaglandins may help to limit or counteract proinflammatory mediators in the skin [6]. For example, prostaglandin E_2 (PGE_2) does not only exert proinflammatory effects relevant for a sunburn reaction, but also has immunosuppressive effects. The expression of cell surface-associated adhesion molecules in human antigen-presenting cells can be inhibited by PGE_2, and this is thought to have profound effects on T cell activation (in particular Th1-like cells) [10]. PGE_2 can also directly act on Th1 cells by suppressing the production of IFN-γ.

Mediator Induction and Connective Tissue Disease

In vitro studies indicate that UVA1 radiation exposure leads to an increase in IL-1 and IL-6 mRNA and protein expression in cultured human dermal fibroblasts, which act in an autocrine manner to induce the expression of collagenase I in these cells [38]. Such a UVA1 radiation-inducible, autocrine loop could be partially responsible for the induction of collagenase I mRNA expression, which has been observed in lesional skin of patients with localized scleroderma following successful high-dose UVA1 therapy [35].

Modulation of Cell Surface Receptors

There is increasing evidence that both UVB and UVA radiation and PUVA treatment can directly affect the expression and function of cell surface receptors, including adhesion molecules, cytokine, and growth factor receptors.

Effects on Adhesion Molecules

A hallmark of UV- or PUVA-responsive skin diseases such as psoriasis, atopic dermatitis, and cutaneous T cell lymphoma, is an increased expression of the adhesion molecule intercellular adhesion molecule (ICAM)-1 on the surface of epidermal keratinocytes [19]. The ICAM-1 molecule is functionally defined by its capacity to serve as a counter-receptor for the lymphocyte function-associated antigen (LFA)-1, which is present on the surface of leukocytes. There is strong in vitro and in vivo evidence that ICAM-1/LFA-1-mediated cell–cell adhesion is an important prerequisite for the generation and maintenance of a variety of inflammatory and immune reactions in the skin. In healthy human skin, keratinocytes express no or only very little ICAM-1 on their surface. This is in sharp contrast to inflamed skin, in which keratinocyte ICAM-1 expression is markedly upregulated upon stimulation of keratinocytes with proinflammatory cytokines, including IFN-γ, TNF-β, and TNF-α [19]. It has therefore been of particular phototherapeutic interest to learn that cytokine-induced ICAM-1 expression may be efficiently inhibited by irradiation of cultured keratinocytes with sublethal doses of UVB or UVA radiation [15, 31]. This anti-inflammatory property of UV radiation may also be observed in vivo [33]. Exposure of human skin to suberythemal doses of UVB radiation was sufficient to effectively suppress upregulation of keratinocyte ICAM-1 expression, which was induced through i.c. injection of recombinant human IFN (rhIFN)-γ. In vitro and in vivo inhibition of ICAM-1 expression was observed only if UVB irradiation preceded cytokine stimulation. In additional studies it was demonstrated that the UVB radiation-induced suppression of ICAM-1 induction was transient in nature, because 24 h after UVB radiation exposure, significant induction of keratinocyte ICAM-1 expression was observed [17, 33]. If UVB irradiation was repeated 24 h after the first exposure, reinduction of ICAM-1 suppression was achieved, indicating that a maximal anti-inflammatory effect required repetitive UVB phototherapy on a day to day basis.

The gene-regulatory mechanisms responsible for this anti-inflammatory effect are poorly understood. Inhbition of cytokine-induced ICAM-1 expression does not depend on the nature of the ICAM-1-inducing cytokine [17]. It is therefore unlikely that UVB radiation interferes with intracellular signal transduction induced by a specific cytokine, but it may very well be that UVB radiation induces a mechanism which in a more general way prevents transcription of inducible genes. The latter possibility is supported by a series of recent observations indicating that UVB radiation also suppresses the upregulation of other cytokine-inducible genes, including HLA class II molecules and IL-7 [12].

Successful PUVA therapy of psoriasis is associated with a marked reduction in keratinocyte ICAM-1 expression in lesional skin [23]. It should be noted, however, that there is currently no convincing evidence that PUVA, similar to UVB or UVA radiation, is capable of directly modulating cytokine-induced or constitutive keratinocyte ICAM-

1 expression. PUVA therapy-induced downregulation of keratinocyte ICAM-1 expression may therefore best be explained by an indirect mechanism, e.g., the reduction of cytokine-producing, skin-infiltrating, inflammatory cells, which could also result in reduced ICAM-1 expression.

In addition to keratinocytes, UVB radiation has been found to significantly suppress adhesion molecule expression in antigen-presenting cells such as monocytes or epidermal Langerhans cells [16, 34]. These downregulatory effects appear to be relatively specific and to mainly affect the ICAM-1 molecule as well as members of the B7 family. UVB radiation-induced inhibition of adhesion molecule expression is of functional relevance, because the resulting alteration of the costimulatory repertoire of antigen-presenting cells appears to cause induction of anergic Th1 cells and preferential activation of Th2 cells.

Cytokine and Growth Factor Receptors as Targets Molecules

Keratinocyte-derived IL-1α is one of the key cytokines in the initiation of cutaneous inflammation, and regulation of keratinocyte IL-1 receptor expression therefore has a major impact on the course of inflammatory reactions in the skin. Human keratinoyctes express two different receptor molecules for IL-1: the IL-1 receptor type I (IL-1RI) and the IL-1 receptor type II (IL-1RII). These molecules markedly differ from a functional point of view, because only IL-1RI serves as a signaling receptor, whereas IL-1RII does not mediate IL-1-induced signals, but, by virtue of its capacity to bind IL-1, functions as a decoy receptor, thus limiting or suppressing IL-1-mediated tissue responses. It was therefore of phototherapeutic interest to learn that UVB radiation regulates IL-1RI and IL-1RII expression differentially in human keratinocytes [11]. Expression of IL-1RII was rapidly and dramatically induced after UVB radiation, whereas at the same time IL-1RI expression was decreased (but at later time points gradually increased). It has therefore been proposed that UVB radiation may limit overshooting responses to IL-1 stimulation of keratinocytes under inflammatory conditions by two complementary mechanisms: (1) increased expression of the decoy receptor IL-1RII and (2) decreased expression of the signaling molecule IL-1RI. Downregulation of the signaling receptor by UVB radiation is not specific for IL-1α, but may also be observed for other cytokines including TNF-α. Accordingly, in vitro exposure of human keratinocytes to sublethal doses of UVB radiation initially decreased mRNA and protein expression of the 55-kDa TNF receptor, which was subsequently followed by TNF receptor reexpression, eventually exceeding baseline levels [36]. Moreover, at time points of decreased TNF receptor expression, TNF responsiveness of UVB-irradiated keratinocytes was significantly reduced. UVB radiation did not affect the release of soluble TNF receptors from human keratinocytes. In a similar manner, UVB or UVA1 radiation also failed to modulate the production of soluble ICAM-1 molecules produced by human keratinocytes [20].

In addition to cytokines, growth factor receptors such as the epidermal growth factor (EGF) receptor appear to be important target molecules for UV radiation as well as PUVA treatment. Modulation of EGF receptor expression and function is thought to be of central importance within the signal transduction cascade relevant for UV radiation-induced gene expression. These studies were mainly directed at analyzing the so-called stress reponse in mammalian cells, and the UV radiation doses used were of no or minor therapeutic relevance. This is in contrast, however, to studies assessing the effects of PUVA treatment on EGF receptor function. In both murine and human cells, PUVA treatment inhibits binding of EGF to its receptors [22]. Since EGF is a growth factor for keratinocytes, it has been proposed that PUVA-induced inhibition of EGF binding might contribute to the beneficial effects induced by PUVA therapy in psoriasis.

Ultraviolet-Induced Apoptosis

Induction of programmed cell death (apoptosis) in pathogenetically relevant cells such as tissue-infiltrating inflammatory cells is currently being regarded as one of the key principles upon which widely used anti-inflammatory reagents such as glucocorticosteroids are based. Recent studies have provided compelling evidence that UVB and UVA (and in particular UVA1) irradiation and PUVA treatment are highly efficient in inducing apoptosis in human cells [4, 25]. T cells, as compared to other cell populations such as monocytes or keratinocytes, have an increased susceptibility towards UV- or PUVA-induced apoptosis [14, 40]. Induction of apoptosis is therefore of particular importance for T cell-mediated skin diseases such as atopic dermatitis, cutaneous T cell lymphoma, and possibly psoriasis. This assumption is supported by recent studies in which high-dose UVA1 phototherapy of patients with atopic dermatitis, after only a few UVA1 radiation exposures, was shown to induce apoptosis in skin-infiltrating Th cells present in eczematous skin [29]. Continuation of high-dose UVA1 therapy was associated with a gradual increase in the number of apoptotic T cells and eventually resulted in reduction of the inflammatory infiltrate and improvement of clinical symptoms. Similarly, successful UVB phototherapy of psoriasis has recently been reported to induce a reduction in the number of skin-infiltrating T cells and susbsequent normalization of keratinocyte morphology [14]. In vitro UVB irradiation is capable of inducing T cell apoptosis, and it has therefore been suggested that reduction of the inflammatory infiltrate is due to UVB phototherapy-induced T cell apoptosis. The in vivo proof for this speculation, however, is still lacking. It is also important to realize that, because of its physical properties, UVB radiation may only affect intraepidermal T cells in a direct manner [3], and it is therefore not surprising that UVB phototherapy mainly reduced the number of intraepidermal, but not intradermal T cells [14].

Induction of T cell apoptosis is thought to represent a key mechanism for PUVA therapy as well [25]. Evidence for the appearance of apoptotic T cells under PUVA therapy has thus far been provided for peripheral blood T cells in patients with Sézary syndrome undergoing extracorporeal photopheresis [40]. Whether systemic or topical PUVA treatment of PUVA-responsive skin diseases such as psoriasis or cutaneous T cell lymphoma leads to the induction of apoptotic T cells within lesional skin is currently not known.

In addition to T cells, phototherapy and photochemotherapy may also have the capacity to induce apoptosis in epidermal and/or dermal dendritic cells and thereby cause depletion of these cell populations from human skin (Fig. 1).

The mechanisms by which UVB irradiation or PUVA treatment induce apoptosis are not well characterized. This is in contrast to UVA1 phototherapy. In a recent study, Morita et al. [29] demonstrated that UVA1 radiation-induced apoptosis in human Th cells is mediated through the FAS and FAS ligand system. In particular, UVA1 irradiation, through the generation of singlet oxygen, leads to a translocation of preformed FAS ligand molecules from the cytoplasm into the cell membrane (early apoptosis) and

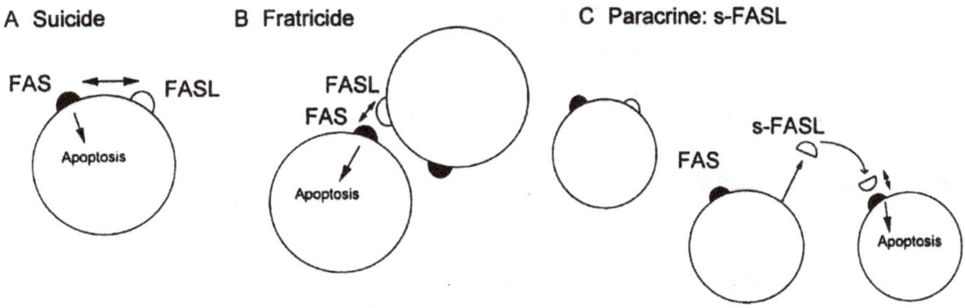

Fig. 2A–C. Potential mechanisms by which T cell apoptosis may be induced. A Suicide. B Fratricide. C Paracrine: soluble FAS ligand (*s-FASL*)

subsequent synthesis of FAS ligand molecules (late apoptosis). Increased cell surface expression of FAS ligand molecules subsequently results in T cell apoptosis via a suicide mechanism involving the autocrine interaction of these newly expressed FAS ligand molecules with constitutively expressed FAS molecules (Fig. 2). Further studies will need to address the possibility that paracrine processes, e.g., by induction of soluble FAS ligand molecules, may contribute to UV- or PUVA-induced apoptosis.

Photobiological Basis of Ultraviolet-Induced Immunomodulation

Several immunomodulatory effects of phototherapeutic relevance, e.g., the induction of IL-10 or the suppression of ICAM-1 induction, may be achieved by both UVB and UVA(1) irradiation. The photobiological mechanisms responsible for these immunomodulatory effects, however, have been found to greatly differ depending on the type of UV radiation used [21].

Similar to antiproliferative effects, immunomodulation induced by UVB radiation appears to result from UVB radiation-induced generation of DNA photoproducts, in particular thymine dimers. UVB radiation-induced suppression of IFN-γ-stimulated keratinocyte ICAM-1 expression was associated with the formation of significant numbers of thymine dimers in UVB-irradiated human skin [33]. Topical application of a DNA repair enzyme encapsulated in liposomes did not only decrease the number of thymine dimer-positive keratinocytes in irradiated skin by about 40%–50%, but completely prevented UVB radiation inhibition of ICAM-1 induction. Esssentially identical results were obtained from in vitro studies in which the role of thymine dimer formation for UVB radiation-induced IL-10 expression in cultured murine keratinocytes was assessed [30]. Exposure of murine keratinocytes (PAM212 cells) to increasing doses of UVB radiation dose-dependently increased both thymine dimer formation and IL-10 protein expression, and treatment of irradiated cells with exogenously supplied DNA repair enzymes was sufficient to partially reduce the number of thymine dimers and at the same time to completely suppress UVB radiation-induced IL-10 protein synthesis. The precise reason for the discrepancy between DNA repair enzyme-induced repair of thymine dimers, which was partial, and prevention of immunomodulatory effects such as IL-10 synthesis or inhibition of ICAM-1 induction, which was always nearly complete, is currently not known. It has been speculated, however, that gene-specific repair mechanisms may explain this phenomenon.

In contrast to UVB radiation, UVA(1) radiation-induced immunomodulatory effects are thought to be based on oxidative mechanisms [21]. In this regard, the generation of singlet oxygen appears to play a prominent role. This conclusion is based on the following three observations: UVA radiation-induced gene-regulatory events, such as the regulation of ICAM-1 or collagenase I expression, could be (1) inhibited by singlet oxygen quenchers, (2) enhanced by means of strategies which allow extension of singlet oxygen half-life, and (3) mimicked by stimulation of nonirradiated cells with singlet oxygen-generating systems [5, 39]. Of central importance for the understanding of these mechanisms is the recent finding that both UVA radiation- and singlet oxygen-induced gene expression are mediated by activation of transcription factor AP2, and that UVA radiation-induced gene expression is controlled by the balance between AP2 and its alternative splice product AP2B [5]. Singlet oxygen, however, is not only an important mediator for UVA radiation-induced gene-regulatory events, but also plays a key role in UVA radiation-induced apoptosis in human Th cells [29].

In contrast to UVB or UVA radiation-induced immunomodulation, the photobiological basis for PUVA-induced immunosuppressive effects has not yet been characterized.

Concluding Remarks

In recent years, substantial progress has been made in identifying and understanding at least some of the mechanisms responsible for the beneficial effects associated with UV radiation and PUVA treatment. These studies provide compelling evidence that phototherapeutic and photochemotherapeutic modalities represent potent immunomodulatory tools. It should be noted, however, that the majority of photoimmunological studies have been performed in vitro, in healthy human skin, or even in animal models (which are not available for most of the UV-responsive skin diseases), and consequently there is a need for further studies focusing on "therapeutic photoimmunology." This is of particular relevance because a single exposure of human skin, e.g., to UVB radiation, has not only anti-inflammatory effects, but at the same time may also cause or enhance skin inflammation. A perfect example for the double-edged nature of UV radiation-induced immunomodulation is the regulation of ICAM-1 expression by UVB radiation [17, 31]. Exposure of cultured human keratinocytes to 100 J/m^2 UVB radiation immediately after irradiation completely prevents cytokine-induced ICAM-1 expression and, from a phototherapeutical point of view, constitutes a beneficial effect. The same UVB dose at later time points, however, upregulates constitutive keratinocyte ICAM-1 expression, and such a proinflammatory activity is thought to contribute to the development of skin lesions in patients with UVB-sensitive photodermatoses. In order to better understand the actual contribution of UV- or PUVA-induced immunomodulatory effects to the therapeutic efficacy of phototherapy and photochemotherapy, it will be necessary to analyze these effects during the therapeutic situation by employing in situ techniques which allow detection and monitoring of immunomodulatory consequences in lesional skin of patients and, most importantly, correlation of these effects with the clinical course of the respective skin disease. This approach will not only lead to a better understanding of the mode of action of phototherapy and photochemotherapy, but also provide valuable insight into the pathogenesis of UV-responsive skin diseases. Based on these studies, it will be possible to make treatment decisions on a rational rather than empirical fundament. It may also be expected that these studies foster the improvement of current phototherapeutic and photochemotherapeutic modalities and the development of new indications which extend beyond the treatment of skin diseases.

Summary

UV irradiation, either alone or in combination with photosensitizing agents, is widely used for the treatment of skin diseases. The efficacy of phototherapeutic and photochemotherapeutic modalities is thought to result, at least in part, from the induction of immunomodulatory effects. In particular, UV radiation was shown (a) to affect the production of soluble mediators, (b) to affect the expression of cell surface receptors, and (3) to induce apoptosis in pathogenetically relevant cells. UVB radiation-induced immunomodulatory effects are limited to the epidermis, whereas UVA radiation affects both epidermal and dermal cell populations. UVB and UVA radiation can exert essentially identical immunomodulatory effects, which, however, result from different photobiological mechanisms.

References

1. Bevilaqua PM, Edelson RL, Gasparro FP (1991) High performance liquid chromatography analysis of 8-methoxypsoralen monoadducts and crosslinks in lymphocytes and keratinocytes. J Invest Dermatol 97:151–155
2. Epstein JH (1968) UVL-induced stimulation of DNA synthesis in hairless mouse epidermis. J Invest Dermatol 52:445–448
3. Everett M, Yeargers E, Sayre R, Olson R (1966) Penetration of epidermis by ultraviolet rays. Photochem Photobiol 5:533–542
4. Godar DE (1996) Preprogrammed and programmed cell death mechanisms of apoptosis: UV-induced immediate and delayed apoptosis. Photochem Photobiol 63:825–830
5. Grether-Beck S, Olaizola-Horn S, Schmitt H, Grewe M, Jahnke A, Johnson JP, Briviba K, Sies H, Krutmann J (1996) Activation of transcription factor AP-2 mediates UVA radiation- and singlet oxygen-induced expression of the human intercellular adhesion molecule-1 gene. Proc Natl Acad Sci USA 93:14586–14591
6. Grewe M, Trefzer U, Ballhorn A, Gyufko K, Henninger HP, Krutmann J (1993) Analysis of the mechanism of ultraviolet B radiation induced prostaglandin E2 synthesis by human epidermoid carcinoma cells. J Invest Dermatol 101:528–531
7. Grewe M, Gyufko K, Schöpf E, Krutmann J (1994) Lesional expression of interferon-g in atopic eczema. Lancet 343:25–26
8. Grewe M, Gyufko K, Krutmann J (1995) Interleukin-10 production by cultured human keratinocytes: regulation by ultraviolet B and ultraviolet A1 radiation. J Invest Dermatol 104:3–6
9. Grewe M, Duvic M, Aragane Y, Schwarz T, Ullrich SE, Krutmann J (1996) Lack of induction of IL-10 expression in human keratinocytes. Reply. J Invest Dermatol 106:1330–1331
10. Grewe M, Klammer M, Stege H, Krutmann J (1996) Involvement of direct and indirect mechanisms in ultraviolet B radiation (UVBR)-induced inhibition of ICAM-1 expression in human antigen presenting cells. J Invest Dermatol 106:933 (abstr)
11. Grewe M, Gyufko K, Budnik A, Berneburg M, Ruzicka T, Krutmann J (1996) Interleukin-1 receptors type I and type II are differentially regulated in human keratinocytes by ultraviolet B radiation. J Invest Dermatol 107:865–870

12. Khan IU, Boehm KD, Elmets CA (1993) Modulation of IFNg-induced HLA-DR expression on the human keratinocyte cell line SCC-13 by ultraviolet radiation. Photochem Photobiol 57:103–106
13. Kripke ML (1981) Immunologic mechanisms in UV radiation carcinogenesis. Adv Cancer Res 34:69–106
14. Krueger JG, Wolfe JT, Nabeja RT, Vallat VP, Gilleaudeau P, Heftler NS, Austin LM, Gottlieb AB (1995) Successful ultraviolet B treatment of psoriasis is accompanied by a reversal of keratinocyte pathology and by selective depletion of intraepidermal T cells. J Exp Med 182:2057–2068
15. Krutmann J, Koeck A, Schauer E, Parlow F, Moeller A, Kapp A, Foerster E, Schoepf E, Luger TA (1990) Tumor necrosis factor b and ultraviolet radiation are potent regulators of human keratinocyte ICAM-1 expression. J Invest Dermatol 95:127–131
16. Krutmann J, Khan IU, Wallis RS, Zhang F, Koehler KA, Rich EA, Ellner JJ, Elmets CA (1990) The cell membrane is a major locus for ultraviolet-B-induced alterations in accessory cells. J Clin Invest 85:1529–1536
17. Krutmann J, Czech W, Parlow F, Trefzer U, Kapp A, Schoepf E, Luger TA (1992) Ultraviolet radiation effects on human keratinocyte ICAM-1 expression: UV-induced inhibition of cytokine induced ICAM-1 mRNA expression is transient, differentially restored for IFN-g versus TNFa, and followed by ICAM-1 induction via a TNFa-like pathway. J Invest Dermatol 98:923–928
18. Krutmann J, Czech W, Diepgen T, Niedner R, Kapp A, Schöpf E (1992) High-dose UVA1 therapy in the treatment of patients with atopic dermatitis. J Am Acad Dermatol 26:225–230
19. Krutmann J (1994) Regulatory interactions between epidermal cell adhesion molecules and cytokines. In: Luger TA, Schwarz T (eds) Epidermal growth factors and cytokines. Dekker, New York, pp 415–432
20. Krutmann J, Elmets CA (eds) (1995) Photoimmunology. Blackwell Science, Oxford
21. Krutmann J, Grewe M (1995) Involvement of cytokines, DNA damage, and reactive oxygen species in ultraviolet radiation-induced modulation of intercellular adhesion molecule-1 expression. J Invest Dermatol 105:67S–70S
22. Laskin JD, Lee E, Yurkow EJ, Laskin DL, Gallo MA (1985) A possible mechanism of psoralen phototoxicity not involving direct interaction with DNA. Proc Natl Acad Sci USA 82:6158–6162
23. Lisby S, Ralfkier E, Rothlein R, Veijsgard GL (1989) Intercellular adhesion molecule-1 (ICAM-1) expression correlated to inflammation. Br J Dermatol 120:479–484
24. Luger TA, Schwarz T (1995) Effects of UV light on cytokines and neuroendocrine hormones. In: Krutmann J, Elmets CA (eds) Photoimmunology. Blackwell Science, Oxford, pp 55–76
25. Marks DI, Fox RM (1991) Mechanism of photochemotherapy induced apoptotic cell death in lymphoid cells. Biochem Cell Biol 69:754–760
26. Morison WL (1993) Photochemotherapy. In: Lim HW, Soter NA (eds) Clinical photomedicine. Dekker, New York, pp 327–346
27. Morita A, Grewe M, Werfel T, Kapp A, Krutmann J (1996) Ultraviolet A1 radiation differentially affects cytokine production by atopen-specific human T-helper cells. Abstract. J Invest Dermatol 106:932
28. Morita A, Grewe M, Ahrens C, Grether-Beck S, Ruzicka T, Krutmann J (1997) Ultraviolet A1 radiation effects on cytokine expression in human epidermoid carcinoma cells. Photochem Photobiol (in press)
29. Morita A, Werfel T, Kapp A, Ahrens C, Stege H, Grewe M, Ruzicka T, Grether-Beck S, Briviba K, Sies H, Krutmann J (1997) High-dose ultraviolet (UV) A1 therapy works through induction of apoptosis in skin-infiltraing T-helper cells. Arch Dermatol Res (abstr) 289:A12
30. Nishigori C, Yarosh DB, Ullrich SE, Vink AA, Bucana CD, Roza L, Krike ML (1996) Evidence that DNA damage triggers interleukin 10 cytokine production in UV-irradiated murine keratinocytes. Proc Natl Acad Sci USA 93:10354–10359
31. Norris DA, Lyons B, Middleton MH, Yohn JY, Kashihara-Sawami M (1990) Ultraviolet radiation can either suppress or induce expression of intercellular adhesion molecule-1 (ICAM-1) on the surface of cultured human keratinocytes. J Invest Dermatol 95:132–138
32. Picot E, Meunier L, Picot-Deheze ML, Peyron JL, Meynadier J (1992) Treatment of psoriasis with a 311nm UVB lamp. Br J Dermatol 127:509–512

33. Roza L, Stege H, Krutmann J (1996) Role of UV-induced DNA damage in phototherapy. In: Hönigsmann H, Jori G, Young AR (eds) The fundamental bases of phototherapy. OEMF spa, Milano, pp 145–152
34. Simon JC, Krutmann J, Elmets CA, Bergstresser PR, Cruz D (1992) Ultraviolet B irradiated antigen presenting cells display altered accessory signaling for T cell activation: relevance to immune responses initiated in the skin. J Invest Dermatol 98:66S–69S
35. Stege H, Berneburg M, Humke S, Klammer M, Grewe M, Grether-Beck S, Dierks K, Goerz G, Ruzicka T, Krutmann J (1997) High-dose ultraviolet A1 (UVA1) radiation therapy for localized scleroderma. J Am Acad Dermatol (in press)
36. Trefzer U, Brockhaus M, Lötscher H, Parlow F, Budnik A, Grewe M, Christoph H, Kapp A, Schöpf E, Luger TA, Krutmann J (1993) The human 55-kd tumor necrosis factor receptor is regulated in human keratinocytes by TNFa and by ultraviolet B radiation. J Clin Invest 92:462–470
37. Volc-Platzer B, Hönigsmann H (1995) Photoimmunology of PUVA and UVB therapy. In: Krutmann J, Elmets CA (eds) Photoimmunology. Blackwell Science, Oxford, pp 265–273
38. Wlascheck M, Heinen G, Poswig A, Schwarz A, Krieg T, Scharfetter-Kochanek K (1994) UVA-induced autocrine stimulation of fibroblasts derived collagenase/MMP-1 by interrelated loops of interkeukin-1 and interleukin-6. Photochem Photobiol 59:550–556
39. Wlaschek M, Briviba K, Stricklin GP, Sies H, Scharfetter-Kochanek K (1995) Singlet oxygen may mediate the ultraviolet A-induced synthesis of interstitial collagenase. J Invest Dermatol 104:194–198
40. Yoo EK, Rook AH, Elenitas R, Gasparro FP, Vowels BR (1996) Apoptosis induction by ultraviolet light A and photochemotherapy in cutaneous T-cell lymphoma: relevance to mechanism of therapeutic action. J Invest Dermatol 107:235–242

Cytokines with Immunosuppressive Capacities

T. A. Luger and M. Böhm

Introduction

The current concept of the regulation of inflammatory and immune responses implies positive and negative signals which are mediated by a complex network of interacting cytokines. In contrast to the large body of data describing upregulating effects of many cytokines on these processes, only few suppressor factors with anti-immmune and anti-inflammatory properties have been identified [86, 93]. In the search for suppressor factors, many investigations have concentrated on the identification of inhibitory cytokines produced by tumors, since release of such factors could represent a potential escape mechanism from immunosurveillance. Accordingly, several tumors including melanoma, basal cell carcinomas, and squamous cell carcinomas were found to release distinct suppressor factors [76, 107, 121].

There is evidence that suppressor cytokines are not only released by tumor cells, but also by a variety of normal cells, e.g., epidermal cells upon exposure to ultraviolet (UV) light, which is a major environmental carcinogen. Accordingly, keratinocytes were found to synthesize and release suppressor factors such as interleukin (IL)-10 after UVB treatment, and increased levels of these mediators have been detected in the circulation of UV-irradiated individuals [83, 93]. These data suggest that locoregional expression and release of suppressor factors are important sequelae in the induction of immunosuppression during tumor development and upon exposure of cells to cancerogens. The following review will concentrate on the characterization of the most important known suppressor cytokines and will discuss their potential role in various diseases in which immunosuppression is pathogenetically involved.

Interleukin-1 Receptor Antagonist

IL-1 receptor antagonist (IL-1ra) belongs to the IL-1 family, which also includes the other IL-1 proteins IL-1α and IL-1β. When present in ten to 100 times excess over IL-1, IL-1ra competes with both IL-1 isoforms for binding to their common receptors. Because it does not cause detectable cell activation, IL-1ra can be regarded as a competitive inhibitor of IL-1 [3, 59, 65]. IL-1ra is a 17-kDa protein and has been shown to be secreted by human monocytes and many other cell types, including keratinocytes [39, 67]. Like both IL-1 forms, it maps to chromosome 2, but has only 19% amino acid sequence homology to IL-1α and 26 % homology to IL-1β respectively [23, 89]. Whereas monocytes mainly produce a secretory form of IL-1ra (sIL-1ra), a nonglycosylated intracellular form (icIL-1ra) with seven additional amino acids at its N terminus appears to be the major IL-1ra form in epithelial cells and vascular smooth muscle cells [5, 67].

Production of sIL-1ra by monocytes is increased as they mature into macrophages as well as upon treatment with granulocyte-macrophage colony-stimulating factor (GM-CSF), IL-4, or IL-13 [4, 71, 144]. Cytokines such as GM-CSF, tumor necrosis factor (TNF)-α, and IL-1 were also found to enhance the production of IL-1ra in polymorphonuclear granulocytes and fibroblasts [4, 89]. In addition, interferon (IFN)-γ upregulates the production of IL-1ra in human macrophages, but downregulates its production in lipopolysaccharide (LPS)-treated human monocytes [34, 135]. Moreover, increased plasma levels of IL-1ra were detected in patients receiving IFN-α or IFN-γ [142]. Thus, induction of IL-1ra may contribute to both the antiviral and the anti-inflammatory effects of interferons. On the other hand, expression of IL-1ra in monocytes was demonstrated to be upregulated by human cytomegalovirus and human immunodeficiency virus (HIV), suggesting that increased production of IL-1ra may contribute to immunosuppression in virus-mediated diseases [78, 149]. There is also evidence that the balance between IL-1 and IL-1ra expression in monocytes may be important in HIV-infected patients, since HIV expression in monocytes is antagonistically regulated by IL-1 and IL-1ra [56]. Interestingly, cisplatinum, which is used successfully in the treatment of a variety of cancers, was found to significantly decrease the synthesis and release of IL-1ra by monocytes, whereas IL-1β production was not affected. Thus, cisplatinum seems to downregulate anti-inflammatory signals in monocytes of cancer patients, which may contribute to its beneficial antitumor effects [2].

In epidermal cells, phorbol esters (PMA) and proinflammatory cytokines such as IL-1α, TNF-α, and IFN-γ have been found to induce production of IL-1ra [33, 62, 87, 117]. In keratinocytes, the expression of icIL-1ra is furthermore upregulated in culture medium containing high concentration of Ca^{2+}, which also promotes their differentiation [13]. In normal human skin, IL-1ra has been immunolocalized mainly in the stratum granulosum, as demonstrated by immunofluorescence studies, and its content in the stratum corneum was enhanced in chronically sun-exposed skin as well as upon UVB irradiation [64, 69]. However, treatment with UVB was found to inhibit the expression of IL-1ra in a human epidermoid carcinoma cell line [90]. Based on these results, investigations were undertaken to examine the expression of IL-1ra in various skin disorders. Decreased levels of IL-1ra were detected in lesional skin of patients with psoriasis. Moreover, polymorphism in the regulatory region of IL-1ra has been postulated to be associated with different types of psoriasis and with the disease severity in systemic lupus erythematosus (LE), lichen sclerosus, or alopecia areata [14, 29, 32, 141]. Elevated serum levels of IL-1ra have been reported in patients with polymyositis or dermatomyositis, which could account for the weak acute phase response in these patients [52].

In view of the well-established proinflammatory and immunomodulating activities of IL-1 and the apparent deregulation of its expression and release during the pathogenesis of many diseases, the therapeutic use of IL-1 antagonists is currently believed to be a promising novel approach [31, 38]. In animal models, the administration of IL-1ra resulted in reduced morbidity or even lethality of several inflammatory diseases, such as immune complex-induced colitis, endotoxin- or TNF-induced shock, bleomycin-induced pulmonary fibrosis, graft-versus-host disease, experimental acute pancreatitis, or experimental allergic encephalomyelitis [30, 46, 98, 109, 110, 114]. Moreover, IL-1ra was found to interfere with tumor progression, as systemic administration of IL-1ra resulted in a significant inhibition of melanoma growth in mice [27, 101]. In contact hypersensitivity (CHS), in which IL-1 functions as a costimulatory signal, IL-1ra was able to significantly inhibit both the sensitization and the elicitation phase [82].

There is evidence from several studies that IL-1 plays an important role in the pathogenesis of rheumatoid arthritis [38]. This notion is supported by the finding that, upon systemic application, IL-1ra is able to suppress experimental arthritis in animals [73]. Moreover, a recent study demonstrated that locoregional overexpression of IL-1ra in synovial cells by gene transfer significantly inhibited the recurrence of arthritis in rats [96]. Preliminary data of a clinical trial using recombinant human IL-1ra (rhuIL-1ra) in patients with rheumatoid arthritis showed that this treatment seems to be effective and safe [21]. Elevated serum levels of anti-inflammatory mediators such as IL-1ra were also found in trauma patients and correlated with the severity of injury and the clinical outcome [45]. Preliminary data of a randomized, placebo-controlled, multicenter trial evaluating the efficacy of IL-1ra treatment in patients with sepsis indicate that human recombinant IL-1ra is safe and may provide a dose-related survival advantage to these patients [49]. However, further clinical trials are required to confirm these findings.

Interleukin-10

Interleukin 10 (IL-10) was originally named cytokine synthesis inhibitor and characterized as a T-helper (Th) lymphocyte type 2-derived cytokine that inhibited the release of cytokines by Th1 cells. Subsequently, a variety of other cells, including B cells and keratinocytes, were identified as producers of IL-10 [40, 103]. In contrast to human IL-10 (hIL-10), murine IL-10 (mIL-10) is species specific and affects only murine cells [103]. Viral homologues of IL-10 are encoded by the Epstein-Barr virus (EBV) and equine herpesvirus type 2. Viral IL-10 (vIL-10), which is encoded by the EBV homologue BCRF-I, shares some, but not all biological activities of IL-10 on mouse and human cells. Both IL-10 and BCRF-1 block synthesis of IFN-γ. Since IFN-γ inhibits the generation and outgrowth of EBV-transformed B cells, IL-10 and its viral homologue may manipulate the immune response raised against virally infected cells, resulting in enhanced survival of the virus [102, 103, 123]. The receptors for IL-10 (IL-10R) were recently cloned. The hIL-10R binds only hIL-10, whereas the mIL-10R binds both human and murine IL-10. Since both hIL-10R and mIL-10R are structurally related to the IFN receptors (IFNR), they belong to the class II subgroup of cytokine receptors [70, 91].

There is clear evidence from several studies that IL-10 is synthesized and released by keratinocytes upon appropriate stimulation. Production of IL-10 in the skin is upregulated upon application of contact allergens, while tolerogens or irritants have no effect [41]. Moreover, UVB-light induces IL-10 production in human as well as murine keratinocytes, and keratinocyte-derived IL-10 appears to be involved in UVB-mediated systemic immunosuppression [44, 120]. On the other hand, both IL-10 and IL-6 are are upregulated upon UV irradiation and both have been shown to induce the production of autoantibodies and thereby may be involved in the UV-mediated exacerbation of autoimmune diseases such as LE [48, 92]. The role of IL-10 in the pathogenesis of LE is further supported by a recent study on patients with LE which demonstrated a correlation between disease activity and the number of IL-10-secreting cells in peripheral blood mononuclear cells (PBMC) [63]. Further evidence for a crucial role of IL-10 in the pathogenesis of autoimmune disorders comes from the observation that IL-10 is sufficient for the development of autoimmune diabetes when an appropriate major histocompatibility complex (MHC) is provided, as demonstrated in a transgenic mouse model [88].

IL-10 inhibits effector functions of Th1 cells and may therefore play a role in determining the class of immune response directed against the particular antigen [103]. This is further supported by recent findings which indicate that IL-10 suppresses the effector phase of CHS and downregulates delayed-type hypersensitivity (DTH) reactions as well as granuloma formation in schistosomiasis [50, 127]. Subcutaneous injection of IL-10 prior to hapten application was found to induce antigen-specific tolerance via inhibition of proinflammatory cytokines such as IL-1, IL-2, TNF-α, IFN-γ and GM-CSF [43]. IL-10 also interferes with the presentation of alloantigens and tumor-associated antigens by Langerhans cells to Th1 cells, resulting in an abrogation of the induction and elicitation of protective tumor immunity as well as induction of hapten-specific tolerance [6, 42, 79]. These findings are in accordance with observations in IL-10-deficient mice demonstrating an enhanced CHS response to contact allergens [7]. Moreover, in dendritic cells, the production of IL-12, which was also found to reverse the UV-mediated inhibition of CHS, was inhibited by IL-10 [80, 128]. It is possible that downregulation of costimulatory molecules such as B7 (CD80/86) are in part responsible for this antigen-presenting defect mediated by IL-10 [19, 25]. This is supported by a recent study showing that IL-10 seems to contribute to the immunologic unresponsiveness in patients with chronic schistosomiasis via the downregulation of B7 expression [77]. In human skin, overexpression of IL-10 was reported in lesions of atopic eczema and was immunohistochemically localized in large mononuclear cells in the dermal infiltrate [111]. Furthermore, IL-10 expression was upregulated in tape-stripped skin, poison ivy dermatitis, and Sézary syndrome, but not in psoriatic skin lesions [108].

In an animal model, IL-10 was shown to prevent lethality to endotoxin by reducing TNF-α secretion [53]. In severe combined immunodeficient (SCID) mice implanted with human fetal thymus and liver, plasma viremia and infection after inoculation with HIV was inhibited upon treatment with IL-10 [81]. Recently, IL-10 was demonstrated to be chemotactic for $CD8^+$ T cells, but to inhibit IL-8-induced $CD4^+$ T lymphocyte migration and to induce long-term antigen-specific anergy of $CD4^+$ T cells [61, 72]. Moreover, IL-10 costimulates thymocytes and mast cells and inhibits the antigen-presenting function of macrophages and B lymphocytes by downregulating MHC class II antigen expression [103]. In addition to being a growth and differentiation factor for human B lymphocytes, IL-10 was also identified as a switch factor for IgG1 and IgG3 synthesis and seems to enhance anti-CD40- and IL-4-induced IgG and IgE production [18, 143]. Since IL-10 upregulates the expression of adhesion molecules such as intercellular adhesion molecule (ICAM)-1 and endothelial leukocyte adhesion molecule (ELAM)-1 on human dermal microvascular endothelial cells, it appears to be one of the mediators responsible for leukocyte accumulation in cutaneous inflammatory reactions [112, 145]. In IL-10-deficient gene-targeted mice, a severe chronic enterocolitis was reported which appears to be predominantly mediated by Th1 $CD4^+$ T cells and antibody responses [35, 84].

The role of IL-10 in tumor pathology is still a matter of controversy. The cytotoxicity of alveolar macrophages and monocytes against the human melanoma cell line A 375 was significantly suppressed by IL-10 [107]. Moreover, in several murine tumor models, IL-10 secretion inhibited cell-mediated antitumoral immune responses [17, 74]. In contrast, systemic application of IL-10 into mice bearing established sarcomas, melanomas, or colorectal carcinomas resulted in tumor rejection and the cured mice were subsequently immune to rechallenge with the same tumor cells. However, in melanoma transfectants bearing vIL-10, an enhanced outgrowth was observed, whereas transfection with mIL-10 resulted in rejection of tumors, suggesting distinct pathways for vIL-10 and mIL-10 [8]. Other studies demonstrated that transfection of IL-10 into murine mammary adenocarcinoma cells or Chinese hamster ovary cells lead to complete tumor rejection upon injection [54, 119]. The rejection correlated with the amount of IL-10 produced by the tumor cells and was mediated by a combined action of $CD8^+$ cells, natural killer (NK) cells, and neutrophils. In addition, it has been reported that IL-10 is differentially expressed in basal versus squamous cell carcinomas, suggesting that overexpression by the latter may represent a potential mechanism of evasion from local T lymphocyte-mediated immune responses [75].

Because of its inhibitory effects on T cell proliferation and cytokine synthesis by stimulated monocytes, IL-10 was recently used to treat mice with collagen-induced arthritis. In this animal model, IL-10 was found to suppress established arthritis, probably by inhibiting the production of proinflammatory cytokines [147]. The immunosuppressive effects of IL-10 were further examined in a murine heterotopic cardiac allograft model. Retroviral-mediated transfer of vIL-10 significantly prolonged allograft survival without the need for conventional systemic immunosuppression [116]. In a human phase I clinical trial, a single bolus injection of IL-10 resulted in a transient neutrophilia and monocytosis. Leukocyte blood count blood fell by 25%, and T cell proliferation was reduced by 50% after stimulation [26]. Additionally, a marked decrease in TNF-α and IL-1β expression of whole blood cells stimulated ex vivo was observed. These findings demonstrate that in vivo administration of IL-10 in humans has potent immunoregulatory functions which are associated with suppressive effects on T cells and downregulation of proinflammatory cytokines.

Transforming Growth Factor-β

The transforming growth factor (TGF)-β family consists of at least five homodimeric polypeptides known as β1–β5 which can influence a variety of biological processes, including cell growth, differentiation, and morphogenesis. TGF-β1 is found in almost any tissue, whereas the expression of the other isoforms is more restricted [121]. The major source of TGF-β1 are activated platelets, but upon appropriate stimulation TGF-β1 is secreted by many different cells, including keratinocytes [100, 121]. Depending on the cell type or culture conditions, the production of TGF-β can be influenced by a number of stimuli, including other growth factors, cytokines, hormones, retinoids, and vitamin D3 [121]. The human TGF-β isoforms are encoded as precursors and are proteolytically processed to yield the final 12.5-kDa residue, which forms disulfate-linked homodimers. All forms of TGF-β are released as biologically inactive precursors due to their association with a glycosylated latency-associated protein (LAP) and a specific binding protein (latent TGF-binding protein) [121, 146]. Activation of the latent complex is a multistep process which is not completely understood and requires direct cell to cell contact, the presence of proteases, and acidic conditions. Activated TGF-β may either bind to its respective receptor or, after reassociation with LAP, adhere to extracellular matrix proteins or other proteins such as α_2-macroglobulin to become a biologically inactive, stored form [121]. The receptors for TGF-β belong to a family of glycoprotein receptors, some of which are present on virtually all cells. Members of this receptor family are TGF-β type-1 to -3 receptors, endoglin (which is expressed at high levels on human vascular endothelial cells), activin A receptor, TSR-1, and AcRI [99].

The multiple biological activities of TGF-β are not species specific. TGF-β is a potent growth inhibitor for many different cell types, including epithelial cells, endothelial cells, fibroblasts, hematopoietic cells, and tumor cells [121]. There is also evidence that TGF-β1 can suppress tumor formation in vivo, but no apparent correlation between the intratumoral expression of TGF-β and the stage of the disease has been found. In light of recent findings, the loss of the growth-inhibitory response to TGF-β due to aberrant receptor expression or alterations in the signal transduction pathways of TGF-β appear to be more important [130].

Regarding its effect on inflammatory responses, TGF-β has been reported to have bidirectional effects. This apparent paradox may be explained by the activation or differentiation state of cells, which determines whether TGF-β exerts pro- or anti-inflammatory effects [146]. During inflammatory reactions, TGF-β turned out to be an important early signal. It causes adhesion and chemotaxis of leukocytes and at higher concentrations stimulates T cells and monocytes to release inflammatory mediators. In addition, TGF-β regulates B cell antibody production, and depending on the presence or absence of other cytokines, different TGF-β isoforms have also been reported to either promote or inhibit T cell proliferation and differentiation [122, 125]. Furthermore, TGF-β is a chemoattractant for macrophages and induces the production of IL-1 and several growth factors. In combination with GM-CSF, TNF- α, and stem cell factor (SCF), TGF-β was found to promote the development of dendritic cells in vitro from hemopoietic progenitor cells [121, 140].

On the other hand, TGF-β turned out to be a potent suppressor of inflammatory reactions. It inhibits the function of differentiated macrophages and blocks the proliferation of $CD4^+$ lymphocytes via inhibition of IL-2. TGF-β suppresses IgM and IgG synthesis, but upregulates IgA production. It may also play a role in the downregulation of allergic inflammation through its capacity to inhibit IgE synthesis and mast cell proliferation [16, 37]. TGF-β also inhibits IL-1R expression, induces synthesis of IL-1ra, and modulates acute-phase protein production [136]. In addition, it has been demonstrated to inhibit various types of T cell-mediated immune responses and was also shown to inhibit antigen presentation of cultured, but not fresh Langerhans cells under some experimental conditions [57, 122]. The immunosuppressing potential of TGF-β1 in vivo was supported by a study revealing that gene transfer therapy with plasmid DNA encoding TGF-β1 prolonged survival of cardiac allografts in mice via altering cytotoxic T cell generation [115].

TGF-β is known to be critically involved in tissue repair, fibrosis, and neovascularization. Accordingly, TGF-β recruits fibroblasts and promotes accumulation of extracellular matrix by stimulating transcription and translation of collagen, fibronectin, and glucosaminoglycans, whereas the degradation of these matrix proteins is inhibited [146]. The crucial role of TGF-β in the pathogenesis of fibrotic diseases is underscored by the finding that many fibrotic diseases exhibit a deregulated expression of TGF-β in situ. Accordingly, increased concentrations of TGF-β have been detected within fibrotic skin lesions and in other fibrotic inflammatory conditions [85, 113]. In allergic inflammation, expression of TGF-β was also found to be related with fibrosis observed in patients with asthma as well as the subendocardial fibrosis associated with the hypereosinophilic syndrome [136, 146]. Moreover, TGF-β has been identified within scleroderma lesions, mostly around blood vessels [85]. These findings have prompted a novel therapeutic approach utilizing strategies to neutralize TGF-β-mediated effects by TNF-β antibodies, IFN-α, IFN-γ, or antisense oligonucleotides. Preliminary animal studies as well as clinical trials in patients with scleroderma, keloids, and hypertrophic scar formation seem to prove the efficacy of this approach [60, 68, 124, 131]. Interestingly, exogenous application of the TGF-β3 peptide was recently demonstrated to reduce scar formation in an animal model. Thus, in contrast to TGF-β1 and -β2, which are implicated in dermal scar formation, TGF-β3 seems to function as an antiscaring agent [132]. This is further supported by a recent study showing that TGF-β1, -β2, and -β3 are differentially regulated during wound healing and that corticosteroids suppressed expression of TGF-β1 and -β2, whereas TGF-β3 was stimulated [51]. The biological importance of TGF-β for the development of normal skin is further supported by murine studies in which the TGF-β1 gene was disrupted. Transgenic animals which do not produce detectable amounts of TGF-β1 are not able to survive because they develop diffuse inflammation of many organs resembling autoimmune disorders [133]. In transgenic mice overexpressing TGF-β1 in the epidermis, the skin of these mice appeared shiny and tautly stretched. The animals were rigid, did not move normally, and died within 24 h after birth [129].

α-Melanocyte-Stimulating Hormone

There is strong evidence from many investigations that neuropeptides are not only produced by neural tissue but also by a wide variety of other cells including inflammatory and epithelial cells. In addition, these peptides though originally characterized as hormones, have recently been recognized as potent regulators of immune and inflammatory reactions. Specific receptors for many neuropeptides have been found to be expressed on immunocompetent cells [15, 24, 118]. Accordingly, proopiomelanocortin (POMC), the precursor for α-, β-, and γ-melanocyte-stimulating hormone (MSH), adrenocorticotropin (ACTH), corticotropin-like intermediate protein (CLIP), β-lipotropin, and β-endorphin, is not exclusively produced in the pituitary gland, but by a number of different cell types [9]. POMC is synthesized as a large prohormone and is post-translationally cleaved by a unique set of proteases called prohormone convertase 1 (PC1) and (PC2) into the active peptide hormones as listed above [20, 97]. Among immunocompetent cells, POMC peptides have been detected in lymphocytes, macrophages, and splenocytes [9, 15]. In addition, POMC gene products such as ACTH, αMSH, and β-endorphin have been identified in several different epidermal cells, including keratinocytes, melanocytes, Langerhans cells, and Thy-1^+ dendritic epidermal cells [47, 95, 104, 126, 148]. Under normal conditions, keratinocytes produce only low levels of POMC peptides, but stimulation with the proinflammatory cytokine IL-1, ultraviolet light, or tumor promotors upregulates mRNA expression of POMC and αMSH release [126, 148].

POMC peptides exert their pleiotropic activities via binding to one of the melanocortin (MC) receptors, which are differentially expressed by several cell types. Five different members of a unique receptor family have been identified which differ in their binding specificity and avidity [9, 105]. So far, the MC1 receptor which binds αMSH and ACTH has been detected on melanocytes, but there is evidence that this receptor is also expressed on both human and murine monocytes [10, 137]. Furthermore, MC1 receptors were detected on human keratinocytes and dermal microvascular endothelial cells [11, 66]. Other receptors (MC2–MC5) are less specific and also bind several other POMC peptides [9]. Thus, complex interactions exist between the different POMC peptides, and their multiple receptors are differentially expressed in various tissues.

POMC gene products have been demonstrated to affect immune and inflammatory reactions in a number of ways. Several studies demonstrate that αMSH antagonizes the effects of proinflammatory cytokines such as IL-1α, IL-1β, IL-6, and TNF-α [24]. Systemic application of αMSH has been found to decrease fever, leukocytosis, and IL-1-induced plasma levels of acute-phase proteins [22]. Recent evidence suggests that αMSH inhibits the binding of IL-1β to the type I IL-1R, indicating that αMSH may function as an IL-1 antagonist [106]. αMSH also downregulates the production of IFN-γ in human lymphocytes and selectively induces the production of IL-10 by monocytes [12, 94]. The C-terminal tripeptide of αMSH is sufficient to cause these immunoinhibiting and anti-inflammatory effects [12, 24]. Thus, a number of proinflammatory cytokines are downregulated by αMSH, whereas anti-inflammatory cytokines such as IL-10 are upregulated by αMSH, suggesting that this peptide may have important functions in the suppression of immune and inflammatory reactions. The immunoregulatory role of αMSH has recently been further supported by the finding that human and murine macrophages are able to produce αMSH and express MC1 receptors which are specific for αMSH [10, 137]. The possible in vivo importance of POMC peptides is supported by the detection of increased serum levels of several of these peptides during the course of chronic inflammatory responses such as adjuvant induced arthritis, acquired immunodeficiency syndrome (AIDS), or atopic eczema. Therefore, POMC peptides also appear to be involved in the downregulation of the inflammatory tissue response [28, 55, 134].

In addition, a regulatory role of POMC peptides in antibody synthesis by B lymphocytes has been reported. Depending on the presence of B-stimulatory cytokines, POMC peptides may either up- or downregulate antibody synthesis. Accordingly, αMSH and ACTH modulate IL-4- and anti-CD40-mediated release of IgE by human PBMC. Most interestingly, the IgE-inducing capacity of POMC peptides seems to be dependent on the presence of monocytes [1]. ACTH and αMSH at physiological concentrations increase IgE synthesis, whereas higher doses of these peptides strongly inhibit IgE synthesis. These findings indicate that POMC peptides may play a role in the pathogenesis of allergic diseases.

There is strong evidence that αMSH functions as an important mediator in cutaneous immune and inflammatory responses such as CHS and irritant dermatitis. Accordingly, systemic administration of αMSH inhibits both the induction and elicitation of CHS responses in mice and induces hapten-specific tolerance. Moreover, these effects were specific for αMSH and were dose dependent with an optimum injection time of 2 h before hapten application. The inhibitory effect of αMSH on CHS may be attributed to its IL-10-inducing effects, since mice treated with αMSH plus anti-IL-10 displayed normal CHS responses compared to untreated controls [58]. In addition, there is evidence that αMSH inhibits the expression of accessory molecules such as B7-2 (CD86) on antigen-presenting cells [10]. These findings indicate that αMSH may be a significant regulatory mediator in cutaneous immune responses in vivo and may function as one of the signals responsible for anergy or tolerance induction.

Recently, the expression of melanocortin receptors was reported on human dermal microvascular endothelial cells and murine brain microvascular endothelial cells [36, 66]. Furthermore, α MSH significantly enhanced the production of the chemokine IL-8 by endothelial cells, whereas the release of proinflammatory cytokines such as IL-1 or IL-6 was not affected [66]. These data indicate that αMSH, which upon stimulation is produced by both inflammatory cells and epithelial cells, may mediate leukocyte–endothelial cell interactions during inflammation by inducing IL-8. Since chemokines such as IL-8 have been recognized as potent angiogenetic factors by their ability to cause endothelial cell chemotaxis in vitro and neovascularization in vivo, αMSH may also function as a regulator of angiogenesis during wound healing or tumorigenesis [138, 139].

Conclusion

Suppressor cytokines deliver crucial signals which are required for the downregulation of immune and inflammatory responses. Their presence is necessary to prevent chronic inflammation and autoimmunity, whereas deregulated expression and release may lead to systemic immunosuppression and even facilitate tumor development. Therefore, future therapeutic strategies can be developed to neutralize suppressor factors in order to reconstitute a functioning immune response in the immunocompromized tumor-bearing host. On the other hand, careful and controlled application of well-characterized suppressor factors may be useful for the treatment of autoimmune and chronic inflammatory diseases.

Summary

We have outlined the biological significance of cytokines with immunosuppressive capacities in this chapter. The biochemical identity, physiology and pathophysiology of IL-1ra, TGF-β, IL-10 and α-MSH were reviewed and the results of the use of these cytokines in animal models were described. Although our present scenario of agonizing and antagonizing cytokines remains incomplete, as novel cytokines are currently being discovered, the concept of suppressor cytokines has already stimulated the initiation of clinical trials in which the potential benefit of these factors in humans are exploited. It is very likely that in the future suppressor cystokines will make an important contribution to our therapeutic armanentarium, similar to other biological response modifiers such as interferons which have already have an established role in the treatment of many diseases.

Acknowledgement. The authors wish to thank Mrs. M.L. Hülsmann for her expert secretarial assistance. This work was supported by grants from the Deutsche Forschungsgemeinschaft (Lu 443/1-3, So 87/11).

References

1. Aebischer I, Stämpfli MR, Zürcher A, Miescher S, Urwyler A, Frey B, Luger TA, White RR, Stadler BM (1994) Neuropeptides are potent modulators of human in vitro immunoglobulin E synthesis. Eur J Immunol 24:1908–1913
2. Arenberg DA, Kunkel SL, Burdick MD, Standiford TJ, Strieter RM (1995) Regulation of monocyte-derived interleukin 1 receptor antagonist by cisplatinum. Cytokine 7:89–96
3. Arend WP, Welgus HG, Thompson RC, Eisenberg SP (1990) Biological properties of recombinant human monocyte-derived interleukin 1 receptor antagonist. J Clin Invest 85:1694–1697
4. Arend WP, Smith MF, Jr., Janson RW, Joslin FG (1991) IL-1 receptor antagonist and IL-1 beta production in human monocytes are regulated differently. J Immunol 147:1530–1536
5. Beasley D, McGuiggin ME, Dinarello CA (1995) Human vascular smooth muscle cells produce an intracellular form of interleukin-1 receptor antagonist. Am J Physiol 269:C961–C968
6. Beissert S, Hosoi J, Grabbe S, Asahina A, Granstein RD (1995) IL-10 inhibits tumor antigen presentation by epidermal antigen presenting cells. J Immunol 154:1280–1286
7. Berg DJ, Leach MW, Kuhn R, Rajewsky K, Muller W, Davidson NJ, Rennick D (1995) Interleukin 10 but not interleukin 4 is a natural suppressant of cutaneous inflammatory responses. J Exp Med 182:99–108
8. Berman RM, Suzuki T, Tahara H, Robbins PD, Narula SK, Lotze MT (1996) Systemic administration of cellular IL-10 induces an effective, specific, and long-lived immune response against established tumors in mice. J Immunol 157:231–238
9. Bhardwaj RS, Luger TA (1994) Proopiomelanocortin production by epidermal cells: evidence for an immune neuro-endocrine network in the epidermis. Arch Dermatol Res 287:85–90
10. Bhardwaj RS, Becher E, Mahnke K, Schwarz T, Luger TA (1995) Modulation of alpha-melanocyte stimulating hormone receptor expression on human monocytes. J Invest Dermatol 104:651
11. Bhardwaj RS, Becher E, Mahnke K, Hartmeyer M, Scholzen T, Schwarz T, Luger TA (1996a) Evidence of the expression of a functional melanocortin receptor 1 by human keratinocytes. J Invest Dermatol 106:817
12. Bhardwaj RS, Schwarz A, Becher E, Mahnke K, Riemann H, Aragane Y, Schwarz T, Luger TA (1996b) Pro-opiomelanocortin-derived peptides induce IL-10 production in human monocytes. J Immunol 156:2517–2521
13. Bigler CF, Norris DA, Weston WL, Arend WP (1992) Interleukin-1 receptor antagonist production by human keratinocytes. J Invest Dermatol 98:38–44
14. Blakemore AI, Tarlow JK, Cork MJ, Gordon C, Emery P, Duff GW (1994) Interleukin-1 receptor antagonist gene polymorphism as a disease severity factor in systemic lupus erythematosus. Arthritis Rheum 37:1380–1385
15. Blalock JE (1994) The syntax of immune-neuroendocrine communication. Immunol Today 15:504–511
16. Borish L, Rosenwasser LJ (1996) Update on cytokines. J Allergy Clin Immunol 97:719–733
17. Bost KL, Bieligk SC, Jaffe BM (1995) Lymphokine mRNA expression by transplantable murine B lymphocytic malignancies. Tumor-derived IL-10 as a possible mechanism for modulating the anti-tumor response. J Immunol 154:718–729
18. Briere F, Servet-Delprat C, Bridon JM, Saint-Remy JM, Banchereau J (1994) Human interleukin 10 induces naive surface immunoglobulin D+ (sIgD+) B cells to secrete IgG1 and IgG3. J Exp Med 179:757–762
19. Buelens C, Willems F, Delvaux A, Pierard G, Delville JP, Velu T, Goldman M (1995) Interleukin-10 differentially regulates B7-1 (CD80) and B7-2 (CD86) expression on human peripheral blood dendritic cells. Eur J Immunol 25:2668–2672
20. Burbach JPH, Wiegant VM (1990) Gene expression, biosynthesis and processing of proopiomelanocortin peptides and vasopressin. In: de Wied D (ed) Neuropeptides: basics and perspectives. Elsevier, Amsterdam, pp 45–103

21. Campion GV, Lebsack ME, Lookabaugh J, Gordon G, Catalano M, the IL-1ra arthritis study group (1996) Dose-range and dose-frequency study of recombinant interleukin-1 receptor antagonist in patients with rheumatoid arthritis. Arthritis Rheum 39:1092–1101
22. Cannon JG, Tatro JB, Reichlin S, Dinarello CA (1986) Alpha melanocyte stimulating hormone inhibits immunostimulatory and inflammatory actions of interleukin 1. J Immunol 137:2232–2236
23. Carter DB, Deibel MR, Jr., Dunn CJ, Tomich CS, Laborde AL, Slightom JL, Berger AE, Bienkowski MJ, Sun FF, McEwan RN et al (1990) Purification, cloning, expression and biological characterization of an interleukin-1 receptor antagonist protein. Nature 344:633–638
24. Catania A, Lipton JM (1993) Alpha-melanocyte stimulating hormone in the modulation of host reactions. Endocr Rev 14:564–576
25. Chang CH, Furue M, Tamaki K (1995) B7-1 expression of Langerhans cells is up-regulated by proinflammatory cytokines, and is down-regulated by interferon-gamma or by interleukin-10. Eur J Immunol 25:394–398
26. Chernoff AE, Granowitz EV, Shapiro L, Vannier E, Lonnemann G, Angel JB, Kennedy JS, Rabson AR, Wolff SM, Dinarello CA (1995) A randomized, controlled trial of IL-10 in humans. Inhibition of inflammatory cytokine production and immune responses. J Immunol 154:5492–5499
27. Chirivi RG, Garofalo A, Padura IM, Mantovani A, Giavazzi R (1993) Interleukin 1 receptor antagonist inhibits the augmentation of metastasis induced by interleukin 1 or lipopolysaccharide in a human melanoma/nude mouse system. Cancer Res 53:5051–5054
28. Chowdrey HS, Lightman SL, Harbuz MS, Larsen PJ, Jessop DS (1994) Contents of corticotropin-releasing hormone and arginine vasopressin immunoreactivity in the spleen and thymus during a chronic inflammatory stress. J Neuroimmunol 53:17–21
29. Clay FE, Cork MJ, Tarlow JK, Blakemore AI, Harrington CI, Lewis F, Duff GW (1994) Interleukin 1 receptor antagonist gene polymorphism association with lichen sclerosus. Hum Genet 94:407–410
30. Cominelli F, Nast CC, Clark BD, Schindler R, Lierena R, Eysselein VE, Thompson RC, Dinarello CA (1990) Interleukin 1 (IL-1) gene expression, synthesis, and effect of specific IL-1 receptor blockade in rabbit immune complex colitis. J Clin Invest 86:972–980
31. Cork MJ, Duff GW (1993) Interleukin one. In: Luger TA, Schwarz T (eds) Epidermal growth factors and cytokines. Dekker, New York, pp 19–48
32. Cork MJ, Tarlow JK, Blakemore AI, Mee JB, Crane AM, Stierle C, Bleehen SS, Duff GW (1993) Psoriasis and interleukin-1. A translation. J R Coll Phys Lond 27:366
33. Corradi A, Franzi AT, Rubartelli A (1995) Synthesis and secretion of interleukin-1 alpha and interleukin-1 receptor antagonist during differentiation of cultured keratinocytes. Exp Cell Res 217:355–362
34. Danis VA, Millington M, Hyland VJ, Grennan D (1995) Cytokine production by normal human monocytes: inter-subject variation and relationship to an IL-1 receptor antagonist (IL-1Ra) gene polymorphism. Clin Exp Immunol 99:303–310
35. Davidson NJ, Leach MW, Fort MM, Thompson-Snipes L, Kühn R, Müller W, Berg DJ, Rennick DM (1996) T helper cell 1-type CD4+ T cells, but not B cells, mediate colitis in interleukin-10 deficient mice. J Exp Med 184:241–251
36. de Angelis E, Sahm UG, Ahmed AR, Olivier GW, Notarianni LJ, Branch SK, Moss SH, Pouton CW (1995) Identification of a melanocortin receptor expressed by murine brain microvascular endothelial cells in culture. Microvasc Res 50:25–34
37. Defrance T, Vanbervliet B, Briere F, Durand I, Rousset F, Banchereau J (1992) Interleukin 10 and transforming growth factor beta cooperate to induce anti-CD40-activated naive human B cells to secrete immunoglobulin A. J Exp Med 175:671–682
38. Duff GW (1994) Cytokines and acute phase proteins in rheumatoid arthritis. Scand J Rheumatol [Suppl] 100:9–19
39. Eisenberg SP, Evans RJ, Arend WP, Verderber E, Brewer MT, Hannum CH, Thompson RC (1990) Primary structure and functional expression from complementary DNA of a human interleukin-1 receptor antagonist. Nature 343:341–346

40. Enk A, Katz SI (1992) Identification and induction of keratinocyte-derived IL-10. J Immunol 149:92–95
41. Enk AH, Katz SI (1992) Early molecular events in the induction phase of contact sensitivity. Proc Natl Acad Sci USA 89:1398–1402
42. Enk AH, Angeloni VL, Udey MC, Katz SI (1993) Inhibition of Langerhans cell antigen-presenting function by IL-10. A role for IL-10 in induction of tolerance. J Immunol 151:2390–2398
43. Enk AH, Saloga J, Becker D, Mohamadzadeh M, Knop J (1994) Induction of hapten-specific tolerance by interleukin 10 in vivo. J Exp Med 179:1397–1402
44. Enk CD, Sredni D, Blauvelt A, Katz SI (1995) Induction of IL-10 gene expression in human keratinocytes by UVB exposure in vivo and in vitro. J Immunol 154:4851–4856
45. Ertel W, Keel M, Bonaccio M, Steckholzer U, Gallati H, Kenney JS, Trentz O (1995) Release of anti-inflammatory mediators after mechanical trauma correlates with severity of injury and clinical outcome. J Trauma 39:879–885
46. Everaerdt B, Brouckaert P, Fiers W (1994) Recombinant IL-1 receptor antagonist protects against TNF-induced lethality in mice. J Immunol 152:5041–5049
47. Farooqui JZ, Medrano EE, Boissy RE, Tigelaar RE, Nordlund JJ (1995) Thy-1+ dendritic cells express a truncated form of POMC mRNA. Exp Dermatol 4:297–301
48. Finck BK, Chan B, Wofsby D (1994) Interleukin 6 promotes murine lupus in NZB/NZWF1 mice. J Clin Invest 94:585–591
49. Fisher CJ Jr, Slotman GJ, Opal SM, Pribble JP, Bone RC, Emmanuel G, Ng D, Bloedow DC, Catalano MA (1994) Initial evaluation of human recombinant interleukin-1 receptor antagonist in the treatment of sepsis syndrome: a randomized, open-label, placebo-controlled multicenter trial. The IL-1RA Sepsis Syndrome Study Group. Crit Care Med 22:12–21
50. Flores Villanueva PO, Zheng XX, Strom TB, Stadecker MJ (1996) Recombinant IL-10 and IL-10/Fc treatment down-regulate egg antigen-specific delayed hypersensitivity reactions and egg granuloma formation in schistosomiasis. J Immunol 156:3315–3320
51. Frank S, Madlener M, Werner S (1996) Transforming growth factors beta1, beta2, and beta3 and their receptors are differentially regulated during normal and impaired wound healing. J Biol Chem 271:10188–10193
52. Gabay C, Gay Croisier F, Roux Lombard P, Meyer O, Maineti C, Guerne PA, Vischer T, Dayer JM (1994) Elevated serum levels of interleukin-1 receptor antagonist in polymyositis/dermatomyositis. A biologic marker of disease activity with a possible role in the lack of acute-phase protein response. Arthritis Rheum 37:1744–1751
53. Gerard C, Bruyns C, Marchant A, Abramowicz D, Vandenabeele P, Delvaux A, Fiers W, Goldman M, Velu T (1993) Interleukin 10 reduces the release of tumor necrosis factor and prevents lethality in experimental endotoxemia. J Exp Med 177:547–550
54. Giovarelli M, Musiani P, Modesti A, Dellabona P, Casorati G, Allione A, Consalvo M, Cavallo F, di Pierro F, De Giovanni C et al (1995) Local release of IL-10 by transfected mouse mammary adenocarcinoma cells does not suppress but enhances antitumor reaction and elicits a strong cytotoxic lymphocyte and antibody-dependent immune memory. J Immunol 155:3112–3123
55. Glinski W, Brodecka H, Glinska-Ferenz M, Kowalski D (1995) Increased concentration of beta-endorphin in the sera of patients with severe atopic dermatitis. Acta Derm Venereol (Stockh) 75:9–11
56. Goletti D, Kinter AL, Hardy EC, Poli G, Fauci AS (1996) Modulation of endogenous IL-1 beta and IL-1 receptor antagonist results in opposing effects on HIV expression in chronically infected monocytic cells. J Immunol 156:3501–3508
57. Grabbe S, Bruvers S, Lindgren AM, Hosoi J, Tan KC, Granstein RD (1992) Tumor antigen presentation by epidermal antigen-presenting cells in the mouse: modulation by granulocyte-macrophage colony-stimulating factor, tumor necrosis factor alpha, and ultraviolet radiation. J Leukoc Biol 52:209–217
58. Grabbe S, Bhardwaj RS, Steinert M, Mahnke K, Simon MM, Schwarz T, Luger TA (1996) Alpha-melanocyte stimulating hormone induces hapten-specific tolerance in mice. J Immunol 156:473–478

59. Granowitz EV, Clark BD, Mancilla J, Dinarello CA (1991) Interleukin-1 receptor antagonist competitively inhibits the binding of interleukin-1 to the type II interleukin-1 receptor. J Biol Chem 266:14147–14150
60. Granstein RD, Flotte TJ, Amento EP (1990) Interferons and collagen production. J Invest Dermatol 95:75S–80S
61. Groux H, Bigler M, de Vries J, Roncarolo M (1996) Interleukin-10 induces a long-term antigen-specific anergic state in human CD4+ T cells. J Exp Med 184:19–29
62. Gueniche A, Viac J, Charveron M, Schmitt D (1994) Effect of gamma-interferon on IL-1 alpha, beta and receptor antagonist production by normal human keratinocytes. Exp Dermatol 3:113–118
63. Hagiwara E, Gourley MF, Lee S, Klinman DM (1996) Disease severity in patients with systemic lupus erythematosus correlates with an increased ratio of interleukin-10: interferon gamma secreting cells in the peripheral blood. Arthritis Rheum 39:379–385
64. Hammerberg C, Arend WP, Fisher GJ, Chan LS, Berger AE, Haskill JS, Voorhees JJ, Cooper KD (1992) Interleukin-1 receptor antagonist in normal and psoriatic epidermis. J Clin Invest 90:571–583
65. Hannum CH, Wilcox CJ, Arend WP, Joslin FG, Dripps DJ, Heimdal PL, Armes LG, Sommer A, Eisenberg SP, Thompson RC (1990) Interleukin-1 receptor antagonist activity of a human interleukin-1 inhibitor. Nature 343:336–340
66. Hartmeyer M, Scholzen T, Becher E, Bhardwaj RS, Fastrich M, Schwarz T, Luger TA (1996) Human microvascular endothelial cells (HMEC-1) express the melanocortin receptor type 1 and produce increased levels of IL-8 upon stimulation with αMSH. J Invest Dermatol 106:809
67. Haskill S, Martin G, Van Le L, Morris J, Peace A, Bigler CF, Jaffe GJ, Hammerberg C, Sporn SA, Fong S et al (1991) cDNA cloning of an intracellular form of the human interleukin 1 receptor antagonist associated with epithelium. Proc Natl Acad Sci USA 88:3681–3685
68. Hein R, Behr J, Hündgen M, Hunzelmann N, Meurer M, Braun-Falco O, Urbanski A, Krieg T (1992) Treatment of systemic sclerosis with gamma-interferon. Br J Dermatol 126:496
69. Hirao T, Aoki H, Yoshida T, Sato Y, Kamoda H (1996) Elevation of interleukin 1 receptor antagonist in the stratum corneum of sun-exposed and ultraviolet B-irradiated human skin. J Invest Dermatol 106:1102–1107
70. Ho ASY, Liu Y, Khan TA, Hsu DH, Bazan JF, Moore KW (1993) A receptor for interleukin-10 is related interferon receptors. Proc Natl Acad Sci USA 90:11267–11271
71. Janson RW, Hance KR, Arend WP (1991) Production of IL-1 receptor antagonist by human in vitro-derived macrophages. Effects of lipopolysaccharide and granulocyte-macrophage colony-stimulating factor. J Immunol 147:4218–4223
72. Jinquan T, Larsen CG, Gesser B, Matsushima K, Thestrup Pedersen K (1993) Human IL-10 is a chemoattractant for CD8+ T lymphocytes and an inhibitor of IL-8-induced CD4+ T lymphocyte migration. J Immunol 151:4545–4551
73. Joosten LAB, Helsen MMA, van de Loo FAJ, van den Berg WB (1996) Anticytokine treatment of established type II collagen induced arthritis in DBA/1 mice. Arthritis Rheum 39:797–809
74. Kambayashi T, Alexander HR, Fong M, Strassmann G (1995) Potential involvement of IL-10 in suppressing tumor-associated macrophages. Colon-26-derived prostaglandin E2 inhibits TNF-alpha release via a mechanism involving IL-10. J Immunol 154:3383–3390
75. Kim J, Modlin RL, Moy RL, Dubinett SM, McHugh T, Nickoloff BJ, Uyemura K (1995) IL-10 production in cutaneous basal and sqamous cell carcinomas. A mechanism for evading the local immune response. J Immunol 155:2240–2247
76. Kim JM, Brannan CI, Copeland NG, Jenkins NA, Khan TA, Moore KW (1992) Structure of the mouse IL-10 gene and chromosomal localization of the mouse and human genes. J Immunol 148:3618–3623
77. King CL, Medhat A, Malhotra I, Helmy A, Khaudary J, Ibrahim S, El-Sherbiny M, Zaky S, Stupi RJ, Brustoski K, Shehata M, Shata MT (1996) Cytokine control of parasite-specific anergy in human urinary schistosomiasis. IL-10 modulates lymphocyte reactivity. J Immunol 156:4715–4721

78. Kline JN, Geist LJ, Monick MM, Stinski MF, Hunninghake GW (1994) Regulation of expression of the IL-1 receptor antagonist (IL-1ra) gene by products of the human cytomegalovirus immediate early genes. J Immunol 152:2351–2357
79. Knop J, Enk AH (1995) Cellular and molecular mechanisms in the induction phase of contact sensitivity. Int Arch Allergy Immunol 107:231–232
80. Koch F, Stanzl U, Jennewein P, Janke K, Heufler C, Kämpgen E, Romani N, Schuler G (1996) High level IL-12 production by murine dendritic cells: upregulation via MHC class II and CD40 molecules and downregulation by IL-4 and IL-10. J Exp Med 184:741–746
81. Kollmann TR, Pettoello Mantovani M, Katopodis NF, Hachamovitch M, Rubinstein A, Kim A, Goldstein H (1996) Inhibition of acute in vivo human immunodeficiency virus infection by human interleukin 10 treatment of SCID mice implanted with human fetal thymus and liver. Proc Natl Acad Sci USA 93:3126–3131
82. Kondo S, Pastore S, Fujisawa H, Shivji GM, McKenzie RC, Dinarello CA, Sauder DN (1995) Interleukin-1 receptor antagonist suppresses contact hypersensitivity. J Invest Dermatol 105:334–338
83. Kripke ML (1990) Photoimmunology. Photochem Photobiol 52:919–924
84. Kuhn R, Lohler J, Rennick D, Rajewsky K, Muller W (1993) Interleukin-10-deficient mice develop chronic enterocolitis. Cell 75:263–274
85. Kulozik M, Hogg A, Lankat Buttgereit B, Krieg T (1990) Co-localization of transforming growth factor beta 2 with alpha 1(I) procollagen mRNA in tissue sections of patients with systemic sclerosis. J Clin Invest 86:917–922
86. Kupper TS (1994) The second decade of epidermal cytokines: an overview. In: Luger TA, Schwarz T (eds) Epidermal growth factors and cytokines. Dekker, New York, pp 293–302
87. Kutsch CL, Norris DA, Arend WP (1993) Tumor necrosis factor-alpha induces interleukin-1 alpha and interleukin-1 receptor antagonist production by cultured human keratinocytes. J Invest Dermatol 101:79–85
88. Lee M, Mueller R, Wicker LS, Peterson LB, Sarvetnick N (1996) IL-10 is necessary and sufficient for autoimmune diabetes in conjunction with NOD MHC homozygosity. J Exp Med 184:2663–2668
89. Lennard AC (1995) Interleukin-1 receptor antagonist. Crit Rev Immunol 15:77–105
90. Lew W, Lee SH, Park YK (1995) Opposing effects of ultraviolet B irradiation on interleukin-1 receptor antagonist and interleukin-1 alpha messenger RNA expression in a human epidermoid carcinoma cell line. Photodermatol Photoimmunol Photomed 11:91–94
91. Liu Y, Wei SHY, Ho ASY, de Waal Malefyt R, Moore KW (1994) Expression cloning and characterization of a human IL-10 receptor. J Immunol 152:1821–1829
92. Llorente L, Zou W, Levy Y, Richaud-Patin Y, Wijdenes J, Alcocer-Varela J, Morel-Fourrier B, Brouet JC, Alarcon-Segovia D, Galanaud P, Emilie D (1995) Role of interleukin 10 in the B lymphocyte hyperactivity and autoantibody production of human systemic lupus erythematosus. J Exp Med 181:839–844
93. Luger TA, Schwarz T (1995) The role of cytokines and neuroendocrine hormones in cutaneous immunity and inflammation. Allergy 50:292–302
94. Luger TA, Schauer E, Trautinger F, Krutmann J, Ansel J, Schwarz A, Schwarz T (1993) Production of immunosuppressing melanotropins by keratinocytes. Ann NY Acad Sci 680:567–570
95. Lunec J, Pieron C, Sherbet GV, Thody AJ (1990) Alpha-melanocyte-stimulating hormone immunoreactivity in melanoma cells. Pathobiology 58:193–197
96. Makarov SS, Olsen JC, Johnston WN, Anderle SK, Brown RR, Baldwin AS Jr, Haskill JS, Schwab JH (1996) Suppression of experimental arthritis by gene transfer of interleukin 1 receptor antagonist cDNA. Proc Natl Acad Sci USA 93:402–406
97. Marcinkiewicz M, Day R, Seidah NG, Chretien M (1993) Ontogeny of the prohormone convertases PC1 and PC2 in the mouse hypophysis and their colocalization with corticotropin and alpha-melanotropin. Proc Natl Acad Sci USA 90:4922–4926
98. Martin D, Near SL (1995) Protective effect of the interleukin-1 receptor antagonist (IL-1ra) on experimental allergic encephalomyelitis in rats. J Neuroimmunol 61:241–245
99. Massague J (1992) Receptors for the TGF-beta family. Cell 69:1067–1070

100. McKenzie RC, Lea RG, Sauder DN (1991) Ultraviolet radiation induces expression of interleukin 8 and transforming growth factor beta in human kertinocytes. J Invest Dermatol 96:610
101. McKenzie RC, Oran A, Dinarello CA, Sauder DN (1996) Interleukin-1 receptor antagonist inhibits subcutaneous B16 melanoma growth in vivo. Anticancer Res 16:437–441
102. Moore KW, Vieira P, Fiorentino DF, Trounstine ML, Khan TA, Mosmann TR (1990) Homology of cytokine synthesis inhibitory factor (IL-10) to the Epstein-Barr virus gene BCRFI. Science 248:1230–1234
103. Moore KW, O'Garra A, de Waal Malefyt R, Vieira P, Mosmann TR (1993) Interleukin-10. Annu Rev Immunol 11:165–190
104. Morhenn VB (1991) The physiology of scratching: involvement of proopiomelanocortin gene-coded proteins in Langerhans cells. Prog Neuro Endo Immun 4:265–267
105. Mountjoy KG, Robbins LS, Mortrud MT, Cone RD (1992) The cloning of a family of genes that encode the melanocortin receptors. Science 257:1248–1251
106 Mugridge KG, Perretti M, Ghiara P, Parente L (1991) Alpha-melanocyte-stimulating hormone reduces interleukin-1 beta effects on rat stomach preparations possibly through interference with a type I receptor. Eur J Pharmacol 197:151–155
107. Nabioullin R, Sone S, Mizuno K, Yano S, Nishioka Y, Haku T, Ogura T (1994) Interleukin-10 is a potent inhibitor of tumor cytotoxicity by human monocytes and alveolar macrophages. J Leukoc Biol 55:437–442
108. Nickoloff BJ, Fivenson DP, Kunkel SL, Strieter RM, Turka LA (1994) Keratinocyte interleukin-10 expression is upregulated in tape-stripped skin, poison ivy dermatitis, and Sezary syndrome, but not in psoriatic plaques. Clin Immunol Immunopathol 73:63–68
109. Norman J, Franz M, Messina J, Riker A, Fabri PJ, Rosemurgy AS, Gower WRJ (1995) Interleukin-1 receptor antagonist decreases severity of experimental acute pancreatitis. Surgery 117:648–655
110. Ohlsson K, Bjork P, Bergenfeldt M, Hageman R, Thompson RC (1990) Interleukin-1 receptor antagonist reduces mortality from endotoxin shock. Nature 348:550–552
111. Ohmen JD, Hanifin JM, Nickoloff BJ, Rea TH, Wyzykowski R, Kim J, Jullien D, McHugh T, Nassif AS, Chan SC et al (1995) Overexpression of IL-10 in atopic dermatitis. Contrasting cytokine patterns with delayed-type hypersensitivity reactions. J Immunol 154:1956–1963
112. Palmetshofer A, Schwarz A, Mahnke K, Bhardwaj RS, Luger TA, Schwarz T (1994) Interleukin-10 affects the expression of adhesion molecules on human dermal microvascular endothelial cells. Exp Derm 3:138
113. Peltonen J, Kahari L, Jaakkola S, Kahari VM, Varga J, Uitto J, Jimenez SA (1990) Evaluation of transforming growth factor beta and type I procollagen gene expression in fibrotic skin diseases by in situ hybridization. J Invest Dermatol 94:365–371
114. Piguet PF, Vesin C, Grau GE, Thompson RC (1993) Interleukin 1 receptor antagonist (IL-1ra) prevents or cures pulmonary fibrosis elicited in mice by bleomycin or silica. Cytokine 5:57–61
115. Qin L, Chavin KD, Ding Y, Woodward JE, Favaro JP, Lin J, Bromberg JS (1994) Gene transfer for transplantation. Prolongation of allograft survival with transforming growth factor-beta. Ann Surg 220:508–518
116. Qin L, Chavin KD, Ding Y, Tahara H, Favaro JP, Woodward JE, Suzuki T, Robbins PD, Lotze MT, Bromberg JS (1996) Retrovirus-mediated transfer of viral IL-10 gene prolongs murine cardiac allograft survival. J Immunol 156:2316–2323
117. Rasmussen HH, Celis JE (1993) Evidence for an altered protein kinase C (PKC) signaling pathway in psoriasis. J Invest Dermatol 101:560–566
118. Reichlin S (1993) Neuroendocrine-immune interactions. N Engl J Med 329:1246–1253
119. Richter G, Kruger Krasagakes S, Hein G, Huls C, Schmitt E, Diamantstein T, Blankenstein T (1993) Interleukin 10 transfected into Chinese hamster ovary cells prevents tumor growth and macrophage infiltration. Cancer Res 53:4134–4137
120. Rivas JM, Ullrich SE (1992) Sytemic suppression of delayed-type hypersensitivity by supernatants from UV-irradiated keratinocytes. An essential role for keratinocyte-derived IL-10. J Immunol 149:3865–3871

121. Roberts AB, Sporn MB (1990) The transforming growth factor-betas. In: Sporn MB, Roberts AB (eds) Handbook of experimental pharmacology. I. Peptide growth factors and their receptors. Springer, Berlin Heidelberg New York, pp 419 472
122. Roberts AB, Sporn MB (1993) Physiological actions and clinical applications of transforming growth factor-beta (TGF-beta). Growth Factors 8:1–9
123. Rode HJ, Janssen W, Rosen Wolff A, Bugert JJ, Thein P, Becker Y, Darai G (1993) The genome of equine herpesvirus type 2 harbors an interleukin 10 (IL10)-like gene. Virus Genes 7:111–116
124. Rowe PM (1994) Clinical potential for TGF-beta. Lancet 344:72–73
125. Ruscetti FW, Palladino MA (1991) Transforming growth factor-beta and the immune system. Prog Growth Factor Res 3:159–175
126. Schauer E, Trautinger F, Köck A, Bhardwaj RS, Simon M, Schwarz A, Ansel JC, Schwarz T, Luger TA (1994) Proopiomelanocortin derived peptides are synthesized and released by human keratinocytes. J Clin Invest 93:2258–2262
127. Schwarz A, Grabbe S, Riemann H, Aragane Y, Simon M, Manon S, Andrade S, Luger TA, Zlotnik A, Schwarz T (1994) In vivo effects of interleukin-10 on contact hypersensitivity and delayed-type hypersensitivity reactions. J Invest Dermatol 103:211–216
128. Schwarz A, Grabbe S, Aragane Y, Sandkuhl K, Riemann H, Luger TA, Kubin M, Trinchieri G, Schwarz T (1996) Interleukin-12 prevents ultraviolet B (UVB)-induced local immunosuppression and overcomes UVB-induced tolerance. J Invest Dermatol 106:1187–1191
129. Sellheyer K, Bickenbach JR, Rothnagel JA, Bundman D, Longley MA, Krieg T, Roche NS, Roberts AB, Roop DR (1993) Inhibition of skin development by overexpression of transforming growth factor beta 1 in the epidermis of transgenic mice. Proc Natl Acad Sci USA 90:5237–5241
130. Serra R, Moses HL (1996) Tumor suppressor genes in the TGF- signaling pathway? Nature Med 2:390–391
131. Shah M, Foreman DM, Ferguson MW (1992) Control of scarring in adult wounds by neutralising antibody to transforming growth factor beta. Lancet 339:213–214
132. Shah M, Foreman DM, Ferguson MW (1995) Neutralisation of TGF-beta 1 and TGF-beta 2 or exogenous addition of TGF-beta 3 to cutaneous rat wounds reduces scarring. J Cell Sci 108:985–1002
133. Shull MM, Ormsby I, Kier AB, Pawlowski S, Diebold RJ, Yin M, Allen R, Sidman C, Proetzel G, Calvin D et al (1992) Targeted disruption of the mouse transforming growth factor-beta 1 gene results in multifocal inflammatory disease. Nature 359:693–699
134. Smith EM, Hughes TKJ, Hashemi F, Stefano GB (1992) Immunosuppressive effects of corticotropin and melanotropin and their possible significance in human immunodeficiency virus infection. Proc Natl Acad Sci USA 89:782–786
135. Sone S, Orino E, Mizuno K, Yano S, Nishioka Y, Haku T, Nii A, Ogura T (1994) Production of IL-1 and its receptor antagonist is regulated differently by IFN-gamma and IL-4 in human monocytes and alveolar macrophages. Eur Respir J 7:657–663
136. Sporn MB, Roberts AB (1992) Transforming growth factor-beta: recent progress and new challenges. J Cell Biol 119:1017–1021
137. Star RA, Rajora N, Huang J, Chavez R, Catania A, Lipton JM (1995) Evidence of autocrine modulation of macrophage nitric oxide synthase by alpha-MSH. Proc Natl Acad Sci USA 92:8016–8020
138. Strieter RM, Polverini PJ, Arenberg DA, Kunkel SL (1995a) The role of CXC chemokines as regulators of angiogenesis. Shock 4:155–160
139. Strieter RM, Polverini PJ, Arenberg DA, Walz A, Opdenakker G, Van Damme J, Kunkel SL (1995b) Role of C-X-C chemokines as regulators of angiogenesis in lung cancer. J Leukoc Biol 57:752–762
140. Strobl H, Riedl E, Scheinecker C, Bello-Fernandez C, Pickl WF, Rappersberger K, Majdic O, Knapp W (1996) TGF-β1 promotes in vitro development of dendritic cells from CD34+ hemopoietic progenitors. J Immunol 157:1499–1507
141. Tarlow JK, Clay FE, Cork MJ, Blakemore AI, McDonagh AJ, Messenger AG, Duff GW (1994) Severity of alopecia areata is associated with a polymorphism in the interleukin-1 receptor antagonist gene. J Invest Dermatol 103:387–390

142. Tilg H, Mier JW, Vogel W, Aulitzky WE, Wiedermann CJ, Vannier E, Huber C, Dinarello CA (1993) Induction of circulating IL-1 receptor antagonist by IFN treatment. J Immunol 150:4687–4692
143. Uejima Y, Takahashi K, Komoriya K, Kurozumi S, Ochs HD (1996) Effect of interleukinn-10 on anti-CD40- and interleukin-4-induced immunoglobulin E production by human lymphocytes. Int Arch Allergy Immunol 110:225–232
144. Vannier E, de Waal Malefyt R, Salazar Montes A, de Vries JE, Dinarello CA (1996) Interleukin-13 (IL-13) induces IL-1 receptor antagonist gene expression and protein synthesis in peripheral blood mononuclear cells: inhibition by an IL-4 mutant protein. Blood 87:3307–3315
145. Vora M, Romero LI, Karasek MA (1994) IL-10 iduces E-selectin on small and large blood vessel endothelial cells. J Exp Med 184:821–830
146. Wahl SM (1993) Regulation of tissue inflammation, repair, and fibrosis by transforming growth factor beta. In: Luger TA, Schwarz T (eds) Epidermal growth factors and cytokines. Dekker, New York, pp 241–252
147. Walmsley M, Katsikis PD, Abney E, Parry S, Williams RO, Maini RN, Feldmann M (1996) Interleukin-10 inhibition of the progression of established collagen-induced arthritis. Arthritis Rheum 39:495–503
148. Wintzen M, Gilchrest BA (1996) Proopiomelanocortin, its derived peptides, and the skin. J Invest Dermatol 106:3–10
149. Zavala F, Rimaniol AC, Boussin F, Dormont D, Bach JF, Descamps Latscha B (1995) HIV predominantly induces IL-1 receptor antagonist over IL-1 synthesis in human primary monocytes. J Immunol 155:2784–2793

Extracorporeal Photochemotherapy

M. Girardi and P. Heald

Introduction

Immunointervention therapies have found a role in the management of many T cell-mediated skin diseases. Extracorporeal photochemotherapy (ECP) has found a role as an immunointervention in the following diseases:

- Cutaneous T cell lymphoma (CTCL)
- Pemphigus vulgaris
- Pemphigus foliaceous
- Graft-versus-host disease (GVHD)
- Psoriatic arthritis
- Scleroderma
- Lupus erythematosus
- Epidermolysis bullosa acquisita (EBA)

ECP is regarded as an immunotherapy because a small portion of the lymphocyte pool (less than 1%) is damaged and then reinfused to induce changes well beyond the effects from deleting that small portion of the peripheral lymphocyte pool.

ECP was initially shown to have a therapeutic impact on CTCL as reported by Edelson in the initial monotherapy trial for erythrodermic disease. After this therapy became available, it was applied in the management of many T cell-mediated cutaneous and noncutaneous diseases. The latter are not discussed in this article, but can be found in the recent literature concerning cardiac and renal transplantation [18, 25, 27].

Constraints

Several factors influence the decision to start ECP. Currently, ECP is available in over 100 centers in the United States and Europe. Since most therapy protocols require treatment schedules over months and years, geographic constraints limit availability of therapy. Most treatment centers perform ECP in an outpatient setting, and an individual treatment session takes 3–3.5 h.

The procedure can be performed through a peripheral vein, preferably with an 18-gauge needle. This constraint limits therapy to those patients with accessible veins. After establishing venous access, the patient undergoes discontinuous pheresis cycles to harvest the lymphocyte rich buffy coat. These cycles may deplete the patient of 200–400 cc of volume, and if their cardiovascular system cannot tolerate this therapy, this cannot be performed. At the completion of the treatment cycle, the reinfusion phase leaves the patient with a net gain of up to 500 cc of fluid. Again, the cardiovascular system must be able to tolerate this fluid challenge for therapy to be performed safely. In patients with mild intolerance of the fluid loading, diuretics can be administered simultaneously to avoid hypervolemia.

The clinical responses to ECP are gradual. This means that the patient should not have rapidly progressive disease. With cardiac transplant patients, the therapeutic results occur rapidly, and in that setting, unstable patients are frequently treated. Eruptive tumor-stage CTCL should be treated with a rapidly acting adjunct such as radiotherapy.

The ECP procedure is currently performed with oral 8-methoxypsoralen (8-MOP). To achieve therapeutic levels of the drug, patients often need to ingest 0.6–0.8 mg/kg and the resulting nausea can complicate therapy. Knobler [14] developed a technique for preparing 8-MOP that can be injected directly into the treatment cassette. UVADEX (Roche Laboratories; Nutley, NJ, USA) is an injectable preparation of 8-MOP that is currently under study for use in ECP.

Regimens for Use

Cutaneous T Cell Lymphoma

As with most therapies that have undergone clinical trials to establish efficacy, the regimens for using ECP reflect the schedules used in the initial multicenter clinical trials. The first version of the lymphocyte photoinactivating device took an entire day to treat a patient, and patients were treated on 2 consecutive days. These 2-day treatment cycles were repeated at 4-week intervals. The results with this schedule of therapy were dramatic in erythrodermic patients. Based on the success of this schedule, patients have subsequently followed the 2-day, 4-weekly regimen.

The results of the initial clinical trials and follow-up studies have shown that, as a monotherapy, ECP can induce a remission in approximately one fourth of the patients treated [12]. One half of the patients with erythrodermic CTCL had a significant partial response, and the remainder had no response or progressive disease. This same proportion of responses was observed in the smaller series of CTCL patients reported by Zic et al. [31], Armus et al. [2], and Bisaccia et al. [3]. The responses of patients with erythrodermic CTCL to ECP can often be dramatic, as shown in Fig. 1.

There have been modifications in the scheduling of ECP treatments that have also met with success. Bowen et al. [4] reported on using a 2-weekly regimen at the initiation of therapy. The patient in that report had hyperleukocytic disease, and after the leukemia improved the patient was put on a 4-week cycle. Several other centers have used this accelerated delivery schedule at the initiation of therapy.

Before ECP is started, patients should be thoroughly evaluated in terms of their tumor burden and peripheral blood status. Patients with tumorous infiltration of the skin and those with hyperleukocytosis are not good candidates for monotherapy with ECP (adjuncts are discussed later). Erythrodermic patients beginning on ECP should be initially re-evaluated after three cycles of therapy. By this point, a trend in their clinical status should be evident. If there are signs of improvement, the therapy should be continued to maximize the therapeutic response. Complete clearing can occur after 6–8 months of gradual improvement. Patients with incomplete responses at 3–6 months should be considered for adjunctive therapy.

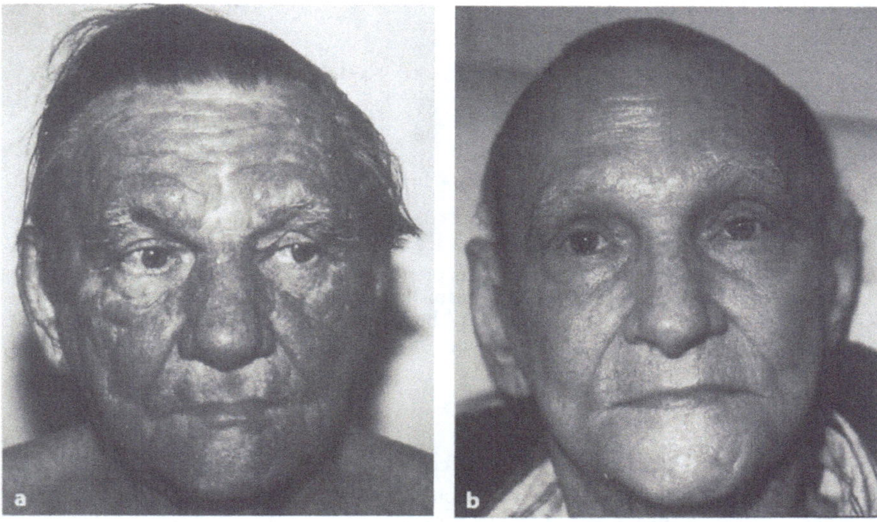

Fig. 1a,b. A patient with erythrodermic cutaneous T cell lymphoma (CTCL) **a** before and **b** after treatment with extracorporeal photochemotherapy (ECP)

In evaluating options of adjunctive therapy, it is worthwhile reviewing all therapies of CTCL. There are three broad categories to choose from: (1) skin-directed therapy, (2) biological response modifiers, and (3) low-dose chemotherapy. In patients with significant tumor burden, a reduction of that tumor burden with a skin-directed treatment can work synergistically with ECP. The skin-directed therapies available are radiotherapy, psoralens and ultraviolet A (PUVA), and topical chemotherapy. Wilson et al. [29] reported that series of patients treated with ECP and total-skin electron beam had improved survival rates when compared to similarly staged patients at the same institution treated with total-skin electron beam therapy alone; one of the patients treated in that series had significant lymph node disease, and the response to therapy is shown in Fig. 2. A not infrequent occurrence is to have patch or plaque lesions of CTCL appear as the erythroderma fades and unmasks them. In that situation, any of the skin-directed therapies can be successful in eliminating these fixed cutaneous lesions.

Biological response modifiers include ECP, interferons, retinoids, antibodies, cytokines, and cytokine-based fusion toxins. Several reports have presented beneficial results of combining biological response modifiers. Rook et al. [24] reported the use of interferon-α with ECP to establish a remission in a patient with advanced CTCL. Lim and Harris [16] utilized retinoid therapy with a resultant beneficial response in a patient on ECP. These preliminary results are encouraging both for helping patients and for increasing our understanding of CTCL. However, the failing immunity of CTCL patients [22] is a direct result of the malignant cells, and a skin-directed therapy often provides a direct debulking effect to help reduce the tumor burden.

The immunosuppressive effects of advancing CTCL are the reasons why traditional high-dose chemotherapy has been unsuccessful in treating CTCL. Low-dose chemotherapy has been employed with beneficial results. Methotrexate at 15–25 mg per week can

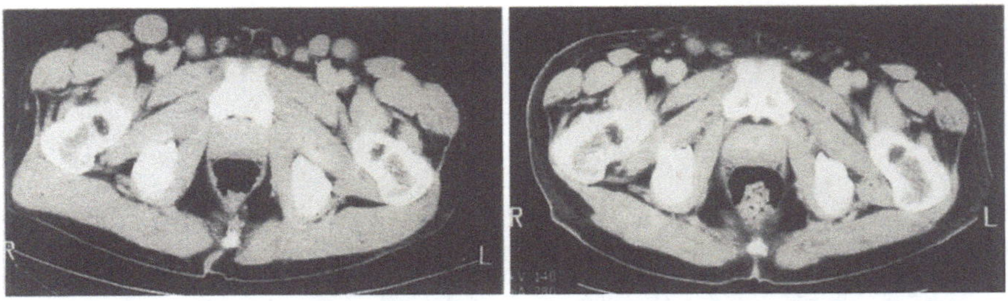

Fig. 2. On the computed tomography (CT) scan, pretreatment inguinal adenopathy is seen (*left*). The patient underwent combined electron-beam therapy/extracorporeal photochemotherapy (ECP) with no direct radiation of lymph nodes. The reduction of tumor burden is demonstrable by the inguinal nodes returning to normal size (*right*)

safely be given to patients on ECP. Oral corticosteroids can be palliative in CTCL patients, but their immunosuppressive effects have been shown to negate the therapeutic effects of ECP in experimental models. These murine systems may not adequately reflect the human system, because Rose et al. [25] reported that cardiac transplantations patients have benefits from ECP while on systemic steroids and cyclosporine.

In summary, ECP should be used as a monotherapy with erythrodermic disease or as part of a multiagent regimen for refractory erythrodermas or those patients with advanced disease. The goal of therapy should be to achieve remission and then gradually to taper treatment. The taper schedule used in the majority of the patients in the initial study was to add a 1-week interval every three cycles of therapy. Once patients achieved 8-week intervals and were clear, they were taken off therapy. These patients with tumor stage CTCL need to continue with their maintenance schedule of skin-directed therapy (typically PUVA at one treatment per week or month).

Patients with an unacceptable response or progressive disease with ECP should have their next line of therapy introduced before discontinuing ECP completely. Flares of CTCL have occurred in patients going off ECP for CTCL.

Treatment of Autoimmune Disorders

CTCL is characterized by a malignant clone of T-helper cells. Many of the so-called autoimmune disorders are likely mediated by an autoreactive population of oligoclonal T cells. Thus the apparent ability of ECP to stimulate an immune response against pathogenic clones of T cells suggests a role for ECP as a immune modifier capable of inducing downregulation of pathogenic T cells in various autoimmune disorders. Clinical studies have demonstrated the potential efficacy of ECP in the treatment of various disorders (see "Introduction").

Pemphigus Vulgaris

Pemphigus vulgaris in an autoimmune disorder whereby the production of antibodies generated against the desmoglein-3 protein component of keratinocyte desmosomal connections leads to blister and erosion formation of cutaneous and mucosal surfaces.

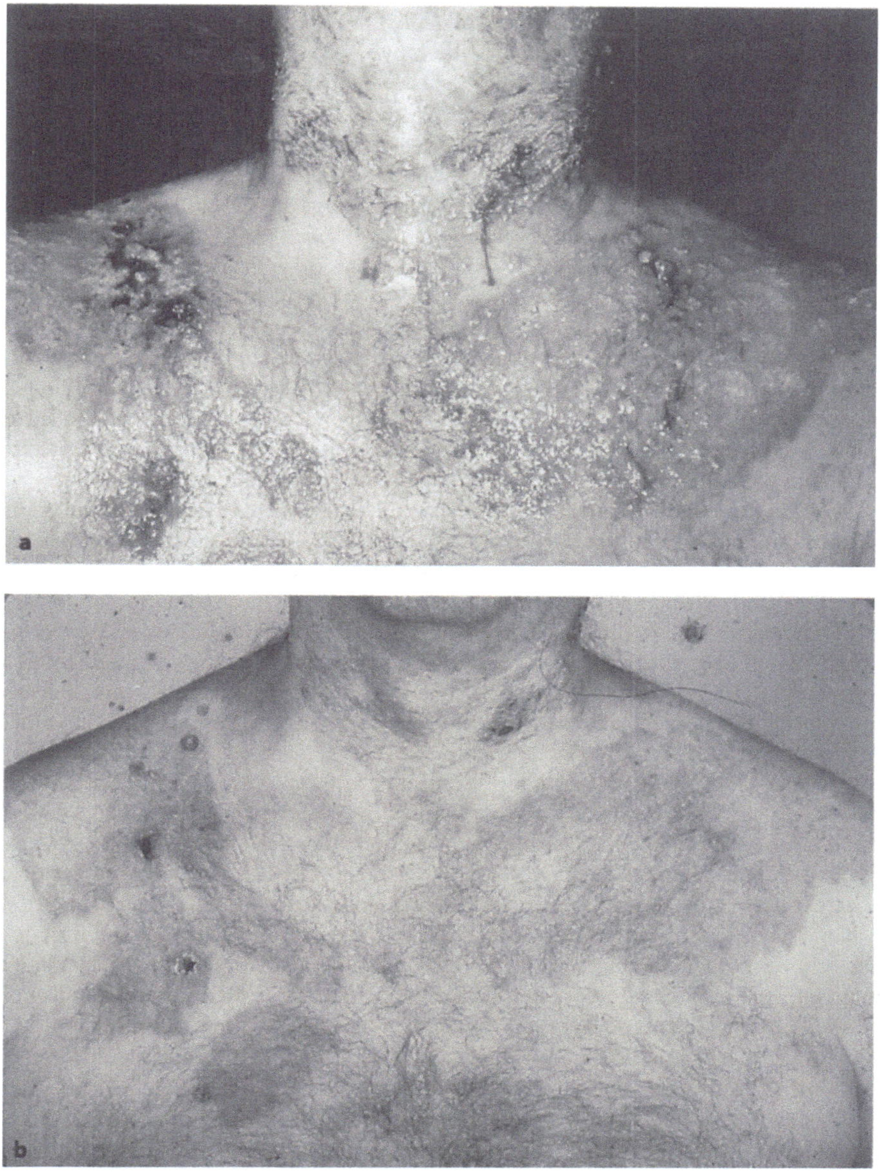

Fig. 3. a Patient with pemphigus vulgaris before starting extracorporeal photochemotherapy (ECP). b After 12 months, most of the lesions have cleared

The majority of patients are adequately controlled with the use of high-dose corticosteroids and often other potent immunosuppressive medications such as azathioprine, cyclosporine, cyclophosphamide, and diaminodiphenylsulfone. However, long-term treatment with these medications is often complicated by side effects, and mortality rates remain around 5 %–15 %, largely due to complications from these drugs. ECP, with its excellent short-term and long-term side effect profile, represents a potential treatment for pemphigus patients failing drug therapy.

A total of six patients with pemphigus vulgaris treated with ECP have been reported in the literature by three different investigative groups. Rook et al. [23] initially reported the efficacy of ECP in a pilot study of four patients with extensive and refractory pemphigus vulgaris, despite large doses of immunosuppressive medications. The patients ranged in age from 61 to 78 years and had an average disease duration of 3.5 years (range, 1–6 years). Patients were treated with ECP on 2 successive days at 4-week intervals and continued to receive prednisone alone or with azathioprine. All four patients showed clinical improvement (see Fig. 3) within the first 6 months of therapy, and all four eventually displayed a drop in antidesmosomal antibody levels. After 36–48 months, three of the four patients demonstrated a complete remission (i.e., no clinical evidence of active disease and undetectable antidesmosome antibody levels), which lasted an average of 19.3 months (range, 7–36 months). Notably, relapses in the three responded to reinitiation of ECP after only three to four monthly cycles. During the study, systemic immunosuppressive medications were discontinued or tapered to lower doses.

Two other cases have been reported in which ECP demonstrated a benefit in pemphigus patients. Liang et al. [15] reported a 31-year-old man with a 4-year history of severe disease resistant to high doses of various combinations of prednisone, gold, cyclosporine, methotrexate, azathioprine, and pulse cyclophosphamide with methylprednisolone. A total of 70% body surface area was involved with pemphigus. After receiving ECP every 2 weeks for seven cycles, the patient ceased forming new lesions, and the frequency of treatment was decreased to every 3 weeks. The patient continued to improve, despite decreasing his immunosuppressive medications, and eventually achieved almost complete healing of all skin lesions. In a case reported by Gollnick et al. [10], a 37-year-old woman with a 5-year history of severe pemphigus was poorly controlled with prednisone, azathioprine, and methotrexate. Furthermore, she had developed corticosteroid-associated side effects of moon facies, diabetes mellitus, osteoporosis, and amenorrhea. After the sixth cycle of ECP, the patient demonstrated a 95% improvement in her skin and mucosal lesions, despite lowering of her azathioprine and prednisolone doses.

None of the six patients discussed above developed serious side effects, immunosuppressive or otherwise, that were attributable to ECP. All patients showed at least some improvement, despite a decrease in their immunosuppressive medications, and five of the six demonstrated marked responses while on ECP. These case reports suggest that ECP may be a very promising potential treatment for pemphigus vulgaris. However, a randomized, controlled study would be needed to define the use of ECP in less severe disease or as a first-line therapy. Nonetheless, ECP represents a viable option for patients with pemphigus vulgaris poorly controlled with, or unable to tolerate, combinations of high-dose immunosuppressive medications.

Scleroderma

Scleroderma is characterized by the abnormal deposition of excessive collagen (i.e., fibrosis) within the skin leading to decreased mobility of joints due to skin tightening. Since there is also frequent sclerosis of visceral organs such as the heart, lungs, gastrointestinal tract, and kidneys, a more accurate term for this condition is systemic sclerosis (SS). Standard treatment for this condition has included d-penicillamine, an inhibitor of collagen cross-linking, as well as globally immunosuppressive medications. The early phase of SS is characterized by a greater inflammatory infiltrate and edema within the dermis. Activated T-helper cells within the infiltrate may stimulate the production of collagen synthesis and subsequent fibrosis via the secretion of certain cytokines. Although collagen in the skin continually undergoes a remodeling process whereby old fibers are reabsorbed and new fibers laid down, the degree to which fibrosis is reversible in patients with SS is unknown. Thus it is perhaps not surprising that ECP for scleroderma has demonstrated the greatest therapeutic effect in patients with relatively recent disease onset.

A randomized, parallel-group, single-blinded, multicenter clinical trial reported by Rook in 1992 [24] demonstrated the safety and efficacy of ECP in the treatment of scleroderma. Seventy-nine patients with SS of an average duration of 1.8 years (maximum, 4 years) and worsening of cutaneous involvement of at least 30% during the preceding 6 months were randomized to receive ECP (treatments every month on 2 consecutive days) or oral d-penicillamine (maximum dose, 750 mg/day) for 6 months. Patients were excluded if they demonstrated significant renal (serum creatinine > 3.0 mg/dl) or pulmonary involvement (carbon monoxide-diffusing capacity less than 50% of normal). Blinded clinical examiners determined a skin score based on skin thickness, percentage of surface area involved, oral aperture, and hand closure. A significant improvement in skin score occurred in 68% (21 of 31) of patients receiving ECP, and 32% (eight of 25) of patients on d-penicillamine, while significant worsening was observed in 10% (n=3) receiving ECP and 32% (n=8) receiving d-penicillamine. The difference between the two groups was statistically significant ($p< 0.02$). Furthermore, adverse reactions in the ECP study group were minimal, and all patients completed the study. In contrast, six patients had to permanently discontinue d-penicillamine due to adverse effects such as renal failure and liver function abnormalities.

Subjects from an independent study by Di Spaltro [7] in which nine patients with SS in an open trial were treated with ECP for 6–21 months demonstrated significant improvement in their skin, musculoskeletal system, functional index, and symptoms including Raynaud's phenomenon, dyspnea, fatigue, dysphagia, and arthralgias. Again, patients were relatively early in their disease onset, with a history of only 6 months to 4 years. However, in separate trials reported by Zachariae et al. [30] (eight patients with SS) and Cribier et al. [5] (seven patients with SS), subjects showed little response or worsening despite treatment with ECP. Average disease duration in both trials was longer than in the randomized multicenter trial discussed above. Furthermore, patients were not excluded on the basis of severe internal organ involvement.

In summary, patients with SS appear most likely to benefit from treatment with ECP if they have recent onset of disease before presumably irreversible chronic fibrotic changes take place. To date, patients with evidence of significant visceral disease involvement (e.g., serum creatinine > 3.0 mg/dl, or carbon monoxide-diffusing capacity less than 50 % of normal) have been excluded from most studies and the results with that group are unknown.

Graft-Versus-Host Disease

GVHD is a frequent complication of allogeneic bone marrow transplantation (BMT). Cutaneous involvement ranges from widespread erythematous eruptions in acute GVHD to lichenoid and sclerodermoid reactions in chronic GVHD. Extensive disease is characterized by multiorgan involvement and can be resistant to high-dose immunosuppressive medications. GVHD is mediated by T cells autoreactive against major and minor histocompatibility self-antigens. That ECP is capable of eliciting an immunoregulatory response against such pathogenic T cells is suggested by the results of several experimental systems, including specific inhibition of skin graft rejection [21] and prevention of stimulatory GVHD in mice [8].

Two cases have been reported to show a benefit of ECP in the treatment of chronic GVHD. Owsianowski et al. [20] reported a 43-year-old woman who developed chronic GVHD with severe sclerodermatous manifestations, including joint contracture, skin ulceration, and liver involvement. Despite treatment with cyclosporin A, corticosteroids, and PUVA, disease was progressive. ECP was performed on 2 consecutive days every 4 weeks. After 3 months of therapy, skin improvement was evident by initiation of reepithelialization of ulcers. Total closure of the ulcers occurred by 24–30 weeks of therapy. Spotty skin softening initially occurring over the thighs led to larger areas of softening up to 30 cm in diameter. Reversal of breast induration was noted after only six cycles of ECP. Furthermore, there was a marked improvement in joint mobility. No side effects of therapy were noted.

Rosetti et al. [26] reported on a 14-year-old boy who developed chronic GVHD following allogeneic bone marrow transplantation for acute lymphoblastic leukemia 9 months previously. The patient no longer tolerated steroids or cyclosporin A due to uncontrolled hypertension, glaucoma, and hypertriglyceridemia. During the 18 months of treatment with ECP (2 consecutive days every 4 weeks), a theumatologist blinded to the mode of treatment observed a gradual improvement in severity skin score of 50 % and extension skin score of 50 %. Furthermore, objective measures of esophageal and pulmonary involvement demonstrated significant improvement. These two cases suggest a potential role of ECP in the treatment of chronic GVHD recalcitrant to standard therapy. The role of ECP in acute GVHD has yet to be addressed.

Systemic Lupus Erythematosus

Systemic lupus erythematosus (SLE) is characterized by abnormal circulating B and T cells and autoantibody production. This results in a variety of cutaneous abnormalities (i.e., photosensitivity, mucosal erosions, discoid lesions) and systemic abnormalities (i.e., renal, hematogical, joint). Disease is usually controlled to some degree with standard therapies including antimalarials, corticosteroids, and other immunosuppressive agents. Studies in two different mouse models suggest that the downregulation of lupus-mediating T cells might be attainable through treatment with ECP.

To test the feasibility of ECP in the treatment of SLE, a pilot study of ten patients was conducted by Knobler et al. [13]. Patients satisfied the American College of Rheumatology criteria for SLE and had disease adequately controlled with low-dose prednisone, chloroquine, azathioprine, and/or cyclophosphamide, but all rebounded with multiple drug-tapering attempts. Strict inclusion criteria resulted in a study population with mild to moderate systemic involvement. Patients were treated on 2 consecutive days every month for 6 months, then every 2 months for another 6 months. In the eight patients who completed the study, disease activity, as measured by the SLE Activity Index Scoring System, dropped from a median of 7 (range, 4–9) down to 1 (range, 0–5). In all patients except one, the dosage of steroids and immunosuppressive medications was reduced during this time. A marked resolution of cutaneous lesions was observed in six patients after 4–6 months of ECP. Laboratory abnormalities showed no difference from baseline. Observed side effects were minor.

In summary, SLE patients with mild disease who are no longer tolerating or who wish to decrease treatment with systemic medications may benefit from treatment with ECP. Subsequent studies with ECP in SLE can be done based on the safety demonstrated in this pilot study. The infusion of photodamaged DNA into patients with antinuclear and anti-DNA antibodies did not lead to any exacerbation of the autoimmune disease.

Psoriatic Arthritis

Psoriatic arthritis represents a distinct inflammatory arthropathy which occurs in about 5 % of patients with psoriasis. An association with certain HLA phenotypes, shifts in the CD4 to CD8 ratios in the peripheral blood, and response to T cell-targeted treatments such as cyclosporin A and DABIL-2 (partial diphtheria toxin conjugated to soluble interleukin-2) are some of the evidence suggesting that psoriasis is a T cell-mediated disorder. In progressive forms of psoriatic arthritis, disease may be poorly responsive to anti-inflammatory, immunosuppressive, and cytotoxic agents.

As reported by Wilfert et al. [28], five patients (aged 26–58 years) with long-standing psoriatic arthritis were treated with ECP every 4 weeks for a total of 20–60 weeks. All medications except for nonsteroidal anti-inflammatory agents were discontinued 4 weeks prior to initiation of ECP. The clinical results were variable. Four of the five patients reported a reduction in pain intensity and a decrease in morning stiffness. Objectively measured parameters of grip strength and swelling improved in three patients. However, no clear improvement in skin disease was detectable. Three patients (aged 29–43 years) with psoriatic arthritis treated with ECP for 1 year were reported by de Misa et al. [6]. Two of the three patients demonstrated moderate improvement in spontaneous pain, morning stiffness, joint swelling, and the laboratory-measured parameter of erythrocyte sedimentation rate (ESR). Skin improvement was not interpretable, since patients continued to receive topical therapy. Side effects in these cases were minimal and included nausea and vasovagal responses.

In summary, treatment of psoriatic arthritis with ECP may help to ameliorate some of the arthropathic symptoms of this disorder in patients recalcitrant to or intolerant of standard therapy. The cutaneous manifestations of psoriasis have not shown a consistent response to ECP therapy.

Epidermolysis Bullosa Acquisita

EBA is a blistering disorder characterized by the production of autoantibodies to anchoring fibrils at the dermal–epidermal junction. Aggressive forms of EBA may be nonresponsive to standard immunosuppressive medications. Miller et al. [19] reported a 31-year-old man with severe EBA refractory to high-dose oral and intravenous-pulsed steroids, various combinations of immunosuppressive medications, and plasmapheresis. After only 3 months of ECP, the patient ceased development of new bullae. Despite tapering of his prednisone, the patient's skin remained disease free over 2 more years. The patient did, however, develop an unexplained cardiomyopathy. Further, more extensive studies are necessary before ECP proves to be an effective treatment option for aggressive forms of EBA.

Monitoring Patients

When ECP is initiated, the therapeutic goals need to be defined and the appropriate parameters measured at the start. In cutaneous lymphoma patients, tumor burden can be assessed by recording skin lesions, flow cytometry, molecular assessment of the peripheral blood, and computed tomography (CT) scans of the lymph nodes. Because the response to ECP is gradual, a periodic assessment of these tumor burden measures should be conducted every 4–8 weeks. Goldman et al. [9] reported on the value of following soluble interleukin-2 receptor levels in the serum. They demonstrated that this parameter decreased as the patients lymphoma responded to ECP. With pemphigus, skin lesions should also be recorded, and the pemphigus antibody titer measured. In scleroderma patients, the skin sclerosis score can be determined along with a biopsy in order to help monitor their disease. Adams et al. [1] reported on the use of imaging to document the scleroderma response to ECP. In each of these situations, it is best at the start by outlining the goal of therapy and the guidelines for when to begin adjunctive therapy.

When there has been a partial response to therapy, ECP can be continued to maintain the improved state. When there has been a complete response to therapy, ECP is tapered gradually by adding 1 week per cycle every 3 weeks. Erythrodermic lymphoma patients treated in this way have maintained their remissions after stopping therapy. For the latter group, the final treatment sessions were conducted every 8 weeks.

ECP-related side effects do not need to be monitored beyond the extent of a physical examination. Repeated studies looking for autoimmune phenomena have not demonstrated any value in the routine monitoring of autoantibodies.

Modifications

The crucial components of ECP have been identified in clinical studies and laboratory models. CD8 T cells are an important component of antitumor responses, since they can give rise to cytolytic T cells. Previous studies have shown that, within patients of the same clinical stage, those with larger populations of CD8 cells in their lesions survive longer. In ECP patients, those with higher CD4 to CD8 ratios in the blood do not respond as well as those with low CD4 to CD8 ratios [12]. CD8 T cells thus appear to be associated with ECP responsiveness, and augmentation of suppressor T cell activity is a desirable goal. CD8 cell interactions with major histocompatibility complex (MHC) class I-expressing antigen-presenting cells can potentially be enhanced. Interferon-γ and interleukin-12 may prove to be useful adjuncts to ECP therapy. Interleukin-2 promotes suppressor T cell activity.

Antigen-presenting cells play a critical role in presenting tumor-associated antigens to suppressor T cells. In the future, it may be possible to increase antigen-presenting cells with cytokine administration. Antigen-presenting cell–CD8 cell interaction could also be boosted if the appropriate tumor-related peptides could be added to the therapy. Augmentation of the antitumor response may be the explanation for why interleukin-2 can induce beneficial responses in patients with CTCL [17]. Administration of interleukin-2 at the time of ECP may also represent the future for expanding immunotherapy with ECP.

In addition to the immunologic pathway, which could be optimized in the future to streamline ECP, it is also possible that delivery of the drug and light could be optimized. The administration of UVA light from a small fiberoptic implanted in the thoracic dust would provide lymphocytes with UVA irradiation, and the patient could ingest psoralens to provide drug for the phototoxic event. Given the range of clinical responses to ECP and the ability to optimize its performance, this progression is inevitable.

Summary

Extracorporeal photochemotherapy (ECP) is an immunointerventive therapy whereby a small portion of the patient's peripheral leukocyte pool is removed, photochemically attenuated, and then intravenously reinfused back into the patient. ECP was initially shown to be beneficial for the treatment of cutaneous T cell lymphoma (CTCL), particularly for erythrodermic disease. More recently, several reports have discribed the potential use of ECP as a therapy for so-called autoimmune diseases such as pemphigus vulgaris, graft-versus-host disease, scleroderma, and others. ECP is now available at over 100 centers in the United States and Europe. A review of the ECP as an immunotherapy for CTCL and autoimmune disorders affecting the skin is presented.

References

1. Adams LB, Park JH, Olsen NJ, Gardner ES, Hernanz-Schulman M, King LE Jr (1995) Quantitative evaluation of improvement in muscle weakness in a patient receiving extracorporeal photopheresis for scleroderma: magnetic resonance imaging and magnetic resonance spectroscopy. J Am Acad Dermatol 33(3):519–522
2. Armus S, Keyes B, Cahill C et al (1990) Photopheresis for the treatment of cutaneous T-cell lymphoma. J Am Acad Dermatol23:898–902
3. Bisaccia E, Berger C, Klainer AS (1990) Photopheresis for the treatment of cutaneous T-cell lymphoma. J Am Acad Dermatol 23:5–11
4. Bowen GM, Steens SR, Dubin HV, Siddiqui J, Cooper KD (1995) diagnosis of Sezary syndrome in a patient with generalized pruritus based on early molecular study and flow cytometry. J Am Acad Dermatol 33(4):678–680
5. Cribier B, Faradji T, Le Coz C, Oberling F, Grosshans E (1995) Extracorporeal photochemotherapy in systemic sclerosis and severe morphea. Dermatology 191(1):25–31
6. de Misa RF, Azana JM, Harto A, Boixeda P, Moreno R, Ledo A (1994) Psoriatic arthritis: one year of treatment with extracorporeal photochemotherapy. J Am Acad Dermatol 30(6): 1037–1038
7. Di Spaltro FX, Cottrill C, Cahill C, Degnan E, Mulford GJ (1993) Extracorporeal photochemotherapy in progressive systemic sclerosis. Int J Dermatol 32(6):417–421
8. Girardi M, Herreid P, Tigelaar RE (1995) Specific suppression of lupus-like graft-versus-host disease using extracorporeal photochemical attenuation of effector lymphocytes. J Invest Dermatol 104(2):177–182
9. Goldman BD, Oh SK, Davis B et al (1993) Serum soluble interleukin 2 receptor levels in erythrodermic cutaneous T-cell lymphoma correlate with response to photopheresis based treatment. Arch Dermatol 129:1166–1170
10. Gollnick HP, Owsianowski M, Taube KM, Orfanos CE (1993) Unresponsive severe generalized pemphigus vulgaris successfully controlled by extracorporeal photopheresis. J Am Acad Dermatol 28(1):122–124
11. Heald P, Knobler R, LaRoche L (1994) Photoinactivated lymphocyte therapy of cutaneous T-cell lymphoma. Dermatol Clin 12(2):443–449

12. Heald PW, Rook A, Perez M et al (1992) Treatment of erythrodermic cutaneous T-cell lymphoma patients with photopheresis. J Am Acad Dermatol 27:427–433
13. Knobler RM, Graninger W, Lindmaier A, Trautinger F, Smolen JS (1992) Extracorporeal photochemotherapy for the treatment of systemic lupus erythematosus. A pilot study. Arthritis Rheum 35(3):319–324
14. Knobler RM, Trautinger F, Graninger W. Macheiner W, Gruenwald C, Neumann R, Ramer W (1993) Parenteral administration of 8-methoxypsoralen in photopheresis. J Am Acad Dermatol 28(4):580–584
15. Liang G, Nahass G, Kerdel FA (1992) Pemphigus vulgaris treated with photopheresis. J Am Acad Dermatol 26(5, 1):779–780
16. Lim HW, Harris HR (1995) Etretinate as an effective adjunctive therapy for recalcitrant palmar/plantar hyperkeratosis in patients with erythrodermic cutaneous T-cell lymphoma undergoing photopheresis. Dermatol Surg 21:597–599
17. Maolleua JP, Baccard M, Flageul, Ryojad M, Laroche L, Verola O, Brandley M, Morel P, Gisselbrecht C (1995) High-dose recombinant interleukin-2 in advanced cutaneous T-cell lymphoma. Arch Dermatol 131(5);574–579
18. Meiser EM, Kur F, Reichenspurner H. Wagner F., Boos KS, Veilhauer S, Weiss M, Rohrbach H, Kreuzer E, Uberfuhr P, Reichart B (1994) Reduction of the incidence of rejetion by adjunct immunosuppression with photochemotherapy after heart transplantation. Transplantation 57(4):563–568
19. Miller JL, Stricklin GP, Fine JD, King LE, Del Carmen Arzubiaga M, Ellis DL (1995) Remission of severe epidermolysis bullosa acquisita induced by extracorporeal photochemotherapy. Br J Dermatol 133:467–471
20. Owsianowski M, Gollnick H, Siegert W, Schwerdtfeger R, Orfanos CE (1994) Successful treatment of chronic graft-versus-host disease with extracorporeal photopheresis. Bone Marrow Transplant 14(5):845–848
21. Perez MI, Edelson RL, LaRoche L, Berger CL (1989) Inhibition of anti-skin allograft immunity by infusions with syngeneic photoinactivated effector lymphocytes. J Invest Dermatol 92: 669–674
22. Rook AH, Heald P (1995) The immunopathogenesis of cutaneous T-cell lymphoma. Hematol Oncol Clin North Am 9(5):997–1010
23. Rook AH, Jegasothy BV, Heald P, Nahass GT, Ditre C, Witmer WK, Lazarus GS, Edelson RL (1990) Extracorporeal photochemotherapy for drug-resistant pemphigus vulgaris. Ann Intern Med 112(4):303–305
24. Rook AH, Freundlich B, Jegasothy BV, Perez MI, Barr WG, Jimenez SA, Rietschel RK, Wintroub B, Kahaleh MB, Varga J (1992) Treatment of systemic sclerosis with extracorporeal photochemotherapy. Results of a multicenter trial. Arch Dermatol 128(3):337–346
25. Rose EA, Barr ML, Xu H, Pepino P, Murphy MP, McGovern MA, Ratner AJ, Watkins JF, Marboe CC, Berger CL, (1992). Photochemotherapy in human heart transplant recipients at high risk for fatal rejection. J Heart Lung Transplant 11(4):746–750
26. Rossetti F, Zulian F, Dall'Amico R, Messina C, Montini G, Zacchello F (1995) Extracorporeal photochemotherapy as single therapy for extensive, cutaneous, chronic graft-versus-host disease. Transplantation 59(1):49–51
27. Sunder-Plassman G, Druml W, Steininger R, Honigsmann H, Knobler R (1995) Renal allograft rejection controlled by photopheresis. Lancet 346(8973):506
28. Wilfert H, Honigsmann H, Steiner G, Smolen J, Wolff K, (1990). Treatment of psoriatic arthritis by extracorporeal photochemotherapy. Br J Dermatol 122(2):225–232
29. Wilson LD, Licata AL, Braverman IM, Edelson RL, Heald PW, Feldman AM, Kacinski BM (1995) Systemic chemotherapy and extracorporeal photochemotherapy and T3 and T4 cutaneous T-cell lymphoma patients who have achieved a complete response to total skin electron beam therapy. Int J Radiat Oncol 32:987–995
30. Zachariae H, Bjerring P, Heickendorff L, Moller B, Wallevik K (1992) Photopheresis and systemic sclerosis. Arch Dermatol 128(12):1651–1653
31. Zic J, Arzubiaga C, Salhany KE et al (1992) Extracorporeal photopheresis for the treatment of cutaneous T-cell lymphoma. J Am Acad Dermatol 27:729–736

Glucocorticosteroids

C.A. Akdis

Introduction

Glucocorticosteroids (also known as glucocorticoids, corticosteroids, and or adrenocorticoids; GC) are potent anti-inflammatory agents that have been used since the 1940s. Of all the pharmaceutical approaches to the treatment of allergic and inflammatory diseases, GC are undoubtedly the most commonly prescribed drugs. Glucocorticoids exist naturally in the body as endogenous hormones. They act by multiple mechanisms on various target cells and elicit pleotropic effects including the control of general inflammatory responses [13]. They influence carbohydrate, protein, and lipid metabolism; water and electrolyte balance; and functions of the immune system, cardiovascular system, kidney, skeletal muscle, nervous system, and other organs and tissues. During an inflammatory response inflammatory cells release numerous mediators. Glucocorticoids decrease the synthesis of most of the inflammatory mediators and dampen inflammation. Recently the molecular mechanism of action of GC became more apparent with the discovery of GC receptors, glucocorticoid response elements (GREs) on DNA, and the interaction of GC with transcription factors. Their clinical efficacy in certain diseases can be better understood in terms of GC action on molecular mediators and cells of inflammation.

Molecular Mechanisms of Action

Glucocorticoid Receptor

GC exert their effects through GC receptors. These exist in the cell cytoplasm as a single molecule in association with various heat-shock proteins (hsp). The current view of the way in which most GC effects are produced is illustrated in Fig. 1. The hormone (GC) is thought to penetrate into the cell where it binds to the specific receptor (R) and forms a GC-R complex. The GC receptor is a heteromer glycoprotein composed of a single steroid and DNA-binding subunit and two 90-kDa hsp [59, 92]. This complex becomes activated, releases hsp, and gains enhanced nuclear binding affinity. In addition to the steroid-binding protein and two hsp 90 monomers, the receptor has been suggested to contain several other components such as 59-kDa and 72-kDa proteins, but the status of these has not yet been established [98]. Activated GC receptor then forms nuclear-bound complex by binding to regulatory GRE [64] associated with certain genes that can activate or inhibit transcription of these genes. The proteins coded by these genes may be enzymes, secretory products, or regulators of various functions including transcription of other genes. The particular genes and proteins regulated by GC depends

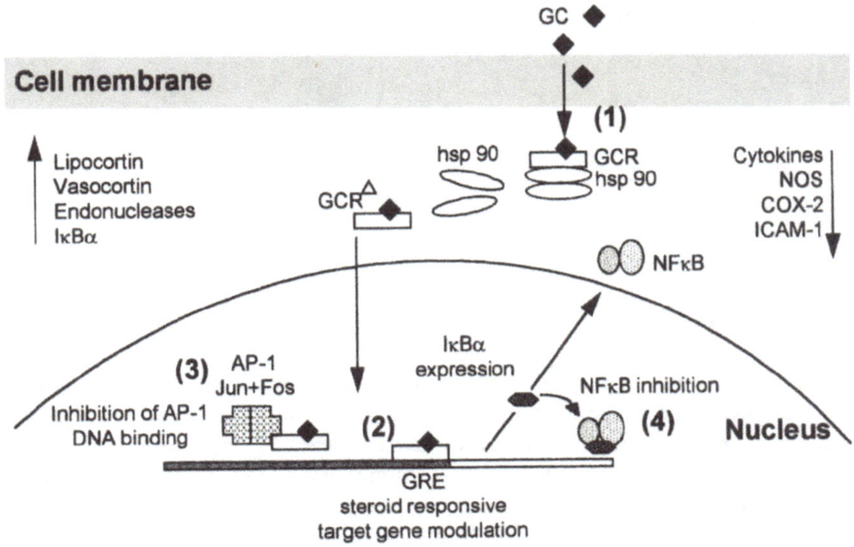

Fig. 1. Molecular mechanism of action of GC. 1, GC penetrate freely into the cell and bind to receptor (*R*) to form a complex (*GCR*). This complex becomes activated (*GCRΔ*), releases hsp, and gains enhanced nuclear binding affinity to regulatory GRE. 2, Activated GC receptor forms a protein-protein complex with the Fos component of transcription factor AP-1 and inhibits AP-1 binding to DNA. *3*, GC up-regulate inhibitor κBα levels, which traps activated NF-κB in inactive cytoplasmic complexes and functions to block nuclear translocation and DNA binding of NF-κB (*4*)

on the affected cell type. For example, a kidney cell may respond very differently than a lymphocyte. The binding of GC to GC receptors can modify the expression of many of genes in a tissue-specific manner. Several aspects of the inflammatory process can be inhibited by GC by increasing or decreasing gene transcription of certain proteins. These genes are the following:

Increased transcription
- Lipocortin
- Vasocortin
- β_2-Adrenoreceptor
- Secretory leukocyte inhibitory protein
- Plasminogen activator inhibitor
- Endonucleases
- Ribonucleases
- Neutral endopeptidase
- Receptors for hormones and cytokines (IL-1 RII)
- Migration inhibitory factor
- Somatostatin

Decreased transcription
- Cytokines (IL-1, IL-2, IL-3, IL-4, IL-5, IL-6, IL-8, IL-11, IL-12, IL-13, TNF-α, GM-CSF, RANTES, MIP-1α, SCF, IFNs)
- Nitric oxide synthase

- Cyclo-oxygenase
- Phospholipase A2
- Endothelin-1
- NK-1 receptors
- Adhesion molecules (ICAM-1)
- Elastase
- Collagenase
- Collagen
- Plasminogen activator

Interaction of Glucocorticoid Receptor with Transcription Factors

GC display their effect on responding cells by activating GC receptors to regulate certain target gene transcriptions [34]. The number of genes per cell which are directly regulated by GC is estimated to be up to 100, and many genes are regulated indirectly by interaction with other transcription factors. Activated GC receptor binds to GRE on the 5'-upstream promoter sequence of steroid-responsive genes. GREs may increase and decrease transcription, resulting in increased and decreased mRNA and protein synthesis. Other transcription factors binding in the vicinity of GRE may affect steroid inducibility.

Transcription Factor Activator Protein-1. Activated GC receptor interacts with other transcription factors which bind to each other via so-called leucine zipper interactions [70]. This interaction was first demonstrated for the collagenase gene induced by tumor necrosis factor (TNF) α and phorbol esters. Collagenase gene is induced by activator protein 1 (AP-1), which is a heterodimer of Fos and Jun oncoproteins. AP-1 binds to DNA from a specific binding site (TPA response element, TGACTCA). GC are potent inhibitors of gene transcription by means of AP-1 activation [40]. Activated GC receptor forms a protein-protein complex with the Fos component of AP-1. This prevents AP-1 binding to DNA and inhibits AP-1 from inducing the relevant inflammatory gene transcription [45].

Nuclear Factor-κB. Similar to their effect on AP-1, recently it has been demonstrated that GC can regulate nuclear factor-kB (NF-kB) [74]. Functional NF-kB binding sites have been found in the promoters of many different genes. These promoter/enhancers include interleukins (IL) 2 and 6, granulocyte-macrophage colony-stimulating factor (GM-CSF), intercellular adhesion molecule (ICAM-1), and MHC class I [10]. NF-κB binding sites are inducible transcriptional regulatory elements that respond to immunological stimuli such as TNF-α, IL-1, lipopolysaccharide, and T cell activation signals. The range of inducers is not limited to that of mediators of immune function; NF-κB is affected by growth factors, UV irradiation, and virus infection as well [10]. GC inhibit NF-κB by two mechanisms. First, several reports indicate that activated GC receptors interact directly with and inhibit NF-κB subunits [74, 81]. A second mechanism was recently reported involving the transcriptional activation of the inhibitory protein called inhibitory κBa (IκBα) gene in response to treatment with GC [8, 82]. GC upregulate IκBa protein levels, which traps activated NF-κB in inactive cytoplasmic complexes and functions to block nuclear translocation and DNA binding of NF-κB.

Role of Lipocortin in Glucocorticoid Actions

Early work on the mechanism of action of GC suggested that at least some of their effects are the consequence of inhibiting eicosanoid release [32]. A steroid-induced protein was discovered to mediate the actions of GC on eicosanoid release [16]. This protein is named lipocortin [29]; the gene has been cloned as lipocortin 1 [103]. Originally lipocortin was discovered in steroid-treated preparations, and after the isolation of the gene it was shown that lipocortin mRNA is induced by steroid treatment [103]. The basic property of all preparations of lipocortin is their ability to inhibit the enzyme PLA_2 and eicosanoid formation, which can be reversed by the addition of arachidonic acid [63]. In various models of inflammation lipocortin has been found to act in the same profile as indomethacin. It is ineffective against platelet-activating factor (PAF), serotonin, and dextran-induced edema but appears to inhibit the eicosanoid-dependent component of inflammation. However, GC are effective in all these models. Lipocortin does not mediate GC-induced inhibition of paw edema in response to injection of PAF, serotonin, or dextran [22]. Thus lipocortin appears to be one of the protein mediators of the inhibition of eicosanoid-mediated inflammation by GC, whereas a number of GC-induced anti-inflammatory effects remain to be explained by other mechanisms and protein mediators.

Glucocorticoid Effect on Cytokines

It is now well established that T cell responses are polarized by the activation of T helper (Th) cell subsets. Th1-type cells secrete IL-2 and interferon (IFN) γ and activate primarily macrophages. These cells are induced particularly during intracellular infections and are responsible for cell-mediated immune responses. In contrast, Th2-type cells produce IL-4, IL-5, IL-6, IL-10, and IL-13 and help B cells to produce antibodies [58]. A significant proportion of the activated T cells display the type-2 Th phenotype in atopic diseases by the secretion of IL-4 and IL-13 which induce IgE switching in B cells [28, 72], and IL-5 is an eosinophil differentiation and survival factor [37, 100]. In contrast, contact hypersensitivity is an inflammation in which Th_1 type cytokines predominate [41]. GC inhibit the transcription of most of the cytokines that are relevant in inflammation without discriminating Th_1 or Th_2 [5, 11, 15, 26, 61]

Cytokine genes are particularly sensitive to the inhibitory effects of GC. In the IL-6 gene four GREs have been identified close to the promoter site, and there is a blocking GRE very close to the start of transcription [75]. Such a negative regulatory GRE consensus sequence exists in the promoter region of only few cytokines, suggesting that GC inhibit transcription via different molecular mechanisms. For example, IL-2 gene transcription is potently inhibited by GC in T cells; however, there is no GRE consensus sequences in the IL-2 promoter region. IL-2 transcription is regulated by a specific nuclear factor of activated T cells (NF-AT), which requires AP-1 for increased transcription. GC appear to inhibit IL-2 transcription by binding to AP-1, thus inhibiting increased transcription due to activated NF-AT [62]. GC also down-regulate some cytokines by affecting the stability of mRNA. This is via enhanced transcription of specific ribonucleases that lead to shortened turnover time of mRNA and has been demonstrated for certain cytokines such as IFN, GM-CSF, IL-1β, IL-3, and IL-6 [44, 65, 91].

Keratinocytes use IL-1α and transforming growth factor (TGF) α for growth in cultures, and they also produce IL-1α and TGF-α. These two cytokines induce the production of themselves in an autocrine loop. It has been proposed that this autocrine loop is hyperactive in psoriasis. GC inhibit the synthesis of both IL-1α and TGF-α keratinocytes and break down the autocrine mechanism [48]. Antagonism of the effects of this autocrine loop may be one of the mechanisms by which GC exert clinically useful effects in psoriasis and other diseases of the skin.

Macrophage migration inhibitory factor (MIF) is known as a T cell, pituitary and macrophage cytokine with proinflammatory activity. MIF and GC appear to be a unique counterregulatory system that functions to control inflammatory and immune responses. In contrast to other cytokines, GC induce MIF production from macrophages [19]. MIF then acts to override GC-mediated inhibition of cytokine secretion by lipopolysaccharide-stimulated monocytes to overcome GC protection against lethal endotoxemia.

GC inhibit not only the synthesis of cytokines but also the effect of cytokines on target cells. This inhibition is mediated mainly through nuclear factors that are inactivated by GC. As in the case of TNF-α receptor signaling in macrophages and that of IL-2 receptor signaling in T cells, cytokine receptor signaling through AP-1 or NF-κB is inhibited by GC [10]. GC also modify the transcription of genes coding surface receptors. IL-1 acts at two types of surface receptors, called IL-1 RI and IL-1 RII. IL-1 RII has no signaling activity but binds IL-1 and therefore acts as a molecular trap. GC are potent inducers of this decoy IL-1 receptor, which leads to release of a soluble form of the receptor and thus reduces the functional activity of IL-1 [76].

Glucocorticoid Effect on Adhesion Molecules

Adhesion molecules play a key role in the trafficking of inflammatory cells to sites of inflammation. The expression of many adhesion molecules on endothelial cells is induced by cytokines, and GC may lead indirectly to reduced expression via their inhibitory effects on cytokines such as IL-1β and TNF-α. IL-4 and IL-13 activate the endothelium to express vascular cell adhesion molecule 1 which has a counterligand very late activation antigen 4 [18, 88]. Cells expressing very late activation antigen 4 include basophils, eosinophils, monocytes, and lymphocytes, but not neutrophils. This appears to be the main mechanism for the trafficking of eosinophils in allergic inflammatory sites, whereas neutrophils are not generally associated with allergic inflammation. As with the nonspecific endothelial activators IL-4 and IL-13, production is inhibited by GC. GC may also have a direct effect on the expression of adhesion molecules such as ICAM-1 and E-selectin at the level of gene transcription [25]. The effect on ICAM-1 expression is presumably through inhibition of NF-κB, which plays a role for the induction of ICAM-1 [99]. ICAM-1 expression is induced by IFN-γ in keratinocyte cultures, and in contrast to other findings, GC do not display a direct inhibitory effect on ICAM-1 expression on keratinocytes [43].

Other Molecules of Glucocorticoid Action

Nitric oxide synthase (NOS) is induced by proinflammatory cytokines resulting in increased nitric oxide production. Nitric oxide may increase blood flow, and plasma exudation in inflamed skin. The induction of inducible form of NOS (iNOS) is potently inhibited by GC [73]. NF-κB appears to be the most important transcription factor for iNOS inhibition [109]. GC also inhibit the induction of the gene coding for inducible cyclo-oxygenase (COX-2) in monocytes and epithelial cells [60]. Another mechanism for suppression of the inflammatory reaction by GC is via stimulation of local somatostatin expression, which occurs in parallel to the inhibition of the local inflammatory mediators [42]. GC reduce the neurokinin-1 receptor [1] and increase the expression of β2-adrenoreceptors [24], each of which may be relevant for their beneficial effects on asthmatic lung inflammation. The effect on neurokinin receptor is through AP-1 inhibition whereas the human β_2-adrenoreceptor has three potential GREs which function to increase the rate of transcription [96]. The major influence of GC on healthy skin decreases the skin tickness by inducing atrophy [38]. GC treatment suppresses the synthesis of both type I and type II collagen in the dermis, which may be responsible for atrophy [9].

Impact of Glucocorticoids on Inflammatory Cells

GC may have both direct and indirect inhibitory actions on several inflammatory cells involved in a wide range of inflammatory conditions of the skin. A brief description is presented below of the role which each cell type may play in inflammation, followed by a synopsis of the effects of GC on the function, proliferation, and regulation of the cell type both in vitro and in vivo.

Lymphocytes

There is considerable evidence that T cells play a role in regulating the cellular composition of the inflammatory cell infiltrate in tissues via cytokines. Mucosal mast cells are under the control of T cells via production of IL-3 [39]. In addition, murine connective tissue mast cells can proliferate under the combined action of IL-3 and IL-4 [36]. T lymphocytes are major sources for a number of cytokines that contribute to the growth and differentiation of effector cells of inflammation. In addition, there is a relationship between T cell activation and erythema nodosum formation [2]. GC effectively inhibit T cell activation and cytokine production both in patients on GC therapy [61] and in an in vivo mouse system [5]

It was surprising and of concern that GC were shown to increase the synthesis of total IgE in various in vitro systems and in vivo; this led to debates on whether potential IgE-enhancing effects of GC conceal detrimental effects to allergic patients undergoing GC treatment [47, 108]. The effect of GC has been analyzed in a human culture system that allows the production of allergen (bee venom phospholipase A_2) specific IgE antibodies from bee venom sensitized individuals [3]. GC selectively inhibited the production of specific IgE and IgG, while the formation of total IgE increased, as in previous reports [47, 108]. The inhibitory effect on specific IgE and IgG production was mediated by T cells since GC did not affect either specific or total IgE and IgG production of purified B cells. The inhibitory effect of GC on specific antibody synthesis was in parallel to suppression of T cell proliferation and cytokine production. Furthermore, GC inhibit the surface expression of accessory molecules such as ICAM-1 and E-selectin [25]. They also induce and regulate T cell apoptosis [112]. Thus, GC most likely reduce antigen-specific IgE and IgG production by inhibition of specific T cell–B cell collabo-

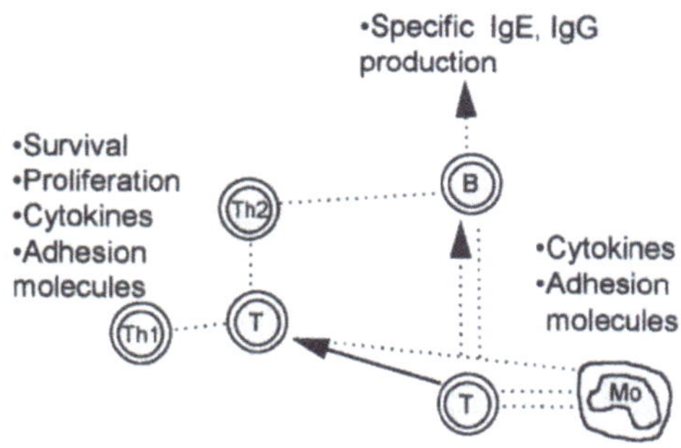

Fig. 2. Effect of GC on antigen-specific immune response. GC inhibit the development of antigen-specific immune response through inhibition of cytokines and adhesion molecules during APC–T cell interaction. They inhibit proliferation, cytokine production, adhesion molecule expression, and induce apoptosis in T cells without Th1–Th2 discrimination. They also down-regulate de novo induced antigen-specific IgE and IgG production of B cells

ration by inhibiting relevant cytokine production and adhesion molecule expression. Together these results suggest that GC affect the interaction between antigen-presenting cells (APC) and T cells in antigen-specific immune responses. Figure 2 describes the negative regulatory effects of GC on T cell, B cell, and monocyte interaction during the development of antigen-specific immune response.

Monocytes and Macrophages

Monocytes and macrophages are "professional" APC with phagocytosis capacity. Upon antigen presentation they induce profound T cell activation, cytokine production and proliferation [4]. Macrophages activate endothelial cells by two main cytokines, IL-1 and TNF-α, which initiate leukocyte recruitment to tissues in inflammation [69]. They also contribute to inflammation with a number of lipid mediators, nitric oxide, enzymes such as elastase, collagenase, and lysozyme, cytokines and by inducing coagulation cascade.

Monocytes and macrophages are the most sensitive cells to anti-inflammatory effects of GC [35]. Administration of GC markedly diminishes the number of circulating monocytes, especially the FcεR-bearing subset in the circulation [56, 105]. They also reduce the number of skin macrophages [14]. The release of all inflammatory mediators is efficiently inhibited by GC [35, 97, 106]. GC inhibit the intracellular killing of various phagocytosed micro-organisms by macrophages, thus showing strong immunosuppressive activity against intracellular micro-organisms [80].

Dendritic Cells

Dendritic cells are mononuclear cells that can present antigen, and which constitute less than 1% of peripheral blood mononuclear cells. They differ from other immunocytes that they are MHC class II positive but lack Fc receptors and specific lymphocyte and monocyte markers. Dendritic cells use IL-4 and GM-CSF as growth factors, and IFN-γ upregulates their MHC class II expression [49, 78]. GC have been shown to down-regulate MHC class II expression in dendritic cells [49] and indirectly inhibit their growth and antigen-presentation capacity by inhibition of T cell cytokines [55]. Langerhans cells are $CD1^+$ dendritic cells in skin and mucosa and possess a high-affinity receptor for IgE. Local steroid treatment decreases the tissue number of $CD1^+$ cells and other HLA-DR positive cells in tissues [33].

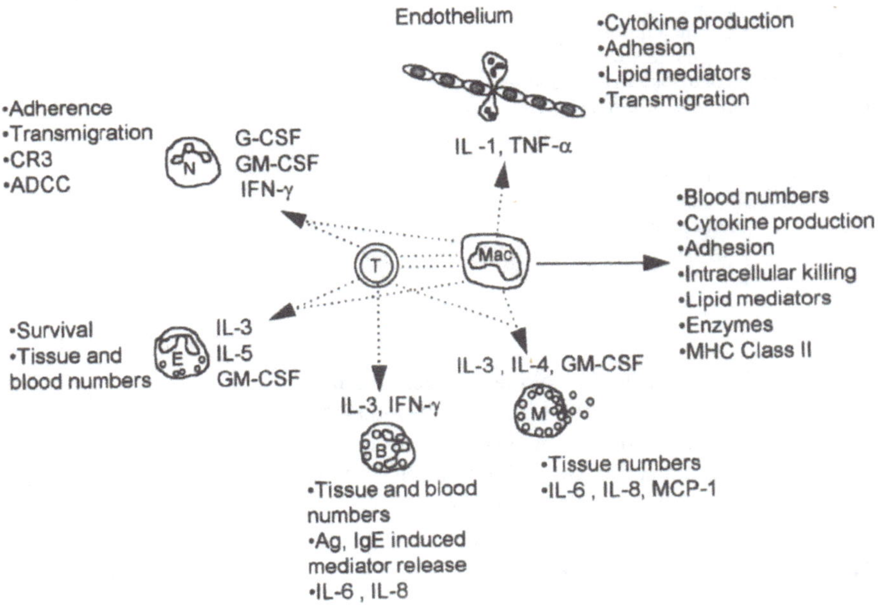

Fig. 3. Impact of glucocortocoids on effector cells of inflammation. Anti-inflammatory effects of GC are mediated by negative regulation of the inflammatory function and mediators of the inflammatory cells: endothelium, macrophage (Mac), mast cell (*M*), basophil (*B*), eosinophil (*E*), and neutrophil (*N*). The inhibition of cytokine production by T cells and macrophages, which regulate priming, activation, and survival of effector cells, displays the dominant anti-inflammatory action of GC

Mast Cells

GC down-regulate inflammatory responses by direct or indirect actions on effector cells of inflammation such as mast cells, basophils, eosinophils, neutrophils, and endothelial cells (Fig. 3). Recent studies demonstrate that mast cells are capable of producing cytokines and chemokines distinct from mast cell chemical mediators. The production of IL-3, IL-4, IL-5, IL-6, IL-8, and TNF-α has been shown in mast cells upon antigen or phorbol ester/calcium ionophore stimulation [39, 50, 83]. Dexamethasone potently suppresses the production of IL-6 and IL-8 from both mast cell and basophil lines [50]. Mast cells are also source for a number of chemokines, including I-309, monocyte chemoatractant protein (MCP) 1, macrophage inflammatory proteins (MIPs) 1α and 1β, and RANTES [90]. Interestingly, prednisolone has been shown to inhibit only mast cell MCP-1 production whereas GC have more distinct and general effects on T cell chemokines [89, 90].

In experimental allergen challenge systems in humans GC are widely agreed to be effective in dampening or completely blocking the appearance of the late-phase reaction following allergen challenge in skin, upper airways, and lungs [54, 67, 71]. Mast cells are responsible for the immediate acute-phase response in these experimental models. GC do not inhibit the release of preformed mediators such as histamine, prostaglandin D_2, leukotrienes B_4 and D_4, and PAF from human mast cells. They do inhibit the vascular permeability response and the mucus secretory response of the target tissues [83]. Most studies have found that oral GC treatment fails to block the acute phase of the experimental allergen challenge response in skin, nose, and lungs [54, 67, 71]. However, topically applied GC preparations have been demonstrated to decrease reaction severity, prevent the physiological response, and reduce mast cell mediators of the acute response to allergen challenge [6, 68].

Basophils

Increased numbers of basophils are visible during late allergic reactions in the skin and upper airways [12, 104]. GC treatment appears to be effective on basophils in many ways. First, GC treatment reduces the number of circulating basophils by more than 80 % [77]. Second, GC inhibit the release of allergen and IgE-dependent histamine and leukotriene C4 in long-term cultured peripheral blood basophils [84, 85]. Third, IL-3 and IFN-γ are two T cell cytokines which play a role on activation and priming of basophils. By blocking the release of IL-3 and IFN-γ from T cells GC can indirectly inhibit basophil priming and release of mediators [86]. Fourth, as with mast cells, basophils have the capacity to produce various cytokines. Dexamethasone inhibits the production of IL-6 and IL-8 from human basophils [50].

GC have been shown to inhibit the local accumulation of basophils during the allergen-induced late-phase reaction in both skin and upper airways [12, 21]. In this respect dexamethasone acts directly on basophils to inhibit the migration caused by C5a, IL-3, and IL-8 [110]. However, basophil adherence in vitro to cultured cytokine activated vascular endothelial cells is not inhibited by GC [17].

Eosinophils

Eosinophils are effector inflammatory cells with the ability to release inflammatory lipid mediators and high-charged cationic proteins. Their inflammatory features are negatively affected by GC in a number of ways. Injection and oral administration of GC causes a marked fall in the number of circulating eosinophils [7, 79]. In addition, GC have a therapeutic effect by reducing or eliminating hypodense eosinophils, which has been associated with hypereosinophilia [46]. During the late phase of allergic reactions GC treatment reduces eosinophil accumulation in the skin and upper respiratory tract. Earlier studies interpreted this effect as possibly due to the inhibition of eosinophil chemotaxis and diapedesis [31]. In the last few years, however, evidence has been accumulated that eosinophilia in allergic disorders is an outcome of increased eosinophil survival or inhibited eosinophil apoptosis [94, 95]. IL-3, IL-5, and GM-CSF are cytokines that have marked effects on eosinophil activation and survival [37, 101]. GC exhibit an antagonistic effect on the viability of eosinophils cultured in the presence of suboptimal concentrations of GM-CSF, IL-3, and IL-5 [37]. GC also inhibit eosinophil survival by decreasing the synthesis of survival factors from T cells (IL-3, IL-5, GM-CSF), macrophages (GM-CSF), and endothelial cells (GM-CSF) [57, 93, 101, 102]. Thus, as discussed repeatedly for all of the other inflammatory cells throughout this chapter, GC display an indirect effect by inhibiting the release or action of cytokines. This has potential importance in their mechanism of anti-inflammatory action.

Neutrophils

Neutrophils are the major cells in the circulating leukocytes and make up some 50–65 % of overall leukocyte pool. Almost twice the number of circulating neutrophils are thought to exist in the capillary marginal pool ready to transmigrate to tissues upon chemotactic stimuli. In their cytoplasmic granules they contain many tissue-destructive proteolytic enzymes. They can produce arachidonic acid metabolites and active oxygen radicals, and phagocytose and kill micro-organisms. Extracellular release of cytotoxic substances by neutrophils can also occur when they are activated through their Fcγ receptors by immune complexes. This may be an important pathogenic mechanism in immune-complex diseases [52].

The GC response pattern of human neutrophils differs from that of other inflammatory cells. Upon a single dose of parenteral steroid most circulating inflammatory cell types decrease in number while the number of neutrophils increases by a factor of 2–4 [7]. Culture of human neutrophils or treatment with GC vivo leads to reduced adherence capacities [23]. This presumably results from the inhibition of complement receptor 3 (CR3) and may explain the demargination of neutrophils seen with GC treatment [66]. IFN-γ increases expression of CR3 and antibody-dependent cell cytotoxic activity (ADCC) in neutrophils. The culture of neutrophils in GC effectively inhibits ADCC activity [66]. In addition, oral steroid treatment inhibits the influx of neutrophils in cutaneous late-phase reactions [53]. The inhibition of neutrophil emigration to tissues is likely to be mediated predominantly via inhibition of local release of the factors that activate endothelium [30, 111]. However, GC does not affect neutrophil release of leukotriene B_4 or lysosomal enzymes [87].

Endothelial Cells

The endothelium was earlier regarded as a passive barrier between circulation and tissues. According to the current view, however, the vascular endothelium comprises active cells that take part in inflammation by production of proinflammatory cytokines, coagulation factors, lipid mediators, and expression of adhesion molecules. Vascular permeability is an important feature of inflammatory edema. GC inhibit inflammatory edema in various ways. First, by suppressing the generation of permeability increasing or vasodilator mediators such as arachidonic acid mediators, nitric oxide, and PAF [107]. Second, they induce the synthesis of a protein called vasocortin that inhibits microvascular permeability responses by an action on endothelium [20]. Third, by leukocyte-endothelial cell interaction inhibition through cytokines such as IL-1, IL-8, and TNF-α and adhesion molecules such as CR3 and CD11/CD18 [27, 107]. Endothelial cells, such as macrophages, are a GC-sensitive cell type. GC inhibit arachidonic acid metabolite formation and MHC class II expression from endothelium, but adhesion glucoproteins such as E-selection are not affected directly [27]

Discussion

Clinical administration of GC began about 50 years ago; however, their molecular mechanism of action has only been understood in the past decade. GC have become the drug of choice in many allergic and inflammatory diseases and are commonly used in organ transplantation and chemotherapy protocols. Unfortunately, the limiting factor in their use are side effects which are important and sometimes life threatening. Higher doses can be introduced to target organ, and some of the side effects can be decreased or eliminated with their topical use as creams, ointments, sprays, and inhalants. The development of GC preparations suitable for topical administration has revolutionized the therapy of a number of common skin diseases. Maibach and Stoughton [51] have classified 20 dermatological disorders that respond to topical GC.

GC are nature's remedy for inflammation as endogenous substances existing in the circulation. The up-regulated and down-regulated genes by GC indicate important targets of anti inflammatory therapy. Many of these genes are also affected by other anti-inflammatory molecules. Although a number of points still remain to be clarified, the known molecular mechanism of action of GC can serve as an area of future studies in the discovery of new anti-inflammatory molecules.

Summary

Glucocorticosteroids are frequently used immunosuppressive and anti-inflammatory agents that act through multiple mechanisms with a wide range of effects in inflammatory or immune mediated components of diseases. This chapter provides an updated outline of the molecular mechanisms by which glucocorticosteroids display anti-inflammatory effects. The molecular mechanism of action is linked to vivo or vitro glucocorticosteroid effects on individual inflammatory cells and experimental inflammation models of the skin and other organs.

Acknowledgements. The author thanks Drs. K. Blaser and H.-U. Simon, Swiss Institute of Allergy and Asthma Research, Davos, Switzerland, for critical review and enlightening suggestions in the writing this chapter and Uludag University, Bursa, Turkey, for continuous support.

References

1. Adcock IM, Peters M, Gelder C, Shiraski H, Brown CR, Barnes PJ (1993) Increased tachykinin receptor gene expression in asthmatic lung and its modulation by steroids. J Mol Endocrinol 11:1–7
2. Akdis CA, Kilicturgay K, Helvaci S, Mistik R, Oral B (1993) Immunological evaluation of erythema nodosum in tularaemia. Br J Dermatol 129:275–279
3. Akdis CA, Blesken T, Akdis M, Alkan SS, Wuthrich B, Heusser C, Blaser K (1997) Induction and differential regulation of bee venom phospholipase A2-specific human IgE and IgG4 antibodies vitro requires allergen-specific and non-specific activation of T and B cells. J Allergy Clin Immunol 99:345–353
4. Akdis CA, Blesken T, Wymann D, Akdis M, Faith A, Blaser K (1996) Allergen conformation dependent T cell cytokine and antibody isotype patterns in bee sting sensitized subjects. J Allergy Clin Immunol 97:246
5. Alkan SS, Akdis CA, Feuerlein D, Gruninger M (1996) Direct measurement of cytokines (IFN-γ IL-4, -5, and -6) from organs after antigenic challenge. Ann NY Acad Sci 796:82–90
6. Andersson M, Pipkorn U (1987) Inhibition of the dermal immediate allergic reaction through prolonged treatment with topical glucocorticosteroids. J Allergy Clin Immunol 79:345–349
7. Athens JW, Haab OP, Raab SO (1961) The total blood, circulating and marginal granulocyte pools and the granulocyte turnover rate in normal subjects. J Clin Invest 40:989–995

8. Auphan N, DiDonato JA, Rosette C, Helberg A, Karin M (1995) Immunosuppression by glucocorticoids: inhibition of NF-κB activity through induction of I-κB synthesis Science 270:286–290
9. Autio P, Oukarinen A, Melkko J, Ristelli J, Ristelli L (1994) Systemic glucocorticoids decrease the synthesis of type I and type II collagen in human skin in vivo, whereas isoretinoin treatment has little effect. Br J Dermatol 131:660–663
10. Baldwin AS (1996) The NF-κB and I-κB proteins: new discoveries and insights. Annu Rev Immunol 14:649–681
11. Barton BE, Jakway JP, Smith SR, Siegel MI (1991) Cytokine inhibition by a novel steroid, mometasone furoate. Immunopharmacol Immunotoxicol 13:251–261
12. Bascom RB, Wachs M, Naclerio RM, Pipkorn U, Galli SJ, Lichtenstein LM (1988) Basophil influx occurs after nasal antigen challenge: effects of topical corticosteroid pretreatment. J Allergy Clin Immunol 81:581–589
13. Basedowsky H, Rey AD, Sorkin H, Dinarello CA (1986) Immunoregulatory feedback between interleukin-1 and glucocorticoid hormones. Science 893:652–654
14. Belsito DV, Flotte TJ, Lim HW, Baer RC, Thoebecke GJ, Gigli I (1982) Effect of glucocorticosteroids on epidermal Langerhans cells. J Exp Med 155:291–302
15. Beutler B, Krochin N, Milsark IW, Luedke C, Cerami A (1986) Control of cachectin (tumor necrosis factor) synthesis: mechanisms of endotoxin resistance. Science 232:977–980
16. Blackwell GJ, Carnuccio R, Di Rosa M, Flower RJ, Parente L, Persico P (1980) Macrocortin: a polypeptide causing the anti-phospholipase effect of glucocorticoids. Nature 287:147–149
17. Bochner BS, Peachell PT, Brown KE, Schleimer RP (1988) Adherence of human basophils to cultured umbilical vein endothelial cells. J Clin Invest 81:1355–1364
18. Bochner BS, Klunk DA, Sterbinsky SA, Coffman RL, Schleimer RP (1995) Interleukin-13 selectively induces vascular cell adhesion molecule-1 (VCAM-1) expression in human endothelial cells. J Immunol 154:799–803
19. Calandra T; Bernhagen J, Metz CN, Spiegel LA, Bacher M, Donnelly T, Cerami A, Bucala R (1995) MIF as a glucocorticoid induced modulator of cytokine production. Nature 377:68–71
20. Carnuccio R, Rosa MD, Guerrasio B, Ialenti A, Sautebin L (1987) Vasocortin: a novel glucocorticoid-induced anti-inflammatory protein. Br J Pharmacol 90:443–445
21. Charlesworth EN, Kagey-Sobotka A, Schleimer RP, Norman PS, Lichtenstein LM (1991) Prednisone inhibits the appearance of inflammatory mediators and the influx of eosinophils and basophils associated with the cutaneous late-phase response to allergen. J Immunol 146: 71–676
22. Cirino G, Peers SH, Flower RJ Browning JL, Pepinsky RB (1988) Human recombinant lipocortin 1 has acute local anti-inflammatory properties in the rat paw oedema test. Proc Natl Acad Sci USA 86:3428–3432
23. Clark RAF, Gallin JI, Fauci AS (1979) Effects vitro prednisone on in vitro eosinophil and neutrophil adherence and chemotaxis. Blood 53:633–641
24. Collins S, Caron MG, Lefkowitz RJ (1988) β-Adrenergic receptors in hamster smooth muscle cells are transcriptionally regulated by glucocorticoids. J Biol Chem 263:9067–9070
25. Cronstein BN, Kimmel SC, Levin RI, Martiniuk F, Weissmann G (1992) A mechanism for the anti-inflammatory effects of corticosteroids: the glucocorticoid receptor regulates leukocyte adhesion to endothelial cells and expression of endothelial leukocyte adhesion molecule-1 and intercellular adhesion molecule-1. Proc Natl Acad Sci USA 89:9991–9995
26. Culpepper JA, Lee F (1985) Regulation of IL-3 expression by glucocorticoids in cloned murine T lymphocytes. J Immunol 135:3191–3197
27. Cybulsky MI, McComb DJ, Dinarello CA, Movat HZ (1987) Mediation by interleukin-1 of neutrophil leukocyte emigration induced by endotoxin. In: Movat HZ (ed) Leukocyte emigration and its sequelae. Karger, Basel, pp 38–50
28. Del Prete G, Maggi E, Paola P, Ghretien I, Tiri A, Macchia D, Banchereau J, De Vries JE, Romagnani S (1988) IL-4 is an essential factor for the IgE synthesis induced vitro by human T cell clones and their supernatants. J Immunol 140:4193–4198
29. Di Rosa M, Flower RJ, Hirata F, Parente L, Russo-Marie F (1984) Nomenclature announcement. Anti-phospholipase proteins. Prostaglandins 28:441–442

30. Doukas J, Hechtinan HB, Shepro D (1988) Endothelial secreted arachidonic acid metabolites modulate polymorphonuclear leukocyte chemotaxis and diapedesis in vitro. Blood 71: 771–779
31. Eidinger D, Wilkinson R, Bose B (1964) A study of cellular responses in immune reactions utilizing the skin window technique. J Allergy 35:77–85
32. Flower RJ (1988) Lipocortin the mechanism of action of glucocorticoids. Br J Pharmacol 94:987–1015
33. Godthelp T, Holm AF, Blom H, Klein-Jan A, Rijntjes E, Fokkens WJ (1995) The effect of flucitasone propionate aqueous nasal spray on nasal mucosal inflammation in perennial allergic rhinitis. Allergy 50 [Suppl 23]:21–24
34. Gronemeyer H (1992) Control of transcription activation by steroid hormone receptors. FASEB J 6:2524–2529
35. Guyre PM, Munck A (1988) Glucocorticoid actions on monocytes and macrophages. In: Schleimer RP, Claman HN, Oronsky AR (eds) Antiinflammatory steroids: basic and clinical aspects. Academic, New York, pp 199–225
36. Hamaguchi Y, Kanakura Y, Fujita Jtakeda S, Nakano T, Tarui S, Honjo T, Kitamura Y (1987) Interleukin 4 is an essential factor for vitro clonal growth of murine connective tissue-type mast cells. J Exp Med 165:268–273
37. Her E, Frazer J, Austen F, Owen WF (1991) Eosinophil hematopoietins antagonize the programmed cell death of eosinophils. Cytokine and glucocorticoid effects on eosinophils maintained by endothelial cell conditioned medium. J Clin Invest 88:1982–1987
38. Iwasaki K, Mishima E, Miura M, Sakai N, Shimao S (1995) Effect of RU 486 on the atrophogenic and antiinflammatory effects of glucocorticoids in skin. J Dermatol Sci 10:151–158
39. Jarrett EEE, Haig DM (1984) Mucosal mast cells vivo and in vitro. Immunol Today 5:115–118
40. Jonat C, Rahmsdorf HJ, Park KK, Cato ACB, Gebel S, Ponta H, Herrlich P (1990) Anti-tumor promotion and anti-inflammation: down modulation of AP-1 (fos/jun) activity by glucocorticoid hormone. Cell 62:1189–1204
41. Kapsenberg ML, Wierenga EA, Stiekerna FEM, Tiggelman AMBC, Bos JD (1992) Th1 lymphokine production profiles of Ni-specific CD4+ T-lymphocyte clones from Ni contact allergic and non allergic individuals. J Invest Dermatol 98:59–63
42. Karalis K, Mastorakos G, Sano H, Wilder RL, Chrousos GP (1995) Somatostatin may participate in the anti-inflammatory actions of glucocorticoids. Endocrinology 136:4133–4138
43. Kashihara-Swami M, Norris DA (1992) The state of differentiation of cultured human keratinocytes determines the level of intercellular adhesion molecule-1 (ICAM-1) expression induced by gamma-interferon. J Invest Dermatol 98:741–747
44. Kern JA, Lamb JR, Reed JL, Daniele RP and Nowell PL (1988) Dexamethasone inhibition of interleukin 1 beta production by human monocytes: post transcriptional mechanism. J Clin Invest 81:237–244
45. Kerrpola TK, Luk D, Curran T (1993) Fos is preferential target of glucocorticoid receptor inhibition of AP-1 activity in vitro. Mol Cell Biol 13:3782–3790
46. Lamas AM, Marcotte GV, Schleimer RP (1989) Human endothelial cells prolong eosinophil survival. Regulation by cytokines and glucocorticoids. J Immunol 142:3978–3984
47. Lane SJ, Kemeny DM (1994) Glucocorticoids and IgE: an vitro paradox. Clin Exp Allergy 24:1001–1004
48. Lee SW, Morhenn WB, Ilnicka M, Eugui EM, Allison AC (1991) Autocrine stimulation of interleukin-1 alpha and transforming growth factor alpha production in human keratinocytes and its antagonism by glucocorticoids. J Invest Dermatol 97:106–110
49. Leszczynski D, Ferry B, Schellekens H, van der Meide PH, Harry P (1986) Antagonistic effects of gamma interferon and steroids on tissue antigenicity. J Exp Med 164:1470–1477
50. Lippert U, Kruger-Krasagakes S, Moller A, Kiessling U, Czarnetzki BM (1995) Pharmacological modulation of IL-6 and IL-8 secretion by the H1-antagonists decarboethoxy-loratadine and dexamethasone by human mast and basophilic cell lines. Exp Dermatol 4:272–276
51. Maibach HI, Stoughton RB (1973) Topical corticosteroids. Med Clin North Am 57:1253–1264
52. Malech HL, Gallin JI (1987) Neutrophils in human diseases. N Engl J Med 317:687–694

53. Mancini RE, Colombi PA, Galli H, Orcivoli L (1961) Effect of glucocorticoids on experimentally induced allergic reactions on human skin. J Allergy 32:471–482
54. Martin GL, Atkins PC, Dunsky EH, Zweiman B (1980) Effects of theophylline, terbutaline, and prednisone on antigen-induced bronchospasm and mediator release. J Allergy Clin Immunol 66:204–212
55. McWilliam AS, Nelson DJ, Holt PG (1995) The biology of airway dendritic cells. Immunol Cell Biol 73:405–413
56. Melewicz FM, Zeiger RS, Mellon MH, O'Connor RD, Spiegelberg HL (1981) Increased peripheral blood monocytes with Fc receptors for IgE in patients with severe allergic disorders. J Immunol 126:1292–1295
57. Metcalf D (1985) The granulocyte-macrophage colony stimulating factors. Science 229:16–22
58. Mosmann TR, Sad S (1996) The expanding universe of T-cell subsets: Th1, Th2 and more. Immunol Today 17:142–146
59. Munck A, Mendel DB, Smith LI, Orti E (1990) Glucocorticoid receptors and actions. Am Rev Respir Dis 141:S2–S10
60. O'Banion MK, Winn VD, Young DA (1992) cDNA cloning and functional activity of a glucocorticoid regulated inflammatory cyclooxygenase. Proc Natl Acad Sci USA 89:4888–4892
61. Oehling AG, Akdis CA, Shapowal A, Blaser K, Schmitz M, Simon H-U (1997) Suppression of the immune system by oral glucocorticoid therapy in bronchial asthma. Allergy 52:144–154
62. Paliogianni F, Raptis A, Ahuja SS, Najjar SM, Boumpas DT (1993) Negative transcriptional regulation of human interleukin 2 (IL-2) gene by glucocorticoids through interference with nuclear transcription factors AP-1 and NF-AT. J Clin Invest 91:1481–1489
63. Parente L, Di Rosa M, Flower RJ, Ghiara P, Meli R, Persico P, Salmon JA, Wood JN (1984) Relationship between the anti-phospholipase and anti-inflammatory effects of glucocorticoid proteins. Eur J Pharmacol 99:233–299
64. Payvar F, Wrange Ö, Carlstedt-Duke J, Okret S, Gustafsson JA, Yamamoto KR (1981) Purified glucocorticoid receptors bind selectively vitro to a cloned DNA fragment whose transcription is regulated by glucocorticoids vivo. Proc Natl Acad Sci USA 78:6628–6632
65. Peppel K, Vinci JM, Baglioni C (1991) The AU-rich sequences in the 3' untranslated region mediate the increased turnover of interferon mRNA induced by glucocorticoids. J Exp Med 173:349–355
66. Petroni KC, Shen L, Guyre PM (1988) Modulation of human polymorphonuclear leukocyte IgG Fc receptors and Fc receptor mediated functions by IFN-gamma and glucocorticoids. J Immunol 140:3467–3472
67. Pipkorn U, Proud D, Lichtenstein LM, Schleimer RP, Peters SP, Adkinson NF Jr, Kagey-Sobotka A, Norman PS, Naclerio RM (1987a) Effect of short-term systemic glucocorticoid treatment on human nasal mediator release after antigen challenge J Clin Invest 80:957–961
68. Pipkorn U, Proud D, Lichtenstein LM, Kagey-Sobotka A, Norman PS, Naclerio RM (1987b) Inhibition of mediator release in allergic rhinitis by pretreatment by topical glucocorticosteroids. N Engl J Med 316:1506–1510
69. Pohlman TH, Stanness KA, Beatty PG, Ochs HD, Harlan JM (1986) An endothelial cell surface factor(s) induced vitro by lipopolysaccharide, interleukin 1, and tumor necrosis factor-a increases neutrophil adherence by a Cdw18 dependent mechanism. J Immunol 136:4548–4553
70. Ponta H, Cato ACB, Herrlich P (1992) Interference of specific transcription factors. Biochim Biophys Acta 1129:255–261
71. Poothullil J, Umemoto L, Dolovich J, Hargreave FE, Day RP (1976) Inhibition by prednisolone of late cutaneous allergic responses induced by antiserum to human IgE. J Allergy Clin Immunol 57:164–167
72. Punnonen J, Aversa G, Cocks BG, Mc Kenzie ANJ, Menon S, Zurawski G, De Waal Melefyt R, and De Vries JE (1993) Interleukin-13 induces interleukin-4 independent IgG4 and IgE synthesis and CD23 expression by human B cells. Proc Natl Acad Sci USA 90:3730–3734.
73. Radomski MW, Palmer RMJ, Moncada S (1990) Glucocorticoids inhibit the expression of an inducible, but not the constitutive nitric oxide synthase in vascular endothelial cells. Proc Natl Acad Sci USA 87:10043–10049

74. Ray A, Prefontaine KE (1994) Physical association and functional antagonism between the p65 subunit of transcription factor NF-kappa B and the glucocorticoid receptor. Proc Natl Acad Sci USA 91:752
75. Ray A, Laforge KS, Sehgal PB (1990) On the mechanisms for efficient repression of the interleukin-6 promoter by glucocorticoids: enhancer TATA box and RNA start site (1 nr motif) occlusion. Moll Cell Biol 10:5736–5746
76. Re F, Muzio M, De Rossi N, Polentarutti N, Giri JG, Mantovani A, Colatta F (1994) The type II receptor as a decoy target for interleukin 1 in polymorphonuclear leukocytes: characterization of induction by dexamethasone and ligand binding properties of the released decoy receptor. J Exp Med 179:739–743
77. Saavedra-Delgado AMP, Mathews KP, Pan PM, Kay DR, Muilenberg ML (1980) Dose response studies of the suppression of whole blood histamine and basophil counts by prednisone. J Allergy Clin Immunol 66:464–471
78. Salusto F, Lanzavecchia A (1994) Efficient presentation of soluble antigen by cultured human dendritic cells is maintained by granulocyte/macrophage colony-stimulating factor plus interleukin 4 and down-regulated by tumor necrosis factor alpha. J Exp Med 179:1109–1118
79. Saunders RH, Adams E (1950) Changes in circulating leukocytes following the administration of adrenal cortex extract (ACE) and adrenocorticotropic hormone (ACTH) in infectious mononucleosis and chronic lymphatic leukaemia. Blood 5:732–741
80. Schaffner A (1985) Therapeutic concentrations of glucocorticoids suppress the antimicrobial activity of human macrophages without impairing their responsiveness to gamma interferon. J Clin Invest 76:1755–1764
81. Scheinman R, Gualberto A, Jewell C, Cidlowski J, Baldwin A (1995) Characterization of mechanisms involved in transrepression of NF-κB by activated glucocorticoid receptors. Mol Cell Biol 15:943–953
82. Scheinman R, Cogswell P, Lofquist A, Baldwin A (1995) Role of transcriptional activation of IκBα in mediation of immunosuppression by glucocorticoids. Science 270:283–286
83. Schleimer RP (1990) Effects of glucocorticosteroids on inflammatory cells relevant to their therapeutic applications in asthma. Am Rev Respir Dis 141:S59–S69
84. Schleimer RP, Lichtenstein LM, Gillespie E (1981) Inhibition of basophil histamine release by antiinflammatory steroids. Nature 292:454–455
85. Schleimer RP, Davidson DA, Peters SP, Lichtenstein LM (1985) Inhibition of basophil leukotriene release by antiinflammatory steroids. Int Arch Allergy Appl Immunol 77:241–243
86. Schleimer RP, Derse CP, Friedman B, Gillis S, Plaut M, Lichtenstein LM, MacGlashan DW Jr (1989) Regulation of human basophil mediator release by cytokines. I. Interaction with anti-inflammatory steroids. J Immunol 143:1310–1317
87. Schleimer RP, Freeland HS, Peters SP, Brown KE, Derse CP (1989) An assessment of the effects of glucocorticoids on degranulation, chemotaxis, binding to vascular endothelium and formation of LTB4 by human neutrophils. J Pharmacol Exp Ther 250:598–605
88. Schleimer RP, Sterbinsky SA, Kaiser J Bickel CA, Klunk DA, Tomioka K, Newman W, Luscinskas FW, Gimbrone MA Jr, McIntyre BW, Bochnar BS (1992) Interleukin-4 induces human eosinophils and basophils but not neutrophils to adhere endothelium: association with expression of VCAM-1. J Immunol 148:1086–1092
89. Schweibert LA, Beck LA, Stellato C, Bickel CA, Bochner BS, Schleimer RP (1996) Glucocorticosteroid inhibition of cytokine production: relevance to antiallergic actions. J Allergy Clin Immunol 97:143–152
90. Selvan RS, Butterfield JH, Krangel MS (1994) Expression of multiple chemokine genes by a human mast cell leukaemia. J Biol Chem 269:13893–13898
91. Shaw G, Kamen R (1986) A conserved AV sequence from the 3' untranslated region of GM-CSF on RNA mediates selective mRNA degradation. Cell 46:659–667
92. Sherman MR, Stevens J (1984) Structure of mammalian steroid receptors: evolving concepts and methodological developments. Annu Rev Physiol 46:83–105
93. Sieff CA (1987) Hematopoietic growth factors. J Clin Invest 79:1549–1557
94. Simon H-U, Blaser K (1995) Inhibition of programmed eosinophil death: a key pathogenic event for eosinophilia? Immunol Today 16:53–55

95. Simon H-U, Yousefi S, Dommann-Scherrer CC, Zimmermann DR, Bauer S, Barandun J, Blaser K (1996) Expansion of cytokine producing CD4–CD8– T cells associated with abnormal Fas expression and hypereosinophilia. J Exp Med 183:1071–1082
96. Strader CD, Sigal IS, Dixon RAF (1989) Structural basis of β-adrenergic receptor function. FASEB J 3:1825–1832
97. Synder DS, Unanue ER (1982) Corticosteroids inhibit murine macrophage Ia expression and interleukin-1 production. J Immunol 129:1803–1805
98. Tai P-KK, Maeda Y, Nakao K, Wakim NG, Duhring JL, Faber LE (1986) A 59-kilodalton protein associated with progestin, estrogen, androgen, and glucocorticoid receptors. Biochemistry 25:5269–5275
99. van De Scolpe A, Caldenhoven E, Stade BG, Koenderman L, Raaijmakers JAM, Johnson JP, van der Saag PT (1994) 12-*O*-Tetradeconyl phorbol-13-acetate and tumor necrosis factor alpha-mediated induction of intercellular adhesion molecule-1 is inhibited by dexamethasone: functional analysis of the human intercellular adhesion molecule-1 promoter. J Biol Chem 269:6185–6192
100. Varney VA, Hamid QA, Gaga M, Ying S, Jacobson M, Frew AJ, Kay AB, Durham SR (1993) Influence of grass pollen immunotherapy on cellular infiltration and cytokine mRNA expression during allergen-induced late-phase cutaneous responses. J Clin Invest 92:644–651
101. Walker C, Virchow JC Jr, Bruijnzeel PLB, Blaser K (1991) T cell subsets and their soluble products regulate eosinophilia in allergic and nonallergic asthma. J Immunol 146:1829–1835
102. Wallen N, Kita H, Weiler D, Gleich GJ (1991) Glucocorticoids inhibit cytokine mediated eosinophil survival. J Immunol 147:3490–3495
103. Wallner BP, Mattaliano RJ, Hession C, Cate RL, Tizard R, Sinclair LK, Foeller C, Chow EP, Browning JL, Ramachandran KL, Pepinsky RB (1986) Cloning and expression of human lipocortin 1, a phospholipase A2 inhibitor with potential anti-inflammatory activity. Nature 320:77–81
104. Warner JA, Pienkowski MM, Plaut M, Norman PS, Lichtenstein LM (1986) Identification of histamine releasing factor(s) in the late phase of cutaneous IgE-mediated reactions. J Immunol 136:2583–2587
105. Wenck U, Speirs N (1957) The effect of cortisone on blood leukocytes and peritoneal fluid cells of mice. Acta Haematol 17:193–201
106. Werb Z (1978) Biochemical actions of glucocorticoids on macrophages in culture. Specific inhibition of elastase, collagenase, and plasminogen activator secretion and effects on other metabolic functions. J Exp Med 147:1695–712
107. Williams TJ, Yarwood H (1990) Effect of glucocorticosteroids on microvascular permeability. Am Rev Respir Dis 141:S39–S43
108. Wu CY, Sarfati M, Heusser C, Fournier S, Rubio-Trujillo M, Peleman R, Delespesse G (1991) Glucocorticoids increase the synthesis of immunoglobulin E by interleukin 4-stimulated human lymphocytes. J Clin Invest 87:870–877
109. Xie Q-W, Kashiwarbara Y, Nathan C (1994) Role of transcription factor NF-κB/Rel in induction of nitric oxide synthase. J Biol Chem 269:4705–4708
110. Yamaguchi H, Hirai K, Nakajima K, Ohtoshi T, Takaishi T, Ohta K, Morita Y, Ito K (1994) Dexamethasone inhibits basophil migration. Allergy 49:371–375
111. Yancey KB, Hammer CH, Harvath L, Renfer L, Frank MM, Lawley TJ (1985) Studies of human C5a as a mediator of inflammation in normal human skin. J Clin Invest 75:486–495
112. Yang Y, Mercep M, Ware CF, Ashwell JD (1995) Fas and activation-induced Fas ligand mediate apoptosis of T cell hybridomas: inhibition of Fas ligand expression by retinoic acid and glucocorticoids. J Exp Med 181:1673–1682

High-Dose Intravenous Immunoglobulins

G. Messer and M. Meurer

Introduction

After the introduction of the ethanol precipitation method by Cohn, human IgG became available in large quantities and made both intramuscular injections and intravenous infusions of IgG possible [1]. In the last decade, the processing of IgG was further optimized and resulted in stabilized immunoreactive preparations which can be used in high concentrations and with a high degree of safety [2]. High-dose intravenous immunoglobulin therapy (IVIG) is administered in primary and secondary immunodeficiencies with suppression of humoral immunity; these include X-linked agammaglobulinemia, hypogammaglobulinemia, common variable immunodeficiency (CVID), severe combined immunodeficiency (SCID), Wiskott-Aldrich syndrome, multiple myeloma, and chronic lymphocytic leukemia. Later, IVIG was also given in diseases with multifactorial host defense defects, such as acquired immunodeficiency syndrome (AIDS), mostly in children, immunodeficiency following myeloablative therapy, and graft-versus-host disease (GVHD).

In 1981, Imbach and coworkers observed a rapid rise in platelet counts within 24 h in children with autoimmune thrombocytopenic purpura upon application of high doses of intravenous IgG [3]. In the following years, many other diseases with underlying autoimmune pathomechanisms were treated with IVIG, almost always in uncon-

Table 1. Intravenous immunoglobulin (IVIG) in controlled, randomized studies

Disease	Patients	Response	References
Bone marrow transplantation	382	+	[7]
Kawasaki syndrome	549	+	[8]
Dermatomyositis	15	+	[9]
Acute ITP of childhood	146	+	[10]
Juvenile rheumatoid arthritis	29	±	[11]
Multiple myeloma	82	+	[12]
Recurrent pregnancy loss	64	–	[13]
	95	+	[14]
Chronic lymphocytic leukemia	34	+	[15]
	42	+	[16]
Multiple sclerosis	20	+	[17]
Graves' ophthalmopathy	40	+	[18]

ITP, immune thrombocytopenic purpura; +, clinical response; ±, limited clinical response; –, no clinical response

trolled trials and with differing results, but with benefits for the patients (for reviews, see [4–6]). Only in the last decade were randomized, controlled studies with IVIG performed and its effectiveness shown [7–18] (Table 1). In many studies, IVIG introduced rapid, albeit transient responses in immunocompromised patients [7, 12, 15, 16], in patients with autoimmune diseases who did not respond to standard therapy regimens [9–11, 13, 14, 17, 18], including the following:

- Fetal-maternal Rh immunization
- Recurrent spontaneous abortions of immune etiology
- Preterm infants (prophylaxis)
- Neonatal sepsis
- Human immunodeficiency virus (HIV) infection (in children)
- Humoral deficiency and immune thrombocytopenic purpura
- Acute and chronic autoimmune thrombocytopenic purpura
- Autoimmune neutropenia
- Autoimmune hemolytic anemia
- Autoimmune coagulopathies
- Insulin-dependent diabetes mellitus
- Autoimmune thyroid disease
- Vasculitis
- Uveitis
- Inflammatory bowel disease
- Polymyositis
- Multiple sclerosis
- Inflammatory demyelinating disease
- Guillain-Barré syndrome
- Myasthenia gravis
- Multifocal motor neuropathy

Clinical relapses and transient characteristics of the immunomodulatory effects were noted when IVIG treatment was discontinued [3, 19–26] (for a review, see [6]). The favorable therapeutic response in children with immune thrombocytopenic purpura (ITP) and with Kawasaki syndrome led to the consensus statement of the National Institute of Health (Bethesda) in 1990 and established IVIG as the standard therapy for these two diseases. For long-term treatment, the therapy is given in cycles of polyclonal IgG infusions on 2–5 consecutive days, which can be repeated every 3–4 weeks or more.

Intravenous Immunoglobulins in Autoimmune Diseases with Skin Involvement

Use of IVIG in autoimmune diseases with cutaneous involvement, such as Kawasaki syndrome [8] (for a review, see [5, 6, 27]), systemic vasculitis [28, 29], systemic lupus erythematosus (SLE; for a review, see [5]), juvenile dermatomyositis [30, 31], dermatomyositis [9, 32], paraneoplastic dermatomyositis [33], rheumatoid arthritis [26, 34], and antiphospholipid syndrome [35, 36], or autoimmune blistering diseases, such as bullous pemphigoid [21, 37–39], pemphigus vulgaris [25, 38–43], pemphigus foliaceus [39, 43], epidermolysis bullosa acquisita [44, 45], and pyoderma gangrenosum [46], has resulted in good therapeutic responses in the majority of patients treated (Table 2).

Table 2. Intravenous immunoglobulin (IVIG) in autoimmune diseases with skin involvement

Type	Disease
Collagen-vascular	Dermatomyositis Juvenile dermatomyositis Paraneoplastic dermatomyositis Rheumatoid arthritis Systemic lupus erythematosus Sjörgren's syndrome Antiphospholipid antibody syndrome
Vasculitis	Kawasaki syndrome ANCA-associated systemic vasculitis Polyarteritis nodosa Pyoderma gangrenosum
Blistering autoimmune	Bullous pemphigoid Pemphigus vulgaris Pemphigus foliaceus Epidermolysis bullosa acquisita

ANCA, antineutrophil cytoplasmic autoantibodies

In Kawasaki syndrome, a vasculitis of medium-sized vessels affecting children, treatment with IVIG alone or in combination with aspirin significantly reduced inflammatory signs and the incidence of coronary artery aneurysms (for a review, see [27]). The benefit from IVIG was also noted in antineutrophil cytoplasmic antibody (ANCA)-associated systemic vasculitides. Jayne et al. [23] treated seven patients with a single course of IVIG (0.4 g/kg body weight per day) for 5 days and observed a positive clinical response in all patients accompanied by significant reductions of ANCA titers and C-reactive protein serum levels; three relapses after 2, 6, and 9 months were reported [23]. In the study published by Richter et al. in 1995 [28], 15 patients with ANCA-positive systemic vasculitis were treated with IVIG (30 g/day) either for 5 consecutive days or with the same protocol given repeatedly once every fourth week. In 6 of the 15 patients, a significant clinical improvement was reported; however, no improvement was seen in patients with eye involvement, pericarditis, or nephritis. In 1995, Boman et al. reported favorable results upon IVIG in one patient with primary systemic vasculitis of the central nervous system and another patient with polyarteritis nodosa [29].

The immunomodulatory potential of IVIG was explored early on in SLE and in patients with Sjögren's disease. A positive effect on the cutaneous vasculitis present in these entities and on peripheral cytopenia, circulating immune complexes, and systemic inflammatory parameters was noted in early reports; however, evaluation of IVIG in SLE in large controlled studies is still lacking. The results of IVIG in SLE patients with renal involvement are not consistent, although a reduction of C1q- and C3-binding immune complexes was reported [47]. It should be noted that, in several patients, worsening of proteinuria and renal function or even the onset of renal disease was reported after IVIG therapy (for a review, see [5]). In women with spontaneous abortions associated with antiphospholipid syndrome, IVIG can result in a decrease in antiphospholipid antibody titers and can have a positive effect on growth retardation in the developing child [35, 36].

Dermatomyositis and polymyositis are autoimmune skin diseases with muscle involvement in which IVIG treatment has been widely applied. Both polymyositis and dermatomyositis can become unresponsive to standard treatment protocols with corticosteroids or may not respond to more experimental regimens such as leukapheresis and plasma exchange. As an alternative, IVIG was evaluated with promising results. Cherin and coworkers reported on 14 patients with recalcitrant polymyositis and six patients with dermatomyositis who were treated either with 1 g/kg for 2 consecutive days or with 0.4 g/kg body weight for 5 days. Significant increase of muscle strength, decrease in mean creatine phosphokinase serum levels, and a steroid-sparing effect were observed in this clinical study [32].

Later, Dalakas et al. proved the efficacy of IVIG in a double-blinded, controlled study of 15 dermatomyositis patients in which (including crossover treatments) 12 patients received 2 g IgG/kg body weight per month. Statistically significant improvement of muscle strength and neuromuscular symptoms and an increase in muscle fiber diameter and in the numbers and diameter of capillaries were measured [9]. The favorable response to IVIG was also shown in patients with juvenile dermatomyositis and paraneoplastic dermatomyositis [30, 31, 33].

The use of IVIG was evaluated in rheumatoid arthritis. Long-term treatment in nine patients with severe rheumatoid arthritis resulted in significant improvement of both subjective and objective parameters, including the Ritchie and the Lee articular index. Concomitantly, reduction of $CD4^+$ $CDw29^+$ to $CD4^+$ $CD45RA^+$ cell ratio was observed. Discontinuation of IVIG after 6 months of treatment was followed by a relapse of rheumatoid arthritis activity within a few weeks [26]. Another study analyzed the efficacy of IVIG in ten patients with rheumatoid arthritis who had been unsuccessfully treated with at least one slow-acting antirheumatic drug prior to the onset of IVIG therapy. In these rheumatoid arthritis patients, IVIG was given in doses of 0.4 g/kg body weight for 3 consecutive days, followed by 0.4 g/kg body weight once per month for 1 year [34]. A delayed clinical improvement starting after 6 months was observed, and decreased serum levels of tumor necrosis factor (TNF)-α and systemic soluble interleukin-2 receptor (sIL-2R) concentrations were found [34]. In seven adult patients with Still's disease, between one and eight IVIG cycles with 1 g/kg body weight for 2 consecutive days were administered. Compared to other therapy regimens, in this uncontrolled study about 50% of patients treated with IVIG improved [48].

In 31 patients with systemic juvenile rheumatoid arthritis, a double-blinded, placebo-controlled multicenter IVIG trial was conducted, with 1.5 g/kg body weight administered every 2 weeks for the first 2 months, followed by monthly infusions of the same dose for up to 6 months [11]. Some clinical improvement in the IVIG group was noted, although without reduction of days with fever or effects on pathologic albumin and hemoglobulin concentrations, platelet counts, and erythrocyte sedimentation rates. The overall efficacy of IVIG in systemic juvenile rheumatoid arthritis was therefore assumed to be only limited [11].

The clinical response of bullous pemphigoid to IVIG was first described in 1985 by Godard et al. [21], who treated nine patients with one cycle of IVIG as single therapy. Eight of the nine patients who received 0.4 g IgG/kg body weight daily for 5 days experienced immediate reduction of pruritus as well as erythematous and urticarial skin lesions. The effect of IVIG in these bullous pemphigoid patients, however, lasted for only about 2 weeks before a rebound made combined therapy with systemic corticosteroids and plasmapheresis necessary [21]. Another publication reports on two patients with bullous pemphigoid who had previously been unsuccessfully treated with pulse therapy receiving high doses of intravenous cyclophosphamide and dexamethasone or dexamethasone alone. IVIG was started; after treatment with 0.4 g IgG/kg body weight per day for 5 days, both patients promptly responded to systemic corticosteroids [37].

The first reports in the literature on the efficacy of IVIG in pemphigus vulgaris were controversial [38, 40, 41]. However, later studies showed an immediate anti-inflammatory effect of IVIG and an improved response of severe pemphigus with mucosal involvement to low-dose standard and adjuvant treatments after IVIG treatment [25, 39, 42, 43]. Two patients with pemphigus foliaceus receiving short-term IVIG had a similar response [39, 43]. Taken together, in these reports 11 out of 14 patients with pemphigus responded favorably to IVIG. The use of IVIG in pemphigus seems to have a steroid-sparing effect and reinstalls the response to low to moderate doses of systemic corticosteroids and adjuvant immunosuppressants given together with IVIG or later. Moreover, reduction of pemphigus autoantibody titer and the CD4 to CD8 lymphocyte ratio points to a direct effect of IVIG on the underlying immune-mediated pathogenesis [25, 39, 43]. Long-term use of IVIG in pemphigus has led to clinical remission [41, 42]; however, a controlled study has not been performed so far.

Therapeutic intervention in epidermolysis bullosa acquisita can be very difficult, particularly in the inflammatory variant resembling bullous pemphigoid. One 16-year-old patient with long-lasting generalized epidermolysis bullosa acquisita who had not responded to systemic corticosteroids, dapsone, and plasmapheresis was treated with IVIG cycles given on 4 consecutive days (0.4 g/kg body weight per day) at 2-week intervals [44]. After a rapid clearance of blistering within several days, a rebound occurred approximately 10 days after the last infusion of the first cycle. Within four cycles, circulating specific autoantibodies to type VII collagen became undetectable, whereas direct immunofluorescence microscopy still demonstrated tissue-bound activity of anti-collagen VII antibodies [44].

In another patient with epidermolysis bullosa acquisita, IVIG was started as long-term treatment in combination with colchicine (2 mg/day), prednisone (12 mg/day), dapsone (100 mg/day), and azathioprine (100 mg/day) [45]. Immunoglobulin infusions (0.4 g/kg body weight per day) were given for 5 consecutive days in nine cycles repeated every 4 weeks. After 3 months, blister formation stopped, and after 9 months the lesions healed and the skin became more resistant to friction [45].

Pyoderma gangrenosum is an uncommon chronic or relapsing vasculitic disease of multiple etiology leading to localized or widespread cutaneous ulcerations. Pyoderma gangrenosum can be associated with ulcerative colitis or other autoimmune diseases and is often extremely recalcitrant to high-dosage immunosuppressive therapy regimens. In one patient with pyoderma gangrenosum, Gupta et al. observed a temporary beneficial effect after IVIG (1 g/kg body weight per day) given in one cycle for 5 days in combination with prednisone (60 mg/day) and cyclosporin A (6 mg/kg body weight per day). Another two courses of IVIG led to slow healing of the pyoderma gangrenosum, which made gradual reduction of the prednisone and cyclosporin A doses possible [46].

A very rare indication for IVIG was a case of dermal erythropoiesis in a newborn child with blueberry muffin rash. Because of extremely high titers of anti-D, the mother was treated with IVIG (0.4 g/kg body weight per day) for 4 days every 2 weeks in combination with plasmapheresis beginning from gestational week 17. The child was treated postpartum with 1 g IgG/kg body weight infusions for 1 day and with 0.5 g/kg body weight for the following 3 days together with double-volume exchange transfusions [49]. Interestingly, this treatment, which is established for Rh incompatibility in pregnant women, resulted in a favorable course in the newborn; no viral or bacterial infections were observed, which otherwise are a major risk when neonatal dermal erythropoiesis is treated with immunosuppressive drugs [49].

Immune-Regulatory Properties of Intravenous Immunoglobulin

The immunologic mechanisms behind the immediate response to IVIG in patients with ITP are mainly due to a blockade of Fc receptors of the reticuloendothelial system (RES) cells by polyclonal IgG. This Fc receptor blockade prevents destruction of antibody-bound platelets [19, 50]. In addition, a reduced clearance of labeled red blood cells by spleen and liver was measured upon IVIG treatment [19] (Table 3).

Rapid anti-inflammatory effects of IVIG can also be explained by blocking of the classical complement activation cascade. Polyclonal IgG preparations reduce or block the activity of complement components C1q, C3, and C4 and inhibit complement-dependent attraction of immunocompetent cells, opsonization by macrophages, and ultimately formation of the membrane attack complex, thus resulting in reduced tissue injury [51–53]. In addition to its effect on acute anti-inflammatory reactions, IVIG may also modulate other immunoregulatory pathways triggered by Fc receptor ligation. The decline of pathophysiologically relevant autoantibody titers such as anti-thrombocytic, anti-factor VIII, or anti-desmoglein antibodies is presumably caused by the presence of anti-idiotypic antibodies in polyclonal IgG preparations pooled from many individuals [54, 55] (for a review, see [6, 56]). A decrease of disease-specific antibody titers upon IVIG was noted in patients with autoimmune coagulopathies, myasthenia gravis, pemphigus vulgaris, epidermolysis bullosa acquisita, antiphospholipid syndrome, and vasculitis [23, 25, 36, 39, 42, 44, 57, 58]. In several autoimmune diseases, including chronic ITP and hemophilia A and B with antibodies to factors VIII and IX, treatment with $F(ab')_2$ fragments [59] (for a review, see [56]) or Fcγ fragments [50] showed effectiveness both in vitro and in vivo.

Moreover, IVIG may have an effect on the cellular immune response; decrease of the CD4 to CD8 ratio with relative increase of $CD8^+$ T lymphocytes [20, 22, 25, 43, 58], potential activation of suppressor $CD8^+$ T cell functions [60, 61], and reduced B cell responses were described both in vivo and in peripheral blood mononuclear cells (PBMC) and B cell lines in vitro [22, 58, 62, 63]. Functionally, blockade of the Fc receptor pathways for IgG – of FcγRI (CD64), FcγRII (CD32), and FcγRIII (CD16) – could lead to reduced activation and secretory capacity of multiple cell types [50, 63]. Increased peripheral $CD8^+$ lymphocytes found upon IVIG may be due to altered regulatory signals by cell-bound or soluble factors. Potent immunomodulators such as interleukin (IL)-1, IL-6, TNF-α, and the membrane-bound IL-2 receptors were found to be downregulated in macrophage and PBMC short-time cultures in vitro in the presence of high doses of IgG [64–67]. Shimozato et al. provided further evidence for a contribution of Fcγ

Table 3. Possible immunologic mechanisms involved in intravenous immunoglobulin (IVIG)

Time	Mechanism
Immediate	Antigen neutralization Neutralization of circulating antibodies Functional blockade of Fc receptors on RES cells Inhibition of complement components Clearance of immune complexes Effects on signal transduction pathways Modulation of gene regulation Modulation of cytokine/antagonist responses Phenotypic changes on lymphocytes
Long-term	Suppression of allo- and autoantibody synthesis Modulation of T and B cell repertoires

RES, reticuloendothelial system

receptor-triggered pathways, showing that the production level of the proinflammatory cytokines IL-1 and TNF-α of lipopolysaccharide (LPS)-stimulated macrophages decreased upon addition of IgG or Fc fragments [65]. Poutsiaka and coworkers reported on the upregulation of the naturally occurring inhibitory molecule IL-1 receptor antagonist (IL-1ra) by IgG [68]; thus it is conceivable that multiple inhibitory effects of IVIG on proinflammatory signals have a strong additional immunoregulatory influence on the control of autoimmune diseases. As the only exception, the cytokine IL-8 was found to be increased both in stimulated PBMC and monocytic cells in the presence of IgG [67, 69].

Additional regulatory effects of IVIG on cellular responses and cytokine levels could be exerted by immunocompetent soluble molecules such as soluble human leukocyte antigens (sHLA), soluble intercellular adhesion molecule (sICAM)-1, and soluble CD4 and CD8 receptors present in the IVIG preparations [70, 71]. However, some of these findings have been questioned because of possible interspecies cross-reactivity of the antibody detection systems used [72].

Finally, evidence was raised for the immunomodulatory action of IgG antibodies against key molecules governing specific and nonspecific immune responses such as multiple cytokines, human leukocyte antigens, and the T cell, CD4, CD5, and CD8 receptors [56, 73–75].

Discussion

Standard therapy regimens with corticosteroids and antiproliferative drugs in autoimmune skin diseases often lead to marked systemic immunosuppression and can cause severe drug-related side effects. Reactivation of mycobacteriae, colonization by bacteriae or fungi, spread of herpes simplex virus, or generalized zoster infections can complicate the clinical situation and may result in severe generalized infections of the skin, pneumonia, or septicemia with a lethal outcome. Prevention of life-threatening infections by IVIG in immunocompromised patients has been demonstrated in large randomized studies with 82 plateau-phase multiple myeloma and 382 bone marrow transplanted (BMT) patients with significant reduction of recurrent infections and GVHD in BMT patients [7, 12]. In addition to direct neutralization of antigen, IVIG posesses considerable potential to block bacterial superantigen-initiated T cell activation, which might be a major trigger of autoimmune reactions [76].

Novel therapeutic modalities should be considered for cutaneous autoimmune diseases not responsive to high doses of systemic corticosteroids and to combination protocols, or complicated by infections or severe side effects. Ample clinical and experimental evidence has now accumulated that IVIG can reduce local and systemic inflammatory reactions of skin and mucous membranes and, in addition, that it can help to maintain or restore the immune surveillance in critical clinical situations.

Disadvantages of IVIG therapy are the high costs of the pooled IgG preparation and the transient mode of the anti-inflammatory immunoregulation. Anaphylactoid reactions are rarely experienced, with the exception of patients with IgA deficiency, who should therefore be excluded. Moreover, the possibility of infections by agents such as hepatitis C virus or HIV cannot be ruled out, even though the risk is extremely low [77, 78]. Concerning the novel risk for transmission of Creutzfeldt-Jacob disease by disease-related prion protein (PrP^{Sc}) [79], definite data are not yet available.

From our experience with IVIG, daily dosages as low as 0.25 g/kg body weight per day can downregulate inflammatory cascades and production of harmful autoantibodies in severe pemphigus when IVIG cycles of 5 days are repeated three times every third or fourth week. No side effects of IVIG were noted; however, after IVIG a much better response to standard therapy regimens became apparent. In dermatomyositis [9], pemphigus vulgaris [41, 42], epidermolysis bullosa acquisita [44, 45], rheumatoid arthritis [26, 34], SLE (reviewed in [5]), and GVHD [7], long-term IVIG alone or in combination with immunosuppressants resulted in definite clinical improvement and decreased the risk for secondary infections. Based on these observations, we would encourage the use of long-term IVIG treatment for severe immune-mediated vasculitis, for pyoderma gangrenosum, for skin ulcerations in rheumatoid arthritis, systemic scleroderma, livedo racemosa, autoimmune overlap syndromes [80],and for rare cases of so-called catastrophic autiphospholipid syndrome, perhaps in combination with anticoagulation.

So far, no influence of IVIG on the antitumor immune response is known; therefore, IVIG could also be considered as treatment for paraneoplastic autoimmune disease such as paraneoplastic pemphigus, dermatomyositis, and bullous pemphigoid in coexistence with tumors.

For long-term treatment of chronic autoimmune diseases such as dermatomyositis, SLE, rheumatoid arthritis, or vasculitis, the extremely high costs of IVIG are a limiting factor. For short-term treatment, IVIG can be used as a crisis intervention protocol in pemphigus vulgaris, autoimmune vasculitis, bullous pemphigoid, or other cutaneous autoimmune diseases recalcitrant to standard therapy regimens or complicated by serious side effects.

Summary

High-dose IVIG is increasingly being considered as an effective treatment modality in various immune-mediated and autoimmune disorders, such as ITP, hemolytic anemia, immune neutropenia, autoimmune coagulopathies, and mucocutaneous lymph node syndrome. Immunomodulatory properties of polyclonal human IgG as a single or adjuvant therapy have led to significant improvement in many organ-specific or systemic autoimmune diseases. This review focuses on experience with IVIG in immune-mediated skin diseases and discusses the current understanding of underlying immunoregulatory mechanisms.

References

1. Cohn EJ, Strong LE, Hughes WL, Mulford DJ, Ashworth JN, Melin M, Taylor HL (1946) Preparation and properties of serum and plasma proteins. I. A system for the separation into fractions of the protein and lipoprotein components of biological issues and fluids. J Am Chem Soc 68:459–475
2. Zuhrie SR, Webster ADB, Davies R, Fay ACM, Wallington TB (1995) A prospective controlled crossover trial of a new heat-inactivated intravenous immunoglobulin. Clin Exp Immunol 99:10–15
3. Imbach P, Barundun S, Baumgartner C, Hirt A, Hofer F, Wagner HP (1981) High-dose intravenous gammaglobulin therapy of refractory, in particular idiopathic thrombocytopenia in childhood. Helv Paediatr Acta 36:81–86
4. Schwartz SA (1990) Intravenous immunoglobulin in autoimmune disorders. J Clin Immunol 10:81–89
5. Ballow M (1991) Mechanisms of action of intravenous immunoglobulin therapy and potential use in autoimmune connective tissue diseases. Cancer 68:1430–1436
6. Dwyer JM (1992) Manipulating the immune system with immune globulin. N Engl J Med 326:107–116
7. Sullivan KM, Kopegky KJ, Jocom J, Fisher L, Buckner D, Meyers JD, Counts GW, Bowden RA, Petersen FB, Witherspoon RP, Budinger MD, Schwartz RS, Appelbaum FR, Clift RA, Hansen JA, Sanders JE, Thomas ED, Storb R (1990) Immunomodulatory and antimicrobial efficacy of intravenous immunoglobulin in bone marrow transplantation. N Engl J Med 323:705–712
8. Newburger JW, Takahashi M, Beiser AS, Burns JC, Bastian J, Chung KJ, Colan SD, Duffy CE, Fulton DR, Glode MP, Mason WH, Meissner HC, Rowley AH, Shulman ST, Reddy V, Sundel RP, Wiggins JW, Colton T, Melish ME, Rosen FS (1991) A single infusion of intravenous gammaglobulin compared to four daily doses in the treatment of acute Kawasaki syndrome. N Engl J Med 324:1633–1639
9. Dalakas MC, Illa I, Dambrosia JM, Soudeidan SA, Stein DP, Otero C, Dinsmore ST, McCrosky S (1993) A controlled trial of high-dose intravenous globulin infusions as treatment for dermatomyositis. N Engl J Med 329:1993–2000
10. Blanchette V, Imbach P, Andrew M, Adams M, McMillan J, Wang E, Milner R, Kaiser A, Barnard D, Bernstein M, Chan KW, Esseltine D, deVeber B, Israels S, Kobrinsky N, Luke B (1994) Randomised trial of intravenous immunoglobulin G, intravenous anti-D, and oral prednisone in childhood acute immune thrombocytopenic purpura. Lancet 344:703–707
11. Silverman ED, Cawkwell GD, Lovell DJ, Laxer RM, Lehman TJ, Passo MH, Zemel LS, Giannini EH (1994) Intravenous immunoglobulin in the treatment of systemic juvenile rheumatoid arthritis: a randomized placebo controlled trial. Pediatric Rheumatology Collaborative Study Group. J Rheumatol 21:2353–2358
12. Chapel HM, Lee M, Hargreaves R, Pamphilon DH, Prentice AG (1994) Randomised trial of intravenous immunoglobulin as prophylaxis against infection in plateau-phase multiple myeloma. Lancet 343:1059–1063

13. The German RSA/IVIG Group (1994) Intravenous immunoglobulin in the prevention of recurrent miscarriage. Br J Obstet Gynaecol 101:1072–1077
14. Coulam CB, Krysa L, Stern JJ, Bustillo M (1995) Intravenous immunoglobulin for treatment of recurrent pregnancy loss. Am J Reprod Immunol 34:333–337
15. Chapel H, Dicato M, Gamm H, Brennan V, Ries F, Bunch C, Lee M (1994) Immunoglobulin replacement in patients with chronic lymphocytic leukaemia: a comparison of two dose regimens. Br J Haematol 88:209–212
16. Boughton BJ, Jackson N, Sim S, Smith N (1995) Randomized trial of intravenous immunoglobulin prophylaxis for patients with chronic lymphocytic leukaemia and secondary hypogammaglobulinaemia. Clin Lab Haematol 17:75–80
17. Achiron A, Barak Y, Goren M, Gabbay U, Miron S, Rotstein Z, Noy S, Sarova-Pinhas I (1996) Intravenous immune globulin in multiple sclerosis: clinical and neuroradiological results and implications for possible mechanisms of action. Clin Exp Immunol 104S:67–70
18. Kahaly G, Pitz S, Müller-Forell W, Hommel G (1996) Randomized trial of intravenous immunoglobulins versus prednisolone in Graves' ophthalmopathy. J Clin Immunol 106:197–202
19. Fehr J, Hofmann V, Kappeler V (1982) Transient reversal of thrombocytopenia in idiopathic thrombocytopenic purpura by high-dose intravenous gamma globulin. N Engl J Med 306: 1254–1258
20. Tsubakio T, Kurata Y, Katagiri S, Kanakura Y, Tamaki T, Kuyama J, Kanayama Y, Yonezawa T, Tarui S (1983) Alteration of T cell subsets and immunoglobulin synthesis in vitro during high dose gamma-globulin therapy in patients with idiopathic thrombocytopenic purpura. Clin Exp Immunol 53:697–702
21. Godard W, Roujeau JC, Guillot B, Andre C, Rifle G (1985) Bullous pemphigoid and intravenous gammaglobulin. Am J Intern Med 83:965
22. Dammacco F, Iodice G, Campobasso N (1986) Treatment of adult patients with idiopathic thrombocytopenic purpura with intravenous immunoglobulin: effects on circulating T cell subsets and PWM induced antibody synthesis in vitro. Br J Haematol 62:125–135
23. Jayne DRW, Davies MJ, Fox CVJ, Black CM, Lockwood CM (1991) Treatment of systemic vasculitis with pooled intravenous immunoglobulin. Lancet 337:1137–1139
24. Dietrich G, Varela FJ, Hurez V, Bouanani M, Kazatchkine MD (1993) Selection of the expressed B cell repertoire by infusion of normal immunoglobulin G in a patient with autoimmune thyroiditis. Eur J Immunol 23:2945–2950
25. Messer G, Sizmann N, Feucht H, Meurer M (1995) High-dose intravenous immunoglobulins for immediate control of severe pemphigus vulgaris. Br J Dermatol 133:1014–1016
26. Tumiati B, Casoli P, Veneziani M, Rinaldi G (1992) High-dose immunoglobulin therapy as an immunomodulatory treatment of rheumatoid arthritis. Arthritis Rheum 35:1126–1133
27. Durongpisitkul K, Gururaj VJ, Park JM, Martin CF (1995) The prevention of coronary artery aneurysm in Kawasaki disease: a meta-analysis on the efficacy of aspirin and immunoglobulin treatment. Pediatrics 96:1057–1061
28. Richter C, Schnabel A, Csernok E, DeGroot K, Reinhold-Keller E, Gross WL (1995) Treatment of anti-neutrophil cytoplasmic antibody (ANCA)-associated systemic vasculitis with high-dose intravenous immunoglobulin. Clin Exp Immunol 101:2–7
29. Boman S, Ballen JL, Seggev JS (1995) Dramatic responses to intravenous immunoglobulin in vasculitis. J Intern Med 238:375–377
30. Collet E, Dalac S, Maerens B, Courtois JM, Izac M, Lambert D (1994) Juvenile dermatomyositis: treatment with intravenous gamma-globulin. Br J Dermatol 130:231–234
31. Lang BA, Laxer RM, Murphy G, Silverman ED, Roifman CM (1991) Treatment of dermatomyositis with intravenous gammaglobulin. Am J Med 91:169–172
32. Cherin P, Herson S, Wechsler B, Piette JC, Bletry O, Coutellier A, Ziza JM, Godeau P (1991) Intravenous immunoglobulin for polymyositis and dermatomyositis. Am J Med 91:162–168
33. Esteve E, Cambie MP, Serpier H, Vanderbroere-Bouquet A, Bellaiche P, Kalis B (1994) Paraneoplastic dermatomyositis: efficacy of intravenous gammaglobulin. Br J Dermatol 131:917–918

34. Muscat C, Bertotto A, Ercolani R, Bistoni O, Agea E, Cesarotti M, Fiorucci G, Spinozzi F, Gerli R (1995) Long term treatment of rheumatoid arthritis with high doses of intravenous immunoglobulins: effect on disease activity and serum cytokines. Ann Rheum Dis 54:382–385
35. Valensise H, Vaquero E, De Carolis C, Stipa E, Perricone R, Arduini D, Romanini C (1995) Normal fetal growth in a woman with antiphospholipid syndrome treated with high-dose intravenous immunoglobulin (IVIG). Prenat Diagn 15:509–517
36. Kwak JY, Quilty EA, Gilman-Sachs A, Beaman KD, Beer AE (1995) Intravenous immunoglobulin infusion therapy in woman with recurrent spontaneous abortions of immune etiologies. J Reprod Immunol 28:175–188
37. Rütter GH, Sunderkötter C, Rütter A, Biel K, Hildebrand A, Mohr C, Luger TA, Kolde G (1994/1995) Intravenöse Immunoglobuline, ein wirksames und gut verträgliches Additivum in der Behandlung therapieresistenter bullöser Autoimmundermatosen. In: Macher E, Kolde G, Bröcker EB (eds) Jahrbuch der Dermatologie 1994/95 – Tumoren und Haut. Biermann, Zülpich, pp 275–288
38. Tappeiner G, Steiner A (1989) High-dosage intravenous gamma globulin: therapeutic failure in pemphigus and pemphigoid. J Am Acad Dermatol 20:684–685
39. Beckers RCY, Brand A, Vermeer BJ, Boom BW (1995) Adjuvant high-dose intravenous gammaglobulin in the treatment of pemphigus and bullous pemphigoid: experience in six patients. Br J Dermatol 133:289–293
40. Hunziker T, Schwarzenbach HR, Krebs A, Nydegger UE, Camponovo F, Hess M (1981) Plasmaaustausch bei Pemphigus vulgaris. Schweiz Med Wochenschr 111:1637–1642
41. Humbert P, Derancourt C, Aubin F, Agache P (1990) Effects of intravenous γ-globulin in pemphigus. J Am Acad Dermatol 22:326
42. Bewley AP, Keefe M (1996) Successful treatment of pemphigus vulgaris by pulsed intravenous immunoglobulin therapy. Br J Dermatol 135:128–129
43. Messer G, Wollenberg A, Stumpenhausen G, Feucht H, Plewig G, Meurer M (1997) High-dose intravenous immunoglobulins in pemphigus vulgaris: a therapeutic option for severe cases. (submitted)
44. Meier F, Sönnichsen K, Schaumburg-Lever G, Dopfner R, Rassner G (1993) Epidermolysis bullosa acquisita: Efficacy of high-dose intravenous immuno-globulins. J Am Acad Dermatol 29:334–337
45. Mohr C, Sunderkötter C, Hildebrand A, Biel K, Rütter A, Rütter GH, Luger TA, Kolde G (1995) Successful treatment of epidermolysis bullosa acquisita using intravenous immunoglobulins. Br J Dermatol 132:824–826
46. Gupta AK, Shear NH, Sauder DN (1995) Efficacy of human intravenous immune globulin in pyoderma gangrenosum. J Am Acad Dermatol 32:140–142
47. Lin RY, Racis SP (1986) In vivo reduction of circulating C1q binding immune complexes by intravenous gammaglobulin administration. Int Arch Allergy Appl Immunol 79:286–290
48. Permal S, Wechsler B, Cabane J, Perrot S, Blum L, Imbert JC (1995) Treatment of Still disease in adults with intravenous immunoglobulins. Rev Med Interne 16:250–254
49. Pizarro A, Elorza D, Gamallo C, Camara CDL, Arrieta R, Contreras F, Casado M (1995) Neonatal dermal erythropoiesis associated with severe rhesus immunization: amelioration by high-dose intravenous immunoglobulin. Br J Dermatol 133:334–335
50. Debre M, Bonnet M-C, Fridman W-H, Carosella E, Philippe N, Reinert P, Vilmer E, Kaplan C, Teillaud J-L, Griscelli C (1993) Infusion of Fcγ fragments for treatment of children with acute immune thrombocytopenic purpura. Lancet 342:945–949
51. Berger M, Rosenkranz P, Brown CY (1985) Intravenous and standard immune serum globin preparations interfere with uptake of 125I-C3 onto sensitized erythrocytes and inhibit hemolytic complement activity. Clin Immunol Immunpathol 34:227–232
52. Basta M, Dalakas MC (1994) High-dose intravenous immunoglobulin exerts its beneficial effect in patients with dermatomyositis by blocking endomysial deposition of activated complement fragments. J Clin Invest 94:1729–1742
53. Qi M, Schifferli JA (1995) Inhibition of complement activation by intravenous immunoglobulins. Arthritis Rheum 38:146

54. Sultan Y, Kazatchkine MD, Maisoneuve P, Nydegger UE (1984) Anti-idiotypic suppression of autoantibodies to factor VIII (antihaemophilic factor) by high-dose intravenous gammaglobulin. Lancet 8406:765–768
55. Mouthon L, Haury M, Lacroix-Desmazes S, Barreau C, Cautinho A, Kazatchkine MD (1995) Analysis of the normal human IgG antibody repertoire: evidence that IgG autoantibodies of healthy adults recognize a limited and conserved set of protein antigens in homologous tissues. J Immunol 154:5769–5778
56. Mouthon L, Kazatchkine MD (1996) Autoantibodies in therapeutic preparations of human IgG (IVIg). In: Peter JB, Shoenfeld Y (ed) Autoantibodies. Elsevier, Amsterdam, pp 91–95
57. Nilsson IM, Berntorp E, Zettervall O (1988) Induction of immune tolerance in patients with hemophilia and antibodies to factor VIII by combined treatment with intravenous IgG, cyclophosphamide, and factor VIII. N Engl J Med 318:947–950
58. Cook L, Howard JF Jr, Folds JD (1988) Immediate effects of intravenous IgG administration on peripheral blood B and T cells and polymorphonuclear cells in patients with myasthenia gravis. J Clin Immunol 8:23–31
59. Sultan Y, Rossi F, Kazatchkine MD (1987) Recovery from anti-VIII:C (antihaemophilic factor) autoimmune disease is dependent on generation of antiidiotypes against anti-VIII:C autoantibodies. Proc Natl Acad Sci USA 84:828–831
60. Leung DY, Burns JC, Newburger JW (1987) Reversal of lymphocyte activation in vitro in the Kawasaki syndrome by intravenous gammaglobulin. J Clin Invest 79:468–472
61. Ballow M, White W, Desbonnet C (1989) Modulation of in vitro synthesis of immunoglobulin and the induction of suppressor activity by therapy with intravenous immune globulin. J Allergy Clin Immunol 84:595–601
62. Stohl W (1986) Cellular mechanisms in the in vitro inhibition of pokeweed mitogen-induced B cell differentiation by immunoglobulin for intravenous use. J Immunol 136:4407–4413
63. Kondo N, Kasahara K, Kameyama T, Suzuki Y, Shimozawa N, Tomatsu S, Nakashima Y, Hori T, Yamagishi A, Ogawa T, Iwata H, Takahashi Y, Takenaka R, Watanabe K, Haga M, Orii T (1994) Intravenous immunoglobulins suppress immunoglobulin productions by suppressing Ca^{2+}-dependent signal transduction through Fcγ receptors in B lymphocytes. Scand J Immunol 40:37–42
64. Andersson JP, Andersson UG (1990) Human intravenous immunoglobulin modulates monokine production in vitro. Immunology 71:372–376
65. Shimozato T, Iwata M, Kawada H, Tamura N (1991) Human immunoglobulin preparation for intravenous use induces elevation of cellular cyclic adenosine 3':5'-monophosphate levels, resulting in suppression of tumour necrosis factor alpha and interleukin-1 production. Immunology 72:497–501
66. Andersson UG, Björk L, Skansen-Saphir U, Andersson JP (1993) Down-regulation of cytokine production and interleukin-2 receptor expression by pooled human IgG. Immunology 79:211–216
67. Andersson U, Bjork L, Skansen-Saphir U, Andersson J (1994) Pooled human IgG modulates cytokine production in lymphocytes and monocytes. Immunol Rev 139:21–42
68. Poutsiaka DD, Clark BD, Vannier E, Dinarello CA (1991) Production of interleukin-1 beta by peripheral blood mononuclear cells is differentially regulated. Blood 78:1275–1281
69. Ruiz de Souza V, Carreno MP, Kaveri SV, Ledur A, Sadeghi H, Cavaillon JM, Kazatchkine MD, Haeffner-Cavaillon N (1995) Selective induction of interleukin-1 receptor antagonist and interleukin-8 in human monocytes by normal polyspecific IgG (intravenous immunoglobulin). Eur J Immunol 25:1267–1273
70. Blascyk R, Westhoff U, Grossewilde H (1993) Soluble CD4, CD8, and HLA molecules in commercial immunoglobulin preparations. Lancet 341:789–790
71. Lam L, Whitsett CF, McNicholl JM, Hodge TW, Hooper J (1993) Immunologically active proteins in intravenous immunoglobulin. Lancet 342:678
72. Perosa F, Rizzi R, Pulpito V, Dammaco F (1995) Soluble CD4 antigen in intravenous immunoglobulin preparations: is it specific? Clin Exp Immunol 99:16–20

73. Hansen MB, Svenson M, Abell K, Yasukawa K, Diamant M, Bendtzen K (1995) Influence of interleukin-6 (IL-6) autoantibodies on IL-6 binding to cellular receptors. Eur J Immunol 25:348–354
74. Kaveri S, Vassilev T, Hurez V, Lengagne R, Lefranc C, Cot S, Pouletty P (1996) Antibodies to a conserved region of HLA class I molecules, capable of modulating CD8 T cell-mediated function, are present in pooled normal immunoglobulin for therapeutic use. J Clin Invest 97:865–869
75. Marchalonis JJ, Kaymaz H, Dedeoglu F, Schlutter SF, Yocum DE, Edmundson AB (1992) Human autoantibodies reactive with synthetic autoantigens from T-cell receptor β chain. Proc Natl Acad Sci USA 89:3325–3329
76. Takei S, Arora YK, Walker SM (1993) Intravenous immunoglobulin contains specific antibodies inhibitory to activation of T cells by staphylococcal toxin superantigens. J Clin Invest 91:602–607
77. Dodd RY (1996) Infectious risk of plasma donations: relationship to safety of intravenous immune globulins. Clin Exp Immunol 104S:31–34
78. Yap PL (1996) The viral safety of intravenous immune globulin. Clin Exp Immunol 104S:35–42
79. Collinge J, Sidle KCL, Meads J, Ironside J, Hill AF (1996) Molecular analysis of prion strain variation and the aetiology of 'new variant' CJD. Nature 383:685–690
80. Bodemer C, Teillac D, Le Bourgeois M, Wechsler B, de Prost Y (1990) Efficacy of intravenous immunoglobulins in sclerodermatomyositis. Br J Dermatol 123:545–551

3 Immunostimulatory Substances and Vaccination Therapies

Interferon-α Therapy in Dermatology

M. Micksche

Introduction

Interferons (IFN) have pleiotropic effects on a variety of biological systems. The antiviral effect led to the discovery of IFN-α and still serves to standardize these cytokine preparations. The antitumoral activity of IFN-α is characterized by inhibition of cell proliferation in vitro and possibly in vivo, by alterations of cell differentiation, and by an interference with oncogen expression and tumor cell growth factor production [1]. The immunomodulating effects of IFN-α, especially the stimulation of cytotoxic effector cells and changes in the expression of membrane antigens on tumor or host cells, seem also to contribute to the therapeutic efficacy (antitumoral, antiviral activity), giving IFN-α a particular place in therapy [1].

In this review, recent advances in the use of IFN in malignant and nonmalignant dermatological diseases are presented.

Malignant Melanoma

In locally advanced and metastatic melanoma results achieved by cytotoxic chemotherapy are still rather disappointing. Studies including large numbers of patients document response rates (RR) of 15–20% obtained with the most effective single agents. Combination chemotherapies improved RR significantly, but have so far not any influence on overall survival (OS) time [2]. Both clinical course (e.g., spontaneous remissions, foudroyant progression, and metastasis formation together with evidence of tumor-associated antigens) and cellular immune reactions against melanoma cells suggest that the clinical behavior of malignant melanoma is influenced by immune mechanisms. Based upon these findings, a broad spectrum of immunotherapeutic methods have been employed in the treatment of malignant melanoma, yet none of them have brought significant results to date in either palliative or adjuvant settings [3].

The introduction of IFN into the treatment of malignant melanoma in 1980 was especially based on the finding that IFN-α has a pronounced immunomodulating activity and additionally exerts a direct antiproliferative effect on melanoma cells in tissue culture.

In clinical trials in patients with inoperable metastatic melanoma, RR (complete plus partial, CR+PR) of 15–30% were achieved by rIFN-α therapy. In responding patients, pulmonary and cutaneous metastases were particularly sensitive to IFN-α therapy. IFN-α doses presently used are in the range of 3–10 MU/m^2, three to five times weekly, given s.c. and often by self-administration [4].

Several attempts have been made at improving therapy results by combining IFN-α with chemotherapeutic agents. Results achieved in phase II studies with a combination of IFN-α + dacarbazine (DTIC; the gold standard in advanced melanoma therapy) were controversial. Reports on increased RR obtained with this combination are contradicted by other studies that do not confirm this advantage of the combination over monotherapy with IFN-α or DTIC [5, 6]. Results of the first randomized study comparing DTIC with DTIC + IFN-α (10 MU) for treatment of metastatic melanoma have been recently published [7]. Combination therapy significantly increased RR, i.e., 53 % vs. 20 %, and also improved median survival times. Other studies currently under way – using this combination therapy at lower IFN-α doses (10 MU) – have not yet shown such pronounced effects [8]. Thus the combination of DTIC and IFN-α is still experimental.

Combination of IFN-α with interleukin (IL)-2 (see also below) has produced remission rates in the range of 10–25 % [9]. The efficacy of this combination requires further assessment by randomized prospective studies.

In preclinical studies, the synergistic antitumoral activity of IFN-α and cis-platinum (CDDP) has been documented. A phase II study has shown that this combination is an apparently active regimen in advanced melanoma, though limited by the nephrotoxicity of CDDP [10]. In order to avoid these side effects, CDDP was replaced by carboplatin, and this combination was evaluated by us in a phase II study in patients with metastatic melanoma [11]. Therapy started with IFN-α on days 1, 3, and 5, and on day 8 carboplatin (400 mg/m^2 i.v.) was given. IFN-α therapy (3 MU/m^2 s.c. three times a week) was continued in weeks 3 and 4. This cycle was repeated every 28 days. Eight of 19 patients showed objective responses (RR, 42 %), five CR, and three PR. Therapy was generally well tolerated, with dose-limiting side effects in 36 out of 175 carboplatin and 34 out of 175 IFN-α cycles [11].

Presently, combinations of IFN-α with other chemotherapies as well as the antioestrogen tamoxifen are being investigated in phase II and III studies. The efficiency of chemotherapy containing CDDP and/or DTIC is reported to be increased by the addition of tamoxifen [12]. Patients with metastatic melanoma randomized for treatment with DTIC alone and DTIC plus tamoxifen had RR of 12 % and 28 %, respectively . Additionally, a significant influence on survival times, i.e., 29 vs. 48 weeks, was documented [13]. Several ongoing studies are investigating whether the addition of tamoxifen to IFN-α and polychemotherapy combinations results in an increase in RR. Preliminary data of the phase II studies point to an increase (up to 50 %) in RR. However, there is evidence that addition of tamoxifen leads to an increased hematological toxicity. So far, randomized studies have not documented that addition of this antiestrogen results in superior therapy [14]. A promising therapy regimen for metastatic melanoma consists of IFN-α (3 MU per day) plus four-drug chemotherapy, i.e., DTIC, vincristin, bleomycin, and lomustine (CCNU). In 45 evaluable patients, an objective response of 62 % (six CR, 22 PR) was documented [15]. Toxicity of this regimen, given mainly on an outpatient basis, seems to be generally tolerable. Most frequent side effects were transient fever, nausea, vomiting, fatigue, and hematological toxicity grades 1 and 2 [15].

Locoregional administration of IFN-α is to some extent effective. In metastatic melanoma, intralesional injection of rIFN-α at a dosage of 10 MU, three times weekly, led to CR in 16 patients and PR in seven, i.e., a RR of 45 %; however, no systemic responses have been observed [16].

The efficiency of adjuvant therapy with rIFN-α after surgery of the primary melanoma in patients with high risk for relapse with or without lymph node metastases is being investigated in randomized studies. The objective is the prolongation of the relapse-free survival (RFS) and OS, a goal which so far has not been achieved with either chemotherapy or immunotherapy.

The ECOG 1684 clinical trial evaluated the efficacy of IFN-α_{2b} as adjuvant therapy [17]. High-risk melanoma patients (n=280) were randomized to receive IFN-α_{2b} (20 MU/m^2 per day i.v. 5 days a week for 4 weeks in an outpatient setting as induction, followed by 10 MU/m^2 per day s.c. three times a week for 48 weeks as consolidation/maintenance) or close observation. IFN-α_{2b} treatment was continued until disease relapse or study completion. Patients were monitored for a period of 0.6–9.6 years, with a median follow-up of more than 6.9 years among 109 survivors. The median RFS for patients receiving IFN-α_{2b} was significantly longer than in patients under observation alone (p=0.005). Furthermore, patients receiving IFN-α_{2b} had a significantly longer OS than patients under observation (p=0.047). The greatest impact on reduction of disease relapse occurred during the initial months of treatment. An aggregate analysis of the node-positive patients in this trial, who appeared to benefit most, as analysis at 4.7 years median follow-up, revealed a highly significant impact of IFN-α_{2b} treatment on RFS (p=0.0004) and OS (p=0.0086) [17]. The IFN-α_{2b} treatment regimen resulted in significant toxicity, but was tolerated by the majority of patients with appropriate intervention, dosage reduction, and/or dosage interruption. The most frequent adverse events included constitutional symptoms (i.e., fever, chills, and flu-like symptoms), leukopenia, and neurotoxicity. Hepatotoxicity was also observed early in the trial as a potentially serious adverse event. Dose delay or reduction was required at least once in 50% of patients during the induction phase of the trial and in 48% of patients during the consolidation/maintenance phase. The majority of treatment withdrawals occurred in the first 4 months of therapy [17].

The World Health Organization (WHO) has conducted the largest study so far and presented its results at the American Society of Clinical Oncology Meeting in 1995. In this study, 444 melanoma patients with regional nodal metastases were randomized to receive low-dose IFN-α (3 MU s.c. three times per week) for 3 years (n=225) or simply to be observed (n=219). In the first report, there was an improvement in disease-free survival (p=0.02) [18], but the last analysis showed no difference in either disease-free survival or OS [19].

The North Central Cancer Treatment Group (NCCTG) recently reported the results of a randomized trial comparing adjuvant therapy with high-dose IFN-α_{2a} (20 MU/m^2 i.m. three times per week for 12 weeks) versus observation in patients with primary tumors of 1.69 mm or with nodal metastases. A total of 262 patients were enrolled, of whom 102 had primary lesions and 160 nodal metastases. For all patients, there was no significant difference in either RFS or OS, although subset analysis showed borderline improvement in OS patients with nodal metastases [20].

Basal Cell Carcinoma of the Skin

Basal cell carcinoma of the skin (BCC) is the most frequent type of skin cancer and is primarily treated by surgery. Due to the partly multifocal origin and the tendency to recur in about 10–15%, frequent surgery may be required, occasionally causing cosmetic problems, particularly in the facial area. Since BCC is easily accessible for local therapy, IFN-α was applied intralesionally at doses of 1.5–4.5 MU three times weekly for 3 months, resulting in tumor remission in more than 80% of the patients [19]. Side effects were minimal. It is assumed that IFN enhances differentiation of these cells, thus reducing their dividing capacity. Consequently, IFN offers a therapeutic alternative in BCC after failure of surgery and radiotherapy or in order to avoid mutilating surgery [21].

Squamous Cell Carcinoma

Localized squamous cell carcinoma (SCC) is a highly curable disease. The traditional methods comprise Mohs micrographic surgery, cryosurgery, radiation therapy, electrodissection, and recently IFN-α combined with retinoids. This latter class of substances inhibits proliferation of tumor cells, promotes their differentiation, and additionally stimulates cellular immune reactions of the host. Lippman et al. [22] reported that the combination of IFN-α with 13-cis-retinoic acid (RA) led to 24% CR and 41% PR in patients with therapy-refractory SCC. Results of studies including larger numbers of patients are required in order to allow recommendation of this combination therapy in individual patients.

Cutaneous T Cell Lymphoma

Cutaneous T cell lymphoma (CTCL), an indolent non-Hodgkin lymphoma, is characterized by a clonal proliferation of T-helper lymphocytes infiltrating the skin. In progressive CTCL, lymph nodes, spleen, liver, and other internal organs are involved. Treatment options are irradiation with electrons, photochemotherapy with PUVA (psoralen ultraviolet A radiation), retinoid therapy, and topical and systemic chemotherapy. However, none of these modalities is curative, and patients frequently relapse or the disease progresses.

Initially IFN-α was given to therapy-refractory patients. As extremely high doses up to 50 MU/m^2 were used, resulting in severe side effects, duration of both treatment and response was short. More recent studies with lower doses document RR of about 60%, particularly in patients in early stages of CTCL. At present, attempts are being made to combine the above IFN-α therapy with the conventional methods mentioned.

In a pilot study, we used the combination of IFN-α (2 MU s.c. three times a week) with 13-cis-RA (1 mg/kg per day) for the treatment of CTCL. With this treatment schedule, stable responses were achieved in 60% of patients. After achievement of remission, doses of both agents were reduced and therapy was thus well tolerated, without any severe side effects [23]. For the combination of PUVA and IFN-α, RR of 90%, a mean duration of response of 28 months, and a median survival of 62 months have been reported [24].

Condylomata Acuminata

In recent years, incidence of condylomata has been rising dramatically. At present, the cooncogenic potential of this human papillomavirus infection is being discussed with regard to the development of cancer of the anogenital tract. Surgery (cryosurgery, electrocauterization, laser therapy) and/or local treatment with podophyllin or cytotoxic agents are commonly used therapies. Despite these locoregional measures, about 40 % of patients relapse repeatedly.

Because of its antiviral and immunostimulating action, IFN-α has been considered an alternative to standard local therapy. Efficiency and good tolerance of intralesional injection therapy with rIFN (1 MU per lesion three times weekly for 3 weeks) have been documented by placebo-controlled studies. In the IFN-α therapy group, a reduction or decrease in the number of lesions was achieved significantly more often than in a placebo group. By IFN-α therapy, an improvement was obtained within 2–4 weeks and maximal response within 4–9 weeks after initiation of therapy. In more than 50 % of the lesions, remission occurred during these 3 weeks of IFN-α treatment. The therapeutic effect was further increased by a second treatment phase (3 MU three times weekly for 3 weeks). CR was achieved in a total of 63 % of condylomata lesions treated [25]. In about 80 % of the patients, short-term side effects (flu-like symptoms), ceasing after 24 h, were reported. A total of 20 % of patients in the placebo group and in the IFN-α group complained of pain, burning, and/or pruritus at the injection site.

The efficiency of systemic application (i.m. or s.c.) of rIFN-α has been also demonstrated. The relatively low incidence of side effects and, especially, the success achieved in a comparative cross-over study suggest that low-dose systemic IFN-α therapy is advantageous in this disease: IFN- α therapy (1.5 and 18 MU, respectively) for 7–14 days led to significant remissions within the following 4 weeks in eight out of 14 patients included in this study [26]. These results document that both local and systemic IFN-α therapy are active in condylomata acuminata.

The efficiency of rIFN-α, applied s.c. in patients with giant condylomata, has also been documented. In a pilot study using increasing and subsequently decreasing doses (1 MU, increased to 15 MU, and then decreased to 1 MU) over a period of 66 days, we documented long-lasting CR of the disease manifestation in five out of seven patients [27]. Despite the high doses of IFN-α, only few side effects appeared. One important aspect of this study was that patients with giant condylomata were spared invasive and mutilating surgery (vulvectomy) by IFN-α therapy. Nevertheless, this treatment modality requires confirmation by larger studies.

Discussion

IFN-α is playing an increasingly important role in treatment of (non)malignant dermatological diseases. In malignant melanoma, it has additive/synergistic effects with mono/combination chemotherapies, as is currently being investigated in phase III studies [28]. It is, therefore, advisable to treat patients within clinical trials. The results of ECOG 1684 provide the first conclusive evidence from a randomized trial in more than 20 years of clinical research that adjuvant IFN-α treatment in high-risk melanoma patients can clearly and significantly alter the natural history of the disease. High-dose IFN-α might be considered for patients with pathologically proven nodal metastases and for patients with other forms of locoregional disease, including in transit disease, satellites, or local recurrence. Results with IFN-γ therapy in melanoma have so far been disappointing. In a recently published study, in particular, adjuvant IFN-γ therapy in high-risk patients improved neither disease-free survival nor OS [29]. IFN-β has not yet been extensively investigated in melanoma patients.

In CTCL, IFN-α therapy with doses in the range of 2–5 MU/m^2, especially in early stages of the disease, results in RR of about 60 %. Combination therapy, especially with PUVA and/or retinoids, seems to be promising, and remission rates of up to 90 % can be achieved. Condylomata acuminata can be treated by local measures; however, relapses occur frequently. This may be explained by the persistence of the viruses in the healthy tissue surrounding the papillomas, but also indicates that surgical removal of the warts is not radical enough. Locally/systemically applied IFN-α appears to be effective.

The role of IFN-α therapy in hemangioma and Kaposi's sarcoma has not been presented in detail; however, it should be emphasized that IFN-α is efficient in both diseases [30, 31] when administered either locally or systemically. Especially in Kaposi's sarcoma, IFN-α alone or in combination with antiretroviral agents is an active substance, resulting in a considerable number of remissions [30]. Among the side effects of IFN-α therapy, the most common are flu-like symptoms (e.g., nausea, vomiting); neutropenia and thrombopenia are clearly dose-dependent, and cardiac and liver toxicity are rare. Side effects are reversible with cessation of IFN-α therapy [30].

IFN-α represents a new class of therapeutic substances, i.e., cytokines, which can be successfully applied in dermatological diseases.

Summary

In more than 15 years of clinical experience with IFN-α (both natural and recombinant), the therapeutic efficiency of this agent in viral, hematological, and oncological diseases has been documented. In metastatic melanoma, IFN-α leads to remission rates of about 20 %. In high-risk melanoma, the success of adjuvant IFN-α therapy is dose-dependent, i.e., only intermediate/high doses for a period of approximately 1 year prevent relapses and increase survival. Patients with BCC and CTCL also respond to IFN-α monotherapy. Results can be improved by including other treatment modalities, such as retinoids; this also holds true for SCC. Treatment of condylomata acuminata with IFN-α is effective. IFN-α, a prototype of a biological response modifier, has a unique spectrum of activities and can be successfully applied in nonmalignant and malignant dermatological diseases.

References

1. Baron S, Tyring SK (1991) The interferons: mechanisms of action and clinical application. JAMA 266:1375–1380
2. Legha SS (1989) Current therapy for malignant melanoma. Semin Oncol 16:34–44
3. Parkinson DR, Veronesi U, Kirkwood JM (1993) Malignant melanoma. Educational Book, ASCO, pp 84–94
4. Kirkwood JM, Ernstoff MS (1990) Role of interferons in the therapy of melanoma. J Invest Dermatol 95:180–184
5. McLeod GRC, Thomson DB, Hershey P (1982) Recombinant interferon alfa-2a in advanced malignant melanoma. A phase I-II study in combination with DTIC. Int J Cancer [Suppl] 1:31–35
6. Kirkwood JM, Ernstoff MS, Giuliano A, Gams R, Robinson WA, Constanzi J, Pouillart P, Speyer J, Grimm M, Spiegel R (1990) Interferon-a-2a and dacarbazine in melanoma. J Natl Cancer Inst 82:1062–1063
7. Falkson CI, Falkson G, Falkson HC (1991) Improved results with the addition of interferon alfa-2b to dacarbazine in the treatment of patients with metastatic malignant melanoma. J Clin Oncol 9:1403–1408
8. Thompson A, Adena M, McLeod GRC et al (1992) Interferon alpha-2a does not improve response or survival when added to dacarbazine in metastatic melanoma: results of a multiinstitutional Australian randomized trial. Proc Am Soc Clin Oncol 11:343
9. Atzpodien J, Körfer A, Franks CR, Poliwoda H, Krichner H (1990) Home therapy with recombinant interleukin-2 and interferon-a2b in advanced human malignancies. Lancet 335:1509–1512
10. Richner J, Cerny T, Mickschc M et al (1990) Phase II study of continuous subcutaneous alpha 2b interferon combined with cisplatin in advanced malignant melanoma. Proc Am Soc Clin Oncol 9:280
11. Kokoschka EM, Klocker J, Loicht U et al (1994) Interferon-a-carboplatin combination therapy for metastatic melanoma: phase II study. Eur J Cancer 30A:2182–2183
12. McClay EF, Mastrangelo MJ, Sprandio JD, Bellet RE, Berd D (1989) The importance of tamoxifen to a cisplatin-containing regimen in the treatment of metastatic melanoma. Cancer 63/7:1292–1295
13. Cocconi G, Bella M, Calabresi F et al (1992) Treatment of metastatic malignant melanoma with dacarbazine plus tamoxifen. N Engl J Med 327:516–523
14. Legha S, Ring S, Bendikian A, Eton O, Plager C, Papadopoulos N, Ensign LG, Benjamin RS (1993) Lack of benefit from tamoxifen added to a regimen of cisplatin, vinblastine, DTIC and alpha interferon in patients with metastatic melanoma (MM). Proc ASCO, abstract 1325
15. Pyrhönen S, Hahka-Kemppinen M, Muhonen T (1992) A promising interferon plus four-drug chemotherapy regimen for metastatic melanoma. J Clin Oncol 10:1919–1926
16. Von Wussow P, Block B, Hartmann F et al (1988) Intralesional interferon-alpha therapy in advanced malignant melanoma. Cancer 61:1071–1074
17. Kirkwood JM, Strawderman MH, Ernstoff MS, Smith, TJ, Borden EC, Blum RH (1996) Interferon alfa-2b adjuvant therapy of high-risk resected cutaneous melanoma: the Eastern Cooperative Oncology Trial EST 1684. J Clin Oncol 14/1:7–17
18. Cascinelli N, Bufalino R, Morabito A et al (19) Results of adjuvant interferon study in WHO melanoma programme. Lancet 343:913–914
19. Cascinelli N (1995) Evaluation of efficacy of adjuvant rIFNa 2A in melanoma patients with regional node metastases. Proc Am Soc Clin Oncol 14:410
20. Creagan E, Dalton R, Ahmann D (1995) Randomized, surgical adjuvant clinical trial of recombinant interferon alfa-2a in selected patients with malignant melanoma. J Clin Oncol 13:2776–2783
21. Greenway HT (1990) Interferon – coming of age. Arch Dermatol 126:1080–1082
22. Lippman SM, Parkinson DR, Itri LM et al (1992a) 13-cis-retinoic acid and interferon-2a: effective combination therapy for advanced squamous cell carcinoma of the skin. J Natl Cancer Inst 84:235–240

23. Knobler R, Trautinger F, Kokoschka EM et al (1991) Synergistic effect of interferon-alpha-2b and retinoids in the treatment of cutaneous T-cell lymphoma. J Am Acad Dermatol 24:247–252
24. Kuzel TM, Roenigk HH, Samuelson E et al (1995) Effectiveness of interferon a -2a combined with phototherapy for mycosis fungoides and the Sézary syndrome. J Clin Oncol 13/1:257–263
25. Eron LJ, Judson F, Tucker S et al (1986) Interferon therapy for condylomata acuminata. N Engl J Med 315:1059–1064
26. Gross G, Ikenbergh H, Roussaki A et al (1986) Systemic treatment of condylomata acuminata with recombinant interferon-alpha-2a: low-dose superior to the high-dose regimen. Chemotherapy 32:537–541
27. Grablowitz D, Micksche M, Söltz-Szöts J (1992) Systemic treatment of extensive condylomata acuminata with interferon. J Am Acad Dermatol 26:1009–1010
28. Micksche M (1994) Interferon alpha therapy in malignant melanoma. Contemp Ther 1:17–23
29. Meyskens FL Jr, Kopecky KJ, Taylor CW, Noyes RD, Tuthill RJ, Hersh EM, Feun LG, Doroshow JH, Flaherty LE, Sondak VK (1995) Randomized trial of adjuvant human interferon gamma versus observation in high-risk cutaneous melanoma: a Southwest Oncology Group study. J Natl Cancer Inst 87/22:1710–1713
30. Dorr RT (1993) Interferon α in malignant and viral diseases: a review. Drugs 45:177–211
31. Folkman J (1989) Successful treatment of an angiogenic disease. N Engl J Med 320:1211–1211

Tumor Necrosis Factors

R. M. Trüeb

Introduction

The observation of a tumor necrosing effect coincident with infection in a patient with a sarcoma of the neck by Coley [1] more than 100 years ago generated much excitement. Pathogenic bacteria and their products ("Coley's toxins") were thought to comprise a potential means of tumor therapy. In animals bearing a tumor, lipopolysaccharide (LPS) was observed to disproportionately destruct the tumor mass [2]. The LPS-induced factor that caused tumor necrosis was identified in 1975 by Carswell et al. [3]. In 1985, Beutler et al. [4] isolated cachectin as a cause of wasting diathesis in chronic infection. The purification of cachectin by Cerami and Beutler led them to realize that cachectin is also a mediator of shock induced by LPS injection in mice and that it is the same molecule as tumor necrosis factor (TNF)-α [5]. The extraordinary advances in molecular cloning and recombinant technology have since not only supplied large quantities of TNF-α for clinical and basic research, but also the means for neutralizing TNF-α by designing effective inhibitors. Over the past few years, it has also become clear that TNF-α is but one member of a family of ligands for several type I integral membrane glycoproteins with distinctive homologous, repetitive domain structures within their extracellular, amino-terminal regions. The prototype members of this family are the receptors for TNF-α and nerve growth factor (NGF). The anticipation that the ligands for the other receptors would also possess cytokine-like activity was validated by the identification of a series of type II membrane proteins with structural homology to TNF-α that bind to and signal through these receptors (Fig. 1; reviewed in [6–8]). Identification of the TNF families of receptors and ligands has made it possible to study the diverse immunological effects generated by the interaction of these receptor and ligand pairs.

Tumor Necrosis Factor Families of Receptors and Ligands

The TNF/NGF family of receptors now has ten members – 55-kD and 75-kD TNF receptors, NGF receptor, lymphotoxin (LT)-β receptor, Fas, CD40, CD27, CD30, 4–1BB, OX40 protein – excluding viral (Shope fibroma, cowpox, myxoma, and vaccinia viruses) and fungal (the fungal ECP1 protein) homologues (reviewed in [6–8]). Each member of this family of type I transmembrane glycoproteins contains a variable number of a characteristic repeating extracellular cysteine-rich motif. Diversity of the cytoplasmic domain structure among the members of the TNF receptor family enables particular responses to ligands which otherwise share similar structures, cell surface targets, and mechanisms of receptor activation.

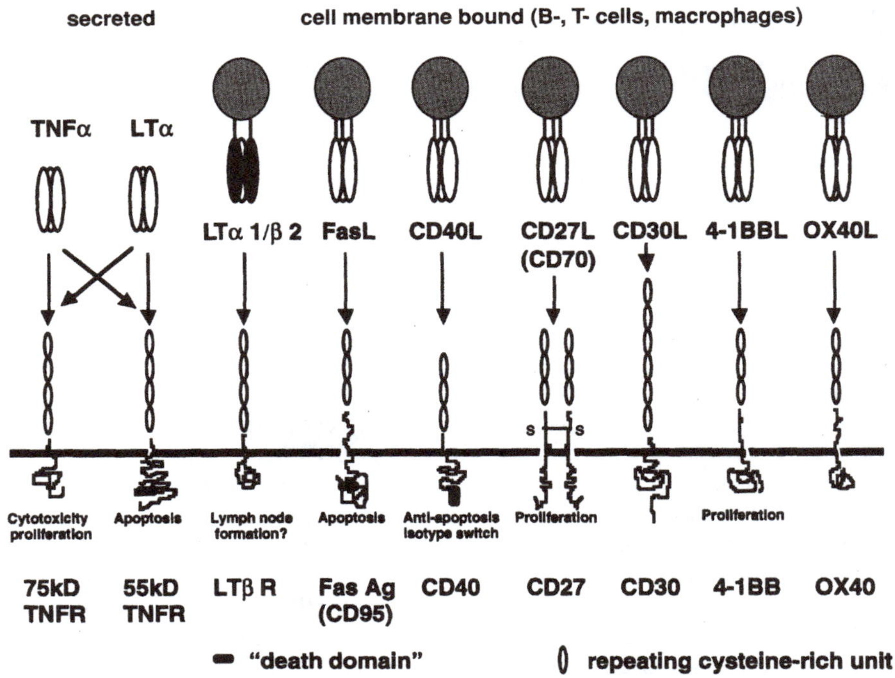

Fig. 1. The tumor necrosis factor (*TNF*) ligand and receptor families. *TNFR*, TNF receptor; *LT*, lymphotoxin. (Adapted from Beutler and van Huffel [6])

The family of ligands for these receptors so far has nine members. Sequence similarities between members of the TNF family of ligands is confined to about 145 residues in the receptor-binding, carboxy-terminal region of the extracellular domains. First, TNF-α and LT-α were shown to be structurally related, and subsequently also the CD40 ligand (CD40L), CD30L, CD27L (CD70), FasL, 4–1BBL, OX40L, and the recently discovered LTβ (reviewed in [6–8]). Although its receptor has homology to the TNF family of receptors, NGF does not exhibit sufficient homology to be regarded as a member of the TNF ligand family. TNF-α and LT-α exert analogous effects on the cell, each capable of binding to two of the TNF receptors (55- and 75-kD TNF receptors), while the other ligands and their receptors interact one on one. However, the different regulatory mechanisms that control the production of TNF-α and LT-α enable particular cytokine actions to occur. Homotrimeric LT-α is entirely secreted; TNF-α is both secreted and able to act as membrane-associated TNF-α, killing target cells by direct cell contact [9]. It also provides a costimulatory signal for B cells [10]. In contrast to TNF-α and secreted LT-α, surface-bound LT-α is distinguished by its ability to form a heterotrimeric cell surface complex with LT-β [11]. This membrane form of LT-α is unique in that it does not retain its transmembrane region, but instead is tethered to the surface via complexation with LT-β [11]. These complexes (LT-β heteromer) are engaged by a specific LT-β receptor (LT-βR) [12]. The soluble form, once considered characteristic of protein hormones, is now acknowledged to be, at least in part, incidental to cytokine function, as exemplified by the TNFs; the ligands for CD40, CD30, CD27, Fas, 4–1BB, OX40, and LT-βR are all predominantly membrane associated and mediate their effects by intercellular contact.

Unraveling Functions of Tumor Necrosis Factor Receptors and Ligands

The identification or creation of mutations that affect the expression or structure of members of the TNF families has given considerable insight into essential functions of several of these proteins.

Naturally occurring mutations affecting the ligand of CD40 have recently been identified as the cause of the human X-linked hyper-IgM syndrome (X-HIM) [13–18], a primary immunodeficiency syndrome characterized by a normal or elevated level of circulating IgM and diminished or absent circulating IgG, IgA, or IgE antibody. Affected children are susceptible to bacterial and opportunistic infections, generally beginning in early infancy. Signaling both through the B7-CD28 and the CD40-CD40L costimulatory pathways plays a central role in the outcome of cognate interactions between T-helper cells and B cells (reviewed in [19]). These molecules stabilize the interaction between the T cell receptor (TCR) and antigen bound to the major histocompatibility complex (MHC) and are involved in lymphokine production, T cell proliferation, and development of T cell effector functions. Ligation of the TCR–CD3 complex with MHC antigen leads to the upregulation of CD40L expression on T cells and its sequential interaction with CD40 on B cells. Signaling via CD40 on the B cell in combination with T cell-derived interleukin (IL)-4 results in the expression of B7 on B cells, whereby these become competent antigen-presenting cells (APCs) and in turn activate T cells by the binding of CD28 to B7. Reciprocal costimulation of T cells by CD40 implies that CD40–CD40L interaction activates not only B cells, but also T cells. In this context, it is noteworthy that X-HIM patients exhibit clinical symptoms implicative of immune dysfunction not restricted to B cells, such as *Pneumocystis carinii* pneumonia and cryptosporidial diarrhea. In addition, dendritic cells have recently been showed to express high levels of functional CD40 [20]: CD40–CD40L interactions enhance dendritic cell survival, enabling prolonged interactions with T cells. Finally, CD40 has been observed on thymic epithelium [21], suggesting a role in T cell development. Such defective T cell development may help to explain the high incidence of autoimmunity in patients with X-HIM.

The lupus-like autoimmune disease of the mouse spontaneous mutants *Lpr* (lymphoproliferation) and *Gld* (generalized lymphoproliferative disease) provides a model for the study of mechanisms of self-tolerance and autoimmunity [22]. *Lpr* and *Gld* are recessive mutations of the Fas [23] and FasL [24] genes, respectively, which lead to progressive lymphadenopathy due to the accumulation of double-negative T cells, an abnormal number of autoreactive $CD4^+$ T cells, production of high-titered autoantibodies, including anti-DNA and rheumatoid factor, and development of immune complex nephritis in the homozygous animals MRL-*lpr/lpr* and MRL-*gld/gld*. However, it is noteworthy that strains other than MRL carrying *lpr* or *gld* mutations develop lymphadenopathy, but not nephritis, suggesting that other "background" genes contribute to the evolution of full-blown autoimmune disease. Wild-type MRL mice develop weak and delayed autoimmune disease, so that *lpr* and *gld* mutations may be considered as severity factors of autoimmunity rather than its cause [25]. Thymic selection seems to occur normally in MRL-*lpr/lpr* mice. In addition, FasL messenger RNA has not been detected in the thymus, suggesting that the Fas system is not involved in thymic T cell development. Therefore, it is probable that the Fas system normally serves to regulate the removal of these cells in the periphery by Fas-mediated apoptosis [26–28]. While apoptosis contributes to central tolerance as a mechanism of cell death in negative selection of thymocytes [29], activation-induced cell death of mature T cells is a regulatory mechanism that may function to control the size of antigen-stimulated clones in the periphery [30]. Interestingly, human cases of Fas deficiency-related autoimmune lymphoproliferative syndrome have recently also been reported [31, 32].

The deletion of genes encoding cytokines or their receptors has been accomplished in the recent past by gene targeting through homologous recombination in embryonic stem cells. Among the members of the TNF receptor and ligand families, deletion of the 55-kDa TNF receptor [33, 34], the 75-kD TNF receptor [35], LT-α [36], and of both the TNF-α and LT-α loci (H.P. Eugster, personal communication) has been achieved. Homozygous deletion of each of these genes has been associated with remarkable phenotypic effects: mice deficient for the 55-kD TNF receptor were highly susceptible to infection by facultative intracellular pathogens such as *Listeria monocytogenes* and resistant to LPS-induced shock [33,34]. Deletion of the 75-kD TNF receptor gene caused a more subtle phenotype, in which dermal scab formation failed to occur in response to repeated intradermal injection of TNF-α [35]. Mice homozygous for the null mutation of LT-α are born without morphologically detectable lymph nodes or Peyer's patches and with disordered splenic architecture [36].

Naturally occurring TNF-α inhibitors, consisting of truncated receptor molecules, lacking the transmembrane or cytoplasmic domains, have been isolated from plasma and urine [37, 38]. These molecules gained interest since they could conceivably be used as antagonists of TNF-α action in vivo. Unfortunately, truncated forms of the TNF receptor are small enough to be efficiently excreted by renal filtration and are therefore short-lived in vivo. By the use of recombinant DNA technology, longer-lived derivatives of such molecules have been produced by the construction of fusion proteins in which the extracellular domain of the TNF receptor is linked to a IgG heavy-chain constant region [39]. These inhibitor molecules have proven more efficient in antagonizing TNF-α action in vivo and have been used successfully by several groups to neutralize TNF-α activity in animal models of endotoxic shock [40–42]. Currently, the gene transfer of analogous fusion proteins introduced into replication-deficient recombinant adenoviral vectors is being used for in vivo blockade of TNF activity for investigational purposes [43–45].

While the biological profile of TNF-α has been outlined in detail since the initial discovery of its apparently disparate triple action as a tumor necrosing factor and a mediator of both cachexia and shock (reviewed in [46]), the roles of the other ligand–receptor pairs within the families of TNF ligands and receptors are just beginning to be elucidated. Although there is a remarkable divergence within the cytoplasmic domains of the members of the TNF receptor family, some of the receptors share the property of generating cytotoxic signals when activated (55-kD TNF receptor, Fas), whereas others promote proliferation (75-kD TNF receptor, CD27, 4–1BB). The observations that have significantly contributed to the understanding of the role of TNF-α in vivo in pathological conditions have been the following: (a) the presence of TNF-α in a given tissue, as judged from detection of TNFα mRNA or TNFα assays, (b) the effects of TNF-α blocking agents, and (c) the effect of TNF-α administration (reviewed in [46]). On the basis of structural homology and observations of in vitro studies, demonstrating that the TNFs are all to some extent involved in proliferation, apoptosis, and costimulation of the immune response (reviewed in [6–8]), it is tempting to speculate on their role by analogy. However, affirmative statements again require three types of observations in vivo: (1) determination of the tissue-specific pattern of expression of the factor in question, as judged by northern blot analysis and in situ hybridization, (2) study of the effect of its inhibition, and (3) study of the effect of its overexpression.

Role of Tumor Necrosis Factors in Autoimmunity

In the past, the possible role of TNF-α in the pathogenesis of autoimmune disease has attracted much attention through features implied in the regulation of the immune response such as MHC linkage, involvement in intrathymic T cell development, and removal of potentially autoreactive clones by apoptosis. MHC linkage of the TNF-α gene made it a particularly attractive candidate mediator of autoimmunity, in as much as allelic polymorphisms within the TNF-α region have been shown to be closely associated with autoimmune prone haplotypes (HLA-A1, HLA-B8, HLA-DR3) [47]. One of the polymorphisms (the uncommon TNF2 allele within the 5' DNA of the TNF locus), reported to occur in individuals with the disease-associated A1, B8, and DR3 haplotypes [47], occupies a region of the TNF-α gene which is believed to be important in regulation of transcription. Whether these associations of TNF-α gene polymorphism with autoimmune disease are due to the products of these alleles directly or to genes in linkage disequilibrium with them is not clear. However, such genetic polymorphisms may be related to cytokine production phenotypes and thus may represent susceptibility and severity factors in the development of chronic inflammatory diseases [48]. Since TNF-α is a MHC-linked gene, questions have been raised as to whether *cis*-acting mutations of the TNF-α gene that interfere with TNF-α synthesis lead to the development of autoimmune disease. Bazzoni and Beutler [49] addressed this question by placing the suspected NZW – New Zealand white mice, the F1 hybrid cross between New Zealand black (NZB) and NZW mice is considered to be the murine model most closely resembling human systemic lupus erythematosus – and NOD (nonbese diabetic mice) TNF-α genes in their normal chromosomal context together with control TNF-α genes by crossing NZW with NZB and NOD with BALB/c mice, respectively. Reverse transcriptase polymerase chain reaction (RT-PCR) analysis showed that the alleles contributed equally to the pool of cytokine messenger RNA, proving that at the pretranslational level the NZW and NOD TNF-α genes are normally expressed. It therefore seems that *cis*-acting mutations affecting the expression of TNF-α genes are not responsible for the development of autoimmunity in the animal models examined. Conversely, *trans*-acting mutations of MHC-linked genes, the products of which are involved in TNF-α synthesis, may be responsible for immune dysregulation. One candidate gene is that encoding NF-κB. The NF-κB gene is closely linked to the TNF-α–LT-α–LT-β gene cluster residing within the class III region of the MHC and has been shown to regulate transcription of a growing list of genes intrinsically linked to a coordinated inflammatory response [50].

Failure of the apoptotic mechanism to remove autoreactive T cells in the periphery also may result in autoimmune disease. The observation of thymic disease in association with autoimmune disease has stimulated many speculations regarding the role of the thymus in the generation of an autoimmune response. The observation of expression of TNF-α [51], CD40 [21], and most recently also of LT-β [52] in the thymus has hinted at the possibility that these factors may influence thymocytic ontogeny, although no such role has yet been substantiated in the respective knockout mice.

With respect to the hypothesis that peripheral tolerance is maintained through a failure of (auto)antigen presentation in the absence of appropriate costimulation (besides Fas-mediated activation-induced cell death), it is conceivable that aberrant expression of a costimulator activates self-reactive T cells, resulting in autoreactivity. The adenoviral TNF inhibitor expression system, and transgenes constitutively expressing the factor in question, under the control of a keratin promoter [53], can be expected to provide valuable models for the study of the in vivo roles of these cytokines in skin immunology. In addition to these transgenic technologies for the functional analysis of the involvement of the TNFs in the immune response, detailed analysis of the expression patterns of these molecules in health and disease will also be necessary to delineate their roles in immune homeostasis and dysregulation.

Perspectives: Therapeutic Impact

As research continues and the immunologic relevance of TNFs becomes clearer, understanding their effects in health and disease has become important for the clinician, inasmuch as potential clinical uses of these factors and their inhibitors are being realized in the treatment of both neoplastic and inflammatory disease.

The rationale for using TNF-α in the treatment of malignant tumors is based on the well-documented antitumor effect of this cytokine. The administration of TNF-α, however, has been hampered by severe systemic side effects. Nonetheless, regional therapy of malignant melanoma by means of isolated perfusion of the limbs provides the means for regional delivery of high doses of recombinant TNF-α with acceptable systemic side effects and a remarkable response rate (91% as compared to 52 % with chemotherapy alone), as reported by Lejeune et al. [54].

Inducing apoptosis in neoplastic cells is emerging as an exciting new approach in the treatment of tumors. Manipulating cell death programs has become an attractive concept for clinical practice, considering the selectivity and stringent control of apoptosis and the absence of injurious effects on the environment [55]. With the current availability of recombinant cytokines (e.g., TNF-α) and antibodies capable of activating cell surface molecules that trigger apoptosis (e.g., anti-Fas), the intralesional treatment of solid tumors with these agents appears promising, especially in combination with chemotherapeutic drugs (biochemotherapy).

Since the original definition of CD30 by the Ki-1 monoclonal antibody, it has shown been that CD30 is not only expressed on Hodgkin and Reed-Sternberg cells in Hodgkin's disease, but also in a subset of non-Hodgkin's lymphoma designated as Ki-1/CD30 anaplastic large cell lymphoma (ALCL). Little is known about the function of the CD30/CD30L system, but there is circumstantial evidence that CD30–CD30L interaction is involved in the immune response and could be responsible for the characteristic inflammatory background of Hodgkin's disease or control of the proliferation of Hodgkin and Reed-Sternberg cells by modulating cytokine secretion or cell–cell interactions (reviewed in [56]). Because of the restricted expression of CD30 in normal human tissue, the CD30 molecule appears to be an ideal target for immunotherapy of Hodgkin's disease or ALCL with specific anti-CD30 antibodies conjugated to cytotoxic agents (immunotoxin therapy) [56]. First results obtained with anti-CD30 immunotoxins in the therapy of patients with Hodgkin's disease refractory to conventional therapies have so far been encouraging [57, 58].

Role of Tumor Necrosis Factors in the Therapy of Autoimmune Disease

During their passage from the bone marrow into the thymus and from there into the periphery, T cells progress through a sequence of developmental stages. Toleragenic mechanisms controlling T lymphocytes are not entirely confined to the intrathymic negative selection of differentiating T cells specific for self peptides (central tolerance). If the self peptide is either not expressed in the thymus or fails to be presented in an appropriate manner, potentially autoreactive T cells may leak out of the thymus into the periphery. Here they either are deleted by the autoantigen (by Fas-mediated activation-induced apoptosis) or ignore the autoantigen on account of the failure of T cells to be activated by autoantigen present on tissue cells that do not appropriately express MHC or costimulatory molecules (reviewed in [59, 60]). An antigenic determinant on a foreign molecule (e.g., a virus) with homology to self peptide may induce a cross-reactive immune response from T cells of the self-reactive repertoire [61]. The primary focus of inflammation initiated by a single such antigenic determinant may lead to the spreading of the immune response to further antigenic determinants on the same or other self molecules at the site of inflammation [62]. The activity of the initiating self-reactive T cell clone and its secretion of cytokines (including TNF-α) in turn propagate further antigen processing. As primed T and B cells enter the site of inflammation, they upregulate the expression of costimulatory molecules (including members of the TNF families of receptors and their ligands). The representation of self-determinants then reaches a point at which a whole array of latent self-determinants become displayed, leading to the generation of an expanded repertoire of autoreactive cells at the site of inflammation ("epitope spreading") [62]. Inasmuch as proinflammatory cytokines (e.g., TNF-α) and costimulatory molecules (e.g., CD40) substantially contribute to the development of this inflammatory autoreactive response in the periphery, cytokine inhibition and costimulatory pathway blockade seem rational approaches to the therapy of autoimmune disease.

For CD40, it has been shown that blocking the CD40L-mediated costimulatory signal from T cells can prevent collagen-induced arthritis in mice [63].

With respect to the Fas/FasL signaling pathway, it would conceptually seem possible to alleviate chronic pathological conditions caused by inappropriate (autoimmunity) or unwanted (transplantation) immune responses by increasing the efficiency of Fas-dependent activation-induced death of T cells in the periphery. Agents performing this function would be in the next generation of immunosuppressive therapy, because they would be directed at eliminating already activated cells without suppressing the activation of new effectors for other challenges [30].

Finally, the concept of virally mediated gene transfer of inhibitors of cytokine activity may ultimately find application in a form of gene therapy wherever cytokine overexpression is recognized to contribute to the development of chronic inflammatory disease [43]. Alternatively, nuclear transcription factors which activate cytokine expression, such as NF-κB, may represent a potential target for intervention in chronic inflammatory disease [64].

Summary

The TNF ligand and receptor families include secreted and transmembrane molecules with sequence homology to TNF-α and its receptors (55- and 75-kD TNF receptors), respectively. While TNF-α is produced by practically all cells involved in the immune response, has protean functions, and is predominantly secreted, other TNF family members (LT-β, Fas, CD40, CD27, CD30, 4–1BB, OX40) apparently have more restricted expression patterns and predominantly exert their effects in a cell–cell contact-dependent manner. Insights into the functions of these molecules have been gained by the identification of natural mutations that affect their expression (CD40, Fas, Fas ligand), in vivo therapy with monoclonal antibodies (TNF-α), and recently by means of suppression of the genes through homologous recombination in embryonic stem cells (55-kD TNF receptor, 75-kD TNF receptor, LT-α, TNF-α /LT-α) or by the use of transgenes overexpressing inhibitor proteins (TNF-α, LT-β). Several members of the TNF families are involved in lymphoid development, lymphocyte costimulation, and apoptosis. As research continues and the imunologic relevance of TNFs becomes clearer, understanding their effects in health and disease has opened up the way for potential clinical uses of TNFs and of their inhibitors in the treatment of endotoxic shock, cancer, and chronic inflammatory disease.

Acknowledgments. This work was supported by the Swiss National Research Foundation.

References

1. Coley WB (1893) The treatment of malignant tumors by repeated inoculations of erysipelas; with a report of ten original cases. Am J Med Sci 105:487–511
2. O'Malley WE, Achinstein B, Shear MJ (1962) Action of bacterial polysaccharide on tumors. II. Damage of sarcoma 37 by serum of mice treated with Serratia marcescens polysaccharide, and induced tolerance. J Natl Cancer Inst 29:1169–1175
3. Carswell EA, Old LJ, Kassel RL et al (1975) An endotoxin-induced serum factor that causes necrosis of tumors. Proc Natl Acad Sci USA 72:3666–3670
4. Beutler B, Mahoney J, Le Trang et al (1985) Purification of cachectin, a lipoprotein lipase-suppressing hormone secreted by endotoxin RAW 264.7 cells. J Exp Med 161:984–995
5. Beutler B, Cerami A (1986) Cachectin and tumor necrosis factor as two sides of the same biological coin. Nature 320:584–588
6. Beutler B, van Huffel C (1994) Unraveling function in the TNF ligand and receptor families. Science 264:667–668
7. Beutler B, van Huffel C (1994) An evolutionary and functional approach to the TNF receptor/ligand family. Ann NY Acad Sci 730:118–133
8. Armitage RJ (1994) Tumor necrosis factor receptor superfamily members and their ligands. Curr Opin Immumol 6:407–413
9. Liu CC, Detmers PA, Jiang SB et al (1989) Identification and characterization of a membrane-bound cytotoxin of murine cytolytic lymphocytes that is related to tumor necrosis factor/cachectin. Proc Natl Acad Sci USA 86:3286–3290

10. Aversa G, Punnonen J, de Vries JE (1993) The 26-kD transmembrane form of tumor necrosis factor a on activated CD4+ T cell clones provides costimulatory signal for human B cell activation. J Exp Med 177:1575–1585
11. Browning JL, Ngam-ek A, Lawton P et al (1993) Lymphotoxin-β: a new member of the TNF family that forms a heteromeric complex with lymphotoxin on the cell surface. Cell 72:847–856
12. Crowe PD, van Arsdale TL, Walter BN et al (1994) A lymphotoxin-β-specific receptor. Science 264:707–709
13. Spriggs MK, Fanslow WC, Armitage RJ et al (1993) The biology of the human ligand for CD40. J Clin Immunol 13:373–380
14. KorthSuer U, Graf D, Mages HW et al (1993) Defective expression of T-cell CD40 ligand causes X-linked immunodeficiency with hyper-IgM. Nature 361:539–541
15. Allen RC, Armitage RJ, Conley ME et al (1993) CD40 ligand gene defects responsible for X-linked hyper-IgM syndrome. Science 259:990–993
16. Disanto JP, Bonnefoy JY, Gauchat JF et al (1993) CD40 ligand mutations in X-linked immunodeficiency with hyper-IgM. Nature 361:541–543
17. Fuleihan R, Ramesh N, Loh R et al (1993) Defective expression of the CD40 ligand in X chromosome-linked immunoglobulin deficiency with normal or elevated IgM. Proc Natl Acad Sci USA 90:2170–2173
18. Aruffo A, Farrington M, Hollenbaugh D et al (1993) The CD40 ligand, gp39, is defective in activated T cells from patients with X-linked hyper-IgM syndrome. Cell 72:291–300
19. Durie FH, Foy TM, Masters SR et al (1994) The role of CD40 in the regulation of humoral and cell-mediated immunity. Immunol Today 15:406–411
20. Caux C, Massacrier C, Vanbervliet B et al (1994) Activation of human dendritic cells through CD40 cross-linking. J Exp Med 180:1263–1272
21. Galy AHM, Spits H (1992) CD40 is functionally expressed on human thymic epithelial cells. J Immunol 149:775–782
22. Singer GG, Carrera AC, Marshak-Rothstein A et al (1994) Apoptosis, Fas and systemic autoimmunity: the MRL-lpr/lpr model. Curr Opin Immunol 6:913–920
23. Watanabe-Fukunaga R, Brannan CI, Copeland NG et al (1992) Lymphoproliferation disorder in mice explained by defects in Fas antigen that mediates apoptosis. Nature 356:314–317
24. Takahashi T, Tanaka M, Brannan CI et al (1994) Generalized lymphoproliferative disease in mice, caused by a point mutation in the Fas ligand. Cell 76:969–976
25. Nagata S, Golstein P (1995) The Fas death factor. Science 267:1449–1456
26. Singer GG, Abbas AK (1994) The Fas antigen is involved in peripheral but not thymic deletion of T lymphocytes in T cell receptor transgenic mice. Immunity 1:365–371
27. Russell JH, Rush B, Weaver C et al (1993) Mature T cells of autoimmune lpr/lpr mice have a defect in antigen-stimulated suicide. Proc Natl Acad Sci USA 90:4409–4413
28. Drappa J, Brot N, Elkon KB (1993) The Fas protein is expressed at high levels on CD4+CD8+ thymocytes and activated mature lymphocytes in normal mice but not in the lupus-prone strain, MRL lpr/lpr. Proc Natl Acad Sci USA 90:10340–10344
29. Golstein P, Ojcius DM, Young DE (1991) Cell death mechanisms and the immune system. Immunol Rev 121:29–65
30. Russel JH (1995) Activation-induced death of mature T cells in the regulation of immune responses. Curr Opin Immunol 7:382–388
31. Rieux-Laucat F, Deist FK, Hivroz C et al (1995) Mutations in Fas associated with human lymphoproliferative syndrome and autoimmunity. Science 268:1347–1349
32. Fisher GH, Rosenberg FJ, Straus SE et al (1995) Dominant interfering Fas gene mutations impair apoptosis in a human autoimmune lymphoproliferative syndrome. Cell 81:935–946
33. Pfeffer K, Matsuyama T, Kündig TM et al (1993) Mice deficient for the 55 kd tumor necrosis factor receptor are resistant to endotoxic shock, yet succumb to L. monocytogenes infection. Cell 73:457–467
34. Rothe J, Lesslauer W, Lötscher H et al (1993) Mice lacking the tumor necrosis factor receptor 1 are resistant to TNF-mediated toxicity but highly susceptible to infection by Listeria monocytogenes. Nature 364:708–802

35. Erickson SL, de Sauvage FJ, Kikly K et al (1994) Decreased sensitivity to tumor-necrosis factor but normal T-cell development in TNF receptor-2-deficient mice. Nature 372:560–563
36. De Togni P, Goellner J, Ruddle NH et al (1994) Abnormal development of peripheral lymphoid organs in mice deficient in lymphotoxin. Science 264:703–707
37. Seckinger P, Isaaz S, Dayer J-M (1989) Purification and serologic characterization of a specific tumor necrosis factor alpha inhibitor. J Biol Chem 264:11966–11973
38. Engelmann H, Aderka D, Rubinstein M et al (1989) A tumor necrosis factor-binding protein purified to homogeneity from human urine protects cells from tumor necrosis factor toxicity. J Biol Chem 264:11974–11980
39. Peppel K, Crawford D, Beutler B (1991) A tumor necrosis factor (TNF) receptor-IgG heavy chain chimeric protein as a bivalent antagonist of TNF activity. J Exp Med 174:1483–1489
40. Mohler KM, Torrance DS, Smith C et al (1993) Soluble tumor necrosis factor (TNF) receptors are effective therapeutic agents in lethal endotoxemia and function simultaneously as both TNF carriers and TNF antagonists. J Immunol 151:1548–1561
41. Van Zee KJ, Kohno T, Fischer E et al (1992) Tumor necrosis factor soluble receptors circulate during experimental and clinical inflammation and can protect against excessive tumor necrosis factor α in vitro and in vivo. Proc Natl Acad Sci USA 89:4845–4849
42. Evans TJ, Moyes D, Carpenter A et al (1994) Protective effect of 55- but not 75-kD soluble tumor necrosis factor receptor-immunoglobulin G fusion proteins in an animal model of Gram-negative sepsis. J Exp Med 180:2173–2179
43. Kolls J, Peppel K, Silva M, Beutler B (1994) Prolonged and effective blockade of tumor necrosis factor activity through adenovirus-mediated gene transfer. Proc Natl Acad Sci USA 91: 215–219
44. Kolls JK, Lei D, Nelson D et al (1995) Adenovirus-mediated blockade of tumor necrosis factor in mice protects against endotoxic shock yet impairs pulmonary host defense. J Infect Dis 171:570–575
45. Trüeb RM, Brown G, van Huffel C et al (1995) Expression of an adenovirally encoded LT-β inhibitor prevents clearance of Listeria monocytogenes in mice. J Inflammation 45:239–247
46. Vassalli P (1992) The pathophysiology of tumor necrosis factors. Annu Rev Immunol 10: 411–452
47. Wilson AG, de Vries N, Pociot F et al (1993) An allelic polymorphism within the human tumor necrosis factor alpha promoter region is strongly associated with the HLA A1, B8 and DR3 alleles. J Exp Med 177:577–580
48. Jacob CO (1992) Studies on the role of tumor necrosis factor in murine and human autoimmunity. J Autoimmun 5 [Suppl A]:133–143
49. Bazzoni F, Beutler B (in press) Comparative expression of TNF-α alleles from normal and autoimmune-prone MHC haplotypes. J Inflammation
50. Bäuerle PA, Baltimore D (1991) The physiology of NF-κB transcription factor. In: Cohen P, Foulkes JG (eds) Molecular aspects of cellular regulation, vol 6. Elsevier, Amsterdam, pp 423–446
51. Giroir BP, Brown T, Beutler B (1992) Constitutive synthesis of tumor necrosis factor in the thymus. Proc Natl Acad Sci USA 89:4864–4868
52. Pokholok DK, Maroulakou IG, Kuprash DV et al (1995) Cloning and expression analysis of the murine lymphotoxin β gene. Proc Natl Acad Sci USA 92:674–678
53. Sharpe AH (1995) Analysis of lymphocyte costimulation in vivo using transgenic and "knock-out" mice. Curr Opin Immunol 7:389–395
54. Lejeune F, Lienard D, Eggermont A et al (1994) Clinical experience with high-dose tumor necrosis factor alpha in regional therapy of advanced melanoma. Circ Shock 43:191–197
55. Thompson CB (1995) Apoptosis in the pathogenesis and treatment of disease. Science 267:1456–1462
56. Falini B, Pileri S, Pizzolo G et al (1995) CD30 (Ki-1) molecule: a new cytokine receptor of the tumor necrosis factor receptor superfamily as a tool for diagnosis and immunotherapy. Blood 85:1–14
57. Falini B, Bolognesi A, Flenghi L et al (1992) Response of refractory Hodgkin's disease to monoclonal anti-CD30 immunotoxin. Lancet 339:1195–1196

58. Renner C, Jung W, Sahin U et al (1994) Cure of xenografted human tumors by bispecific monoclonal antibodies and human T cells. Science 264:833–835
59. Mamula MJ, Craft J (1994) The expression of self antigenic determinants: implications for tolerance and autoimmunity. Curr Opin Immunol 6:882–886
60. Miller JFAP, Flavell RA (1994) T-cell tolerance and autoimmunity in transgenic models of central and peripheral tolerance. Curr Opin Immunol 6:892–899
61. Fujinami RS, Oldstone MBA (1985) Amino acid homology and virus: mechanisms for autoimmunity. Science 230:1043
62. Lehmann PV, Sercarz EE, Forsthuber T et al (1993) Determinant spreading and the dynamics of the autoimmune T cell repertoire. Immunol Today 14:203–208
63. Durie FH, Fava RA, Foy TM et al (1993) Prevention of collagen-induced arthritis with an antibody to gp39, the ligand for CD40. Science 261:1328–1330
64. McCay IA, Winyard P, Leight IM et al (1994) Nuclear transcription factors: potential targets for new modes of intervention in skin diseases. Br J Dermatol 131:591–597

Cytokines and Cytokine Gene Transfer in Cancer Treatment

D. Schadendorf

Introduction

It is generally accepted that the spontanous generation of cancer cells is a common event and that the immune system ensures strict surveillance with the detection and elimination of these cells. In order to fight cancer, the idea of using the destructive power of immunologic reactions is easily visualized in autoimmune diseases and by the rejection of allografts in transplantation medicine. A number of clinical observations in human malignant melanoma suggest that a particularly vigorous immune response occurs [18, 28, 29, 31]. It is believed that the immune attack against melanoma cells may be responsible for the occurrence of spontanous melanoma regressions and for the concomittant destruction of melanocytes in benign lesions, leading to clinical phenomena such as halo nevi, uveitis, and vitiligo in melanoma patients. In addition, tumor dormancy with a prolonged interval between the occurrence of the primary tumor and melanoma metastases has been interpreted as indicating the existence of specific, immunologic antitumor effector mechanisms. These observations, together with anecdotal and clinical reports of tumor regressions following bacterial infections or more specific immune interventions, suggest that melanoma is a good model with which to evaluate the various strategies of immune therapy [28, 29, 31].

The extensive search for tumor-specific antigens using serological reagents and monoclonal antibodies turned out, however, not to be successful in most instances, since antigens detected were not tumor specific. In recent years, it became increasingly clear that T lymphocytes may play a critical role in antitumor immune responses and surveillance [5, 19, 28]. Furthermore, $CD8^+$ T lymphocytes derived from melanoma lesions or the peripheral blood were shown to be capable of mediating impressive tumor regressions in vivo [17, 34].

$CD8^+$ T cells recognize short peptides that arise within any cell by proteolysis of cellular proteins and are then transported to the cell surface in association with class I HLA molecules. It is believed that $CD8^+$ cells do not respond to complexes of self HLA molecule and self peptide, but are activated to lyse affected cells upon detection of foreign HLA molecules or self HLA molecules presenting foreign or altered peptides [41]. The availability and further characterization of such tumor-specific T cell clones in recent years has led to the identification of several melanoma-associated antigens (reviewed in [5, 19]). For most of these antigens, only one or two short nonapeptides have been identified which are recognized by specific, predominantly $CD8^+$ T cell lines in a HLA-restricted manner [33]. Melanoma-associated tumor antigens can be divided into three major groups: (1) tissue-restricted differentiation antigens, such as tyrosinase, gp100/Pmel 17, gp75/TRP-1 (tyrosinase-related protein), or Melan A/MART-1 (melanoma antigen recognized by T cells), which are also detectable in normal melanocytes, (2) oncofetal antigens, such as the MAGE, BAGE, and GAGE gene families, which are expressed in melanomas and in other epithelial carcinomas, but not in normal tissues except testis, and (3) unique tumor antigens characterized by tumor-specific point mutations detected in β-catenin and cyclin-dependent kinase 4 (CDK4) by specific T cell lines (reviewed by [19]).

However, before specific cytotoxic T lymphocyte (CTL) clones can be activated to lyse target cells, an educational process called "priming" of naive CTL precursors needs to be initiated. For priming of naive T cells, the sole presentation of peptides in the HLA context is insufficient and leads to anergy of T lymphocytes; thus costimulatory signals such as the expression of adhesion molecules, e.g., CD54, CD58, and B7, need to be presented in parallel to the HLA-peptide complex by the antigen-presenting cells (APC) in order to efficiently prime naive T cells. In addition, secretion of cytokines such as interleukin (IL)-12 or interferon (IFN)-γ favor the generation of a cytolytic T-helper (Th)-1 responses ([25]; Fig. 1).

State of the Art

Cytokines

Standard forms in cancer therapy such as surgery, radiation, and chemotherapy, although effective in some instances, often fail to cure affected patients. Melanoma in its advanced stage has a high mortality rate because of the high resistance to conventional therapies [1, 13]. Alternative treatment strategies are therefore urgently needed. The experience of the last few decades, however, using agents for nonspecific stimulation of the immune system, e.g., Camille-Guérin bacillus (BCG), *Corynebacterium parvum*, levamisole, IFN, and many others, was disappointing, since the clinical effects observed were only rare and random without therapeutic benefit for most of the patients (reviewed in [28, 31]). Consequently, at the beginning of 1980s several groups developed more intense approaches to stimulate the immune system based mainly on the T cell growth factor IL-2. IL-2 is known to activate lymphocytes and natural killer (NK) cells to kill tumor cells upon coculture. Although cell lysis mediated by IL-2 was not restricted to cancer cells, the cytokine has been used extensively in both animal models and melanoma patients. It has been injected both intratumorally and systemically, causing not only impressive regressions but also dramatic side effects [47]. By 1990, it had become clear that the infusion of in vitro activated cells or the application of IL-2 alone was not sufficient to cure melanoma patients and that a successful immune response was dependent on the activation of an appropriate set of immune effector functions.

The central role of cytokines and the importance of local cytokine concentrations was discovered to play a pivotal role in regulating T cell function and, furthermore, distinct subsets of $CD4^+$ T cells were distinguished by their different pattern of secreted cytokines (reviewed by [25]; Fig. 1). Such T cell subsets were termed Th-1-secreting IFN-, tumor necrosis factor (TNF)-, and granulocyte-macrophage colony-stimulating factor (GM-CSF) and Th-2-secreting IL-3, IL-4, IL-5, IL-10, and IL-13. The development of the appropriate T-helper subset is crucial, because an improper T-helper response can lead to exacerbation and progression of the disease. $CD8^+$ T cells often secrete a Th-1-like cytokine pattern now classified as T_{C1} cells; however, there is now increasing

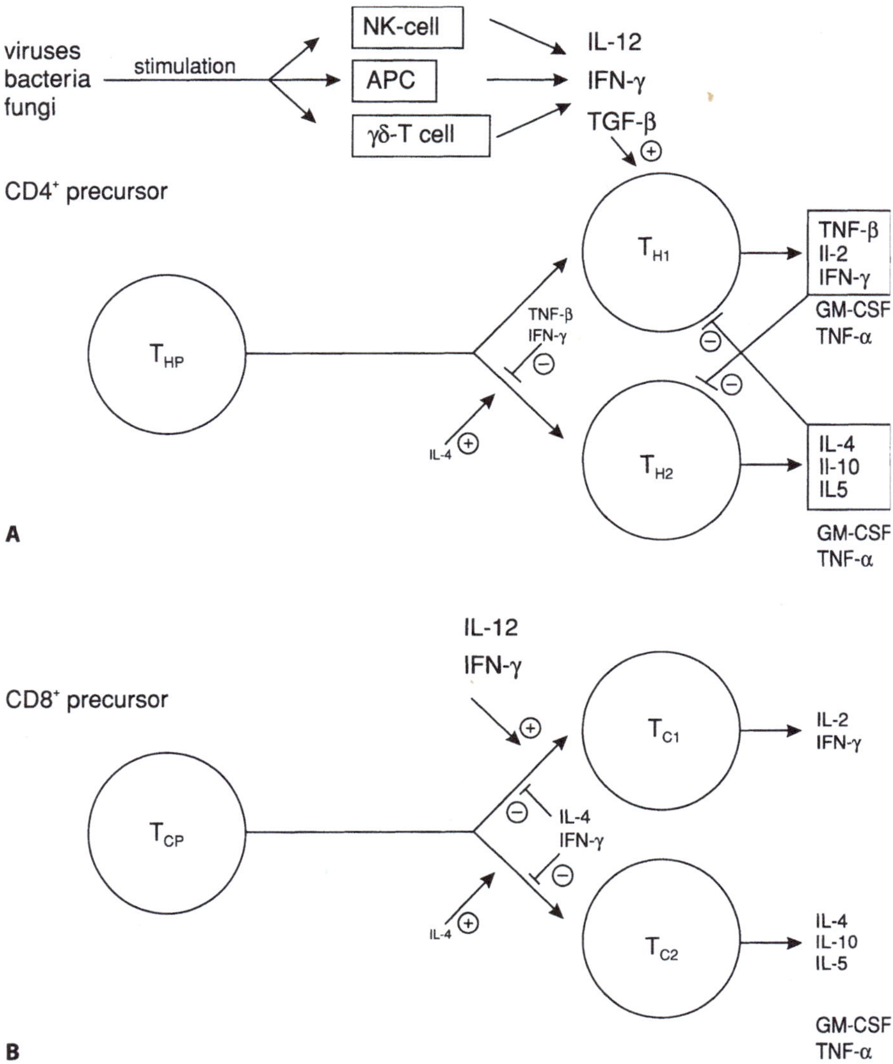

Fig. 1 A,B. T cell subsets and differentiation patterns of **A** $CD4^+$ and **B** $CD8^+$ T cells. $CD4^+$ and $CD8^+$ T cells differentiate from naive precursors (T_{HP}), which secrete interleukin (IL)-2 but not IL-4 or interferon (*IFN*)-γ, into T_{H1}/T_{C1} or T_{H2}/T_{C2} cells. Differentiation of $CD4^+$ and $CD8^+$ T cells is regulated by enhancing (+) and suppressive (–) acting cytokines. LT, lymphotoxin; T_C, T cytotoxic; T_H, T helper; *NK*, natural killer; *APC*, antigen-presenting cell; *TGF*, transforming growth factor; *GM-CSF*, granulocyte-macrophage colony-stimulating factor

evidence for the existence of Th-2-like $CD8^+$ T cells (T_{C2} cells) in humans and in mice. $CD4^+$ and $CD8^+$ subsets can be derived under similar conditions: IL-12 and IFN- encourage the differentiation of precursors into Th-1 or T_{C1} cells, whereas IL-4 induces Th-2 and T_{C2} cells (reviewed in [25]). Therefore, the induction of a Th-1 response with subsequent cell-mediated, delayed-type hypersensitivity (DTH) reaction is one of the goals of therapeutic cytokine administration.

In addition, it is well established that melanoma cells themself secrete a number of cytokines [8], having a great impact on biological behavior including proliferation, metastasis, and immune response. We now know that a deficit of cellular immune response against melanoma cells and antigens is due to several factors that inhibit or impair the induction of an antitumor immune response, including a lack of costimulatory signals, downregulation of major histocompatibility complex (MHC) molecules [35], or the release of immunosuppressive mediators such as transforming growth factor (TGF)-β and IL-10 [8]. Both cytokines are produced in large quantities by human melanoma cells, causing impairment of antigen presentation and T cell activation [3].

Taken together, under physiological conditions cytokines are important mediators of short-range signals involved in the complex interaction of host and tumor as well as in the regulation of the cell-mediated antitumor response. Therefore, interference and modulation of the cytokine network leading to an altered cytokine concentration in the tumor surroundings and a changed tumorigenicity may be promising ways of inducing a systemic immune response towards the tumor.

Animal Models

The dream harbored by tumor immunologists of being able to protect people and to cure patients from cancer by vaccination is an old one. Recent work has supported the concept and feasibility of such an idea in various animal models. Pioneering work by Tepper and coworkers [42] showed that, after transfection of the IL-4 gene, tumor cells were rejected in an animal tumor model, and work by Fearon and colleagues [11] demonstrated that, after gene transfer, cytokines can bypass some of the costimulatory signals in order to cause tumor rejection. Since then, numerous cytokines have been tested in such models for their capacity to inhibit tumor growth and metastasis formation (reviewed in [4, 7, 10, 30]). Surprisingly, a large variety of cytokines were able to induce a local immune response leading to tumor rejection (Table 1). However, certain cytokines are active in some, but not all animal tumor models (reviewed in [4, 7, 10, 30]). At present, it is not clear whether a change in immunogenicity is responsible for the rejection. It is currently thought that the local concentration of cytokine surrounding the tumor cells (Fig. 2A) leads to an influx of immunocompetent cells such as T cells, NK cells, and APC (Fig. 2B): tumor cells destroyed by the inflammatory reaction at the vaccination site are taken up by APC and subsequently presented in the lymph node (LN) to appropriate T cells (Fig. 2C). After priming of a tumor-specific anti-immune response in the LN, a sufficient number of tumor-specfic T cells ($CD4^+$ and $CD8^+$) circulate into the peripheral blood, leading to the destruction of remaining tumor cells in the entire organism (Fig. 2D). Effects on tumor growth after cytokine gene transfer into tumor cells of various histological origin are summarized in Table 1. Cytokines differed in their effects with regard to the effector cells attracted, and sometimes the effects were dependent on the tumor model used. In tumor models studied more

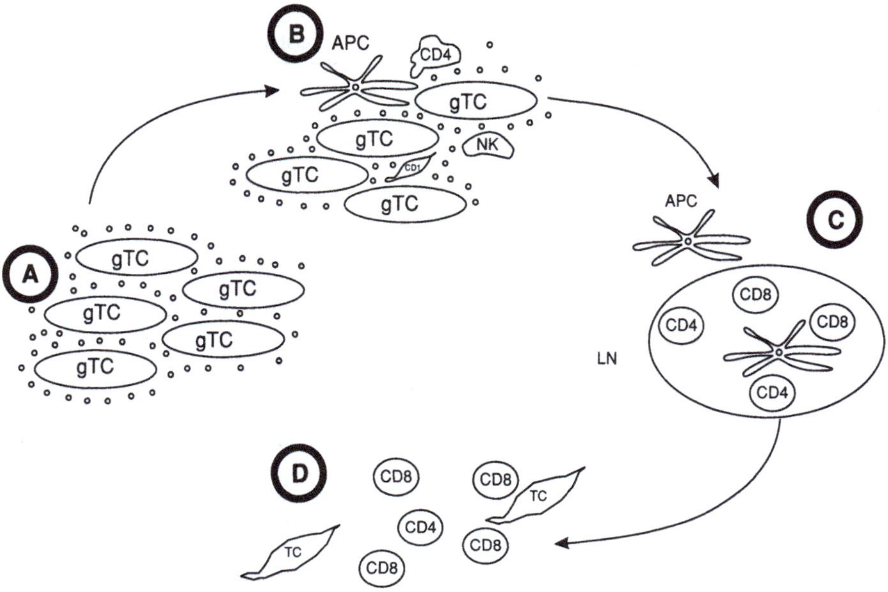

Fig. 2A–D. Induction of systemic antitumor immunity via vaccination with cytokine gene-modified tumor cells. **A** Gene-transfected tumor cells (*TC*) constantly secrete the genetically inserted cytokine and **B** cause a local influx of immunological effector cells such as natural killer cells (*NK*), T cells ($CD4^+$, $CD8^+$), and antigen-presenting cells (*APC*), leading to a local inflammation at the site of vaccination and subsequent destruction of the gene-altered tumor cells. **C** Subsequently, proteins of the destructed tumor cells are taken up by APC, which present the antigens in the context of major histocompatibility complex (MHC) molecules after migration into the lymph node (*LN*). **D** Tumor-specific T cells ($CD4^+$, $CD8^+$) generated in the LN circulate in the body and eliminate tumor cells at distant locations

carefully, dose dependency became visible in several cases, as did the need for $CD8^+$ T cells for tumor eradication and long-term tumor immunity.

Other possible explanations for the tumor-inhibitory effects observed in the animal models include growth retardation by altered tumor cell surroundings caused by the cytokine-secreting tumor cells, differences in transfection efficacy and cytokine levels after transfection, and increased immunogenicity of live tumor cell vaccines as used in most animal models versus irradiated or mitomycin-treated tumor cells. A major question in human gene therapeutic approaches is also whether genetically modified tumor cells are able to induce a systemic (T cell-mediated) immune response that is strong enough to detect and destroy distant, nonmodified tumor cells (reviewed in [4, 7, 10, 30]).

Somatic Gene Therapy – Clinical Trials

At the time of writing (December 1995), roughly 220 trials using so-called gene therapies have been approved worldwide since 1990 (reviewed in [14, 23, 32, 39]). Almost 15% of these studies have no therapeutic intent and are gene-marking trials. The majority

Table 1. Animal tumor models used to evaluate the effects of cytokine gene transfer (reviewed in Columbo and Forni 1994; Blankenstein 1994; Pardoll 1995; Dalgleish 1996; Schadendorf et al. 1997)

Cytokine	Tumor cells used	Tumor inhibtion	Comments
IL- 1α	NIH-3T3, B16F10, MBT-2	+ or –	
IL-2	J558L, B16F10, TS/A, X63-Ag, 4T07, CT26, CMS-5, P815, LCC, YAC-1, MCA-102, 3LL-D122, MBT-2, HSNLV, RAT-1, Line 1	+	Dose-dependent effect; CD8 cells essential for tumor eradication
IL-3	Line 1, YAC-1	+	CD4-dependent tumor rejection, systemic tumor immunity
IL-4	J558L, B16F10, LLC, RENCA, CHO, K485	+ Blocked by IFN-γ and eos neutralizing antibodies	Macrophages and Eos strongly enriched in tumor infiltrate; systemic tumor immunity, CD8 cells essential for tumor eradication
IL-5	J558L, B16F10, TS/A	–	Strong eosinophilic tumor infiltrate
IL-6	J558L, B16F10, TS/A, 3LL-D122, MCA-207	– or + (3LL)	Monocytic, neutrophilic tumor infiltrate
IL-7	J558L, TS/A, FSA, 203-glioma	+	Dose-dependent effect: tumor infiltrate: CD4/CD8$^+$ mixture, Eos, macrophages CD4$^+$: prevented initial tumor growth CD8$^+$: tumor eradication
IL-10	TS/A, CHO	– or + (CHO)	
IL-12	B16F10, RENCA, M5076	+	Dose dependent effect: CD8 cells essential for tumor eradication
IL-13	3LL-D122, P815	+	Monocytic and neutrophilic tumor infiltrate
IFN-α	B16, 3C1-8	+	T cell-dependent tumor rejection
IFN-γ	J558L, B16F10, TS/A, C1300, CMS-5, SP-1, CT-26, MCA-101, MBT-2, 3LL-D122		Dose dependent effect: CD8 cells essential for tumor eradication
TFN-α	J558L, B16F10, TS/A, 1591-RE, MCA-205, MCA-102, EB, EBS	+ or –	Tumor infiltrates heterogenous: tumor rejection metiated by CD4, CD8, or macrophages dependent on model system
G-CSF	C26	+	Via IFN-γ (?); neutrophilic tumor infiltrate; no systemic tumor immunity
M-CSF	J558L	–	
MCF	B16, CHO	+	
GM-CSF	B16F10, TS/a, MBT-2, R3327	+	Dose-dependent effect, T cell-dependent systemic tumor immunity

Tumor cell lines used: *colon:* C26, CT26, SP-1; *melanoma:* B16, B16F10, 1591-RE; *fibrosarcoma:* CMS-5, MCA-101, MCA-102, MCA-207, HSNLV (rat), FSA; *mastocytoma:* P815; *plasmocytoma:* J558L, X63-Ag; *lung carcinoma:* 3LL-D122, Lcc; line 1; *leukemia/lymphoma:* 3C1-8, YAC-1; *bladder carcinoma:* MBT-2; *mammary carcinoma:* TS7A, K485; *renal carcinoma:* RENCA; *neuroblastoma:* C1300; *prostate carcinoma:* R3327.
CHO, Chinese hamster ovary cells; *IL*, interleukin; *IFN*, interferon; *TNF*, tumor necrosis factor; *CSF*, colony-stimulating factor; *GM-CSF*, granulocyte-macrophage CSF; *Eos*, eosinophiles

Table 2. Somatic gene therapy: approved and ongoing clinical trials up to December 1995 (reviewed in Gilboa and Lyerly 1994; Vielweg and Gilboa 1995; Schmidt-Wolf and Schmidt-Wolf 1995; Möller and Schadendorf 1997)

Target gene	Trials (*n*)	Comments
Marker genes	37	NeoR
Cytokines / adhesion molecules		
IL-1RA	1	Rheumatoid arthritis
IL-2	22	MM, RCC, NSCLC, breast, ovary, prostate
IL-4	3	MM, glioblastoma
IL-7	3	MM, RCC, colon
IL-12	2	MM, head and neck, breast
GM-CSF	7	MM, RCC, prostate
TNF-α	2	Cancer
IFN-β	1	Glioblastoma
IFN-γ	2	MM
IL-2 + IFN-γ	1	Prostate
IL-2 + B7	1	MM
CD80 / B7	1	MM
HLA-B7 + β_2-microglobulin	17	MM, RCC, breast, colorectal, head and neck
MDR-1	6	Cancer (breast, ovary, myeloma)
Protooncogenes		
(antisense c-*myc*, c-*fos*, K-*ras*, *erbB2*)	4	Cancer (prostate, breast, ovary, pancreas)
Tumor suppressor genes (p53)	5	Cancer (head and neck, MM, liver, NSCLC)
Tumor-associated antigens	9	PSA, CEA (x6), MAGE-1, E1A
Growth factors		
VEGF	2	Arterial diseases
EGF	1	Wound healing
Antisense IGF-1	1	Glioblastoma
Antisense TGF-β_2	1	Glioblastome
Suicide genes		
Thymidine kinase (TK)	26	HIV, ovary (x5), glioblastoma (x7), MM prostate
Cystosine deaminase	2	Breast, hepatic metastases
Others		
HIV	17	
Genetically determined diseases	38	Mucoviscidosis (CFTR x20)
Miscellaneous	10	

IL, interleukin; *GM-CSF*, garnulocyte-macrophage colony-stimulating factor; *TNF*, tumor necrosis factor; *IFN*, interferon; *EGF*, endothelial growth factor; *VEGF*, vascukar EGf; *TGF*, transforming growth factor; *MM*, malignant melanoma; *RCC*, renal cell carcinoma; *NSCLC*, non-small cell lung cancer; *HIV*, human immunodeficiency virus; *PSA*, prostate-specific antigen; *CEA*, carcino-empryonic antigen; *CFTR*, cystic fibrosis transporter regulator

(65%) of the trials are designed to treat cancer (Table 2). Two third of the protocols utilize murine retroviral vectors, whereas a subset of investigators (17%) use adenoviral vectors or liposomes (10%) for gene delivery. The injection of naked DNA for gene delivery and the use of other viral vectors such as adeno-associated viruses or ballistic gene transfer techniques are currently not commonly in practice.

Roughly 110 clinical gene therapy trials for the treatment of patients suffering from metastatic cancer had been approved or initiated by the end of 1995 (Table 2). The great majority of investigators used immunization strategies with cytokine gene-modified tumor cells (Table 2), the majority being aimed at the treatment of metastatic melanoma followed by the treatment of patients suffering from renal cell carcinomas. Almost one third of the clinical protocols involving cytokine gene transfer use IL-2 for cell transduction (Table 2). However, almost all cytokines that have been shown to be effective in tumor rejection in animal models, such as TNF-, IL-4, IL-7, IFN-, GM-CSF, and IL-12, are being tested in clinical phase I studies.

At the Virchow Clinic in Berlin, a clinical phase I study has been initiated aimed at inducing T cell-mediated cytotoxicity and tumor immunity by vaccination of metastatic melanoma patients [36]. The study was designed to alter autologous melanoma cells by genetic manipulation in order to attract immunologically competent cells to the tumor and to elicit systemic antitumor immunity. Therefore, melanoma metastases from melanoma patients who have failed to respond to other therapies are surgically removed and melanoma cells are expanded in vitro. Subsequently, autologous melanoma cells are transfected in three phases with either the full-length human IL-7, GM-CSF, or IL-12 gene. Patients are vaccinated s.c. with 5×10^{-6} to 5×10^{-7} autologous cells in weeks 1, 2, 3, and 6. In parallel, DTH reactivity is recorded and extensive immunological monitoring, including flow cytometry, NK and lymphokine-activated killer (LAK) activitity, and CTL analysis, is performed. The cytokine gene transfer protocol uses a newly developed gene transfer technology which combines ballistic transfer of biological molecules and magnetic cell sorting [37]. Evaluation of the first ten patients immunized with autologous IL-7 gene-modified melanoma cells demonstrated the safety, lack of toxicity, and feasibility of such an approach; however, no major clinical response was achieved [24]. Eight of ten patients completed the initial three s.c. vaccinations with IL-7 gene-modified cells in Berlin and were eligible for immunological evaluation. Nonspecific cytotoxicity (NK and LAK activity) increased upon vaccination in four out of eight and seven out of eight patients, respectively. Furthermore, peripheral blood lymphocytes were found to contain an an increased number of tumor-reactive T cells after immunization. The number of tumor-reactive and cytolytic T cell lines was significantly higher after vaccination, as determined by a limited dilution analysis in seven patients. Furthermore, in three out of six patients, the frequency of cytolytic microcultures increased between 2.6- and 28-fold. The magnitude of the T cell reactivity was found to be highly associated with the patients' Karnofsky index and recall antigen skin reactivity before vaccination. In conclusion, vaccination of patients with advanced melanoma using autologous, IL-7 gene-modified melanoma cells induced immunological changes that can be interpreted as an increased antitumor immune response even in far advanced, terminally ill patients. Since immunological modulation was most pronounced in patients with a good physical condition, the authors suggested that therapy using IL-7 gene-modified tumor cells might be especially beneficial in patients with minimal tumor load [24].

Besides utilizing autologous tumor cells for gene transfer and vaccination, clinical trials are underway using allogeneic tumor cell lines for vaccination (reviewed in [14, 23, 32, 39]). This approach requires relatively less extensive cell preparations and allows for easier standardization, although the benefit of a strong allogeneic reaction in such an immunization approach has not been sufficiently evaluated. Furthermore, other investigators are using autologous tumor cells admixed with autologous or allogeneic, cytokine gene-modified fibroblasts for immunization [21,43]. In addition to the use of cytokine gene-modified tumor cells in numerous clinical protocols, studies are in progress in which tumor cells have been altered genetically to express the costimulatory molecule B7, and melanoma patients are currently being immunized with such altered cells. B7 has been shown to mediate tumor repression in mice by several groups [14,46]. In addition, intratumoral injection of naked DNA using a retroviral vector encoding a foreign HLA molecule, HLA-B7, has been shown to have some efficacy in reducing the size of injected metastases [27].

Discussion

Recently, cytokine gene transfer into tumor cells has been shown to mediate tumor regression and antimetastatic effects in several animal models via immunomodulation. Consequently, a number of clinical protocols have been developed to treat cancer patients with cytokine gene-modified tumor cells. Based on the experimental model systems described above, the potent tumor-inhibitory capacity of cytokine-transfected tumor cells causing tumor rejection seems to answer the question of whether cytokine gene-transfected tumor cells are useful for vaccination.

However, it has to be borne in mind that not only do the molecules used for gene modification differ widely among studies, but also vaccination strategies are not comparable. Furthermore, most of the experimental models have not been analyzed for the induction of systemic and protective antitumor immune responses. Only a few recent studies have tried to evaluate the impact of cytokine gene transfer itself in the induction of antitumor immunity [2, 7, 16]. It became clear that tumor immunity in animal systems was crucially associated with the ability to replicate tumor cells used for vaccination [2]. Irradiation or mitomycin-treated cells reduced protective immune responses to 10–30 % of immunized mice. Transduction and immunization with multiple cytokine genes did not elicit synergistic effects [16]. In addition, most of the tumor systems described used viral expression vectors which encode additional viral proteins and which might consequently have costimulatory effects essential for eliciting the systemic antitumor response [4]. The optimal dose for vaccination is currently not known, and a study by Blankenstein and coworkers demonstrated that tumor cells mixed with a classical adjuvant such as *Corynebacterium parvum* were as effective in raising protective immunity as cytokine-transfected tumor cells, an effect which became particularly obvious when using higher numbers of tumor cells for challenging [16]. Recently, the combination of cytokine genes such as IL-7 and the costimulatory B7 molecule seemed to significantly enhance the antitumor effect [6]. In conclusion, experimental tumor models using gene-modified tumor cells demonstrated the antitumor effects of various cytokines and point to the need for CTL induction for long-term tumor immunity. Although these results are encouraging since they show the feasibility of the approach, there is still a long way to go before we can image tumor-specific treatment of patients leading to a curative T cell response.

In the last few years, a number of clinical protocols primarily using irradiated, autologous tumor cells or fibroblasts have been approved and initiated. Based on the clinical data reports collected by the Gene Therapy Working Groups in Europe and at the National Institutes of Health (NIH), approximately 1000 patients have currently been treated by the gene transfer methodology without serious adverse events. In particular, there have been no reports of replicating retroviruses in any patients. Ex vivo gene transfer has resulted in numerous cell types being gene modified, and gene transfer has been documented in situ in tumor cells. Furthermore, immunological responses to the genetically altered cells have been observed in cancer and human immunodeficiency virus (HIV) patients. However, gene therapy has recently come under criticism [9, 20, 45], primarily because of the lack of published results. Indeed, only three reports on clinical gene therapy trials dealing with nonhematological neoplasms have been published so far, and only one of these used cytokine (IL-2) gene-modified tumor cells for therapy of glioblastoma (reviewed in [9]). In consequence, more basic biological studies of gene therapy were called for, since cures have not yet been achieved in patients [20, 45].

A number of questions remain open and have only partly been addressed in animal studies, including the immunogenicity of gene-modified tumor cell vaccines and whether this is affected by irradiation or mitomycin treatment. The mechanism of action of gene-modified tumor cells causing tumor immunity and tumor regression is still under discussion, and further work is necessary. Furthermore, the dose of gene-modified cells and/or the cytokine levels needed for effective vaccinations is presently unclear, with a bell-shaped response curve suggested in some models and a linear relationship in others ([38], reviewed in [30]). Thus the optimal immunization schedule and route is not yet known and needs to be explored systematically. Another critical point which needs to be addressed is our immunological understanding with regard to "physiological" cytokine levels, e.g., the cytokine levels needed to effectively stimulate the immune system. The mechanisms involved in tumor suppression are not well understood and possibly interfere with vaccination effects at distant sites of the metastatic disease or in mounting an immune response, including immunological memory. The safety of retroviral vector constructs and subsequent vector generation needs careful attention, especially when using such genetically modified vaccines in future adjuvant therapeutic settings; lastly, evaluation of immunological end points (e.g., analysis of precursor frequency, CTL, DTH) requires standardization, since methodology, reliability, and reproducibility in the evaluation of such parameters is still difficult, if not impossible to compare.

Although gene therapy of human melanoma is still in the early stages, various approaches are currently being clinically tested. At present, it seems safe to conclude that gene therapy strategies involving cytokine gene-modified tumor cells can influence the immunological tumor–host relationship; however, in most cases the response seems not to be strong enough to completely erradicate the tumor in patients who have had a high level of pretreatment and are metastatically far advanced. Optimizing vaccination strategies and vector systems and the application and further improvement of gene therapy treatment modalities will require close cooperation between theoretical scientists and clinicans in order to make an significant impact on the clinical course of patients suffering from melanoma. In recent years, retrospective analyses have shown that immunological strategies such as application of monoclonal antibodies or vaccination with tumor cell extracts or total cell lysates in colonic cancer or melanoma patients might improve patients' clinical outcome (reviewed in [10, 15, 22]).

Overall, only a few communications reporting on gene therapy approaches in humans are currently being published; however, our findings and initial data published by others demonstrate an in vivo immunomodulation after autologous tumor cell vaccination in terminally ill patients. Vaccination with cytokine gene-modified tumor cells might prove to be especially useful in the adjuvant setting because of the low tumor load, and efficacy might be further increased by using other vector systems, such as recombinant BCG for antigen and cytokine expression, which has recently been shown to further improve vaccination effects [26, 42].

Summary

Tumor immunology has made great progress in recent years. It has led to the identification of various tumor-associated antigens, particularly in malignant melanoma, which are recognized in conjunction with the appropriate HLA molecule by cytolytic T cells. Moreover, recent animal studies have indicated that a potent protective immune response can be generated in vivo using cytokine gene-modified tumor cells. Locally secreted cytokines from genetically modified tumor cells, such as IL-2, IL-4, IL-7, IL-12, and GM-CSF, have been shown to mediate tumor rejection and long-term antitumor immunity. Based on these successful animal studies, various clinical protocols for the treatment of human cancer, predominantly using cytokine gene modifications, have been initiated in recent years. However, only very few results from those trials have been published so far.

Acknowlegdement. D.S. is a Heisenberg Fellow of the Deutsche Forschungsgemeinschaft (DFG). Work in the laboratory was generously supported by the DFG, the Deutsche Krebshilfe – Dr. Mildred Scheel-Stiftung, and the Sandoz-Stiftung. The continuous support and encouragement of Prof. Beate M. Henz is highly appreciated.

References

1. Ahmann DL, Creagan ET, Hahn RG, Edmonson JH, Bisel HF, Schaid DJ (1989) Complete responses and long-term survivals after systemic chemotherapy for patients with advanced malignant melanoma. Cancer 63:224–227
2. Allione A, Consalvo M, Nanni P, Lollini P L, Cavallo F, Giovarelli M, Forni M, Gulino A, Colombo MP, Dellabona P, Hock H, Blankenstein T, Rosenthal FM, Gansbacher B, Bosco MC, Musso T, Gusella L, Forni G (1994) Immunizing and curative potential of replicating and nonreplicating murine mammary adenocarcinoma cells engineered with interleukin (IL)-2, IL-4, IL-6, IL-7, IL-10, tumor necrosis factor a, GM-CSF, and gamma-interferon gene or admixed with conventional adjuvants. Cancer Res 54:6022–6026
3. Beissert S, Hosoi J, Grabbe S, Asahina A, Granstein RD (1995) IL-10 inhibits tumor antigen presentation by epidermal antigen-presenting cells. J Immunol 154:1280–1288
4. Blankenstein T (1994) Increasing tumour immunogenicity by genetic modification. Eur J Cancer 30A:1182–1186
5. Boon T, Gajewski TF, Coulie PG (1995) From defined human tumor antigens to effective immunization. Immunol Today 16:334–336
6. Cayeux S, Beck C, Aicher A, Dörken B, Blankenstein T (1995) Tumor cells cotransfected with interleukin-7 and B71 genes induce CD25 and CD28 on tumor-infiltrating T lymphocytes and are strong vaccines. Eur J Immunol 25:2325–2331
7. Colombo MP, Forni G (1994) Cytokine gene transfer in tumor inhibition and tumor therapy: where are we now? Immunol Today 15:48–51
8. Columbo MP, Maccalli C, Mattei S, Melani C, Radrizzani M, Parmiani G (1992) Expression of cytokine genes, including IL-6, in human malignant melanoma cell lines. Melanoma Res 2:181–189

9. Culver KW (1996) Measuring success in clinical gene therapy research. Mol Med Today 6:234–236
10. Dalgleish A (1996) The case for therapeutic vaccines. Melanoma Res 6:5–10
11. Fearon ER, Pardoll DM, Itaya T, Golumbek P, Livitsky HI, Simons JW, Karasuyama H, Vogelstein B, Frost P (1990) Interleukin-2 production by tumor cells bypasses T helper function in the generation of an antitumor response. Cell 60:397–403
12. Friedmann T (1996) Human gene therapy – an immature genie, but certainly out of the bottle. Nature Med 2:144–147
13. Garbe C (1993) Chemotherapy and chemoimmunotherapy in disseminated malignant melanoma. Melanoma Res 3:291–299
14. Gilboa E, Lyerly HK (1994) Specific active immunotherapy of cancer using genetically modified tumor vaccines. Biol Ther Cancer Updates 4 (6):1–16
15. Hersey P (1994) Melanoma vaccines – current status and future prospects. Drugs 47: 373–382
16. Hock H, Dorsch M, Kunzendorf U, Überla K, Qin Z, Diamantstein T, Blankenstein T (1993) Vaccinations with tumor cells genetically engineered to produce different cytokines: effectivity not superior to a classical adjuvant. Cancer Res 53:714–716
17. Kawakami Y, Eliyahu S, Delgado CH, Robbins PF, Sakaguchi K, Appella E, Yannelli JR, Adema GJ, Miki T, Rosenberg SA (1994) Identification of a human melanoma antigen recognized by tumor-infiltrating lymphocytes associated with in vivo tumor rejection. Proc Natl Acad Sci USA 91:6458–6462
18. Mackensen A, Carcelain G, Viel S, Raynal M-C, Michalaki H, Triebel F, Bosq J, Hercend T (1994) Direct evidence to support the immunosurveillance concept in a human regressive melanoma. J Clin Invest 93:1391–1402
19. Maeurer MJ, Storkus WJ, Kirkwood JM, Lotze MT (1996) New treatment options for patients with melanoma: review of melanoma-derived T-cell epitope-based peptide vaccines. Melanoma Res 6:11–24
20. Marshall E (1995) Gene therapy's growing pain. Science 269:1050–1055
21. Mertelsmann R, Lindemann A, Boehm T, Brennscheidt U, Franke B, Kulmburg P, Lahn M, Mackensen A, Rosenthal FM, Veelken H (1995) Pilot study for the evaluation of T-cell-mediated tumor immunotherapy by cytokine gene transfer in patients with malignant tumors. J Mol Med 73:205–206
22. Mitchell MS (1996) Immunotherapy of melanoma. J Invest Dermatol Symp Proc 1:215–218
23. Möller P, Schadendorf D (1997) Somatic gene therapy and its implication for the treatment of malignant melanoma. Arch Dermatol Res
24. Möller P, Sun YS, Dorbic T, Möller H, Makki A, Jurgovsky K, Schroff M, Henz BM, Wittig B, Schadendorf D Vaccination with IL-7-gene modified autologous tumor cells enhances tumor-specific T cell precursor frequency and modulates cytokine secretion in patients with advanced malignant melanoma – a clinical phase I study (submitted)
25. Mosman TR, Sad S (1996) The expanding universe of T-cell subsets: TH1, TH2 and more. Immunol Today 17:138–146
26. Murray PJ, Aldovini A, Young RA (1996) Manipulation and potentiation of antimycobacterial immunity using recombinant Bacille Calmette-Guerin strains that secrete cytokines. Proc Natl Acad Sci USA 93:934–939
27. Nabel GJ, Nabel EG, Yang ZY, Fox BA, Plautz GE, Gao X, Huang I, Shu S, Gordon D, Chang AE (1993) Direct gene transfer with DNA liposome complexes in melanoma: expression, biologic activity, and lack of toxicity in humans. Proc Natl Acad Sci USA 90:11307–11311
28. Oettgen HF, Old LJ (1991) The history of cancer immunotherapy. In: deVita VT, Hellman S, Rosenberg SA (eds) Biologic therapy of cancer, principles and practice. Lippincott, Philadelphia, pp 87–96
29. Old LJ (1981) Cancer immunology: the search for specificity – GHA Clowes Memorial Lecture. Cancer Res 41:365
30. Pardoll DM (1995) Paracrine cytokine adjuvants in cancer immunotherapy. Annu Rev Immunol 13:399–415

31. Parkinson DR, Houghton AN, Hersey P, Borden EC (1992) Biologic therapy for melanoma. In: Balch CM, Houghton AN, Milton GW, Sober AJ, Soong SJ (eds) Cutaneous melanoma. Lippincott, Philadelphia, p 522
32. Parmiani G, Colombo MP (1995) Somatic gene therapy of human melanoma: preclinical studies and early clinical trials. Melanoma Res 5:295–301
33. Rammensee HG, Falk K, Rötzschke O (1993) Peptides naturally presented by MHC class I molecules. Annu Rev Immunol 11:213–244
34. Robbins PF, El-Gamil M, Kawakami Y, Rosenberg SA (1994) Recognition of tyrosinase by tumor-infiltrating lymphocytes from a patient responding to immunotherapy. Cancer Res 54:3124–3126
35. Ruiter DJ, Mattijssen V, Bröcker E-B, Ferrone S (1991) MHC antigens in human melanomas. Semin Cancer Biol 2:35–45
36. Schadendorf D, Czarnetzki BM, Wittig B (1995) Clinical protocol – interleukin-7-, interleukin-12-, and GM-CSF gene transfer in patients with metastatic melanoma. J Mol Med 73: 473–477
37. Schadendorf D, Henz BM, Wittig B (1996) Interleukin 7 trials for melanoma treatment. Mol Med Today 2:143–144
38. Schmidt W, Schweighofer T, Herbst E, Maas G, Berger M, Schilcher F, Schaffner G, Birnstiel ML (1995) Cancer vaccines: the interleukin 2 dosage effect. Proc Natl Acad Sci USA 92:4711–4715
39. Schmidt-Wolf GD, Schmitt-Wolf IGH (1995) Cytokines and clinical gene therapy. Eur J Immunol 25:1137–1140
40. Schmidt-Wolf IGH, Neubauer A, Finke S, Csipai M, Wittig B, Huhn D (1994) Interleukin-7 gene transfer in patients with metastatic colon carcinoma, renal carcinoma, melanoma or with lymphoma. Hum Gene Ther 5:1161–1168
41. Sherman LA, Chattopadhyay S (1993) The molecular basis of allorecognition. Annu Rev Immunol 11:385–402
42. Stover CK, de la Cruz VF, Fuerst TR, Burlein JE, Benson LA, Bennett LT, Bansal GP, Young JF, Lee MH, Hatfull GF, Snapper SB, Barletta RG, Jacobs WR Jr, Bloom BR (1991) New use of BCG for recombinant vaccines. Nature 351:456–460
43. Tahara H, Lotze M, Robbins PD, Storkus WJ, Zitvogel L (1995) IL-12 gene therapy using direct injection of tumors with genetically engineered autologous fibroblasts. Hum Gene Ther 6:1607–1624
44. Tepper RI, Pattengale PK, Leder P (1989) Murine interleukin 4 displays potent anti-tumor activity in vivo. Cell 57:503–512
45. Touchette N (1996) Gene therapy: not ready for prime time. Nat Med 2:7–8
46. Vieweg J, Gilboa E (1995) Considerations for the use of cytokine-secreting tumor cell preparations for cancer treatment. Cancer Invest 13:193–201
47. Whittington R, Faulds D (1993) Interleukin-2 – a review of its pharmacological properties and therapeutic use in patients with cancer. Drugs 46:446–514

Development of a DNA Vaccine Against Malignant Melanoma

K. Moelling, B. Strack, M. Nawrath, J. Heinrich, C. Döhring, S. N. Wagner, and J. Pavlovic

DNA Vaccine – Historical Background

Within the last 3 years, DNA vaccines have entered the scene as a radically new approach to prophylaxis of infectious disease. Surprisingly, if injected intramuscularly, the DNA is expressed in vivo much more efficiently than would have been predicted from tissue culture DNA transfections. Antibody responses and major histocompatibility complex (MHC) class I-restricted cytotoxic T cell responses (CTL) have been observed.

The method was described decades ago but remained unnoticed. In 1960, it was shown that Shope rabbit papillomavirus DNA induced papillomas in rabbit skin. In 1990, Wolff et al. [1] demonstrated direct gene transfer into mouse muscle in vivo. They used a reporter gene coding for chloramphonicol acetyltransferase (CAT) under the control of a long terminal repeat (LTR) or a cytomegalo virus (CMV) immediate-early promoter. Enzyme activity persisted for at least 60 days post injection. This experiment was designed as a control for various liposomes as DNA carriers. The naked DNA without the liposomes proved to be more efficient, which was a big surprise. The DNA remained in an episomal state, and its stability was presumably due to the low proliferation state of muscle cells, the myocytes. Several improvements of the effect have been investigated, such as buffer composition, agents to facilitate uptake, structure of the DNA, linear versus circular DNA structure, different promoters, and routes of injection. CMV promoter and retroviral LTR promoters appeared to lead most consistently to high levels of expression. Particular interest was given to gene guns for intradermal DNA injections, in which ballistically accelerated microscopic gold particles are used to penetrate cell membranes without killing the cell. Penetration of the dermis ranges from 0.1 to 5 mm, depending on the projectile force.

Historically, antibodies against the DNA-coded human growth hormone have been described [2]. An important study was then published in the journal *Science*, in which influenza A viral DNA was used as a vaccine. The major antibody response against influenza in natural infections is directed against the surface protein hemagglutinin (HA), which varies significantly among different influenza strains. Ulmer et al. [3] used a plasmid DNA instead, which codes for the nucleoprotein (NP) of influenza A, a major target of CTL responses which undergoes much less interstrain variability. Indeed, the vaccinated mice survived a challenge with a lethal virus dose and protection was achieved even against distantly related virus strains. The CTL response persisted for at least 13 months. DNA vaccination against hepatitis B virus has shown promising results, which is superior to the presently available recombinant vaccine, with a single DNA injection.

A DNA vaccination has also been described against human immunodeficiency virus (HIV) [4]. Mice immunized with a plasmid DNA coding for the *env* gene of HIV developed an immune response against tumor cells constitutively expressing the envelope gene of HIV as neoantigen. Treatment of naive mice with those cells resulted in tumor growth and lethality, whereas vaccinated mice survived. Antibody production and CTL response were detected [4]. A DNA plasmid for human use was developed based on a publication by David Weiner and colleagues [4]. The original construct was not adequate for application in humans because of the presence of viral genes, e.g. the LTR, that are potentially hazardous for people. The final DNA vaccine construct was developed in close contact with the US Food and Drug Administration (FDA). The company Apollon produced the good manufacturing practice (GMP) material for human use. Preclinical and toxicology studies in mice, rabbits, and chimpanzees were supported by the National Institutes of Health (NIH) because of their extreme interest in the approach. A phase I/II clinical trial to determine the safety of a DNA vaccine was approved by the FDA in June 1995, and the first patients were immunized immediately. A phase I/II clinical trial received approval for Switzerland in September 1995. It was applied to the first four volunteers in February 1996.

The first protocol was designed as a safety study of DNA vaccine for HIV-1-infected individuals, but a trial has since been initiated in 1996 in the United States which involves healthy volunteers.

Successful DNA immunization has been achieved in animal models against many infectious agents, such as human and bovine herpes viruses, rabies virus, measles virus, hepatitis B and C viruses, human papillomaviruses, and malaria. Significant titers of neutralizing antibodies in addition to CTL responses were documented. DNA vaccination mimics a virus infection and is similar to a live attenuated vaccine – without safety hazards. However, a systematic comparison of the relative potency of DNA vaccines versus other live attenuated viral or recombinant proteins plus adjuvant vaccines in standardized animal models is still lacking.

Recently, a first DNA vaccine has been developed against cancer. A DNA plasmid coding for carcinoembryonic antigen (CEA) protected against challenge by CEA-transduced colon carcinoma cells [5]. A phase I/II clinical trial for colon and breast cancer patients was approved with CEA DNA vaccine by the Recombinant DNA Advisory Committee (RAC) in the United States in 1995.

Mechanism of Immune Response

Several possible models for priming the MHC class I-restricted CTL response by intramuscular DNA injections are being discussed by researchers in the field [6]. Naked DNA may be presented directly to the cytotoxic $CD8^+$ T cells by the transduced muscle cells. However, muscle cells are not professional antigen-presenting cells (APC) and lack costimulatory signals required to initiate immune responses. In addition, if transfected, myocytes simply die, there is only a small probability that this results in immune response. The role of some marrow-derived APC has not been adequately evaluated in this context. APC infiltrate the site of injection and might play an important role. These APC would also be able to pick up locally released antigens, e.g., from dying myocytes, and present them via MHC class II-restricted $CD4^+$cell priming to B cells as well. These APC may travel to the draining lymph nodes and present antigenic peptides to both B

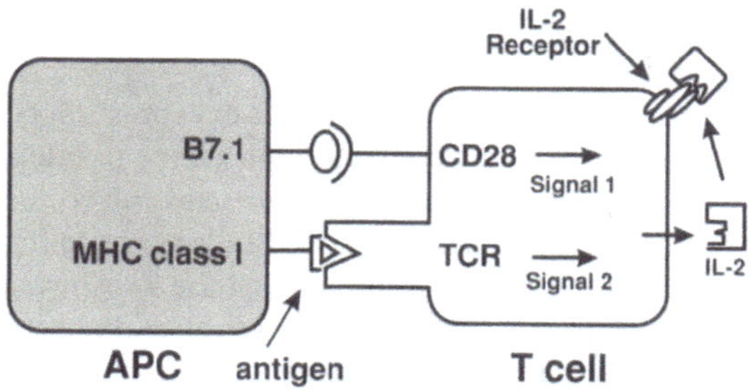

Fig. 1. Model of T-cell costimulation by B7.1. A professional antigen-presenting cell (APC) exhibits two surface receptors, the major histocompatibility complex (*MHC*) class I molecule for peptide antigen presentation and the costimulator B7.1, which binds to CD28 on the T cell to transduce signal 1. Signal 2 is activated upon recognition of the T cell receptor (*TCR*), and the peptide is presented. This leads to T cell activation, interleukin (*IL*)-2 production etc. Tumor cells often lack B7.1 and only express an antigen

and T cells. Yet another model envisages direct DNA uptake by the bone marrow-derived APC infiltrating muscles followed by classical MHC class I processing and costimulation by B7.1, leading to CTL activation (Fig. 1).

As an argument in favor of the model involving APC, one may quote results by Ertl and colleagues which demonstrated that coinjection of granulocyte-macrophage colony-stimulating factor (GM-CSF) with the DNA enhances both humoral and cellular immune responses [7]. GM-CSF stimulates the differentiation of hematopoetic progenitors into professional APC. Furthermore, it induces differentiation of dentritic cells. Their presence in the dermis may explain the possibility of vaccinating with DNA by intradermal injection.

Malignant Melanoma Antigens

Specific immunotherapy has previously been designed to enhance the immunogenic response of patients to their own tumor. Many attempts to develop active immunotherapies against cancer have involved extracts from cancer cells or gene-modified tumor cells to increase their immunogenicity. Several genes encoding tumor-associated antigens in malignant melanoma cells have been identified recently, such as melanoma antigen MAGE-1, MAGE-3, tyrosinase, MART-1 (melanoma antigen recognized by T cells), gp100, and p75 [8, 9]. MART and gp100 have been described to be recognized by CTL from melanoma patients and appear to be involved in tumor regression. These antigens are thus excellent candidates for the development of antigen-specific vaccines. A very recent paper describes the development and characterization of recombinant adenovirus-encoding MART-1 and gp100 for cancer therapy. These viral vector-based vaccines protect mice from challenge with a syngeneic gp100-expressing murine melanoma cell line [8]. It should be noted, however, that, as in the case of CEA, the tumor-associated antigens are not restricted to the tumor cells, but are also expressed in normal melanocytes, retina, and testis.

Construction of a gp100 (pmel17) Expression Plasmid

Vectors for DNA vaccination should allow high levels of expression of the target protein in mammalian cells, but should not be able to replicate or to integrate into the host chromosome. For expression of gp100 (pmel17), we used the vector VR1012 (Fig. 2), which originated from Vical Co. (San Diego). VR1012 is very similar to the vector V1J constructed by Montgomery et al. [11], but contains the kanamycin (Km) resistance gene instead of the ampicillin resistance gene for selection in bacteria. The origin of replication of the high copy-number plasmid pUC18 allows the production of large amounts of VR1012 DNA in *Escherichia coli*. The expression of the target gene is directed by a combination of the human CMV immediate-early (IE1) promoter/enhancer region, including the intron A sequence, with the bovine growth hormone (BGH) polyadenylation signal. This combination turned out to be very efficient for gene expression in mouse muscle [10, 11]

We inserted the human gp100 (pmel17) cDNA fragment [12] into the *Sal*I and *Not*I restriction sites of the VR1012 multiple cloning site (Fig. 2). After transfection of the resulting plasmid VR1012pmel17 into the murine melanoma cell line K1735-M2 [13], expression of the protein was analyzed by means of immunofluorescence using the monoclonal antibody HMB45 (kindly provided by S. Wagner, Essen, Germany) [14]. This antibody does not allow detection of gp100 (pmel17) in immunoblots, but only in immunofluoresence. Transfected cells were shown to express high amounts of the protein, resulting in the typical speckled expression pattern (data not shown).

After expression, the gp100 (pmel17) protein is transported into the melanosomes, where it is anchored in the membrane of these organelles. In order to optimize the presentation of an antigen to the immune system, the signal sequence of the tissue plasminogen activator (TPA) protein has recently been applied in some cases. This signal sequence would allow secretion of the protein, which might improve the amount of antigen available for processing and presentation by professional APC in a MHC class II-dependent manner.

As was recently shown by Zhai et al. [8], immunization with adenovirus expressing the human gp100 (pmel17) gene could protect C57BL/6 mice from murine melanoma B16-F1 challenge when administered intradermally. This may be due to the pronounced homology between the human and the murine gp100 (pmel17) protein sequences. However, if used in murine preclinical studies, the human cDNA clone is a neoantigen, because it originates from a different species. This could provoke an immune response which would not normally occur with a self-antigen. The RAC rejected the CEA DNA vaccine protocol of D. Curiel in the first round because the preclinical mouse studies were performed solely with the human CEA and had to be repeated with the murine equivalent. It is therefore considered essential to construct a murine gp100 (pmel17) expression vector.

Effects of Cytokines and the B7.1 Costimulator on DNA Vaccine

Cytokines which are known to stimulate the immune response are intended to be applied in combination with gp100 (pmel17). The cDNA of the murine cytokines interleukin IL-2, IL-7, IL-12, and GM-CSF are planned to be inserted into the expression vector VR1012 and applied for immunization in combination with VR1012 pmel17.

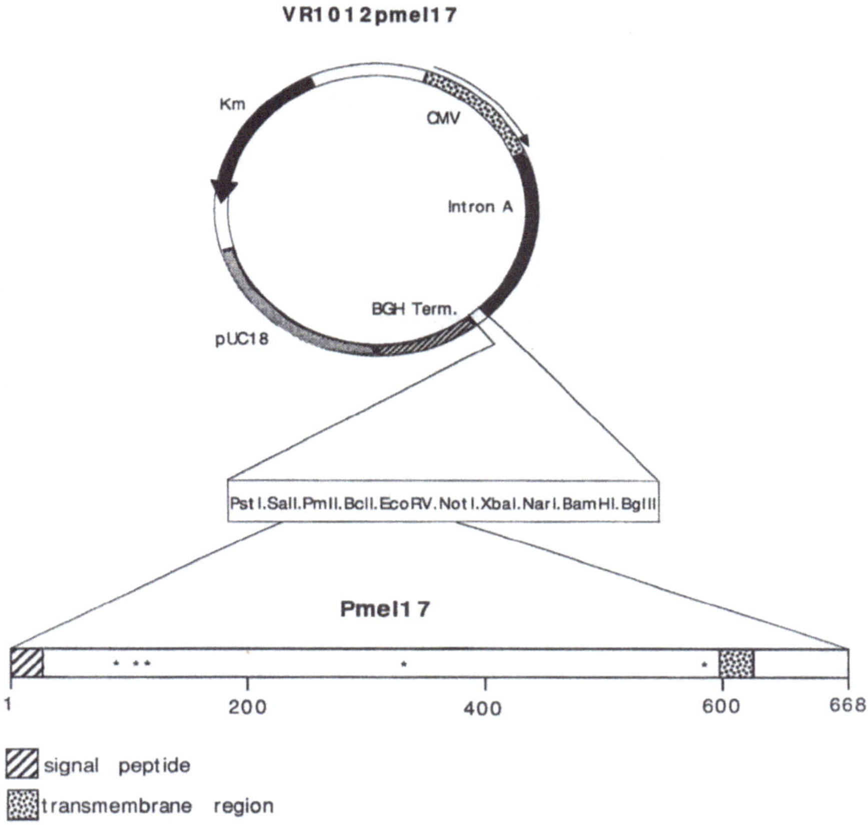

Fig. 2. Construction of the gp100 (pmel17) expression plasmid. Construction of the gp100 (pmel17) expression plasmid. A DNA plasmid with a multicloning site contains the *CMV* promoter, an intron A sequence, the terminator of bovine growth hormone (*BGH*), and a kanamycin resistance marker (*Km*) on a puc18 backbone. gp100 is cloned into the plasmid. Asterisks indicate N-glycosylation sites

While cytokines are not necessarily required to be expressed in the same cell together with gp100 (pmel17), in the case of the costimulatory molecule B7.1, coexpression is absolutely required (see below). Expression of two genes on one DNA plasmid is envisaged to be performed using internal ribosomal entry sites (IRES). This is based on analysis of various vectors described in the literature. We intend to introduce the IRES of poliovirus [15], which was kindly provided by Dr. H. Hauser (Braunschweig, Germany), into the multiple cloning site of VR1012 pmel17 next to the pmel17 gene. Insertion of the cytokine cDNA 3' into the IRES would allow coordinated translation of the two genes from one transcription unit. Since not all dicistronic expression constructs gave rise to levels of expression equivalent to the monocistronic counterparts, something which was caused by differences in half-lives of the mRNA, it may be necessary to test both possible arrangements of the genes within the dicistronic expression vector.

The dicistronic VR1012 vector containing the polioviral IRES will be used to establish coexpression of gp100 (pmel17) and B7.1. The cDNA encoding the murine B7.1 was kindly provided by Dr. G. Freeman (Boston, USA). B7.1 expression can be tested by means of an anti-mB7-1 monoclonal antibody, which is available from Pharmigen (San Diego).

Generation of Tumor Cell Lines Expressing Human gp100 (pmel17)

The mouse melanoma cell line K1735-M2 is known to express MHC class I and class II molecules and has recently been used in a malignant melanoma study [16]. This cell line, which is syngeneic to the C3H/HeN mouse, was established by Dr. I.Y. Fidler (M.D. Anderson Cancer Research Center, Houston) [13]. The line was used to generate stably transfected tumor cell lines for challenge experiments. For that purpose, we cotransfected VR1012 pmel17 and as a control VR1012 with the plasmid pX343 (kindly provided by Dr. H. Diggelmann, Lausanne, Switzerland), conferring hygromycin B resistance into K1735-M2 cells by using lipofectamine as carriers [17]. After hygromycin B selection, the cells were tested for gp100 (pmel17) expression employing indirect immunofluorescence with the HMB-45 antibody (data not shown). The VR1012 pmel17-transfected K1735-M2 cells were shown to exhibit the speckled expression pattern, whereas the VR1012-transfected cells showed only a slight, diffuse staining.

Another possibility for a mouse melanoma cell line is the murine B16-F1 line (ATCC CRL 6323). This line overexpresses the murine gp100 (pmel17) and therefore does not need to be stably transfected. It is derived from C57BL/6 mice and needs to be tested in challenge experiments using mice with this specific genetic background. Overexpression of gp100 (pmel17) in this line has been verified in a preliminary experiment by indirect immunofluorescence using the HMB45 antibody, which is cross-reactive for human and murine gp100 (pmel17).

Expression of gp100 (pmel17) in Mouse Muscle

A prerequisite for a DNA vaccine is its ability to mediate high levels of expression of the target protein in the muscle. In order to test the expression of gp100 (pmel17) in the mouse muscle, we injected VR1012 pmel17 into the quadriceps of the hindlegs of nude mice. After explantation of the muscle and fixation, pmel17 expression was analyzed by means of immunohistochemical methods. High-level expression of pmel17 can be detected in the muscle cells, resulting in a speckled pattern similar to the expression pattern obtained with stably transfected K1735-M2 cells (data not shown).

Efficacy of DNA Vaccination in Mice

The efficacy of the DNA vaccination can be tested by DNA vaccination of mice prior to tumor challenge [4] or by DNA vaccination of mice that carry preexisting tumors.

C57BL/6 or C3H mice were vaccinated following established protocols [4] by intramuscular injection of 50–100 μg VR1012 pmel17 plasmid DNA into the quadriceps of the hindlegs. VR1012 pmel17 alone or in combination with cytokine expression plasmids (see below) was injected into two to four sites of the same muscle. To enhance the efficacy of uptake of the DNA into the target cells, the DNA was applied in the presence of so-called facilitators such as bupivacaine that have been previously shown to enhance

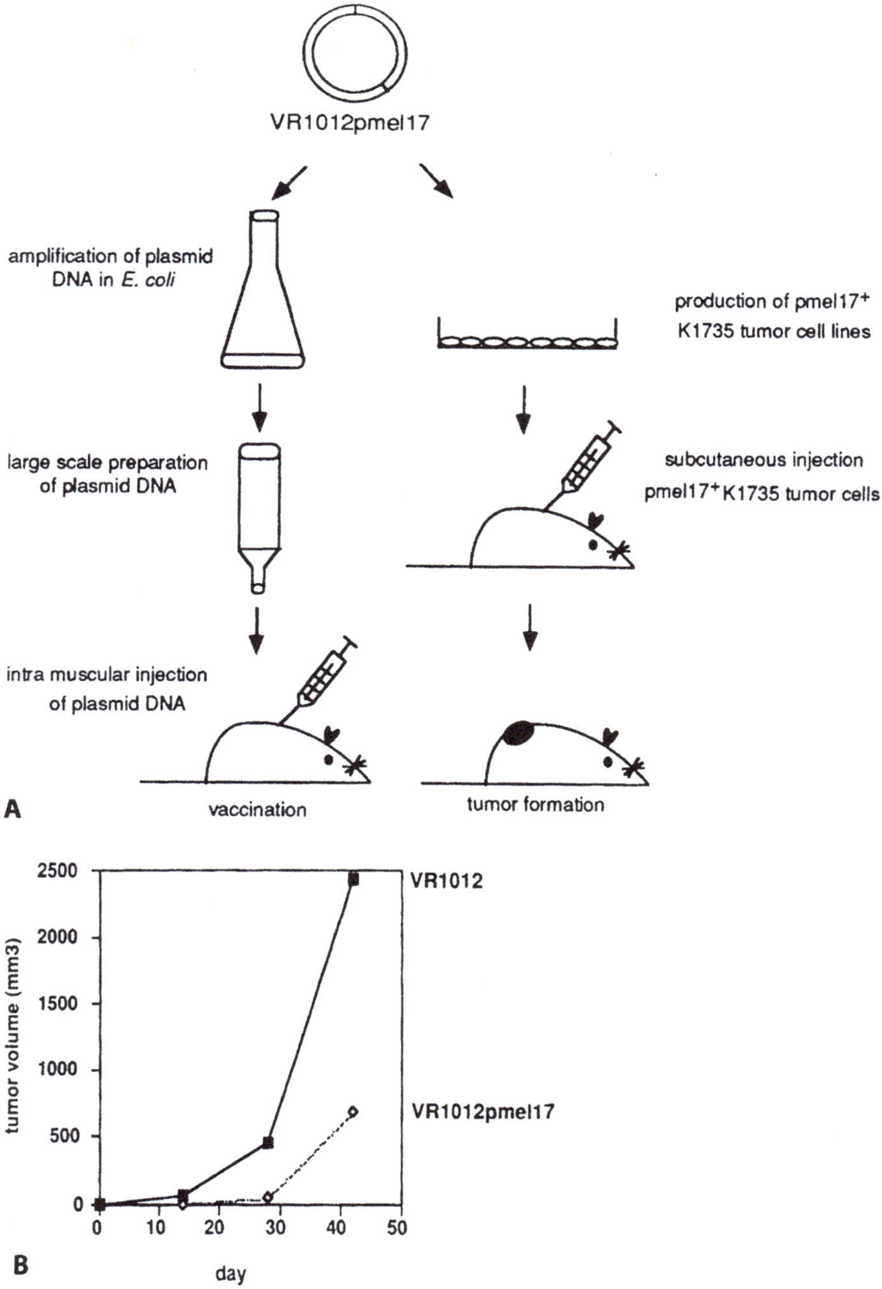

Fig. 3 A, B. Vaccination of gp100 (pmel17). Vaccination of gp100 (pmel17). **A** Plasmid DNA is produced, purified, and injected into mice for vaccination. In parallel, the melanoma cell line K1735 is stably transfected with gp100. The cells are injected into syngeneic mice. Mice pretreated with DNA vaccine should not develop a tumor, while naive mice will develop a tumor. **B** Tumor formation measured in C3H mice with immunization (VR1012 pmel17) and without (VR1012)

the efficacy of the DNA uptake into muscle cells [4]. The mice were boosted once 4–6 weeks after the initial immunization.

Immunized animals were challenged with $1{\times}10^6$ syngeneic melanoma cells by subcutaneous injection 10–20 days following the booster. In the case of C3H mice, K1735-M2 cells stably transfected with human gp100 (pmel17) vector were used. To assess the specificity of the vaccination, some mice were challenged with K1735-M2 cells transfected with the empty vector as a control. In the case of C57BL/6 mice or perforin-deficient mice (see below), naive B16-F1 melanoma cells expressing high levels of endogenous mouse gp100 (pmel17) were injected. Preliminary results are shown in Fig. 3.

In order to evaluate DNA vaccination of mice that carry preexisting tumors, the mice were first injected with $1{\times}10^6$ syngeneic melanoma cells, either K1735-M2 expressing gp100 or B16–F1, and the tumors were allowed to develop. As soon as the tumors reached a volume of approximately 500 ml, the tumors were resected and the animals vaccinated with plasmid DNA following the protocol described above. Preliminary results indicate some delay in onset of tumor formation. In future experiments, $1\text{–}5{\times}10^6$ γ-irradiated melanoma cells expressing murine cytokines (see above) will be injected into the tumor site. If we observe complete remission of the tumor, we will rechallenge these mice with various syngeneic tumor cells that do not express gp100 (e.g., the cell line EL4 for C57BL/6 mice as a control for B16-F1) [18] to test the specificity of the vaccine for gp100.

Future Aspects and Efforts to Increase Efficacy

Immunological Parameters

Following immunization, animals have been tested for the induction of a humoral response to gp100. To that end, serum of animals immunized with gp100 DNA or control DNA was tested for presence of antibodies directed against gp100 by immunofluorescence analysis or western blotting.

To test for a specific cellular response, lymphocytes isolated from spleen of immunized mice will be tested for the presence of gp100-specific $CD4^+$ cells and $CD8^+$ cells. Specific $CD4^+$ cells will be detected by employing lymphocyte proliferation assays, and $CD8^+$ cells by CTL killing assays. We will also look for the presence of tumor-infiltrating lymphocytes (TIL) in the tumors by immunohistochemical methods, and in some experiments we will isolate the TIL from the tumor and test for their specificity for gp100 (pmel17). These experiments will be carried out in collaboration with the Institute of Dermatology, University Hospital of Zurich.

Combination of DNA Vaccine with gp100 (pmel17)-Specific Cytotoxic T Lymphocyte Epitope Peptides

Five different antigenic epitopes of human Gp100 (pmel17) protein were recently identified which can be recognized by TIL of different melanoma patients when presented by the MHC class I subtype HLA-A2.1 [19–21]. In order to generate a T-helper response, we intend to apply the VR1012 DNA together with synthetic peptides spanning the antigenic epitopes. Uptake of the peptides by professional APC and presentation of the antigen via MHC class II molecules would stimulate $CD4^+$ T-helper cells, which subsequently activate $CD8^+$ pre-CTL by IL-2 production.

Cytokine Combination Therapy in Mice

In various mouse tumor model systems, cytokines such as IL-2, IL-7, GM-CSF, and IL-12 have demonstrated profound antitumor effects in ex vivo therapy [22–25]. Moreover, Ertl and coworkers have shown that DNA vaccination against rabies with plasmid expressing the viral glycoprotein and GM-CSF was more effective than the plasmid expressing the glycoprotein alone [7]. We will construct vectors expressing the cytokines IL-2, IL-7, IL-12, and GM-CSF. IL-12 is composed of two chains which need to be expressed at equal molar amounts on one plasmid (see above). Therefore, a dicistronic construct employing an IRES sequence will be made that encodes both chains on one transcript. Mice will be immunized with vectors expressing cytokines in combination with the gp100 (pmel17) plasmid. As indicated above, we will immunize animals with preexisting tumors and naive animals that will be challenged with B16-F1 melanoma cells following immunization. An alternative approach for combination therapy is to immunize animals with preexisting tumors by intramuscular injection of gp100 (pmel17) DNA and then to inject irradiated autologous tumor cells expressing and secreting the above-listed cytokines into the tumor site. The rationale of this experiment is to support activation of gp100 (pmel17)-specific TIL directly at the tumor site. Retroviral vectors expressing the above-listed cytokines have either been constructed at our institute or are otherwise available.

Combination with Costimulator B7.1 Plasmid DNA

Recognition of the MHC class I presented antigen by the T cell receptor (TCR) is not sufficient for T cell activation. Professional APC (Fig. 1) provide a costimulatory molecule, B7.1, on their surface. Costimulation results from interaction of the CD28 molecule on the T cell surface with the ligand B7.1 on the surface of the APC (reviewed by June et al. [26]). Coexpression of B7.1 and gp100 (pmel17) in the muscle cell may therefore mimic the situation present on the surface of a professional APC.

The dicistronic expression vector permitting coordinated expression of gp100 (pmel17) and B7.1 (see above) will be injected into C57BL/6 mice for immunization. Syngeneic B16-F1 tumor cells will be used for challenge experiments.

Discussion

DNA vaccines hold great promise for protection against infections. The efficiency of this approach for tumor prevention is much less proven and may be less promising because the immune response against modified self-antigens may be low. However, the methodology is very new and has not yet been fully evaluated. One surprising observation was that the levels of DNA per injection should actually be lowered instead of being increased, e.g., down to 10 mg instead of more than 100 mg per injection per mouse. Furthermore, the time period between boosts has been too short in many initial protocols. Combinations with peptides or cytokines or the expression of polyepitopes is still at an early stage.

The method may even have broader applications than protection against infectious agents or cancer. In addition to recent developments of tuberculosis vaccines, a form of treatment against allergy has been investigated [27–29]. Furthermore, the search for the relevant epitopes may be performed by injection of full expression libraries and subsequent screening for the immune response and identification of the relevant epitope, as has been exemplified in the case of *Mycoplasma pulmonaris* [30].

DNA vaccination will be much simpler and cheaper than conventional peptide vaccines, since the production of DNA for clinical use is simpler, and different vaccines should be produced by similar protocols. In addition, DNA vaccines can be easily transported to third-world countries without refrigeration. Combinations of various vaccines can be envisaged, which are also a great advantage. The safety of the methods is considered to be very high. Integration events of DNA vaccines into the chromosome have been tested by high-resolution polymerase chain reaction (PCR) technologies, and the probability of a tumor-promoting event by DNA integration has been determined to be below the statistical events leading to a mutation within the life-time of an individual [31]. Based on these safety considerations, clinical trials have been initiated in healthy volunteers with DNA vaccines against HIV and influenza A. The results will be important for the future of this field.

Summary

The human gp100 (pmel17) is a tumor-associated antigen present in a subset of human melanoma cells. A DNA plasmid expressing gp100 (pmel17) cDNA has been developed. The DNA plasmid has been characterized for high and long-lasting levels of antigen expression, as evidenced in stably transfected K1735-M2 cells, a mouse melanoma cell line. Efficacy of DNA vaccination is being analyzed by intramuscular injection of DNA and subsequent challenge of the pretreated syngeneic mice with gp100-expressing K1735-M2 cells or the B16-F1 melanoma cell line naturally expressing gp100. The efficiency of the DNA vaccine is also being tested in tumor-bearing mice to mimic the natural situation in patients. Increase of immunogenicity of the gp100 DNA vaccine is being pursued by combination of the DNA with melanoma-specific CTL epitope peptides, coexpression of immune modulators such as GM-CSF, IL-2, and IL-7, or the costimulatory molecule B7.1. The cellular immune response is monitored by CTL assays, lymphocyte proliferation tests, and immunohistochemical staining. Mice deficient for certain immunologic parameters, such as perforin or fas knockout mice, should afford some degree of understanding of the underlying molecular mechanism of a DNA tumor vaccine.

References

1. Wolff JA, Malone RW, Williams P, Chong W, Acsadi G, Jani A, Felgner PL (1990) Direct gene transfer into mouse muscle in vivo. Science 247:1465–1468
2. Tang DC, DeVit M, Johnston SA (1992) Genetic immunization is a simple method for eliciting an immune response. Nature 356:152–154
3. Ulmer JB, Donnelly JJ, Parker SE, Rhodes GH, Felgner PL, Dwarki VJ, Gromkowski SH, Deck RR, DeWitt CM, Friedman A et al (1993) Heterologous protection against influenza by injection of DNA encoding a viral protein. Science 259:1745–1749
4. Wang B, Ugen, KE, Srikantan V, Agadjanyan MG, Dang K, Refaeli Y, Sato AI, Boyer J, Williams WV, Weiner DB (1993) Gene inoculation generates immune responses against human immunodeficiency virus type 1. Proc Natl Acad Sci USA 90:4156–4160
5. Conry RM, LoBuglio AF, Loechel F, Moore SE, Sumerel LA, Barlow DL, Curiel DT (1995) A carcionembryonic antigen polynucleotide vaccine has in vivo antitumor activity. Gene Ther 2:59–65

6. Pardoll DM, Beckerleg AM (1995) Exposing the immunology of naked DNA vaccines. Immunity 3:165–169
7. Xiang Z, Ertl HCJ (1995) Manipulation of the immune response to a plasmid-encoded viral antigen by coinoculation with plasmids expressing cytokines. Immunity 2:129–135
8. Zhai Y, Yang JC, Kawakami Y, Spiess P, Wadsworth SC, Cardoza LM, Couture LA, Smith AE, Rosenberg SA (1996) Antigen-specific tumor vaccines. J Immunol 156:700–710
9. Anichini A, Mortarini R, Maccalli C, Squarcina P, Fleischhauer K, Mascheroni L Parmiani G (1996) Cytotoxic T cells directed to tumor antigens not expressed on normal melanocytes dominate HLA-A2.1-restricted immune repertoire to melanoma. J Immunol 156:208–217
10. Manthorpe M, Cornefert–Jensen F, Hartikka J, Felgner J, Rundell A, Margalith M, Dwarki V (1993) Gene therapy by intramuscular injection of plasmid DNA: studies on firefly luciferase gene expression in mice. Hum Gene Ther 4:419–431
11. Montgomery DL, Shiver JW, Leander KR, Perry HC, Friedman A, Martinez D, Ulmer JB, Donnelly JJ, Liu MA (1993) Heterologous and homologous protection against influenza a by DNA vaccination: optimization of DNA vectors. DNA Cell Biol 9:777–783
12. Wagner SN, Wagner C, Höfler H, Atkinson MJ, Goos M (1995) Expression cloning of the cDNA encoding a melanoma-associated Ag recognized by mAb HMB-45 – identification as melanocyte-specific Pmel17 cDNA. Lab Invest 73 (2):229–235
13. Fidler IT, Hart IR (1981) Biological and experimental consequences of the zonal composition of solid tumors. Cancer Res 41:3266–3267
14. Smoller BR, McNutt NS, Hsu A (1988) HMB-45 recognizes stimulated melanocytes. J Cutan Pathol 16: 49–53
15. Dirks W, Wirth M, Hauser H (1993) Dicistronic transcription units for gene expression in mammalian cells. Gene 128:247–249
16. Townsend SE, Allison JP (1993) Tumor rejection after direct costimulation of CD8+ cells by B7-transfected melanoma cells. Science 259:368–379
17. Komine M, Freedberg IM, Blumenberg M (1994) Interleukin-1 alpha is released during transfection of keratinocytes. J Invest Dermatol 103:580–582
18. Townsend SE, Su FW, Atherton JM, Allison JP (1994) Specificity and longevity of antitumor immune responses induced by B7-transfected tumors. Cancer Res 54:6477–6483
19. Kawakami Y, Eliyahu S, Delgado CH, Robbins PF, Sakaguchi, K, Appella E, Yannelli JR, Adema GJ, Miki T, Rosenberg SA (1994) Identification of a human melanoma antigen recognized by tumor-infiltrating lymphocytes associated with in vivo tumor rejection. Proc Natl Acad Sci USA 91:6458–6462
20. Cox AL, Skipper J, Chen Y, Henderson RA, Darrow TL, Engelhard VH, Hunt DF, Slingluff CL (1994) Identification of a peptide recognized by five melanoma-specific human cytotoxic T cell lines. Science 264:716–719
21. Castelli C, Storkus WJ, Maeurer MJ, Martin DM, Huang BN, Pramanik BN, Nagabhushan TL, Parmiani G, Lotze MT (1995) Mass spectrometric identification of naturally processed melanoma peptide recognized by CD8+ cytotoxic T cells. J Exp Med 181:363–368
22. Gansbacher B, Zier K, Daniels B, Cronin K, Bannerji R, Gilboa E (1990) Interleukin 2 gene transfer into tumor cells abrogates tumorigenicity and induces protective immunity. J Exp Med 172:1217–1224
23. Dranoff G, Jaffee E, Lazenby A, Golumbek P, Levitsky H, Brose K, Jackson V, Hamada H, Pardoll D, Mulligan C (1993) Vaccination with irradiated tumor cells engineered to secrete murine granulocyte-macrophage colony-stimulating factor stimulates potent, specific, and long lasting anti-tumor immunity. Proc Natl Acad Sci USA 90:3539–3543
24. Hock H, Dorsch M, Diamantstein T, Blankenstein T (1991) Interleukin 7 induces CD4+ T cell-dependent tumor rejection. J Exp Med 174:1291–1298
25. Tahara H, Zitvogel L, Storkus WJ, Zeh III HJ, McKinney TG, Schreiber RD, Gubler U, Robbins PD, Lotze MT (1995) Effective eradication of established murine tumors with IL-12 gene therapy using a polycistronic retroviral vector. J Immunol 154:6466–6474
26. June CH, Bluestone JA, Nadler LM, Thompson CB (1994) The B7 and CD28 receptor families. Immunol Today 15:321–331

27. Huygen K, Content J, Denis O, Montgomery DL, Yawman AM, Deck RR, DeWitt CM, Orme IM, Baldwin S, D'Souza C, Drowart A, Lozes E, Vandenbussche P, Van Vooren JP, Liu MA, Ulmer JB (1996) Immunogenicity and protective efficacy of a tuberculosis DNA vaccine. Nat Med 2:893–898
28. Tascon RE , Colston MJ, Ragno S, Stavropoulos E, Gregory D, Lowrie DB (1996) Vaccination against tuberculosis by DNA injection. Nat Med 2:888–892
29. Hsu CH, Chua KY, Tao MH, Lai YL, Wu HD, Huang SK, Hsieh KH (1996) Immunoprophylaxis of allergen-induced immunoglobulin E synthesis and airway hyperresponsiveness in vivo by genetic immunization. Nat Med 2:540–544
30. Barry MA, Lai WC, Johnston SA (1995) Protection against mycoplasma infection using expression-library immunization. Nature 377:632–635
31. Kurth R (1995) Risk potential of the chromosomal insertion of foreign DNA. Ann NY Acad Sci 772:140–151

Low Molecular Weight Cytokine Inducers

P. Stütz and E. Liehl

Introduction

Skin is in many ways a unique immunological organ acting as a primary interface between the host and the outside environment. It provides an important barrier function against intruding antigens and an efficient defense system against infections. Skin with an impaired barrier function, as seen, for example, in atopic dermatitis, is prone to chronic inflammation and infection [19].

The intercellular communication of the skin is essentially an immune surveillance system capable of detecting a multitude of antigenic threats to the host's survival and of orchestrating the repair of wounds. It is mediated by cytokines of skin-associated lymphoid tissues and adhesion molecules and their receptors and coreceptors. Although the pathogenesis of skin diseases such as psoriasis and atopic dermatitis and the complex process of wound healing are far from being well understood, monitoring of cytokine kinetics during different states of a skin disease is a useful diagnostic tool [12] and may pave the way to designing novel therapies.

Epidermal cytokines, particularly those produced by keratinocytes, have been studied in great detail over the last few years [22, 38]. It is now well established that dendritic cells, endothelial cells, fibroblasts, macrophages, mast cells, and T cells can contribute their genuine sets of cytokines to the stimulation of keratinocytes, resulting in an even more complex number and/or amplified levels of mediators. External factors such as ultraviolet (UV) light, microorganisms, phorbolesters (croton oil), or retinoids can also play a major role in these processes. Eventually, adhesion molecules may become induced, and cell activation, differentiation, and proliferation is affected positively or negatively. Furthermore, new cells from the circulation may be called in by chemokines [37]. Conversely, systemic effects may spread from the skin into the circulation.

Homeostasis in this highly complex system is provided by the fact that skin cells can secrete immunostimulatory cytokines, e.g., tumor necrosis factor (TNF), interleukin (IL)-1, IL-2, and IL-12, and immunosuppressive cytokines, e.g., transforming growth factor (TGF)-β or IL-10, while other cytokines such as IL-6 [29] or interferon (IFN)-γ may exert mixed functions [22, 38]. Receptors on target cells are up- and downregulated in parallel. In inflammatory diseases, this balance is shifted; for instance, in psoriatic lesional skin, reduced levels of IL-10 were found in comparison to normal skin [25]. In eczematous lesions of atopic dermatitis patients, increased levels of IFN-γ mRNA levels were observed, which may have been induced by IL-12 [9]. Because of this highly redundant system, it is not surprising that there are no reports on the successful treatment of skin diseases with recombinant cytokines so far (the gene therapy approach is excluded here), wound healing being no exception. A more holistic approach by applying a combination of cytokines would probably be more effective. This is, however, limited by their different pharmacokinetic profiles and volumes of distribution and by prohibitively high therapy costs.

Cytokine-producing skin cells are directly or indirectly involved in hyperproliferative and inflammatory events of a disease [15]. There is little doubt that, at least in psoriasis and atopic dermatitis, the disease state is sustained by activated T cells infiltrating the inflamed areas. Restoration of normal Th-1 to Th-2 ratios or regulation at the level of antigen-presenting cells (APC) may be a therapeutic approach [28]. Therapy with immunosuppressive drugs such as cyclosporin A has been shown to be at least transiently effective [34]. Unfortunately, this compound has an inherent risk for systemic side effects, and topical treatment has not been successful. Furthermore, immunosuppressive therapy can render people more sensitive to infections or may delay wound healing.

Therapeutic problems associated with recombinant cytokines could theoretically be overcome by the alternative concept of applying cytokine inducers, e.g., synthetic low molecular weight compounds that are capable of inducing a potentially synergistic combination of cytokines at physiological levels within the reach of target cells. Tempting as this concept may appear at first sight, designing a rational scheme for the identification and development of appropriate compounds for clinical use poses a problem. Fortunately, nature has already provided us with powerful chemical lead structures, cell wall components of bacteria and fungi, which have no chemical counterparts in mammalian organisms. It is probably because of their unique structure that they are highly stimulatory to immune cells. Of these, the most powerful cytokine inducers have been derived from murein (muramyl peptides), the cell wall backbone found in all bacteria, and endotoxin (lipopolysaccharide, LPS) characteristic of gram-negative bacteria.

Therapeutic Rationales for Cytokine Inducers

So far, cytokine inducers have mainly been investigated in tumor patients. The concept of cytokine inducers in skin diseases has not yet been validated clinically. This chapter is, therefore, highly speculative. We would like to put forward the following therapeutic rationales, based on the existing literature:

- Platelet-derived growth factor (PDGF) [30], TNF-α [8], IL-6 [23], TGF-α and -β [31], and other mediators have been reported to play a role in wound healing [30, 31]. In a rabbit dermal ulcer model, significant augmentation of wound healing by a single application of PDGF-BB (the recombinant homodimeric product of the c-sis gene of PDGF), epithelial growth factor (EGF), basic fibroblast growth factor (bFGF), or TGF-β was achieved [26]. We conclude that topical administration of a low molecular weight compound stimulating the release of a combination of these cytokines at physiological levels might speed up the process of epithelialization more efficiently than a single cytokine. There are no reports in the literature about such an approach.
- Compounds inducing IL-1 receptor antagonist (IL-1ra) and/or hematopoietic growth factors – e.g., granulocyte colony-stimulating factor (G-CSF), granulocyte-macrophage CSF (GM-CSF), IL-6, and IL-12 [24] – and/or stimulating phagocytosis may eradicate skin infections in diseases such *as atopy.*

- In atopic dermatitis, high levels of IgE and the dysregulation of Th-1/Th-2 cell-derived cytokines are involved in the causal chain of the disease [28]. Thus it is fair to assume that a compound with the capacity to normalize these conditions would be beneficial in patients. This may be possible by inducing the correct set of cytokines, for example.
- In psoriasis, an inducer of immunosuppressive cytokines or factors counteracting inflammatory and proliferative cell responses may be effective.

In the following, in vitro and in vivo data concerning representative compounds pioneering the above concepts are presented.

Low Molecular Weight Cytokine Inducers Under Investigation

Muramyl Peptide Derivatives

The minimal substructure analogue as a cytokine inducer is muramyl dipeptide (MDP; Fig. 1). This compound (and most analogues) acts like B cell mitogen and potentiates many effects of LPS [1, 18, 35]. Subcutaneous injections of MDP into guinea pigs aggravated delayed-type hypersensitivity (DTH) reactions because of its capacity to induce the release of proinflammatory cytokines [27]. Consequently, pyrogenic activity as the main side effect has precluded extensive use in humans.

There are numerous reports about chemical modifications of this lead structure in order to obtain compounds with a more desirable clinical profile. To date, clinical experience exists with the following representative compounds.

Highly Lipophilic Analogues

Romurtide. This compound (Muroctasin, MDP-LYS-L18, Daiichi Seiyaku Co., Ltd., Japan; Fig. 1). has the ability to induce colony-stimulating activity and to stimulate hematopoietic progenitor cell proliferation [44]. In vivo, it enhances nonspecific resistance to infection [32]. Due to an accelerated hematopoietic recovery, cancer patients could receive chemotherapy at shorter intervals [10, 42].

Muramyl Tripeptide Phophatidylethanolamide. This compound (MTP-PE, CGP-19835, Ciba-Geigy, Switzerland) has been used as a liposomal formulation for tumor therapy, particulary in patients with Kaposi's sarcoma or osteosarcoma. In vitro, it activates the tumoricidal properties in monocytes from cancer patients [14]. In 30 patients with metastasizing melanoma, it induced elevated serum TNF-a levels and monocyte activation, but without objective clinical response [20].

More Polar Muramyl Dipeptide Analogues

Representatives of this class behave differently in a number of assays. Two prototype compounds are discussed here: GMDP and SDZ 282.150.

GMDP. This compound (Allergan, USA, Peptec UK, USA; Fig. 1) is the orally active disaccharide analogue of MDP originally discovered by Russian researchers, bearing an additional (1β→4)-*N*-acetylglucosaminyl moiety. Its spectrum of biological activity is

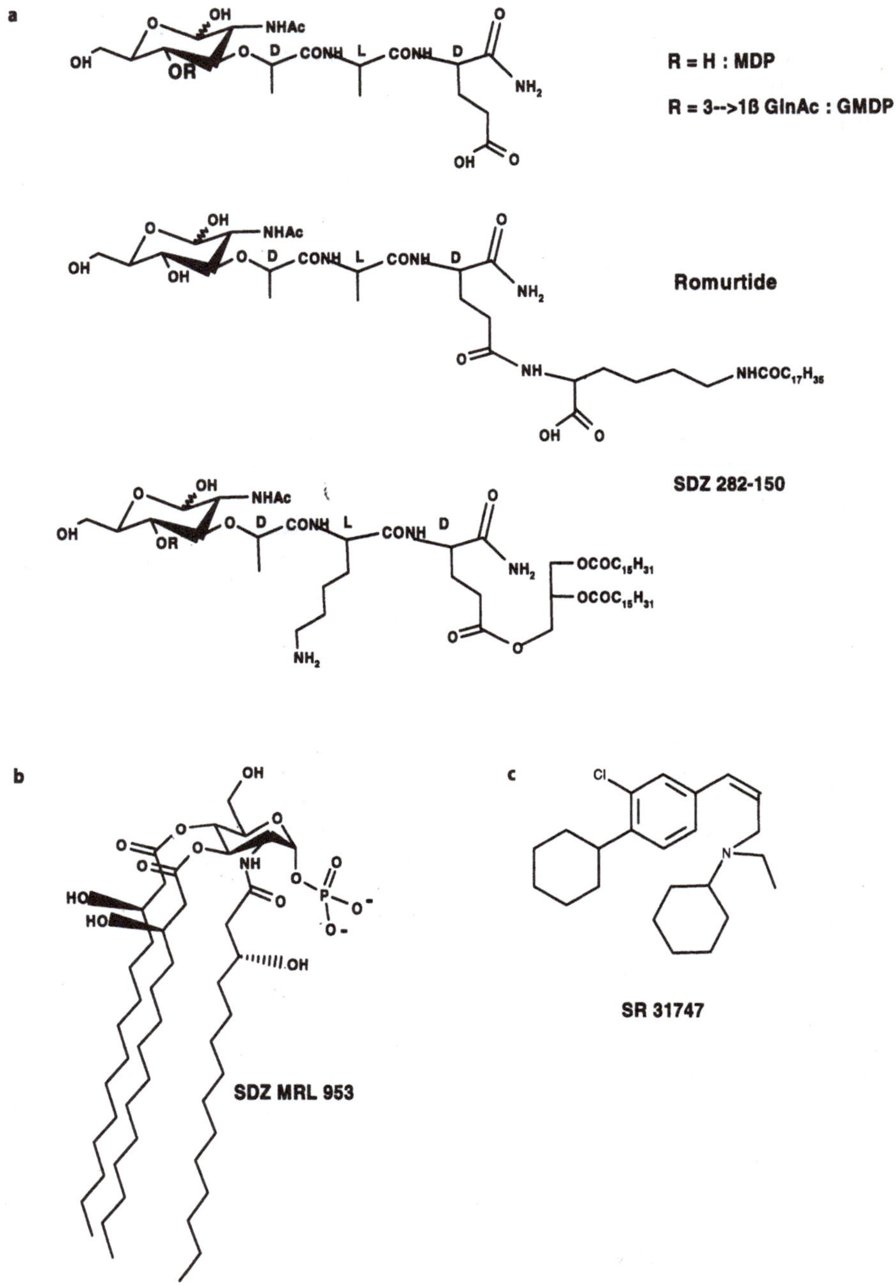

Fig. 1a–c. Chemical structures of representative cytokine inducers. **a** Muramyl dipeptide (*MDP*). **b** Lipid A analogue. **c** Sigma agonist

particularly striking. While it induces colony-stimulating activity and the proinflammatory cytokines TNF and IL-1 in vitro [35], it has recently been claimed to also be effective in psoriatic patients at dosages of 10–20 mg/day p.o. [43]. This was apparently an accidental discovery in the clinics, for which a preclinical rationale cannot be given to date.

The only in vivo effect described in this patent that may correlate with the known antipsoriatic effect of UVB is a downregulation of ATPase-positive epidermal dendritic cells in the mouse ear upon topical application. On the other hand, it did not induce Langerhans cells to migrate to draining lymph nodes as UVB does [41].

SDZ 282.150. This MDP analogue (MDP(Lys)GDP, Sandoz, Switzerland; preclinical standard, Fig. 1), a diacylglycerolester with an inserted l-lysyl between the l-alanyl and d-isoglutamine moieties, has no capacity at all to induce the mRNA of TNF-α, IL-1β, IFN-γ, or inducible nitrogen oxide synthase (iNOS) in thioglycolate-elicited, peritoneal mouse macrophages, in contrast to MDP as a control. Instead, it inhibited their LPS-induced induction in a dose-dependent manner. This effect was reversed by cycloheximide, indicating a post-translational event as the mechanism of action. Intriguingly, this compound synergized with IFN-γ in the production of proinflammatory cytokines in these cells [45]. The potential of this compound to induce immunosuppressive cytokines such as TGF-β or IL-10 was not investigated.

The anti-inflammatory activity observed in vitro was substantiated in a mouse model of allergic contact dermatitis (J. Meingassner, unpublished observation) upon oral and topical treatment. The results of this experiment are given below. Unfortunately, no information is available about the performance of GMDP in this model.

Groups of eight female NMRI mice (10–12 weeks of age) kept under standard conditions were sensitized on the shaved abdomen with 100 µl of an oxazolone solution (Sigma, St. Louis, MO, USA; 2 % in acetone). After 7 days, they were challenged with 10 µl of an oxazolone solution (2%, topical testing; 0.5%, systemic testing) on the inner surface of the right ear. The unchallenged ears served as controls. Twenty-four hours after the challenge, the difference in pinnal weights was determined as a measure of the inflammatory edema. For topical treatment, 10 µl of the dissolved test compound or the vehicle (ratio of dimethylacetamide-amide to acetone to ethanol, 2:4:4 by volume) was applied at the challenged site once, 30 min after the challenge. Systemic treatment was given by three oral doses as aqueous solution 3 days, 2 days, and 1 day before the challenge. Activity was calculated as percentage inhibition of edema relative to vehicle-treated animals.

To the best of our knowledge, SDZ 282-150 is the first MDP derivative for which an anti-inflammatory effect after p.o. and topical treatment has been shown in an animal model (Table 1). At this point, it not clear whether this effect is due to cytokine induction. Subsequent testing in other experimental settings may show whether this or a similar compound can be profiled against existing standards in skin diseases.

Lipid A Partial Structure Analogues

Lipid A is a lipophilic glucosamine disaccharide 1,4'-diphosphate that provides anchoring of LPS to the outer cell membrane of gram-negative bacteria. It is a very potent immunostimulant with the ability to induce the production of a wide range of cytokines

Table 1. Anti-inflammatory activity of SDZ 282-150 expressed as inhibition of pinnal swelling after oral and topical treatment.

Treatment	Pinnal weight Mean	SD	Inhibition of pinnal swelling (%)	Animals (*n*)
SDZ 282-150				
3x50 mg/kg p.o.	16.9	3.6	31*	16
Vehicle	24.5	3.6		16
1x30 mM topical	15.6	6.5	41*	16
1x10 mM topical	15.1	3.1	43*	8
1x3 mM topical	30.2	4.0	−14	8
Vehicle	26.6	5.7		16
Dexamethazone				
1x10 mM topical	7.4	2.4	72**	8
1x3 mM topical	9.4	4.2	68**	16
1x1 mM topical	9.4	4.2	68**	24
1x0.25 mM topical	14.2	7.1	51**	24
1x0.10 mM topical	16.7	5.6	44**	24
1x0.004 mM topical	23.0	11.4	21***	8

The activity of the standards is given for comparison.
* $p < 0.01$; ** $p < 0.001$; *** Not significant

and mediators from monocytes/macrophages. It has, however, essentially no therapeutic window because of its inherent endotoxic side effects due to a concomitant overstimulation of the immune system. Of the numerous efforts to design analogues that could be useful in the clinic, a brief account on the minimal substructure analogue, SDZ MRL 953, is given (Fig. 1).

The main pharmacological effects of this compound appear to be mediated via induction of therapeutically beneficial cytokines from monocytes/macrophages, such as G-CSF, M-CSF, and IL-6. Concurrently, stimulation of the reticuloendothelial system leads to efficient phagocytosis and intracellular killing of pathogenic microorganisms and to cytotoxicity against tumor cells [21]. Unlike LPS, very little, if any noxious cytokines such as TNF-α or IL-1β are produced [13]. This is brought about by a mode of action more specific than that of LPS, since it apparently does not participate in CD14-mediated signaling [7]. In animal models, it induced granulocytosis and early hematopoietic recovery after cytoreductive treatment [39] and induced resistance to bacterial and fungal infections [17], including synergism with antibiotics [16]. Like LPS, it inhibited tumor growth in various tumor models [11] and prevented endotoxin shock on prophylactic treatment [17]. When tested i.v. in tumor patients as a liposomal formulation, a dose-dependent induction of G-CSF, IL-1ra, IL-6, and IL-8 levels and very little TNF-α was seen, with a mean effective dose (MED) of 18 mg/kg. Repeated daily doses led to an efficient downregulation of G-CSF and TNF-α, without affecting neutrophil counts, and to a partial reduction of IL-6 levels in the circulation [7, 13].

To date, there are no reports on the activity of this lipid A analogue in skin diseases.

Sigma Ligands

In recent years, there has been a vast amount of research with regard to compounds binding to sigma receptors in the brain. Of these ligands, receptor antagonists have been proposed as leading candidates for the treatment of psychotic disorders, whereas agonists may worsen symptoms [36]. Su et al. [40] discovered that human monocytes also expressed these receptors. Later, they were also found in mouse lymphocytes [4].

In a recent study, Paul et al. [33] described a new sigma ligand, SR 31747 (Fig. 1), that binds specifically to human and rat lymphocytes. This appears to be the most potent competitive molecule for type-1 and -2 ligands, but there was also evidence that lymphocytes may contain a new subtype of receptor.

SR 31747 is immunosuppressive in vitro and in vivo. It inhibits the proliferative response of mitogens on mouse and human lymphocytes and prevents both graft-versus-host disease and DTH reaction in mice. This indicates that the sigma receptor recognized by SR 31747 is coupled to a biological function in lymphocytes [5].

In mechanistic studies, it was shown that this compound has the ability to down-regulate the production of LPS-induced IL-1, TNF-α, and IL-6 in mice in a dose-dependent manner [6]. More interestingly, this blockade of proinflammatory cytokines was accompanied by an upregulation of the immunosuppressive cytokine IL-10. For comparison, dexamethasone or cyclosporine did not change IL-10 levels significantly [2]. In other experiments, SR 31747 protected mice against lethality induced by staphylococcal enterotoxin B. Protection correlated with inhibition of the serum levels of IL-2, IL-4, GM-CSF, IL-6, and TNF-α, and an enhanced production of IL-10 [3].

Discussion

The cytokine network in the skin has been an intensive area of research over the last few years. However, apart from the progress made regarding the diagnostic role of cytokines during the progression of certain skin diseases and in wound healing, therapeutic success stories with recombinant cytokines are still lacking.

Given the already established complexity of intracellular communication, it is reasonable to assume that compounds with the ability to effectuate the release of a cytokine cocktail that can eventually correct the shifted balance of mediators in skin diseases into normal homeostasis could represent a very efficient therapeutic approach. Unfortunately, our knowledge about the signaling cascades and their mutual influence at the transcriptional level is still far from complete. This means that the biological properties of cytokine inducers that could correct the disease state cannot yet be deduced. The whole approach may be obscured by the induction of still unknown mechanisms by the cytokine inducer, so that some trial and error in the clinic must be admitted in order to identify therapeutically useful, more physiological disease-modifying drugs.

Clinical research with MDP derivatives such as GMDP in psoriasis may provide us with useful feedback information about the design of even more useful follow-up compounds on a rational basis. Comparison of this compound in preclinical models with standards might show whether or not SDZ 282-150 represents a step forward in this direction.

Compounds stimulating nonspecific resistance to infection should encourage clinicians to perform prophylactic studies in atopic dermatitis patients repeatedly suffering from streptococcal and staphylococcal infections. SDZ MRL 953 and Romurtide may already be candidates worth trying in order to prove the principle. Likewise, they may prevent infections in burns and accelerate wound healing if topically applied in a bioavailable formulation.

Selective inducers of immunosuppressive cytokines have not yet been identified to the best of our knowledge. However, the recently described sigma agonist SR 31747, which has the capacity to upregulate LPS-induced IL-10 and to concomitantly downregulate γ-IFN, IL-6, and TNF-α levels, may be an interesting step in this direction, even though the role of the sigma receptor in lymphocytes and macrophages is not yet understood. If proof of the principle of this type of compound can be shown in humans, it might be justified to also test dermatological indications.

To date, it is still uncertain whether cytokine inducers can be designed for skin diseases in a tailor-made fashion so that homeostasis of the cytokine network is ultimately restored. However, we may be at the beginning of a new era and may miss important opportunities if we do not develop concepts in this direction.

Summary

In recent years, much progress has been made in the investigation of the cytokine network of the skin. However, therapeutic applications with recombinant cytokines in skin diseases are still missing. This chapter discusses the novel concept of exploiting the potential of low molecular weight cytokine inducers in skin diseases. Such compounds have the ability to induce the release of a combination of potentially synergistic cytokines at physiological levels and within the reach of target cells. While proof of the concept involved in such compounds is still lacking in skin diseases, this approach might be superior to systemic administration of unphysiologically high concentrations of recombinant cytokines. Current knowledge about representative compounds of bacterial origin, i.e., muramyl peptides and lipid A analogues, and of a synthetic sigma ligand is briefly summarized.

References

1. Baschang G (1989) Muramylpeptides and lipopeptides: studies towards immunostimulants. Tetrahedron 45:6331–6360
2. Bourrié B, Bouaboula M, Benoit JM, Derocq JM, Esclangon M, Le Fur G, Casellas P (1995) Enhancement of endotoxin-induced interleukin-10 production by SR 31747A, a sigma ligand. Eur J Immunol 25:2882–2887
3. Bourrié B, Benoit JM, Derocq JM, Esclangon M, Thomas C, Le Fur G, Casellas P (1996) A sigma ligand, SR 31747A, potently modulates Staphylococcal enterotoxin B-induced cytokine production in mice. Immunology 88:389–393
4. Carr DJ, De Costa BR, Radesca L, Blalock JE (1991) Functional assessment and partial characterization of [3H] (+)-pentazocine binding sites on cells of the immune system. J Neuroimmunol 35:153–165
5. Casellas P, BourriP B, Canat X, Carayon P, Buisson I, Paul R. BreliPre JC, Le Fur G (1994) Immunopharmacological profile of SR 31747: in vitro and in vivo studies on humoral and cellular responses. J Neuroimmunol 52:193–203
6. Derocq JM, BourriP B, SPgui M, Le Flur G, Casellas P (1995) In vivo inhibition of endotoxin-induced pro-inflammatory cytokines production by the sigma ligand SR 31747. J Pharmacol Exp Ther 272:224–230

7. Engelhardt R, Foster C, Golenbock D, Hildebrandt J, Landmann R, Mayer P, Stern A, Stütz P (1995) SDZ MRL 953, a lipid A analog as selective cytokine inducer. In: Levin C, Alving R, Munford R, Redl H (eds) Bacterial endotoxins. Lipopolysaccharides from genes to therapy. Wiley-Liss, New York, pp 549–565 (Progress in clinical and biological research, vol 392)
8. Fahey TJ III, Turbeville T, McIntyre K (1995) Differential TNF expression by wound fibroblasts compared to normal fibroblasts in response to LPS. J Surg Res 58:759–764
9. Grewe M, Walther S, Gyufko K, Czech W, Schöpf E, Krutmann J (1995) Analysis of the cytokine pattern in situ in inhalant allergen patch test reactions of atopic dermatitis patients. J Invest Dermatol 105:407–410
10. Hiraoka A, Masaoka T, Satoh T, Ota K, Oyama A, Horiuchi A, Hasegawa H, Takegawa Y, Hata K (1988) Hematological response to the new synthetic muramyl dipeptide derivative muroctasin after chemotherapy in patients with malignant lymphoma. Arzneimittelforschung/Drug Res 38:1499–1501
11. Jeannin JF, Onier N, Lagadec P, von Jeney N, Stütz P, Liehl E (1991) Antitumor effect of synthetic derivatives of lipid A in an experimental model of colon cancer in the rat. Gastroenterology 101:726–733
12. Kapp A (1993) The roles of cytokines in the psoriatic inflammation. J Dermatol Sci 5:133–142
13. Kiani A, Tschiersch A, Gaboriau E, Seiz A, Knopf HP, Stütz P, Färber L, Haus U, Galanos C, Mertelsmann R, Engelhardt R (1996) Downregulation of the proinflammatory cytokine response to endotoxin by pretreatment with the non-toxic lipid A analog SDZ MRL 953 in cancer patients (submitted)
14. Kleinerman ES, Murray JL, Snyder JS, Cunningham JE, Fidler IJ (1989) Activation of tumoricidal properties in monocytes from cancer patients following intravenous administration of liposomes containing muramyl tripeptide phosphatidyl ethanolamine. Cancer Res 49: 4665–4670
15. Kondo S, Sauder DN (1995) Epidermal cytokines in allergic contact dermatitis. J Am Acad Dermatol 33:786–800
16. Lam C, Schütze E, Liehl E, Stütz P (1991a) Effect of SDZ MRL 953 on the survival of mice with advanced sepsis that cannot be cured by antibiotics alone. Antimicrob Agents Chemother 35:506–511
17. Lam C, Schütze E, Hildebrandt J, Aschauer H, Liehl E, Macher I, Stütz P (1991b) SDZ MRL 953, a novel immunostimulatory monosaccharidic lipid A analog with an improved therapeutic window in experimental sepsis. Antimicrob Agents Chemother 35:500–506
18. Lederer E (1988) Natural and synthetic immunomodulators derived from the mycobacterial cell wall. In: Bizzini B, Bonmassar E (eds) Advances in immunomodulation. Pythagora, Roma-Milan, pp 9–36
19. Leyden JJ, MarpleRR, Kligman AM (1974) Staphylococcus aureus in the lesions of atopic dermatitis. Br J Dermatol 90:525–530
20. Liebes L, Walsh CM, Chachoua A, Oratz R, Richards D, Hochster H, Peace D, Marino D, Alba S, Le Sher D, Blum RH, Vilcek J (1992) Modulation of monocyte functions by muramyl tripeptide phosphatidylethanolamine in a phase II study in patients with metastatic melanoma. J Natl Cancer Inst 84:694–699
21. Liehl E, Lam C, Mayer P, Schütze E, Bahr G, Grobmüller, Stütz P, Hildebrandt J (1993) SDZ MRL 953, a new cytokine inducing agent and stimulant for non-specific immunity. In: Levin J, Alvin R, Munford R, Stütz P (eds) Endotoxin research series, vol 2. Bacterial endotoxin: recognition and effector mechanisms. International Congress Series 1020. Excerpta Medica, Amsterdam, pp 399–413
22. Luger T, Schwarz T (eds) (1994) Epidermal growth factors and cytokines. Dekker, New York
23. Mateo RB, Reichner JS, Albina JE (1994) Interleukin-6 activity in wounds. Am J Physiol 266:R1840–1844
24. Metzger DW, Raeder R, Van Cleave VH, Boyle MD (1995) Protection of mice from group A streptococcal skin infection by interleukin 12. J Infect Dis 171:1643–1645
25. Mussi A,Bonifati C, Carducci M, Viola M, Tomaselli R, Sacerdoti G, Fazio M, Ameglio F (1994) IL-10 levels are decreased in psoriatic lesional skin as compared to the psoriatic lesion-free and normal skin suction blister fluids. J Biol Regul Homeost Agents 8:117–120

26. Mustoe TA, Pierce GF, Morishima C, Deuel TF (1991) Growth factor-induced acceleration of tissue repair through direct and inductive activities in a rabbit dermal ulcer model. J Clin Invest 87:694–703
27. Nagao S, Kawabata Y,Kitano M, Suzuki K, Nishikawa T, Takada H (1995) Modifications of delayed-type hypersensitivy reactions by muramyldipeptide in guinea pigs. FEMS Immunol Med Microbiol 11:231–245
28. Nickoloff BJ, Turka LA, Mitra RS, Nestle FO (1995) Direct and indirect control of T-cell activation by keratinocytes. J Invest Dermatol 105:25S–29S
29. Ohta Y, Nishiyama S, Nishioka K (1994) In situ expression of interleukin-6 in psoriatic epidermis during treatment. J Dermatol 21:301–307
30. Ono I, Gunji H, Zhang JZ, Mauyama K, Kaneko F (1995a) A study of cytokines in burn blister fluid related to wound healing. Burns 21: 352–355
31. Ono I, Gunji H, Zhang JZ, Mauyama K, Kaneko F (1995b) Studies on cytokines related to wound healing in donor site wound fluid. J Dermatol Sci 10: 241–245
32. Otani T, Une T, Osada Y (1988) Stimulation of non-specific resistance to infection by muroctasin. Arzneimittelforschung/Drug Res 38:969–976
33. Paul R, Lavastre S, Floutard D, Floutard R, Canat X, Casellas P (1994) Allosteric modulation of peripheral sigma binding sites by a new selective ligand, SR 31747. J Neuroimmunol 52: 183–192
34. Prens EP, van Joost T, Hegmans JP, 'tHooft-Benne K, Ysselmuiden OE (1995) Effects of cyclosporine on cytokines and cytokine receptors in psoriasis. J Am Acad Dermatol 33: 947–953
35. Rakhmilevich AL, Rakhimova MS, Andronova TM, Bovin MV (1989) In vitro immunostimulated effect of muramyldipeptide, glucosaminyl-muramyldipeptide and their synthetic derivatives. Antibiot Khimioter 34:586–589
36. Schoenwald RD, Barfknecht CF, Shirolkar-S, Xia E (1995) The effects of sigma ligands on protein release from lacrimal acinar cells: a potential agonist/antagonist assay Life Sci 56: 1275–1285
37. Schroeder JM (1995) Cytokine networks in the skin. J Invest Dermatol 105:20S–24S
38. Stoof T, Boorsma D, Nickoloff B (1994) Keratinocytes and Immunological Cytokines. In: Leigh I, Lane B, Watt F (eds) The keratinocyte handbook. Cambridge University Press, Cambridge, pp 365–399
39. Stütz P, Bahr G, Hildebrandt J, Lam C, Liehl E, Macher I, Mayer P, Schütze E (1995) Antimicrobial properties and cytokine release by an LPS-mimetic lipid A analog. In: Tellado JM, Forse RA, Solomkin JS (eds) Modulation of the inflammatory response in severe sepsis. Karger, Basel, pp 167–178 (Progress in surgery, vol 20)
40. Su TP, London ED, Jaffe JH (1988) Steroid binding at sigma receptors suggests a link between endocrine, nervous and immune systems. Science 240:219–221
41. Takashima A (1995) UVB-dependent modulation of epidermal cytokine network: roles in UVB-induced depletion of Langerhans cells and dendritic epidermal T cells. J Dermatol 22:876–887
42. Tsubura E, Nomura T, Niitani H, Osamura S, Okawa T, Tanaka M, Ota K, Nishikawa H, Masaoka T, Ogura T, Kozuru M, Hara N, Hara K, Ichimaru M Taktsuki K (1988) Restorative activity of muroctasin on leukopenia associated with anticancer treatment. Arzneimittelforschung/Drug Res 38:1070–1074
43. World Patent WO 96/01645 (1996) The use of muramyl peptide compounds (GMDP)
44. Yamaguchi F, Akasaki M, Tsukada W (1988) Induction of colony-stimulating factor and stimulation of stem cell proliferation by injection of muroctasin. Arzneimittelforschung/Drug Res 38:980–983
45. Zunic M, Bahr G, Dukor P, Lam C (1996) In vitro anti-inflammatory active of a synthetic derivative of muramyl dipeptide: downregulation of pro-inflammatory cytokines and iNOS. Skin Pharmacol 9:168

4 Clinical Aspects of Immunosuppression and Immunostimulation

4.1 Dermatoses Treated with Immunosuppressives 217
4.2 Dermatoses Treated with Immunostimulatory Drugs and Vaccination Therapies 293
4.2.1 Infections 293
4.2.2 Neoplasms 321
4.2.3 Strategies for Immunointervention in Malignant Melanoma 357

Autoimmune Bullous Diseases

D. Zillikens and L.A. Diaz

Autoimmune bullous diseases comprise a group of skin diseases characterized by the formation of spontaneous blisters either within the epidermis or subepidermally.

Pemphigus

The pemphigus group of diseases (Table 1) is characterized by intraepidermal blisters. Patients with pemphigus exhibit autoantibodies in their serum that bind to cell surface molecules of the keratinocyte. These autoantibodies are pathogenic and induce loss of epidermal cell–cell adhesion [1], a process termed acantholysis. By both direct and indirect immunofluorescence (IF), these autoantibodies bind the intercellular spaces of the epidermis, producing a typical staining pattern. This group of diseases includes pemphigus vulgaris (PV), pemphigus foliaceus (PF), drug-induced pemphigus, and paraneoplastic pemphigus.

Pemphigus Vulgaris

PV is the most common form of pemphigus in North America and Europe. In PV, the immune response is directed to desmoglein-3, a desmosomal glycoprotein of the cadherin family. Clinically, PV is characterized by flaccid blisters that readily rupture leaving erosions on the skin and mucous membranes. Erosions may increase in size, leaving large denuded areas. Commonly, PV begins in the mouth. The histopathologic hallmark of PV is a suprabasilar acantholytic blister. Pemphigus vegetans is a variant of PV and most commonly occurs in axillae and in the groin.

The aim of therapy should be to remove the autoantibodies from the patient's blood and skin. The following clinical signs may help to evaluate the response to therapy: (a) the presence/absence of the Nikolsky sign, (b) the number of new lesions formed per week, and (c) the rate of healing of existing lesions. In the initial phase of the treatment, pemphigus antibody titers should be tested every 4–6 weeks. When clinical remission has been achieved, direct IF will help in the decision of when to stop therapy. A total of 80% of patients with negative direct IF remained disease free for 5 years after cessation of therapy [37].

Before the availability of corticosteroids in the 1950s, approximately 75% of pemphigus patients died from their disease, most commonly within 1 year [32]. Over subsequent decades, mortality dropped to around 10% [8]. Currently, the major cause of death in these patients are treatment-induced side effects.

The mainstay of treatment of PV continues to be corticosteroids. Prednisone is most widely used, and the initial dosage is 1–2 mg/kg per day, depending on disease severity.

Table 1. Autoimmune bullous diseases with intraepidermal blisters

	Deposits by direct immunofluorescence	Auotantigen
Pemphigus vulgaris	Intercellular IgG > C3	Desmoglein-3 (130 kDa)
Pemphigus foliaceus	Intercellular IgG > C3	Desmoglein-1 (160 kDa)
Drug-induced pemphigus	Intercellular IgG > C3	Desmoglein-1 or -3 (some patients)
Paraneoplastic pemphigus	Intercellular IgG > C3 At the BMZ, C3 > IgG	Desmoplakin-1 (250 kDa), Desmoplakin-2 (210 kDa), BP230, and 190- and 170-kDa proteins (unknown)
IgA pemphigus	Intercellular IgA	Desmocollin-1

BMZ, basement membrane zone

The disease activity is considered to be controlled when no new blisters develop and 80 % of preexisting blisters have healed. In our experience, it is only rarely necessary to employ dosages of prednisone higher that 100 mg per day. Once control is achieved, corticosteroids are reduced gradually every 2 weeks [8]. If corticosteroids cannot be tapered completely, they are kept at the lowest possible level to prevent flares. Several immunosuppressive agents, including cyclophosphamide, azathioprine, methotrexate, and cyclosporine, have been used in the treatment of PV. The rationale for the use of these drugs is to reduce the dose of corticosteroids and hence their side effects. Although there is widespread belief that these immunosuppressants result in a steroid-sparing effect, there is no objective data to support this assumption. No controlled studies have been published comparing the effectiveness and side effects of corticosteroids given alone with corticosteroids used in combination with immunosuppressants.

Cyclophosphamide is an effective immunosuppressant. It is usually given orally at a dosage of 1–2 mg/kg per day. Pulse intravenous cyclophosphamide (given on day 1) with concomitant pulse intravenous corticosteroids (given on days 1–3) has been proposed as an alternative therapy in resistant cases of PV [35, 36]. According to the clinical and serological response, this cycle is repeated every 2–4 weeks. Oral maintenance therapy with systemic steroids and cyclophosphamide is then used. Side effects of cyclophosphamide, including hemorrhagic cystitis, infertility, and the potential induction of bladder malignancies, must be closely monitored.

Azathioprine is another immunosuppressive agent commonly used as an adjuvant to corticosteroids in the therapy of PV. The dosage used is 2 mg/kg per day, and its major side effects include bone marrow suppression, hepatotoxicity, and the potential to induce malignancies. When concomitantly using azathioprine or other immunosuppressants along with glucocorticosteroids, it must be remembered that the induction of a leukopenia may be masked by the steroids.

Methotrexate has been used as an adjuvant agent in PV in those patients with side effects to cyclophpsphamide and azathioprine. Some studies suggest a high incidence of severe and fatal infections and impairment of cutaneous healing.

Cyclosporine, when used as the sole therapy, is of limited value in controlling pemphigus. In combination with glucocorticosteroids, cyclosporine appears to have a steroid-sparing effect [31], but the experience with this combination is limited.

Other types of adjuvant therapy in PV include gold and, for very severe cases, plasmapheresis, photopheresis, and high-dose intravenous gammmaglobulins. *Gold* has been used either alone or in combination with corticosteroids. It is administered as an intramuscular injection (gold sodium thiomalate or aurothioglucose) or as an oral preparation (auranofin), which may be less effective. Side effects occur in about 30% of patients and include nausea, allergic reactions, renal and bone marrow toxicity, and liver necrosis. Currently gold is used only rarely. *Plasmapheresis* should be used in combination with corticosteroids and immunosuppressants, most favorably cyclophosphamide, in order to suppress the rebound increase in autoantibody production. One study demonstrated a high mortality rate due to sepsis in PV patients undergoing plasmapheresis combined with moderate doses of corticosteroids [24]. *Extracorporal photopheresis* has also been used to treat PV patients; however, the experience with this treatment modality is only limited. In some patients previously resistant to therapy, reductions in concurrent medications were possible [38]. Encouraging results have recently been reported for the use of high-dose *intravenous γ-globulin* as an adjuvant treatment in recalcitrant PV [6, 47]. In addition to corticosteroids and immunosuppressants, γ-globulins were given at a dosage of 300 mg/kg per day on 5 consecutive days. This cycle was repeated every 4 weeks according to the clinical response [47]. Intravenous γ-globulins appear to be ineffective if used alone [42]. The high cost of γ-globulins is a disadvantage of this therapy.

Pemphigus Foliaceus

In PF, the immune response is directed to desmoglein-1, which is also a desmosomal glycoprotein. PF is characterized by an acantholytic blister at the level of the stratum granulosum, and patients present with fragile blisters that rupture easily, producing erosions, crusting, and scaling. In contrast to PV, the mucous membranes are usually spared, and lesions are most commonly on the face, neck, and trunk. There is an endemic form of PF found in certain areas of Brazil, Colombia, and Tunisia. Substantial epidemiologic evidence suggests that endemic PF may be precipitated by an environmental factor [15, 25]. Pemphigus erythematosus represents a variant of PF with features of systemic lupus erythematosus in the same patient.

Compared with PV, PF is a more benign disease and can usually be treated with less aggressive therapy. The majority of patients respond to 0.5–1 mg prednisone/kg per day. Once remission has been accomplished, the doses of prednisone can be reduced gradually. In addition, sun protection and topical fluorinated corticosteroids are usually helpful. Some patients with a more severe form of the disease may require more aggressive treatment, as outlined for PV.

Other drugs that have been reported to be helpful in the therapy of PF include dapsone, antimalarials, and a combination of tetracycline and niacinamide. *Dapsone*, at a dosage of 200–300 mg/day, was found to be effective in mild forms of PF, whereas the majority of patients with severe disease did not respond to this drug [5]. Side effects of such high doses of dapsone are not uncommon, and cimetidine or vitamin E may be administered along with dapsone to decrease its toxicity [14]. *Antimalarials* such as hydroxychloroquine (200 mg/day) were reported to be useful as steroid-sparing agents in PF [28]. The combination of oral tetracycline (2 g/day) and niacinamide (1.5 g/day) with a topical corticosteroid was recently described as useful in some patients with PF [11]. This regimen, however, has been unsuccessful in our patients.

Drug-Induced Pemphigus

Occasionally, pemphigus may be induced or triggered by drugs. The drugs most commonly implicated in inducing this disease are D-penicillamine and captopril. These patients usually present with the clinical picture of PF and less frequently PV [50]. Antibodies to desmoglein-1 and desmoglein-3 have been detected in sera from patients with drug-induced pemphigus [29]. This disease is usually transient and resolves shortly after the drug has been discontinued, especially in those patients that lack evidence of circulating antibodies. However, some cases follow a chronic course, and it appears that in these patients idiopathic pemphigus has been precipitated by the drug.

Paraneoplastic Pemphigus

Paraneoplastic pemphigus is a recently described blistering disorder that arises exclusively in the context of a neoplasm, most commonly a non-Hodgkin's lymphoma [2]. In addition to polymorphous skin lesions, patients develop prominent, painful mucous membrane ulcerations. When associated with a malignancy, the course of this disease is almost always fatal. If a benign tumor (i.e., Castleman's tumor) is the underlying neoplasm and is removed, paraneoplastic pemphigus responds to treatment with corticosteroids and may resolve completely [9].

Intercellular IgA Dermatosis ("IgA Pemphigus")

Close to 30 patients with intercellular IgA deposits have been reported and summarized in a recent review [44]. Clinically and pathologically, these patients present with two different forms: (1) a subcorneal pustular dermatosis and (2) an intraepidermal neutrophilic dermatosis. Recent data suggest that the autoantibodies in the subcorneal pustular dermatosis type of the disease bind to both human and bovine desmocollin-1, whereas the autoantigen in the other subtype awaits further elucidation [18, 26]. Intercellular IgA dermatosis is associated with an IgA gammopathy in 20% of cases. It usually has a benign course and is managed with dapsone or etretinate [44, 49]. In more resistant cases, corticosteroids alone or in combination with immunosuppressive agents have been used successfully [44]. The concept of this disease is still preliminary and its relationship to pemphigus is not yet completely clarified.

Subepidermal Autoimmune Bullous Diseases

Based on recent studies from France and Germany, the most common subepidermal autoimmune disease is bullous pemphigoid (BP), followed by cicatricial pemphigoid (CP), herpes gestationis (HG), linear IgA disease (LAD), and epidermolysis bullosa acquisita (EBA) ([7, 52]; Table 2).

Table 2. Autoimmune bullous diseases with subepidermal blisters

	Deposits by direct immunofluorescence	Autoantigen
Bullous pemphigoid	C3 > IgG at the BMZ	Hemidesmosomal proteins BP230 and BP180
Herpes gestationis	C3 > IgG at the BMZ	BP180
Cicatricial pemphigoid	IgG > C3 < IgA at the BMZ	BP180, laminin-5 in some cases
Epidermolysis bullosa acquisita	IgG > C3 at the BMz	290 kDa (type VII collagen)
Linear IgA disease	IgA at the BMZ	97-kDa protein
Dermatisis herpetiformis	IgA in dermal papillae	Unknown

BMZ, basement membrane zone

Bullous Pemphigoid

BP is a disease of the elderly characterized by tense, subepidermal blisters. Intertriginous areas are most commonly involved, whereas mucous membranes are usually not affected [53]. Two hemidesmosomal proteins, BP230 and BP180, have been identified as primary targets of BP antibodies [16, 21, 30, 40, 41]. Our laboratory has recently developed the first animal model of BP involving the passive transfer of anti-BP180 antibodies into neonatal mice [23, 33]. The animals develop a subepidermal blistering disease that is dependent upon complement activation and neutrophilic infiltration [34]. In contrast to pemphigus, BP is often a self-limited disease [32], and it may be sufficient to treat the patient symptomatically for a limited period of time.

Systemic corticosteroids are still most commonly used for therapy of generalized BP, but the required dosage necessary to control the disease is lower than in PV (0.5 mg prednisone/kg per day). Corticosteroids are often combined with other immunosuppressants in resistant cases of BP. In this group of elderly patients, commonly suffering from various other medical problems, the complications of systemic corticosteroids may be especially severe. Patients may succumb to side effects of the treatment rather than to the disease itself. As a result, efforts have been made to find alternatives to the use of systemic corticosteroids.

BP may respond well to dapsone or sulfonamides, in combination with either topical or systemic corticosteroids. The required dosage of dapsone is usually 100 mg/day, and therapy is initiated with 50 mg/day [43]. Another regimen, proposed for the treatment of localized forms of BP, consists of the sole use of clobetol propionate cream, followed by tapering with less potent topical corticosteroids over a period of several months [45]. Several authors have proposed the use of oral tetracycline or a combination of tetracycline and niacinamide to treat BP. A recent randomized trial comparing the combination of tetracycline and niacinamide with prednisone found the combination at least as effective as the corticosteroid treatment [19]. An excellent response was also reported with the following regimen: 500 mg oxytetracycline q.i.d. and 400 mg niacinamide t.i.d.; in addition, during the blistering stage of the disease, topical clobetasol propionate was applied. After cessation of new blister formation (1–4 weeks), the topical corticosteroid was discontinued, and tetracycline and niacinamide were tapered [27]. Cyclosporin, intravenous γ-globulin, high-dose pulse therapy with intravenous corticosteroids, and plasmapheresis have all been proposed as treatment alternatives. These regimens are not necessary for the therapy of routine BP cases [53].

Herpes Gestationis

HG usually begins in pregnancy, but patients may also first present during the post-partum period [46]. In 1993, it was shown that HG and BP autoantibodies react with a common immunodominant site on the extracellular domain of the BP180 antigen [22].

In mild cases of HG, topical corticosteroids and an antihistamine to relieve pruritus may be sufficient. In more severe cases and during postpartum exacerbations, prednisone (20–40 mg/day) may be necessary initially and tapered later [39]. Prolonged and therapy-resistant forms of HG have been reported, but are rare.

Cicatricial Pemphigoid

CP predominantly involves mucous membranes and is characteristically associated with scarring. Recent evidence suggests that subepidermal blisters in CP may be triggered by autoantibodies against either BP180 or laminin-5 [4, 17]. CP is difficult to treat, and spontaneous remissions are rare [3]. For CP cases involving only the oral mucosa, treatment may be limited to topical steroids, intralesional steroids, or short courses of systemic corticosteroids. Some patients may respond to dapsone at dosages of 100–150 mg/day [3]. If the eyes or larynx are involved, a more aggressive regimen is warranted, and the use of high doses of glucocorticosteroids in combination with immunosuppressants has been reported to be effective [10]. Of the various immunosuppressive agents available, cyclophosphamide has been shown to be most effective [20].

Epidermolysis Bullosa Acquisita

EBA is characterized by subepidermal blisters and autoantibodies to type VII collagen, the major component of anchoring fibrils. There are three different skin manifestations of the disease: (1) a noninflammatory form of EBA, affecting trauma-prone areas of the skin, (2) a generalized inflammatory blistering eruption, and (3) a CP-like disease mainly affecting mucous membranes.

All forms of EBA are difficult to treat. Systemic corticosteroids alone or in combination with azathioprine or cyclophosphamide are not effective in controlling the disease. Some patients may respond to dapsone [51]. More encouraging reports have been published for the use of cyclosporin A. In addition, a small number of patients have been successfully treated with colchicine or extracorporal photopheresis [13].

Linear IgA Disease and Dermatitis Herpetiformis

LAD and dermatitis herpetiformis (DH) are rare IgA-mediated disorders. LAD may affect children and adults. The adult form may be precipitated by various drugs, most commonly vancomycin. The juvenile form of LAD is also termed chronic bullous disease of childhood. Both forms of LAD are characterized by linear deposits of IgA at the basement membrane zone (BMZ). In DH, in contrast, IgA is found in the tips of the dermal papillae.

Both LAD and DH are usually responsive to dapsone. Alternatively, sulfapyridine or sulfamethoxypyridazine are also effective. LAD of childhood is often a self-limited disease, and most patients enter remission within 2 years [48]. LAD of adulthood may be complicated by severe scarring of the mucous membranes and may then cause similar treatment problems as CP.

Subepidermal Autoimmune Bullous Diseases with Antibodies to 105- or 200-kDa Proteins of the Basement Membrane Zone

Recently, a new pemphigoid-like disease with autoantibodies to a 105-kDa protein of the BMZ has been reported. The patient's condition responded well to systemic corticosteroids [12]. Another report described a subepidermal bullous disease with clinical features of BP and erythema multiforme and nonscarring mucous membrane involvement. The immune response was directed against a 200-kDa protein of the BMZ, and the disease was responsive to tetracycline and niacinamide [54].

Outlook

The past 15 years have seen significant progress in our understanding of the immunopathology of some autoimmune bullous diseases, including PV, PF, BP, and EBA. In these diseases, the autoantigens have been characterized at the molecular level, and recombinant proteins are now available representing either the full length or portions of these autoantigens. These recombinant proteins are currently used for mapping studies of the relevant B and T cell epitopes in these diseases. This may offer the possibility for more specific treatment modalities, including the induction of immunological tolerance to the relevant autoantigens.

Passive transfer mouse models are available for PV, PF, and BP. The clinical, histological, and immunopathological findings in these mice duplicate the findings in the human disease. These animal models greatly facilitate studies aimed at further dissecting the pathophysiology of blister formation in these diseases. They should prove useful in studying drugs which are able to modulate local events at the site of blister formation.

Summary

Autoimmune bullous diseases comprise a group of skin diseases characterized by spontaneous blister formation and production of autoantibodies against keratinocyte cell surface proteins or constituents of the BMZ of the skin. The blisters in these disorders are located either within the epidermis or subepidermally. The autoantigens in most of these diseases have been characterized at the molecular level; however, little is yet known about the factors that initiate the production of autoantibodies. Therapy is therefore directed at controlling the resulting pathologic events rather than at the primary cause. The mainstay of treatment for most of these diseases still consists in the use of systemic corticosteroids. The availability of recombinant forms of some of the autoantigens may open up the way for more specific treatment modalities in the future, including the induction of immunological tolerance.

Acknowledgment. This work was supported by U.S. Public Service Grants RO1-AR32599 and R37-AR32081 and training grant T32-AR07577 from the National Institutes of Health and by a VA Merit Review Grant (LAD). Dr. Zillikens is the recipient of a Research Grant from the Deutsche Forschungsgemeinschaft (Zi 439/2-1).

References

1. Anhalt GJ, Labib R, Voorhees JJ, Beals TF, Diaz LA (1982) Induction of pemphigus in neonatal mice by passive transfer of IgG from patients with the disease. N Engl J Med 306:1189–1196
2. Anhalt GJ, Kim SC, Stanley JR, Korman NJ, Jabs DA, Kory M, Izumi H, Ratrie H, Mutasim D, Ariss-Abo L, Labib RS (1990) Paraneoplastic pemphigus. An autoimmune mucocutaneous disease associated with neoplasia. N Engl J Med 323:1729–1735
3. Axt M, Wever S, Bayer G, Bogdan S, Hashimoto T, Bröcker EB, Zillikens D (1995) Cicatricial pemphigoid – a problem to treat. Hautarzt 46:620–627
4. Balding SD, Prost C, Diaz LA, Bernard P, Bedane C, Aberdam D, Giudice GJ (1996) Cicatricial pemphigoid antibodies react with multiple sites on the BP180 extracellular domain. J Invest Dermatol 106:141–146
5. Basset N, Guillot B, Michel B, Meynadier J, Guilhou JJ (1987) Dapsone as initial treatment in superficial pemphigus. Arch Dermatol 123:783–785
6. Beckers RCY, Brand A, Vermeer BJ, Boom BW (1996) Adjuvant high-dose intravenous gammaglobulin in the treatment of pemphigus and bullous pemphigoid: experience in six patients. Br J Dermatol 133:289–293
7. Bernard P, Vaillant L, Labeille B et al (1995) Incidence and distribution of subepidermal autoimmune bullous skin disease in three French regions. Arch Dermatol 31:48–521
8. Bystryn JC, Steinman NM (1996) The adjuvant therapy in pemphigus. Arch Dermatol 132:203–212
9. Camisa C, Helm TN (1993) Paraneoplastic pemphigus is a distinct neoplasia-induced autoimmune disease. Arch Dermatol 129:883–886
10. Caux FA, Giudice GJ, Diaz LA, Fairley JA (1996) Cicatricial pemphigoid. J Geriatr Dermatol 4:42–46
11. Chaffins ML, Collison D, Fivenson DP (1993) Treatment of pemphigus and linear IgA dermatosis with nicotinamide and tetracycline: a review of 13 cases. J Am Acad Dermatol 28:998–1000
12. Chan LS, Fine JD, Briggaman RA, Woodley DT, Hammerberg C, Drugge RJ, Cooper KD (1993) Identification and partial characterization of a novel 105-kDalton lower lamina lucida autoantigen associated with a novel immune-mediated subepidermal blistering disease. J Invest Dermatol 101:262–267
13. Chan LS, Chen M, Woodley DT (1996) Epidermolysis bullosa acquisita in the elderly: clinical manifestation, diagnosis, and therapy. J Geriatr Dermatol 4:47–52
14. Coleman MD (1993) Dapsone: mode of action, toxicity and possible strategies for increasing patient tolerance. Br J Dermatol 129:507–513
15. Diaz LA, Sampaio SAP et al (1989) Endemic pemphigus foliaceus (fogo selvagem). II. Current and historic epidemiologic studies. J Invest Dermatol 92:4–12
16. Diaz LA, Ratrie III H, Saunders WS, Futamura S, Squiquera HL, Anhalt GJ, Giudice GJ (1990) Isolation of a human epidermal cDNA corresponding to the 180-kD autoantigen recognized

by bullous pemphigoid and herpes gestationis sera. Immunolocalization of this protein to the hemidesmosome. J Clin Invest 86:1088–1094
17. Domloge-Hultsch, Gammon WR, Briggaman RA, Gil SG, Carter WG, Yancey KB (1992) Epiligrin, the major human keratinocyte ligand, is targeted in both an acquired autoimmune and an inherited subepidermal blistering disease. J Clin Invest 90:1628–1633
18. Ebihara T, Hashimoto T, Iwatsuki K, Takigawa M, Ando M, Ohkawara A, Nishikawa T (1991) Autoantigens for IgA anti-intercellular antibodies of intercellular IgA vesiculopustular dermatosis. J Invest Dermatol 97:742–745
19. Fivenson DP, Breneman DL, Rosen GB, Craig SH, Cardone S, Mutasim D (1994) Nicotinamide and tetracycline therapy of bullous pemphigoid. Arch Dermatol 130:753–758
20. Foster CS (1986) Cicatricial pemphigoid. Tr AM Ophth Soc 84:527–663
21. Giudice GJ, Emery DJ, Diaz LA (1992) Cloning and primary structural analysis of the bullous pemphigoid autoantigen, BP180. J Invest Dermatol 99:243–250
22. Giudice GJ, Emery DJ, Zelickson BD, Anhalt GJ, Liu Z, Diaz LA (1993) Bullous pemphigoid and herpes gestationis autoantibodies recognize a common non-collagenous site on the BP180 ectodomain. J Immunol 151:5742–5750
23. Giudice GJ, Liu Z, Diaz LA (1995) An animal model for bullous pemphigoid: what can it teach us? Proc Assoc Am Phys 107:237–241
24. Guillaume JC, Roujeau JC, Morel P et al (1988) Controlled study of plasma exchange in pemphigus. Arch Dermatol 124:1659–1663
25. Hans-Filho G, dos Santos V, Katayama JH et al (1996) An active focus of high prevalence of Fogo Selvagem on an Amerindian reservation in Brasil. J Invest Dermatol 107:68–75
26. Hashimoto T, Amagai M, Garrod DR, Nishikawa T (1996) Human Desmocollin 1 (Dsc1) is an autoantigen for subcorneal pustular dermatosis type of intercellular IgA vesiculopustular dermatosis (IgA pemphigus). J Invest Dermatol 106:832
27. Hornschuh B, Hamm H, Wever S, Hashimoto T, Schröder U, Bröcker EB, Zillikens D (1997) Treatment of 16 patients with bullous pemphigoid with oral tetracycline and niacinamide and topical clobetasol. J Am Acad Dermatol 36:101–103
28. Hymes SR, Jordon RE (1992) Pemphigus foliaceus: use of antimalarial agents as adjuvant therapy. Arch Dermatol 128:1462–1464
29. Korman NJ, Eyre RW, Zone J, Stanley JR (1991) Drug induced pemphigus: autoantibodies directed against the pemphigus antigen complexes are present in penicillamine and captopril-induced pemphigus. J Invest Dermatol 96:273–276
30. Labib RS, Anhalt GJ, Patel HP, Mutasim DF, Diaz LA (1986) Molecular heterogeneity of the bullous pemphigoid antigens as detected by immunoblotting. J Immunol 136:1231–1235
31. Lapidoth M, David M, Ben-Amitai D, Katzenelson V, Lustig S, Sandbank M (1988) The efficacy of combined treatment with prednisone and cyclosporine in patients with pemphigus: preliminary study. J Am Acad Dermatol 30:752–757
32. Lever WF (1965) Pemphigus and pemphigoid. Thomas, Springfield
33. Liu Z, Diaz LA, Troy JL, Taylor AF, Emery DJ, Fairley JA, Giudice GJ (1993) A passive transfer model of the organ-specific autoimmune disease, bullous pemphigoid, using antibodies generated against the hemidesmosomal antigen, BP180. J Clin Invest 92:2480–2488
34. Liu Z, Giudice GJ, Swartz SJ, Fairley JA, Till GO, Troy JL, Diaz LA (1995) The role of complement in experimental bullous pemphigoid. J Clin Invest 95:1539–1544
35. Pandya AG, Sontheimer RD (1992) Treatment of pemphigus vulgaris with pulse intravenous cyclophosphamide. Arch Dermatol 128:1626–1630
36. Pasricha JS, Thanzama J, Khan UK (1988) Intermittent high-dose dexamethason-cyclophosphamide therapy for pemphigus. Br J Dermatol 119:73–77
37. Ratnam KV, Pang BK (1994) Pemphigus in remission. Value of direct immunofluorescence in management. J Am Acad Dermatol 30:547–550
38. Rook AH, Heald PW, Nahass GT et al (1989) Treatment of autoimmune disease with extracorporal photochemotherapy: pemphigus vulgaris: preliminary report. Yale J Biol Med 62: 647–652
39. Shornick JK (1987) Herpes gestationis. J Am Acad Dermatol 17:539–556

40. Stanley JR, Hawley-Nelson P, Yuspa SH, Shevach EM, Katz SI (1981) Characterization of bullous pemphigoid antigen: a unique basement membrane protein of stratified epithelia. Cell 24:897–903
41. Stanley JR, Tanaka T, Mueller S, Klaus-Kovtun V, Roop D (1988) Isolation of a complementary DNA for bullous pemphigoid antigen by use of patients' autoantibodies. J Clin Invest 82:1864–1870
42. Tappeiner G, Steiner A (1989) High-dosage intravenous gamma globulin: therapeutic failure in pemphigus and pemphigoid. J Am Acad Dermatol 20:684–685
43. Venning VA, Millard PR, Wojnarowska F (1989) Dapsone as first line therapy for bullous pemphigoid. Br J Dermatol 120:83–92
44. Wallach D (1992) Intraepidermal IgA pustulosis. J Am Acad Dermatol 27:993–1000
45. Westerhof W (1989) Treatment of bullous pemphigoid with topical clobetasol propionate. J Am Acad Dermatol 20:458–461
46. Wever S, Burger M, Langfritz K, Hashimoto T, Nishikawa T, Bröcker EB, Zillikens D (1995) Herpes gestationis. Clinical spectrum and diagnostic options. Hautarzt 46:158–164
47. Wever S, Zillikens D, Bröcker EB (1996) Successful treatment of refractory mucosal lesions in pemphigus vulgaris using intravenous gammaglobulin as an adjuvant therapy. Br J Dermatol 135:862–863
48. Wojnarowska F, Marsden RA, Bhogal B, Black MM (1988) Chronic bullous disease of childhood, childhood cicatricial pemphigoid, and linear IgA disease of adults. A comparative study demonstrating clinical and immunopathological overlap. J Am Acad Dermatol 19:792–805
49. Zillikens D, Miller K, Hartmann AA, Burg G (1990) IgA pemphigus foliaceus: a case report. Dermatologica 181:304–307
50. Zillikens D, Zentner A, Burger M, Hartmann, AA, Burg G (1993) Penicillamine-induced pemphigus foliaceus. Hautarzt 44:167–171
51. Zillikens D, Erhard E, Prost C, Hashimoto T, Nishikawa T, Bröcker EB (1994) Inflammatory epidermolysis bullosa acquisita. Hautarzt 45:166–170
52. Zillikens D, Wever S, Roth A, Weidenthaler-Barth B, Hashimoto T, Bröcker EB (1995) Incidence of autoimmune subepidermal blistering diseases in a region of central Germany. Arch Dermatol 131:957–958
53. Zillikens D, Giudice GJ, Diaz LA (1996a) Bullous pemphigoid. An autoimmune blistering disease of the elderly. J Geriatr Dermatol 4:35–41
54. Zillikens D, Kawahara Y, Ishiko A, Shimizu H, Mayer J, Rank CV, Liu Z, Giudice GJ, Tran HH, Marinkovich MP, Bröcker EB, Hashimoto T (1996b) A novel subepidermal blistering disease with autoantibodies to a 200-kDa antigen of the basement membrane zone. J Invest Dermatol 106:1333–1336

Rheumatic Disease Group

R. M. Trüeb

Introduction

In the recent past, advances in both basic and clinical research have considerably contributed to our understanding of the cellular and molecular events that lead to autoimmune disease. The importance of genetic susceptibility [1], i.e., particular alleles of major histocompatibility complex (MHC) class II molecules [2], and environmental factors, i.e., molecular mimicry of autoantigens by microbes [3] and microbial superantigens [4], as well as the central role of T cells [5] in the pathogenesis of autoimmune disease is well appreciated, and modern immune-based therapy would thus ideally be directed towards early events in the pathological process. Results obtained using animal models of antigen-induced autoimmune disease, e.g., collagen-induced arthritis and experimental allergic encephalomyelitis, have resulted in optimism that this will eventually be possible. It must be borne in mind, however, that in this type of experimental animal model it is simple to intervene in the development of autoimmune disease, since the induction events (immunization with defined autoantigens) are designed by the investigator. In contrast, in autoimmune disorders of the rheumatic disease group, including lupus erythematosus (LE), systemic sclerosis, dermatomyositis (DM), and polyarteritis nodosa (PAN), we do not know whether a specific autoantigen initiated the disease, nor do we know the time point at which the antigenic challenge occurred. The processes resulting in autoimmune disease begin well before we see the patient, and we as clinicians are faced only with late-term manifestations of the immunologic events that lead to clinical disease. Thus the current therapy of these diseases is essentially limited to chemical immunosuppresssion with corticosteroids and cytotoxic drugs, such as azathioprine, cyclophosphamide, and methotrexate. The introduction of cyclosporine represents major progress compared with substances formerly used in terms of cellular selectivity, inasmuch as cyclosporine does not depress bone marrow hemopoesis and acts selectively on the production of well-defined cytokines [6]. However, significant side effects occur, and the lymphokines in question are involved in a number of immune reactions other than the targeted process [7].

Another important issue to address when dealing with the therapy of autoimmune diseases with cutaneous manifestations is the extent and severity of disease. Attention in therapeutic studies has predominantly focused on the severe forms of disease. With the recognition of distinct benign variants (subsets) limited to the skin, i.e., chronic cutaneous (discoid) LE (DLE), subacute cutaneous LE (SCLE), localized cutaneous sclerosis, amyopathic DM, benign cutaneous PAN, the dermatologist in particular is confronted with the decision whether to use less aggressive therapeutic modalities.

Current Therapy of Cutaneous Rheumatic Diseases

Lupus Erythematosus

LE is a heterogenous autoimmune disorder associated with polyclonal B cell activation with diverse patterns of autoantibody production resulting from an interplay of genetic factors, environmental triggers, and hormonal influences. Although the etiology of LE is still poorly understood, much has been learned about the pathogenetic mechanisms leading to disease, its various clinical patterns, and prognosis. LE can affect one or more vital internal organs (systemic LE, SLE) and the skin (cutaneous LE), producing considerable morbidity and mortality depending on the severity of the cutaneous manifestations and systemic involvement, respectively. LE-specific skin lesions (as defined by the specific histopathologic features of LE) occur in the form of acute cutaneous LE (ACLE), SCLE, and DLE. While ACLE occurs in active SLE and is more often seen by the rheumatologist, SCLE and DLE are predominantly managed by the dermatologist alone. DLE occurs most frequently as an isolated clinical finding, whereas approximately half of the patients with SCLE meet the American College of Rheumatology's criteria for SLE. However, they generally have a more benign form of systemic disease, with only 15% major organ involvement [8].

The therapeutic regimen chosen for the treatment of a patient with LE depends on the type and extent of skin lesions and whether or not there is life-threatening systemic disease. Initially, attention in therapeutic studies has centered on the severe forms of SLE, and the results of such studies were extrapolated to all forms of SLE, thereby unnecessarily submitting patients with more benign forms of LE to aggressive and potentially toxic treatment [9]. Because of the heterogeneous nature of LE, its tendency to spontaneous remissions and exacerbations, and the multitude of possible internal organ involvement, a cornerstone of therapy entails a thorough diagnostic evaluation of the patient and reassessment over time. Where there is underlying systemic disease (SLE), effective communication among physicians of the various medical specialities involved is mandatory for proper management of the patient.

ACLE lesions in the context of active SLE usually respond to the systemic immunosuppressive therapy that is required to control the underlying SLE disease, but antimalarial drugs (hydroxychloroquine, chloroquine) are also frequently used with success to treat both lesions of the skin and musculoskeletal complaints [10]. Sunscreens and topical corticosteroids are cornerstones of therapy in cutaneous LE. In addition, antimalarial drugs are the first line of systemic therapy in patients with SCLE or DLE. Dapsone and the synthetic retinoids are second-line agents with particular effectivity in the treatment of bullous SLE [11] and hypertrophic DLE [12], respectively. Both systemic corticosteroids (0.5–1.5 mg oral prednisone/kg per day) and cytotoxic drugs (azathioprine, methotrexate, cyclophosphamide) are third-line agents reserved for patients with severe disease or disease unresponsive to the less toxic forms of therapy. Particularly azathioprine (1–2 mg/kg per day) has been reported to be of benefit in patients with refractory cutaneous disease [13] and in the treatment of more benign forms of SLE where exposure to the potential toxicities of more aggressive therapy is not justified [9]. The use of cyclophosphamide should be limited to patients with organ-threatening disease who fail to respond to corticosteroids. The superiority of parenteral cyclophosphamide (monthly for at least 6 months in doses of 0.75–1.0 g/m^2)

plus steroids over steroids alone has been documented in well-designed controlled trials only for lupus nephritis, but not for any other manifestation of SLE [9]. Evolving therapies that still have an experimental character in the management of both SLE and cutaneous LE include recombinant interferon (INF)-α_{2a} [14, 15] and the recent use of anti-CD4 monoclonal antibodies [16, 17] (see below).

Scleroderma

Scleroderma denotes the process of thickening, induration, and decrease of elasticity of the skin due to an excessive dermal deposition of collagen and other extracellular matrix proteins. Two main forms of scleroderma are recognized: (1) localized scleroderma (morphea) and (2) systemic sclerosis. While the former refers to a sclerotic process that is limited to the skin, the latter is characterized by distinct features of cutaneous and internal organ involvement. Despite comprehensive definitions based on the clinical expression of the disease, the etiology of scleroderma is still unknown, and studies on its pathogenesis have only very recently shown progress. Genetic susceptibility, immune mechanisms, vascular damage, and a deranged collagen metabolism all appear to play a role. Moreover, scleroderma is the systemic autoimmune disease most frequently associated with chemicals (polyvinyl chloride, silica, organic solvents, vapor of epoxy resins, contaminated Spanish rapseed oil, L-tryptophan) as etiologic agents [18]. The greatest attention has been given to immune phenomena, such as T cell activation and the production of highly specific autoantibodies, including anticentromere, anti-DNA-topoisomerase I (Scl-70), and anti-fibrillarin (Scl-34) antibodies. The histopathologic finding of perivascular dermal inflammatory infiltrates, predominantly T-helper cells with monocytes and macrophages, in the early phase of scleroderma suggests a major role of these cells in disease induction. Elevation of both interleukin (IL)-2 and soluble IL-2 receptor levels as markers of T cell activation were found to be associated with disease activity [19,20]. T-helper lymphocyte activation results in secretion of cytokines which stimulate both fibroblasts and B cells. Polyclonal B cell activation leads to increased production of multiple autoantibodies. In addition, vascular changes may be due to an immunologic injury and occur early, preceding the development of sclerosis [21]. Endothelial damage leads to platelet adhesion and aggregation with consecutive release of mediators such as platelet-derived growth factor (PDGF) [22] and transforming growth factor (TGF)-β [23], which modulate fibroblast activity.

While numerous substances have been used in the therapy of scleroderma, none have been proven to be effective in curing the disease. Current management of patients with scleroderma is mainly symptomatic, supportive, and aimed at preventing or treating complications arising both from skin and internal organ involvement. With respect to the pathogenetic pathways leading to sclerosis, therapeutic agents are grouped into (a) drugs with anti-inflammatory/immunosuppressive activity, (b) vasoactive agents, and (c) substances that influence the connective tissue metabolism [24]. Ideally, one should interfere early in the events leading to sclerosis: To this end, early diagnosis is required, before sclerosis has become established. In general, active immunosuppression shortly after the onset of any immune-mediated process is most effective. After the disease has become established, with substantial loss of function or scarring of affected organs, or parts thereof, the ability to intervene becomes progressively less effective [25].

Immunosuppressive treatment is recommmended in those patients with systemic sclerosis showing active inflammatory disease (clinically and/or histologically) and in those patients with accompanying myositis, arthritis, serositis, or interstitial lung disease. Therapy with oral prednisone, initially at a dosage of 100 mg/day, gradually tapered over 4 weeks to a minimal maintenance dose, has been proposed in patients who clinically demonstrate progression of disease [26]. In patients with serious inflammatory organ involvement, cyclophosphamide (2 mg/kg per day) is added [26]. A good symptomatic response is often noted to such a therapy, but there is no proven evidence that sclerosis of skin and internal organs and hence also prognosis of the disease are positively influenced. As a result of this problem, the physician must choose between attempting organ-saving therapy and exposing the patient to a toxic regimen with limited hope of benefit. More recently, cyclosporine has been used in the treatment of both systemic sclerosis [24] and localized cutaneous sclerosis [28]. Nephropathy remains a major concern in its use for the treatment of systemic sclerosis [28], while cyclosporine use seems justified in the therapy of disabling pansclerotic morphea [29].

Vasoactive therapy primarily involves the use of calcium channel blockers (nifedipine) in the treatment of Raynaud's phenomenon and of angiotensin-converting enzyme inhibitors (enalapril) in the prevention and treatment of renal crises and malignant hypertension.

The sclerotic stage of disease remains the least amenable to therapy. Major problems in studying drug efficacy in the treatment of cutaneous sclerosis are that there are only few objective criteria for studying disease activity and that the optimal time to study the therapeutic effect is limited. An agent that may be effective early in disease cannot be expected to be beneficial in the sclerotic end stage of disease. Moreover, sclerosis, as measured by skin scores, increases during the first few years of disease, reaches a peak, and then gradually declines as the affected skin becomes atrophic with time. The most popular among the agents that affect collagen production has probably been D-penicillamine. While this agent was shown to reduce cutaneous involvement and ameliorate pulmonary function in two retrospective studies [30, 31], a more recent, prospective study failed to demonstrate effectivity of D-penicillamine in arresting disease progression [32]. D-penicillamine also was shown to cause considerable side effects in up to 47% of patients treated in this way, necessitating interruption of therapy in 29% [33]. Taking into account the fact that hydroxylation of prolyl residues is essential for the biosynthesis of collagen, a rational approach to inhibit this process would be to inhibit this enzymatically (prolylhydroxylase) catalyzed step. Several drugs have been recognized to exert this effect (e.g., diphenylhydantoin, penicillin) [34], and others have been developed in vitro for this purpose [35, 36]. Further progress may result in improved agents with less toxicity that specifically inhibit collagen production in vivo. Interestingly, penicillin, traditionally used in Europe in the treatment of scleroderma, has a structure similar to prolylhydroxylase inhibitors. Therapy with repeated intravenous penicillin G infusions (10 million IU/day for 14–21 days) appears to have some beneficial effect, especially when administered in early phases of scleroderma, but there have been no clinical studies proving its efficacy. With respect to antibiotic therapy of scleroderma, the role of *Borrelia* infection in the pathogenesis of localized cutaneous sclerosis is questionable, inasmuch as high-titer antibodies to *B. burgdorferi* in patients with morphea can be demonstrated only in geographic areas with a high prevalence of

Borrelia infection, while no relationship between morphea and *Borrelia* infection is found in countries where the prevalence of *Borrelia* infection is low [37].

The anatomical colocalization of inflammatory cells and activated fibroblasts in the early stages of scleroderma or of TGF-β with alpha1(I) procollagen mRNA in tissue sections of patients with systemic sclerosis [38] indicates the impact of cytokines and growth factors released from the inflammatory cells on the activation of fibroblasts: TGF-β was shown to increase collagen gene expression up to ten times, acting via the nuclear factor-1 site in the promoter region [39]. Hopefully, combination of our understanding of disease-specific patterns of gene expression with knowledge of the structural interactions between nuclear transcription factors and their target sequences will provide the means to design agents that specifically target the limited subset of genes aberrantly expressed in disease [40]. With the awareness of the downregulating activitiy of INF-γ on collagen biosynthesis [41], the effect of recombinant INF-γ in the treatment of systemic sclerosis has been studied in an open trial. At the end of a 12-month treatment period, significant improvement of both the cutaneous abnormalities and pulmonary function was noted [42]. Further studies should address the question of whether a specific antifibrotic effect resulting in clinical benefit is feasible through selective inhibition of collagen gene expression.

Dermatomyositis

DM is one of the least common of the rheumatic diseases. Untreated muscle disease can produce severe and long-term disabilities, and the active cutaneous lesions of DM can cause considerable discomfort from intractable pruritus. In approximately 10% of patients, the cutaneous manifestations of DM are present for many years in the absence of clinical and enzymatic evidence of muscle disease (amyopathic DM) [43]. In childhood DM, a higher frequency of systemic vascular lesions and subcutaneous calcification can cause great morbidity and mortality, while adult DM may be the first indication of an occult malignancy (paraneoplastic DM) [44]. Thus individual patient management depends on the severity of the skin and muscle disease, the presence or absence of multisystem involvement, and the presence or absence of underlying malignancy.

Treatment of DM remains predominantly empiric. Systemic corticosteroids are the first-line therapy in most patients, resulting in an improved lifestyle and prognosis in more than 50% of cases. The earlier the therapy with corticosteroids is begun after disease onset, the better the overall prognosis [45]. Prednisone (0.5–1.5 mg/kg per day) is usually given orally until there is significant improvement of muscle strength testing, normalization of muscle enzyme levels, and improvement of cutaneous lesions. This usually requires up to 2 months of full-dose therapy. Once patients improve, the corticosteroid dose is tapered by 10% every 2 weeks. In unresponsive, acutely ill patients, especially in the management of juvenile DM, intravenous pulse therapy with methylprednisone (1 g/day for 3–5 consecutive days) has been advocated [46]. If there is no response to high-dose oral corticosteroid therapy after 2 months (in approximately 25% of patients) or if the patient is intolerant to corticosteroids, other immunosuppressive agents are started. Various uncontrolled studies have used methotrexate (10–50 mg/week) [47], azathioprine (1–2 mg/kg per day) [48], cyclophosphamide (1–2 mg/kg per day) [48], and, more recently, cyclosporine (5 mg/kg per day) [49].

In some patients, the condition resists all therapies and the patient remains physically disabled. In these patients, high-dose intravenous γ-globulin therapy has been used with success [50, 51], including a double-blind, placebo-controlled study [50]: eight out of 12 patients (including the crossovers) who received γ-globulin in this study also experienced marked improvement of the cutaneous lesions of DM. In contrast to polymyositis, where activated $CD8^+$ cytotoxic T cells directed against hitherto unidentified muscle-specific autoantigens are believed to be responsible for the muscle injury [52], in DM a humoral-based mechanism of intramuscular microangiopathy with perivascular $CD4^+$ T cells and B cells and microvascular deposits of immunoglobulin and complement has been suggested to be pathogenetic [53]. In spite of these distinct characteristics, however, DM has traditionally not been treated separately, but as a part of the inflammatory myopathy group. Recent work has now suggested that the administration of γ-globulin to patients with active DM can arrest the ongoing complement-dependent immune damage to the muscle by intercepting the assembly and deposition of the C5b-C9 membranolytic attack complex on the endomysial capillaries through the formation and inactivation of C3b-containing complexes [54, 55], offering a rational basis for this mode of therapy. Moreover, intravenous γ-globulin therapy offers a safe and effective treatment of DM with infrequent and mild side effects. Nevertheless, the high cost of immunoglobulin may affect its long-term use as a maintenance therapy.

Polyarteritis Nodosa

The syndromes of PAN include (a) classic PAN, (b) microscopic polyangiitis, and (c) benign cutaneous PAN [56, 57]. Differences in the cutaneous presentations between these subsets are a consequence of different sizes of involved vessels, with classic PAN and benign cutaneous PAN primarily involving medium-sized and small arteries, while microscopic polyangiitis comprises small vessels with or without involvement of medium-sized arteries. Benign cutaneous PAN is distinguished by the lack of severe systemic manifestations. Whether or not it represents a distinct vasculitic syndrome is less important than the awareness that patients with benign cutaneous PAN generally do not require aggressive therapy [58]. The association of the PAN syndromes with a variety of underlying conditions must be taken into consideration. Systemic PAN has been associated with drug abuse [59], human immunodeficiency virus (HIV) infection [60], parvovirus B19 infection [61], and hairy cell leukemia [62]. Benign cutaneous PAN has been associated with inflammatory bowel disease [63, 64]. Both systemic and cutaneous PAN have been associated with chronic hepatitis B antigenemia [65, 66] and, especially in the pediatric patient group, are known to occur after β-streptococcal upper respiratory infection [67].

Untreated systemic PAN has an extremely poor prognosis, with a 5-year survival rate of scarcely over 10% [68]. The introduction of corticosteroid therapy has significantly improved the prognosis, and favorable therapeutic results have been reported with the combination of prednisone (1 mg/kg per day) with cyclophosphamide (2 mg/kg per day). Overall, the 5-year survival rate reported in five large series from 1967 to 1995 was between 55% and 63% [69]. The course of benign cutaneous PAN is typically chronic and with a good prognosis. Therapy should be tailored to the needs of the patient for control of symptoms and should not be aggressive [58]. Therapeutic agents that have been proposed include nonsteroidal anti-inflammatory agents, pentoxifylline [70], corticosteroids alone (at an initial dosage of between 20 and 60 mg oral prednisone per day, depending on the severity of symptoms [71]), and low-dose methotrexate (7.5–15 mg weekly) [72]. In PAN syndromes associated with identifiable underlying conditions, more specific therapies should be aimed at, such as INF-α and plasma exchange in hepatitis B-associated PAN [73], intravenous immunoglobulin in PAN-like vasculitis associated with chronic parvovirus B19 infection [61], INF-α in hairy cell leukemia-associated PAN [74], and sulfasalazine therapy in benign cutaneous PAN associated with inflammatory bowel disease [63].

Perspectives: Strategies for a More Selective Intervention in Autoimmune Diseases

The emphasis of current research is directed at the regulation of dysfunctional immune responses. Immunosuppressives, cytokine antagonists, and antibodies against lymphocyte subgroups or against cytokines and their receptors are part of the repertoire. More attractive alternatives are strategic therapy modalities which intervene early in the pathological process, such as the modulation of antigen presentation or the induction of tolerance against autoantigens.

From Increased Cellular Selectivity to Increased Antigen Specificity

Present immunosuppressive therapy restrains the whole immune system for the deviation of a limited number of lymphocytes. The ideal immunosuppressive agent would be one that selectively checks immunopathological lymphocytes while sparing others (cellular selectivity). With the immune system continuously inactivating self-reactive lymphocytes in order to maintain self-tolerance, it should be possible to "tune in" to this process and reprogram the immune system toward restitution of self-tolerance.

In autoimmune disease, a prime therapeutic focus is the peripheral T cell pool containing activated autoreactive T cells. Support for this view is provided by histologic evidence of activated T cells at the sites of pathology and the requirement for (dysregulated) T cell help in the activation of B cells [75]. While it is difficult to target antigen-specific T cells, it appears at least feasible to target freshly activated T cells. Such T cells selectively express high-affinity IL-2 receptors offering targets for chimeric IL-2 toxin conjugates (immunotoxins) [76]. Anti-CD4 monoclonal antibodies are particularly interesting, since most of them show efficacy in the range of limited direct toxicity. In the model of collagen-induced arthritis in DBA/1 mice [77] and in the spontaneous LE syndrome seen in the (NZBxNZW) F1 mouse [78, 79], disease progression was blocked through the use of anti-CD4 monoclonal antibodies. In human disease, monoclonal antibody therapy has been used in rheumatoid arthritis [80, 81], psoriasis [82, 83], SLE [16], and most recently in the treatment of severe cutaneous LE [17]. However, CD4 antibody treatment may induce a dose-related long-term $CD4^+$ lymphopenia. An alternative is to exploit the T cell antigen encounter with antigen by letting that encounter become a tolerogenic one. This idea is based on studies in mice in which anti-CD4 antibodies were used to elicit tolerance to antigen by the administration of both anti-CD4 antibodies and antigen within a limited time window [84]. The induction of tolerance did not depend on $CD4^+$ T cell depletion. Treatment with nondepleting monoclonal anti-CD4 in the presence of antigen induces a state of anergy in the T cell

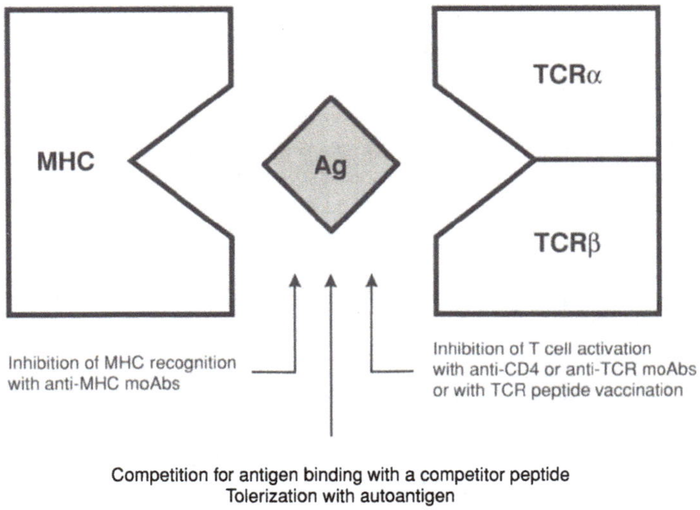

Fig. 1. Trimolecular complex of the major histocompatibility complex (*MHC*), antigenic peptide (*Ag*), and T cell receptor (*TCR*), each representing a separate target for immunointervention: (1) inhibition of MHC recognition by the use of monoclonal antibodies (*moAbs*) directed against the MHC gene product or antagonists competing for antigen binding into the peptide groove; (2) tolerization by the use of the autoantigen itself; (3) inhibition of T cell activation with monoclonal antibodies to CD4 or to the TCR itself, or through TCR peptide vaccination. (Adapted from [86])

population, which can be sustained by repeated exposure to antigen, which, in the case of autoimmune disease, might be adequately provided by natural presentation of autoantigen [85].

Ideally, one would like to intervene specifically in the pathogenic autoimmune reaction responsible for the disease onset or its maintenance (antigen specificity). Assuming that autoimmune diseases are probably generated much in analogy to the normal immune response, investigators have focused their attention on the inductive trimolecular complex consisting of the MHC, antigenic peptide, and T cell receptor (TCR) (Fig. 1). In this complex, the TCR encounters the inducing antigen in association with MHC gene products on the surface of the professional antigen-presenting cell (APC). This trimolecular complex offers attractive sites for potential intervention in blocking further events ultimately resulting in autoimmune disease [86]:

- *MHC antagonist peptides.* Peptides bound to MHC molecules on the surface of APC are the ligand for specific TCR. A given individual expresses a limited number of MHC molecules. To ensure that T cell response can be generated against any antigen, these must therefore bind a large variety of different peptides. One consequence of the low specificity of peptide-MHC interactions is that peptides of different sequences might compete for antigen presentation by a given MHC molecule to T lymphocytes. A striking characteristic of human autoimmune diseases is the increased frequency of certain HLA class II alleles (and to a lesser extent of HLA class I alleles) in affected individuals. Therefore, modulation of T cell activation by antagonizing the binding of antigenic peptides to MHC molecules is able to prevent the induction of experimental autoimmune disease, and this could lead to a new generation of immunosuppressive agents [87].

- *TCR-based immunotherapy (TCR vaccination).* Before having direct access to the autoantigen, it is possible to act at the TCR level on determinants that are related to antigen specifity. The rationale for using synthetic peptides corresponding to germline TCR sequences (TCR peptides) in experimental autoimmune disease evolved from two key findings: (1) It is possible to vaccinate against induced autoimmune diseases using attenuated pathogenic T cell clones, and (2) certain TCR V region genes, including Vβ fragments, are overutilized by pathogenic T cells responsive to autoantigen [88]. Vβ-orientated therapy has been used successfully in experimental allergic encephalomyelitis both with anti-Vβ monoclonal antibodies and anti-Vβ peptide sensitization [89].
- *Oral tolerization.* The oral administration of soluble antigen has long been recognized as a method of inducing antigen-specific peripheral tolerance and has recently been used for the modulation of autoimmune diseases such as experimental allergic encephalomyelitis and rheumatoid arthritis [90, 91]. One of the primary mechanisms of active cellular suppression is via the secretion of suppressive cytokines, such as TGF-β, IL-4, and IL-10 after antigen-specific triggering. In this sense, the gut-associated lymphoid tissue is unique, as it favors the induction of T-helper-2 (Th2) cells (as opposed to Th1 cells) that secrete these cytokines. These clones are structurally identical to Th1 disease-inducing clones in TCR usage, MHC restriction, and epitope recognition, but suppress rather than induce disease [92].

Immunointervention Through Costimulatory Pathway Blockade

The two-signal model of T lymphocyte triggering describes T cell receptor occupancy by the MHC-peptide complex as the first signal for T cell activation [93], while the second, costimulatory signal provided by the APC is critical in determining whether recognition of antigen by T cells leads to T cell activation or (clonal) anergy. Several receptor-ligand pairs can provide costimulatory signals resulting in lymphokine production, T cell proliferation, and development of T cell effector functions [94]. The interaction of B7 molecules on APC with CD28 antigens on T cells prevents the induction of anergy. It has also been proposed that autoreactive cells might even be activated by encountering tissues that aberrantly express such costimulatory molecules [95, 96]. Both in vitro and in vivo studies using antagonists directed against costimulatory molecules have inspired great interest in the manipulation of costimulatory pathways for therapeutic purposes [97–99]. Specifically, methods regulating these pathways may provide new strategies for controlling autoimmune diseases.

Intervention in the Cytokine Cascade of the Inflammatory Response

In a normal immune response, $CD4^+$ T lymphocytes differentiate into effector populations that produce restricted sets of cytokines and perform specific functions [100]. These populations are polarized into Th1 lymphocytes, which play a major role in delayed-type hypersensitivity responses by secreting IL-2 and IFN-γ, and Th2 lymphocytes, which are involved in antibody-mediated responses by secreting IL-4, IL-5, and IL-10. Autoimmune diseases can be similarly subdivided into those mediated by Th1-

type cells with primarily inflammatory manifestations and those mediated by Th2-type cells whose manifestations are secondary to autoantibody-containing immune complexes. As the Th1 and Th2 subpopulations interact and cross-regulate each other [101], one approach to the immunotherapy of certain inflammatory autoimmune disease might involve the antigen-specific modulation of an immune response from one dominated by excessive activity of Th1-like T cells to one dominated by the protective cytokines produced by Th2-like T cells (cytokine-induced immune modulation) [102].

Even though cytokines critically enhance immune responses, a possible central cytokine in a given autoimmune disease has not been identified. If it were to be found, it would offer the possibility of interfering locally with its production or interfering with its activity. Soluble cytokine receptors provide a natural source of highly selective cytokine inhibitors. The association of an IgG heavy chain to cytokine receptors in the form of chimeric molecules has been an effective approach in the stable expression of these soluble receptor molecules, which are otherwise small enough to be efficiently excreted by renal filtration and therefore short-lived in circulation [103, 104]. It has been demonstrated that fusion proteins in which the soluble part of the tumor necrosis factor (TNF) receptor is linked to a IgG heavy chain constant region can protect against the effect of excessive TNF production in vivo [105]. In addition, injection of a soluble IFN-γ receptor-Ig construct was shown to delay appearance of autoantibodies to double-stranded DNA, onset of kidney damage, and mortality in (NZB/NZW) F1 mice that otherwise spontaneously develop a fatal SLE-like syndrome [106].

With respect to cytokine antagonism, endogenous production of cytokine inhibitors would seem more convenient than intermittent administration of purified recombinant protein. Recently, replication-incompetent adenoviral vectors encoding chimeric TNF receptor-Ig constructs were engineered. Animals transduced with inhibitor virus produced large quantities of inhibitor protein in vivo [107, 108]. Expression of the adenovirally transmitted 55-kDa TNF receptor-Ig construct protected mice against endotoxic shock [109]. The concept of virally mediated gene transfer of cytokine inhibitors may ultimately find application in a form of gene therapy. Originally conceived as a strategy to treat hereditary disease, it is now recognized that gene therapy generally represents a powerful approach to deliver any therapeutic protein for local and/or systemic use [110].

Summary

At present, treatment of systemic autoimmune diseases is essentially confined to immunosuppressive agents. These include systemic corticosteroids and the cytotoxic drugs azathioprine, cyclophosphamide, and methotrexate. These are effective in controlling the course of these chronic inflammatory diseases. However, the occurrence of relapses after the treatment is stopped and the risks of toxicity and long-term over-immunosuppression have prompted the search for more selective strategies of intervention. Major efforts are directed towards therapies with increased cellular selectivity or antigen specificity. Cyclosporine, intravenous immunoglobulin, and monoclonal antibodies (anti-CD4) currently constitute the main clinical orientation. At the experimental level, strategies are directed towards peptide therapy (MHC antagonism, TCR vaccination) and tolerance induction to the autoantigen (oral tolerization). Alternatively, manipulation of costimulatory pathways (anti-gp39, CTLA4Ig) and intervention in the cytokine cascade of the inflammatory response by means of cytokine-induced immune modulation or cytokine inhibition (soluble cytokine receptor-Ig fusion proteins) are strategies with a therapeutic potential. As for the limited forms of cutaneous autoimmune disease, it is important to recognize these distinct subsets with their typically favorable prognosis in which less aggressive therapeutic modalities can be used.

References

1. Merriman TR, Todd JA (1995) Genetics and autoimmune disease. Curr Opin Immunol 7:786–792
2. Trüeb RM (1995) Autoimmune-disease-associated MHC class-II molecules. Hautarzt 46: 225–227
3. Fujinami RS, Oldstone MBA (1985) Amino acid homology and virus: mechanisms for autoimmunity. Science 230:1043
4. Friedman SM, Tumang JR, Crow MK (1993) Microbial superantigens as etiopathogenic agents in autoimmunity. Rheum Dis Clin North Am 19:207–222
5. Miller JFAP, Flavell RA (1994) T-cell tolerance and autoimmunity in transgenic models of central and peripheral tolerance. Curr Opin Immunol 6:892–899
6. Fairley JA (1990) Intracellular targets of cyclosporine. J Am Acad Dermatol 23:1329–1334
7. Valdimarsson H (1990) Immunity during cyclosporine therapy. J Am Acad Dermatol 23: 1294–1300
8. David KM, Thornton JC, Davis B et al (1984) Morbidity and mortality in patients with subacute cutaneous lupus erythematosus. J Invest Dermatol 82:408
9. Urowitz MB (1993) Is aggressive therapy necessary for systemic lupus erythematosus? Rheum Dis Clin North Am 19:263–270
10. The Canadia Hydroxychloroquine Study Group (1991) A randomized study of the effect of withdrawing hydroxychloroquine sulfate in systemic lupus erythematosus. N Engl J Med 324:150–154
11. Ruzicka T, Goerz G (1991) Dapsone in the treatment of lupus erythematosus. Br J Dermatol 104:53–56
12. Green SG, Piette WW (1987) Successful treatment of hypertrophic lupus erythematosus with isotretinoin. J Am Acad Dermatol 17:364–368
13. Callen JP, Spencer LV, Burruss et al (1991) Azathioprine: an effective, corticosteroid-sparing therapy for patients with recalcitrant cutaneous lupus erythematosus or with recalcitrant cutaneous leukocytoclastic vasculitis. Arch Dermatol 127:515–522
14. Nicholas JF, Thivolet J, Kanitakis J et al (1990) Response of discoid and subacute cutaneous lupus erythematosus to recombinant interferon alpha 2A. J Invest Dermatol 95 [Suppl]: 142S–145S
15. Martinez J, de Misa RF, Torrelo A et al (1992) Low-dose intralesional interferon alpha for discoid lupus erythematosus. J Am Acad Dermtol 26:494–496
16. Hiepe F, Volk HD, Apostoloff E et al (1991) Treatment of severe systemic lupus erythematosus with anti-CD4 monoclonal antibody. Lancet 338:1529–1530
17. Prinz JG, Meurer M, Reiter C et al (1996) Treatment of severe cutaneous lupus erythematosus with a chimeric CD4 monoclonal antibody, cM-T412. J Am Acad Dermatol 34:244–252
18. Silman AJ (1991) Epidemiology of scleroderma. Ann Rheum Dis 50:846–853
19. Fiocco U, Rosada M, Cozzi L et al (1993) Early phenotypic activation of circulating helper memory T cells in scleroderma: correlation with disease activity. Ann Rheum Dis 52:272–277
20. Zillikens D, Blum C, Dummer R et al (1992) Serum levels of soluble interleukin-2 receptor in systemic and circumscribed scleroderma. Dermatology 184:233–234
21. Tuffanelli DL (1989) Systemic scleroderma. Med Clin North Am 73:1167–1180
22. Pandolfi A, Florita M, Altomare G (1989) Increased plasma levels of platelet-derived growth factor activity in patients with progressive systemic sclerosis. Proc Soc Exp Biol Med 191:1–4
23. Border WA, Ruoslahti E (1992) Transforming growth factor beta in disease: the dark side of tissue repair. J Clin Invest 90:1–7

24. Krieg T, Meurer M (1988) Systemic scleroderma. Clinical and pathophysiologic aspects. J Am Acad Dermatol 18:457–481
25. Steinberg AD, Krieg AM, Takashi T, Gourley MF (1992) Timing of immunosuppression in the natural history of autoimmune disease. J Autoimmunity 5 [Suppl A]:197–203
26. Sollberg S, Hunzelmann N, Roux M, Krieg T (1994) Therapy of systemic sclerosis. Z Haut Geschlechtskr 69:6–14
27. Clements PJ, Lachenbruch PA, Sterz M et al (1994) Cyclosporine in systemic sclerosis. Results of a forty-eight-week open safety study in ten patients. Arthritis Rheum 37:30–32
28. Worle B, Hein R, Krieg T, Meurer M (1990) Cyclosporin in localized and systemic scleroderma – a clinical study. Dermatology 181:215–220
29. Peter RU, Ruzicka T (1991) Low-dose cyclosporin A in the treatment of disabling morphea. Arch Dermatol 127:1420–1421
30. Steen VD, Owens GR, Redmont G et al (1985) The effect of D-penicillamine on pulmonary findings in systemic sclerosis. Arthritis Rheum 28:882–888
31. DeClerk LS, Dequeker J, Francx L, Demedts M (1987) D-penicillamine therapy and interstitial lung disease in scleroderma: a long-term follow-up study. Arthritis Rheum 30:643–650
32. Wollheim F, Akesson A (1989) Treatment of systemic sclerosis in 1988. Semin Arthritis Rheum 18:181–188
33. Steen VD, Blair S, Medsger TA (1986) The toxicity of D-penicillamine in systemic sclerosis. Ann Intern Med 104:699–705
34. Asboe-Hansen G (1982) Treatment of generalized scleroderma with inhibitors of collagen synthesis. Int J Dermatol 21:159–161
35. Uitto J, Ryhaenen L, Tan EML (1985) Increased procollagen production by scleroderma fibroblasts in culture and its inhibition by the analogues of proline. In: Black CM, Myers AR (eds) Current topics in rheumatology: systemic sclerosis (scleroderma). Gower, London, pp 204–207
36. Krieg T, Horlein D, Wiestner M (1978) Aminoterminal extension peptides from type I procollagen normalize excessive collagen synthesis of scleroderma fibroblasts. Arch Dermatol Res 263:171–180
37. Bagot M, Revuz J (1990) Jessner-Kanof lesion and Borrelia infection. J Am Acad Dermatol 23:772–773
38. Kulozik M, Hogg A, Lankat-Buttgereit B, Krieg T (1990) Co-localization of transforming growth factor β2 with alpha1(I) procollagen mRNA in tissue sections of patients with systemic sclerosis. J Clin Invest 86:917–922
39. Rossi P, Karsenty G, Roberts AB et al (1988) A nuclear factor 1 binding site mediates the transcriptional activation of type I collagen promoter by transforming growth factor-beta. Cell 52:405–414
40. McKay IA, Winyard P, Leigh IM et al (1994) Nuclear transcription factors: potential targets for new modes of intervention in skin disease. Br J Dermatol 131:591–597
41. Jimenez SA, Freundlich B, Rosenbloom J (1984) Selective inhibition of human diploid fibroblast collagen synthesis by interferons. J Clin Invest 74:1112–1116
42. Hein R, Behr J, Hündgen M et al (1992) Treatment of systemic sclerosis with g-interferon. Br J Dermatol 126:496–501
43. Euwer RL, Sontheimer RD (1993) Amyopathic dermatomyositis: a review. J Invest Dermatol 100 [Suppl]:124S–127S
44. Sigurgeirsson B, Lindelof B, Edhag O et al (1992) Risk of cancer in patients with dermatomyositis or polymyositis: a population based study. N Engl J Med 326:363–367
45. Fafalak RG, Peterson MG, Kagen LJ (1994) Strength in polymyositis and dermatomyositis: best outcome in patients treated early. J Rheumatol 21:643–648
46. Malleson PN (1990) Controversies in juvenile dermatomyositis. J Rheumatol [Suppl] 23:1–6
47. Zieglschmid-Adams ME, Pandya AG, Cohen SB, Sontheimer RD (1995) Treatment of dermatomyositis with methotrexate: presentation of ten cases and review of the literature. J Am Acad Dermatol 32:754–757
48. Bohan A, Peter JB, Bowman RL, Pearson CM (1977) Computer-assisted analysis of 153 patients with polymyositis and dermatomyositis. Medecine 56:255–286

49. Grau JM, Herrero C, Casademont J et al (1994) Cyclosporine A as first choice therapy for dermatomyositis. J Rheumatol 21:381–382
50. Cherin P, Herson S, Wechsler B et al (1991) Efficacy of intravenous gammaglobulin therapy in chronic refractory polymyositis and dermatomyositis:an open study with 20 adult patients. Am J Med 91:162–168
51. Dalakas MC, Illa I, Dambrosia JM et al (1993) A controlled trial of high-dose intravenous immune globulin infusions as treatment for dermatomyositis. N Engl J Med 329:1993–2000
52. Engel AG, Arahata K (1984) Monoclonal antibody analysis of mononuclear cells in myopathies. II. Phenotypes of autoinvasive cells in polymyositis and inclusion body myositis. Ann Neurol 16:209–215
53. Emslie-Smith AM, Engel AG (1990) Microvascular changes in early and advanced dermatomyositis: a quantitative study. Ann Neurol 27:343–356
54. Basta M, Dalakas MC (1994) High-dose intravenous immunoglobulin exerts its beneficial effect in patients with dermatomyositis by blocking endomysial deposition of activated complement fragments. J Clin Invest 94:1729–1735
55. Lutz HU, Stammler P, Jelezarova E et al (1996) High doses of immunoglobulin G attenuate immune aggregate-mediated complement activation by enhancing physiologic cleavage of C3b in C3bn-IgG complexes. Blood 88:184–193
56. Braverman IM (1981) The angiitides. Skin signs of systemic disease, 2nd edn. Saunders, Philadelphia, pp 378–452
57. Jennette JC, Falk RJ, Andrassy K et al (1994) Nomenclature of systemic vasculitides. Proposal of an International Consus Conference. Arthritis Rheum 37:187–192
58. Moreland LW, Ball GV (1990) Cutaneous polyarteriitis nodosa. Am J Med 88:426–430
59. Citron BP, Halpern M, McCarron M et al (1970) Necrotizing angiitis associated with drug abuse. N Engl J Med 283:1003–1011
60. Calabrese LH (1991) Vasculitis and infection with the human immunodeficiency virus. Rheum Dis Clin North Am 17:131–147
61. Finkel TH, Toeroek TJ, Ferguson PJ et al (1994) Chronic parvovirus B19 infection and systemic necrotising vasculitis: opportunistic infection or aetiological agent? Lancet 343:1255–1258
62. Komadina KH, Houk RW (1989) Polyarteritis nodosa presenting as recurrent pneumonia following splenectomy for hairy-cell leukemia. Semin Arthritis Rheum 18:252–257
63. Gudbjsrnsson B, HSllgren R (1990) Cutaneous polyarteritis nodosa associated with Crohn's disease. Report and review of the literature. J Rheumatol 17:386–390
64. Chiu G, Rajapakse CNA (1991) Cutaneous polyarteritis nodosa and ulcerative colitis. J Rheumatol 18:769–770
65. Trepo CG, Zuckerman AJ, Bird RC, Prince AM (1974) The role of circulating hepatitis B antigen/antibody immune complexes in the pathogenesis of vascular and hepatic manifestations in polyarteritis nodosa. J Clin Pathol 27:863–868
66. Van de Pette JEW, Jarvis JM, Wilton MA, MacDonald DM (1984) Cutaneous periarteritis nodosa. Hepatitis B surface antigen-containing immune-complexes and polymorphonuclear-leukocyte lysosomal enzyme release. Arch Dermatol 120:109–111
67. Sheth AP, Olson JC, Esterly NB (1994) Cutaneous polyarteritis nodosa of childhood. J Am Acad Dermatol 31:561–566
68. Leib ES, Restivo C, Paulus HE (1979) Immunosuppressive and corticosteroid therapy of polyarteritis nodosa. Am J Med 67:941–947
69. Fortin PR, Larson MG, Watters AK et al (1995) Prognostic factors in systemic necrotizing vasculitis of the polyarteritis nodosa group – a review of 45 cases. J Rheumatol 22:78–84
70. Calderon MJ, Landa N, Aguirre A, Diaz-Perez JL (1993) Successful treatment of cutaneous PAN with pentoxifylline. Br J Dermatol 128:706–708
71. Chen K (1989) Cutaneous polyarteritis nodosa: a clinical and histopathological study of 20 cases. J Dermatol 16:429–442
72. Jorizzo L, White WL, Wise CM et al (1991) Low-dose weekly methotrexate for unusual neutrophilic vascular reactions: cutaneous polyarteritis nodosa and Behet's disease. J Am Acad Dermatol 24:973–978

73. Guillevin L, Lhote F, Sauvaget F et al (1994) Treatment of polyarteritis nodosa related to hepatitis B virus with interferon-alpha and plasma exchanges. Ann Rheum Dis 53:334–337
74. Carpenter MT, West SG (1994) Polyarteritis nodosa in hairy cell leukemia: treatment with interferon-alpha. J Rheumatol 21:1150–1152
75. Gleichmann E, van Elven EH, van der Veen JP (1982) A systemic lupus erythematosus (SLE)-like disease in mice induced by abnormal T-B cell cooperation. Preferential formation of autoantibodies characteristic for SLE. Eur J Immunol 12:152–159
76. Strom TB, Anderson PL, Rubin-Kelley VE et al (1990) Immunotoxins and cytokine fusion proteins. Semin Immunol 2:467–479
77. Ranges GE, Sriram S, Cooper SM (1985) Prevention of type III collagen-induced arthritis by in vivo treatment with anti-L3T4. J Exp Med 162:1105–1110
78. Wofsy D, Seaman WE (1985) Successful treatment of autoimmunity in NZB/NZW F1 mice with monoclonal antibody to L3T4. J Exp Med 161:378–391
79. Wofsy D, Seaman WE (1987) Reversal of advanced murine lupus in NZB/NZW F1 mice by treatment with monoclonal antibody to L3T4. J Immunol 138:3247–3251
80. Burmester GR, Emmrich F (1993) Anti-CD4 therapy in rheumatoid arthritis. Clin Exp Rheumatol 11 [Suppl 9]:5139–5145
81. Van der Lubbe PA, Reiter C, Breedveld FC et al (1993) Chimeric CD4 monoclonal antibody cM-T412 as a therapeutic approach to rheumatoid arthritis. Arthritis Rheum 36:1375–1379
82. Prinz JC, Meurer M, Dadonna P et al (1991) Chimeric CD4 monoclonal antibody in treatment of generalized pustular psoriasis. Lancet 338:320–321
83. Thivolet J, Nicolas JF (1994) Immunointervention in psoriasis with anti-CD4 antibodies. Int J Dermatol 33:327–332
84. Benjamin RJ, Waldmann H (1986) Induction of tolerance by monoclonal antibody therapy. Nature 320:449–451
85. Waldmann H, Qin S, Cobbold S (1992) Monoclonal antibodies as agents to reinduce tolerance in autoimmunity. J Autoimmun 5 [Suppl A]:93–102
86. Fathman CG (1992) Immunotherapy of rheumatic diseases based on understanding genetic predisposition to the development of these diseases. Rheum Dis Clin North Am 18:915–926
87. Aichele P, Kyburz D, Ohashi P et al (1994) Peptide-induced T cell tolerance to prevent autoimmune diabetes in a transgenic mouse model. Proc Natl Acad Sci USA 91:444–448
88. Vandenbark AA, Chou YK, Bourdette DN et al (1992) T cell receptor peptide therapy for autoimmune disease. J Autoimmun 5 [Suppl A]:83–92
89. Kumar V, Sercarz EE (1993) The involvement of T cell receptor for peptide-specific regulatory CD4+ T cells in recovery from antigen-induced autoimmune disease. J Exp Med 178:909–916
90. Trentham DE, Dynesisus-Trentham RA, Orav EJ et al (1993) Effects of oral administration of type II collagen on rheumatoid arthritis. Science 261:1727–1730
91. Weiner HL, Friedman A, Miller A et al (1994) Oral tolerance: immunologic mechanisms of treatment of animal and human organ-specific autoimmune diseases by oral admninistration of autoantigens. Annu Rev Immunol 12:809–837
92. Chen Y, Kuchroo VK, Inobe J et al (1994) Regulatory T cell clones induced by oral tolerance: suppression of autoimmune encephalomyelitis. Science 265:1237–1240
93. Mueller DL, Jenkins MK, Schwartz RH (1989) Clonal expansion versus functional clonal inactivation: a costimulatory signalling pathway determines the outcome of T-cell antigen receptor occupancy. Annu Rev Immunol 7:445–480
94. Clark EA, Ledbetter JA (1994) How B and T cells talk to each other. Nature 367:425–428
95. Harlan DM, Hengartner H, Huang ML et al (1990) Mice expressing both B7 and viral glycoprotein on pancreatic beta cells along glycoprotein-specific transgenic T cells develop diabetes due to a breakdown of T-lymphocyte unresponsiveness. Proc Nat Acad Sci USA 248:1349–1356
96. Guerder S, Meyerhoff J, Flavell R (1994) The role of the T cell costimulator B7-1 in autoimmunity and the induction and maintenance of tolerance to peripheral antigen. Immunity 1: 155–166
97. Boussiotis VA, Gribben JG, Freeman GJ et al (1994) Blockade of the CD28 costimulatory pathway: a means to induce tolerance. Curr Opin Immunol 6:797–807

98. Durie FH, Fava RA, Foy RM et al (1993) Prevention of collagen-induced arthritis with an antibody to gp39, the ligand for CD40. Science 261:1328–1330
99. Finck BK, Linsley PS, Wofsy D (1994) Treatment of murine lupus with CTLA4Ig. Science 265:1225–1227
100. Mosmann TR, Coffman RL (1989) THl and TH2 cells: different patterns of lymphokine secretion lead to different functional properties. Annu Rev Immunol 7:145–173
101. Powrie F, Correa-Oliveira R, Mauze S et al (1994) Regulatory interactions between DC45RBhigh and CD45RBlow $CD4^+$ T cells are important for the balance between protective and pathogenic cell-mediated immunity. J Exp Med 179:589–600
102. Racke MK, Bonomo A, Scott DE et al (1994) Cytokine-induced immune deviation as a therapy for inflammatory autoimmune disease. J Exp Med 180:1961–1966
103. Capon DJ, Chamow SM, Mordenti J et al (1989) Designing CD4 immunoadhesins for AIDS therapy. Nature 337:525–531
104. Traunecker A, Schneider J, Kiefer H et al (1989) Highly efficient neutralization of HIV with recombinant CD4-immunoglobulin molecules. Nature 339:68–70
105. Van Zee KJ, Kohno T, Fischer E et al (1992) Tumor necrosis factor soluble receptors circulate during experimental and clinical inflammation and can protect against excessive tumor necrosis factor a in vitro and in vivo. Proc Natl Acad Sci USA 89:4845–4849
106. Ozmen L, Roman D, Fountoulakis M et al (1995) Experimental therapy of systemic lupus erythematosus: the treatment of NZB/W mice with mouse soluble interferon-gamma receptor inhibits the onset of glomerulonephritis. Eur J Immunol 25:6–12
107. Kolls J, Peppel K, Silva M et al (1994) Prolonged and effective blockade of tumor necrosis factor activity through adenovirus-mediated gene transfer. Proc Natl Acad Sci USA 91:215–219
108. Trüeb RM, Brown G, van Huffel C et al (1995) Expression of an adenovirally encoded LT-β inhibitor prevents clearance of Listeria monocytogenes in mice. J Inflamm 45:239–247
109. Kolls JK, Lei D, Nelson D et al (1995) Adenovirus-mediated blockade of tumor necrosis factor in mice protects against endotoxic shock yet impairs pulmonary host defense. J Infect Dis 171:570–575
110. Setoguchi Y, Jaffe HA, Danel C et al (1994) Ex vivo and in vivo gene transfer to the skin using replication-deficient recombinant adenovirus vectors. J Invest Dermatol 102:415–421

Atopic Dermatitis

U. Reinhold

Introduction

Atopic dermatitis (AD) is a chronic inflammatory skin disease frequently associated with bronchial asthma and/or allergic rhinitis in the patient or a member of the immediate family. The etiopathogenesis of the inflammatory skin lesions is largely unknown. Clinical observations and recent research results, however, point to a dysfunction in the cellular immunoregulation [11]. AD patients are more susceptible to bacterial, viral, and mycotic skin infections. From a clinical point of view, this indicates a localized defect in the immune system. Patients with certain primary immune defects (such as Wiskott-Aldrich syndrome, ataxia teleangiectasia, hyper-IgE syndrome, or X-chromosomal hypogammaglobulinemia) may show eczematous skin lesions that cannot be distinguished from those of AD. These diseases and AD have further been observed to show a characteristic rise in the level of serum IgE. In addition to increased IgE synthesis, multiple abnormalities, including decreased number of circulating $CD8^+$ T cells and $CD16^+$ natural killer (NK) cells, impaired autologous mixed lymphocyte reactions, and depressed granulocyte and monocyte chemotaxis, have been described in AD patients. AD is characterized by strongly elevated IgE levels compared to other atopic diseases, and a proportion of this IgE is specific for antigens, which may act as exacerbating factors in the disease. Antigen-induced exacerbations may be mediated by either antigen presentation by Langerhans cells to T cells or cutaneous mast cell mediator release. This assumption is further supported by the finding that patients with AD may show eczematous patch-test reactions to aeroallergens. The results indicate that IgE-mediated contact hypersensitivity to aeroallergens may play an important role in the pathogenesis of AD. These pathogenic conceptions are closely associated with elevated IgE synthesis. According to recent research, the regulation of the IgE response is mediated by cell–cell interactions and by specific mediators secreted by regulatory T cells. On the basis of experimental in vitro findings, it was shown that IgE synthesis is especially regulated by certain cytokines, including interleukin (IL)-4 and interferon (IFN)-γ; IL-4 promotes and IFN-γ inhibits its production. Mosmann and Coffman [13] demonstrated that murine T-helper cells are composed of at least two nonoverlapping subsets that can be distinguished on the basis of their patterns of cytokine secretion. One subset (Th1) produces IL-2 and IFN-γ, whereas the other T cell subset (Th2) secrets IL-4 and IL-5, but does not secrete IL-2 and IFN-γ. In humans, the majority of normal T-helper cell clones exhibit a mixed pattern of cytokine secretion, but Th2-like T cells have been described and seem to a play a significant role in the pathogenesis of AD. Based on these results, modulation of the immune system has been considered as one of the most attractive approaches for therapy of AD patients.

Therapeutic Approaches

Glucocorticosteroids

Topical glucocorticosteroids are one of the mainstays in the treatment of inflammatory skin lesions of AD. The longest remissions and the best control of the disease are obtained by use of gradually decreasing concentrations of topical corticosteroids. The period of treatment depends on the severity and the extent of the skin disease. Application of topical corticosteroids should be stopped before the typical local side effects, e.g., skin atrophy, appear. Systemic corticosteroid therapy is also very effective in suppressing skin inflammation and itching; however, its use is limited to a subgroup of severe, intractable AD patients [30]. This is related to the possibility of serious adverse effects, including hypothalamic-pituitary-adrenal axis suppresion, glucose intolerance, osteoporosis, cataracts, and infectious diseases. Systemic administration of glucocorticoids causes striking effects on the immune system, including inhibitory effects on T cell proliferation and cytokine secretion, impairment of antigen-processing activity of dendritic cells, and inhibitory effects on eosinophils and mediator release of mast cells. However, relatively little is known about the specific mechanism by which systemic corticosteroids influence the impaired immune system in AD. One of the major problems with systemic glucocorticoid therapy in AD is the prolonged nature of the disease, which increases the probability that the continued use of the drug will be required once therapy has started. The possibility of early transfer to alternate-day regimens has received widespread support, since it has been demonstrated that a number of harmful side effects can be avoided using alternate-day steroids. However, cataract formation, growth retardation, and osteoporosis are not prevented by the alternate-day regimen. Other therapeutic regimens such as single, high-dose IV application of methylprednisolone (20 mg/kg per day for 3 days) may represent a novel and safe therapeutic approach in severe AD [4].

Cyclosporin A

Cyclosporin A (CsA) is a potent immunosuppressive agent that selectively affects T-helper cells without suppressing the bone marrow, an effect which is commonly seen with other immunosuppressive drugs. CsA has become the drug of choice to prevent organ rejection, including kidney, liver, and heart transplants. Furthermore, CsA has been proven to be of considerable therapeutic benefit in the treament of certain dermatologic diseases. It is highly efficacious in psoriasis and may be of benefit in treating bullous dermatoses, collagen vascular disorders, and neutrophilic dermatoses. A number of open and placebo-controlled studies [25, 32] have showed that CsA is also of therapeutic benefit in AD. The mechanism of CsA-mediated improvement in AD is unclear, but does not seem to be related to the improvement of classical atopy-related parameters such as elevated IgE levels and immediate and late-phase cutaneous responses to environmental antigens, including house dust mite antigen. Recent results suggest that CsA acts primarily by inhibiting interactions among antigens, antigen-presenting cells, and T cells present in inflammatory skin lesions. Furthermore, improvement of AD by CsA therapy has been shown to be associated with increased IFN-γ production [29] and downregulation of IL-5 production, indicating that T cell-eosinophilic inflammation plays a central role in the pathogenesis of chronic skin inflammation [9].

Short-term treatment with CsA at 5 mg/kg per day has been found to be highly effective in most cases of severe AD, and tachyphylaxis has not been observed. However, after stopping CsA therapy, the disease relapsed in the majority of patients. Therefore, long-term treatment is necessary to maintain clinical improvement. CsA therapy appears to be associated with minimal adverse side effects and toxicity provided that CsA whole blood levels and clinical parameters are monitored regularly and the appropriate laboratory examinations performed. Monitoring should include serum creatinine, urea, bilirubin, liver enzymes, potassium, uric acid, and blood pressure estimations. In addition, direct glomerular filtration rate measurement should be carried out during long-term treatment. Furthermore, patients should be monitored for skin infections and cutaneous malignancy following overexposure to solar radiation. Present data indicate that the dose of CsA required to control inflammatory skin lesions in AD is lower than that required to achieve remission and that the therapeutic index can be further improved by alternative dosing strategies. Intermittent maintenance therapy with 5 mg/kg every fifth day showed better results compared to a continuous dose of 1 mg/kg [5]. Long-term, low-dose CsA treatment may induce permanent remission in selected patients [27]. Although the efficacy of CsA in AD has been shown in double-blind, placebo-controlled studies, the drug is not licensed for this indication in any country. Nephrotoxicity will prevent CsA from becoming a first-line treatment for AD, and the drug should only be given to adult patients with severe, therapy-resistant forms of the disease. For these patients, however, CsA may greatly improve the qualitiy of life, and the therapeutic risks need to be weighed carefully against those of other available treatments such as long-term systemic corticosteroids and high-dose ultraviolet A (UVA) therapy.

Interferons

A constant finding in 60–80% of AD patients is their defective regulation of IgE synthesis. Serum IgE levels are strongly elevated compared to other atopic diseases. Several studies showed that lesional skin of AD patients contains a major T cell subset exhibiting Th2-like activities. Skin-infiltrating T cells were shown to be particularly responsive to IL-4 and to secrete large amounts of IL-4, IL-5, and IL-10, but very little IFN-γ [21]. IL-4 is a potent inducer of IgE production, IL-5 induces eosinophilia , and IL-10 depresses delayed-type hypersensitivity reactions. Thus there is evidence to suggest that an abnormal cytokine secretion pattern of T cells may account for enhanced levels of IgE and eosinophils observed in these patients. As a consequence, IgE has been detected on the surface of Langerhans cells and dendritic cells in AD lesions, which appears to result from binding of circulating IgE on high-affinity IgE receptors expressed on antigen-presenting cells. The present data indicate that the passive binding of antigen-specific IgE on Langerhans cells may play a significant role in the pathogenesis of contact hypersensitivity to aeroallergens observed in AD patients.

The apparent implication of an overproduction of IL-4 and other Th2-related cytokines in the pathogenesis of AD led to search for novel treatment strategies by altering the balance bewteen Th1 and Th2 activities. These approaches include in vivo application of cytokines such as IFN, which have been shown to exert significant Th2-antagonistic effects in vitro and in vivo.

Interferon-α

Interferon-α has been shown to inhibit IL-4-induced IgE production by normal B cells as well as spontaneous IgE production of peripheral blood mononuclear cells (PBMC) from AD patients in vitro [18]. Results from in vivo application of IFN-α in patients with hyper-IgE syndrome revealed objective reduction of eczematous skin lesions as well as reduction of elevated serum IgE levels [31]. Eight patients with severe AD were treated with IFN-α α_{2b}, given by subcutaneous injection three times a week over a period of 6–14 weeks. Results reported showed no changes in eczema or IgE levels, although IFN-α_{2b} treatment significantly decreased blood eosinophils [17]. Another study showed a moderate improvement in four out of eight AD patients after application of IFN-α_{2b} for a period of 4 weeks. Only one out of eight patients showed a clinical improvement after 2 months. In contrast, Torrelo et al. [35] observed markedly clinical improvement after 4 weeks of IFN-α_{2a} treatment (3.0×10^6 IU three times a week) in five out of 13 AD patients. Consistent with the findings of other investigators, no change in serum IgE levels during and after IFN-α therapy was observed. However, a signifcant reduction in IgE receptor-mediated basophil histamine release was noted in AD patients treated with IFN-α_{2a} for 21 days [15].

Interferon-γ

In vitro experiments carried out by our group showed that mononuclear cells of patients with a severe form of AD secreted IFN-γ at a reduced rate after mitogenic stimulation [19, 20]. Reduced in vitro IFN-γ secretion was negatively correlated with serum IgE and IgG_4 concentrations. These results have been confirmed by a large group of other investigators. Furthermore, there is evidence that reduced IFN-γ secretion in AD may be related to a post-transcriptional defect [24, 34]. PBMC isolated from AD patients were shown to be unable to generate normal IL-12-induced IFN-γ responses, which may be due to the excess production of IL-4 and IL-10 detectable in these patients. In addition, acute and chronic AD skin lesions had significantly greater number of cells that were positive for IL-4 and IL-5 mRNA, but not for IFN-γ mRNA, as compared to normal skin and uninvolved skin of AD patients [6, 21]. Since IFN-γ acts as a suppressive factor for IL-4-mediated IgE response, it seems possible that reduced IFN-γ secretion may account for enhanced levels of IgE observed in AD patients. Furthermore, defective secretion of IFN-γ is likely to have several other consequences in terms of immunologic regulation. Immunologic abnormalities in AD include a low NK activity, low or absent expression of HLA class II antigens on keratinocytes, and reduced antiviral activity. The apparent preferential expression of Th2 over Th1 cells in AD has formed a rational basis for the in vivo application of IFN-γ in these patients.

IFN-γ has been used successfully in the therapy of a number of conditions associated with immune abnormalities, including chronic granulomatous disease, Job syndrome, and lepromatous leprosy. Treatment of a child with Omenn's syndrome associated with congenital immunodeficiency and abnormal expression of Th2-like T cells downregulated in vivo expression of IL-5 and IL-10, abrogated hypereosinophilia, and resulted in a significant clinical improvement [26].

In vivo application of IFN-γ in AD was first described by Boguniewicz et al. [1]. Fourteen patients with chronic severe AD were treated daily with subcutaneous IFN-γ at three successive dose levels (10 μg/m^2, 50 μg/m^2, and 100 μg/m^2) for 5 days, with 2 days off between each dose level. Decreases of clinical severity were observed at all three different dose levels after 3 weeks of therapy. However, worsening of skin inflammation and pruritus occurred shortly after cessation of treatment. Another group of eight patients received 50 μg/m^2 IFN-γ daily for 6 weeks. Daily treatment with 50 μg/m^2 over a period of 6 weeks resulted in a significant clincial improvement, with patients remaining stable after maintenance therapy with 50 μg/m^2 IFN-γ three times per week. Immunomonitoring during this trial revealed no reduction of elevated IgE serum levels, whereas spontaneous IgE production in vitro was inhibited in patients receiving IFN-γ therapy. Furthermore, enhanced IL-4 production and IL-4 receptor expression by PBMC from AD patients was downregulated after IFN-γ application in vivo [23]. The efficacy of IFN-γ in patients with severe refractory AD was further documented in uncontrolled studies [14] and in a double-blind, placebo-controlled trial. Eighty-three patients were randomized to receive IFN-γ or placebo at a dosage of 50 μg/m^2 daily for 12 weeks. The percentage of patients showing more than 50 % improvement in the physician's overall response evaluations was significantly greater in the IFN-γ-treated group than in the placebo group. The mean eosinophil count was significantly reduced, whereas a nonsignificant increase in serum IgE levels occurred in the active treatment group.

We treated 14 patients with severe AD with IFN-γ for a period of 6 weeks. Subcutaneous injections of IFN-γ were given on 5 days for the first week of treatment, followed by three injections per week for another 3 weeks, followed by two injections for the last 2 weeks [22]. Eight patients (57 %) showed marked clinical improvement during systemic IFN-γ therapy. Four of these patients showed continuous improvement 3 months after treatment was discontinued. No major adverse effects during or after therapy were observed. The earliest changes, in most patients apparent within the first week of treatment, were alleviation of itching. We were not able to find a statistically significant reduction in total serum and antigen-specific serum IgE levels during and after IFN-γ treatment. However, in agreement with other investigators, we found significantly reduced spontaneous IgE production in vitro after 6 weeks of therapy. Furthermore, we observed a signifcant elevation in IgG_2 serum levels during IFN-γ therapy. In conclusion, preliminary results have clearly shown that IFN-γ therapy results in reduced clinical severity of chronic refractory AD. Although the mechanisms of its action in AD is not well understood, the encouraging therapeutic results suggest the need for further controlled clinical trials.

Thymic Hormones

Thymopoetin is a polypeptide hormone of the thymus, originally purified from bovine thymus extract by its effect on neuromuscular transmission. It is secreted by thymic epithelial cells and has been shown to influence both the differentiation of thymocytes and the function of mature T cells. A synthetic pentapeptide corresponding to the amino acids 32–36 (Arg-Lys-Asp-Val-Tyr) carries the full hormone activity of thymopoietin despite its extremely short half-life of only 30 s. Immunoregulatory in vitro effects of thymopentin include enhanced T cell proliferation in response to alloantigens and mitogens and induction and increase of mitogen-induced IFN-γ secretion.

There are several reports indicating that thymopentin application may have immunomodulatory effects in vivo. Clinical and immunological improvement by thymopentin therapy was approved in primary immunodeficiencies such as DiGeorge syndrome, pluriorificial pyoderma vegetans, chronic mucocutaneous candidosis, and hyperimmunoglobuin E syndrome. Furthermore, several open studies [10] and two double-blind, placebo-controlled clincial trials have demonstrated favorable results of thymopentin therapy in AD patients. One hundred AD patients were randomized to receive either thymopentin (50 mg) or placebo, administered as daily subcutaneous injections for 6 weeks [12]. However, patients were permitted to use topical steroids during the study. A significant reduction from baseline in the total severity score was observed throughout the study for both the placebo-treated and the thymopentin group, respectively. Thymopentin-treated patients demonstrated progressive improvement exceeding the placebo effect, and the reduction in their total severity scores was statistically significant compared to the reduction in the placebo-treated group at week 6. No significant differences between the two groups in the duration of topical corticosteroids were observed. Another randomized, placebo-controlled study evaluating the efficacy of thymopentin in AD patients showed a significantly greater improvement in thymopentin-treated patients compared to those receiving placebo [33]. Thymopentin (50 mg) or placebo were given three times weekly for 12 weeks. As in other studies, patients were permitted to use topical corticosteroids and antihistamines during the study. The authors report that the severity index, based 70% on the total severity score and 30% on the cutaneous surface involved, decreased significantly in the thymopentin-treated group compared with the placebo-treated group. However, there was no statistically significant difference in the total severity score between the two groups.

The current results indicate that thymopentin therapy is relatively safe in AD patients. Confirmation of therapeutic results in further studies, including optimal dose and frequency, is necessary to validate these observations. The mechanism of action is unclear, but there is evidence that thymopentin may increase production of IFN-γ and may decrease production of IL-4, plasma histamine, histamine-releasing factor, and respiratory burst activities of polymorphonuclear leukocytes [8].

Phosphodiesterase Inhibitors

There is substantial evidence to suggest that atopic diseases are associated with increased leukocyte cyclic adenosine monophosphate (cAMP)-phosphodiesterase (PDE) activity [7]. Functional consequences of increased PDE activity and subsequent increased degradation of cAMP in AD patients may include elevated prostaglandine E_2 (PGE_2) production by AD monocytes. It has been hypothesized that increased PGE_2 production in AD monocytes is strongly related to the abnormal Th2-like cytokine response observed in these patients. PGE_2 increases IL-4 production by atopic T cells, whereas IFN-γ production is decreased in the presence of this agent in vitro. Furthermore, low IFN-γ secretion by PBMC from AD patients in vitro can be increased by the removal of monocytes or addition of the PGE_2 synthesis inhibitor indomethacin [2,16]. On the other hand, IFN-γ is able to inhibit PDE activity by itself, which has been suggested as a possible mechanism of clincial improvement in IFN-γ-treated AD patients in vivo [28]. The development of new cAMP-specific PDE inhibitors has opened up a new therapeutic strategy for the treatment of AD patients. Ro20-1724, a specific

PDE IV inhibitor, has been shown to significantly downregulate elevated IL-4 and IL-5 secretion [3] and IgE production in PBMC derived from AD patients. Preliminary clinical results suggest that new high-potency PDE inhibitors may also be active on inflammatory skin lesions in AD patients via topical administration.

Summary

There is substantial evidence to support defective immunoregulatory mechanisms in the pathogenesis of AD. It has been well documented that T cells from AD patients produce increased amounts of IL-4, IL-5, and IL-10 and have a decreased capacity to produce IFN-γ, indicating a preferential expression of Th2-related cytokines. Chronic skin inflammation has been shown to improve significantly with short-term immunosuppressive therapy, including corticosteroids and CsA. The excellent response to CsA treatment may justify long-term, low-dose CsA treatment in severe forms of AD, which may result in long-term or permanent remission of inflammatory skin lesions. Clincial studies suggest that several new immunomodulatory drugs, including IFN and thymus hormones, may also be beneficial in treating AD patients. The potential therapeutic role of these agents should be further evaluated.

References

1. Boguniewicz M, Jaffe HS, Izu A, Sullivan MJ, York D, Geha RS, Leung DYM (1990) Recombinant gamma interferon in treatment of patients with atopic dermatitis and elevated IgE levels. Am J Med 88:365–369
2. Byron KA, Liberatos S, Varigos GA, Wootton AM (1992) Interferon-gamma production in atopic dermatitis: a role for prostaglandins? Int Arch Allergy Immunol 99:50–55
3. Crocker IC, Townley RG, Khan MM (1996) Phosphodiesterase inhibitors suppress proliferation of peripheral blood mononuclear cells and interleukin-4 and -5 secretion by human T-helper type 2 cells. Immunopharmacology 31:223–235
4. Galli E, Chini L, Moschese V, Paone F, Fraioli G, Rossi P (1994) Methylprednisolone bolus: a novel therapy for severe atopic dermatitis. Acta Paediatr 83:315–317
5. Granlund H, Erkko P, Sinisalo M, Reitamo S (1995) Cyclosporin in atopic dermatitis: time to relapse and effect of intermittent therapy. Br J Dermatol 132:106–112
6. Hamid Q, Boguniewicz M, Leung DYM (1994) Differential in situ cytokine gene expression in acute versus chronic atopic dermatitis. J Clin Invest 94:870–876
7. Hanifin JM, Chan SC (1995) Monocyte phosphodiesterase abnormalities and dysregulation of lymphocyte function in atopic dermatitis. J Invest Dermatol 105:84S–88S
8. Hsieh KH, Shaio MF, Liao TN (1992) Thymopentin treatment in severe atopic dermatitis-clinical and immunological evaluations. Arch Dis Child 67:1095–1102
9. Ishii E, Yamamoto S, Hamasaki Y, Miyazaki S (1996) Production of interleukin-5 and the suppressive effect of cyclosporin A in childhood severe atopic dermatitis. J Pediatr 128: 152–155
10. Jullien D, Nicolas JF, Frappaz A, Thivolet J (1993) Alpha interferon treatment in atopic dermatitis. Acat Derm Venereol (Stockh) 73:130–132
11. Leung DYM, Geha RS (1986) Immunoregulatory abnormalities in atopic dermatitis. Clin Rev Allergy 4:67–86
12. Leung DYM, Hirsch RL, Schneider L, Moody C, Takaoka R, Li SH, Meyerson LA, Mariam SG, Goldstein G, Hanifin JM (1990) Thymopentin therapy reduces the clinical severity of atopic dermatitis. J Allergy Clin Immunol 85:927–933
13. Mosmann TR, Coffman RL (1987) Two types of mouse helper T-cells clone. Immunol Today 8:223–227

14. Musial J, Milewski M, Undas A, Kopinski P, Duplaga M, Szczeklik A (1995) Interferon-gamma in the treatment of atopic dermatitis: influence on T-cell activation. Allergy 50:520–523
15. Nielsen BW, Reimert CM, Hammer R, Schiotz K, Thestrup-Pedersen K (1994) Interferon therapy for atopic dermatitis reduces basophil histamine release, but does not reduce serum IgE or eosinophilic proteins. Allergy 49:120–128
16. Ostlere LS, Mallett RB, Kaminski A, Kaminski ER, Pereira RS, Holden CA (1995) Gamma-interferon production in atopic dermatitis shows differential modification by phosphodiesterase and prostaglandin inhibition. Br J Dermatol 133:1–5
17. Paukkonen K, Fraki J, Horsmanheimo M (1993) Interferon-alpha treatment decreases the number of blood eosinophils in patients with severe atopic dermatitis. Acat Derm Venereol (Stockh) 73:141–142
18. Pene J, Rousset F, Briere F, Chretien I, Paliard X, Banchereau J, Spits H, de Vries JE (1988) IgE production by normal human lymphocytes is induced by interleukin-4 and suppressed by interferons g and a and prostaglandin E2. Proc Natl Acad Sci USA 85:6880–6884
19. Reinhold U, Pawelec G, Wehrmann W, Herold M, Wernet P, Kreysel HW (1988) Immunoglobulin E and immunoglobulin G subclass distribution in vivo and relationship to in vitro generation of interferon-gamma and neopterin in patients with severe atopic dermatitis. Int Arch Allergy Appl Immunol 87:120–126
20. Reinhold U, Wehrmann W, Kukel S, Kreysel HW (1990) Evidence that defective interferon-gamma production in atopic dermatitis is due to intrinsic abnormalities. Clin Exp Immunol 79:374–379
21. Reinhold U, Kukel S, Goeden B, Neumann U, Kreysel HW (1991) Functional characterization of skin-infiltrating lymphocytes in atopic dermatitis. Clin Exp Immunol 86:444–448
22. Reinhold U, Kukel S, Brzoska J, Kreysel HW (1993) Systemic interferon gamma treatment in severe atopic dermatitis. J Am Acad Dermatol 29:58–63
23. Renz H, Jujo K, Bradley KL, Domenico J, Gelfand EW, Leung DYM (1992) Enhanced IL-4 production and IL-4 receptor expression in atopic dermatitis and their modulation by interferon-gamma. J Invest Dermatol 99:403–408
24. Rinas U, Horneff G, Wahn V (1993) Interferon-gamma production by cord-blood mononuclear cells is reduced in newborns with a family history of atopic disease and is independent from cord blood IgE-levels. Pediatr Allergy Immunol 4:60–64
25. Salek MS, Finlay AY, Luscombe DK, Allen BR, Berth-Jones J, Camp RDR, Graham-Brown RAC, Khan GK, Marks R, Motley RJ, Ross JS, Sowden JM (1993) Cyclosporin greatly improves the quality of life of adults with severe atopic dermatitis. A randomized, double-blind, placebo-controlled trial. Br J Dermatol 129:422–430
26. Schandené L, Ferster A, Mascart-Lemone F, Crusiaux A, Gérard C, Marchant A, Lybin M, Velu T, Sariban E, Goldman M (1993) T helper type 2-like cells and therapeutic effects of interferon-g in combined immunodeficiency with hypereosinophilia (Omenn's syndrome) Eur J Immunol 23:56–60
27. Sepp N, Fritsch PO (1993) Can cyclosporin A induce permanent remission of atopic dermatitis? Br J Dermatol 128:213–216
28. Shi-hua L, Chan SC, Kramer SM, Hanifin JM (1993) Modulation of leukocyte cyclic AMP phosphodiesterase activity by recombinant interferon-γ: evidence for a differential effect on atopic monocytes. J Interferon Res 13:197–202
29. Shiohara T, Sagawa Y, Nagashima M (1994) An unexpected increase in circulating IFN-γ by cyclosporin A in atopic patients: a discrepancy between in vitro and in vivo events. Acta Derm Venereol (Stockh) 74:20–21
30. Sonenthal KR, Grammer LC, Patterson R (1993) Do some patients with atopic dermatitis require long-term oral steroid therapy? J Allergy Clin Immunol 91:971–973
31. Souillet G, Rousset F, de Vries JE (1989) Alpha-interferon treatment of patients with hyper IgE syndrome. Lancet 17:1384
32. Sowden JM, Berth-Jones J, Ross J, Motley RJ, Marks R, Finlay AY, Salek MS, Graham-Brown RAC, Allen BR, Camp RDR (1991) Double-blind, controlled, crossover study of cyclosporin in adults with severe refractory atopic dermatitis. Lancet 338:137–140

33. Stiller MJ, Shupack JL, Kenny C, Jondreau L, Cohen DE, Soter NA (1994) A double-blind, placebo-controlled clinical trial to evaluate the safety and efficacy of thymopentin as an adjunctive treatment in atopic dermatitis. J Am Acad Dermatol 30:597–602
34. Tang ML, Varigos G, Kemp AS (1994) Reduced interferon-gamma (IFN-gamma) secretion with increased IFN-gamma mRNA expression in atopic dermatitis: evidence for a post-transcriptional defect. Clin Exp Immunol 97:483–490
35. Torrelo A, Harto A, Sendagorta E, Czarnetzki BM, Ledo A (1992) Interferon-α therapy in atopic dermatitis. Acata Derm Venerol (Stockh) 72:370–372

Psoriasis – Mediation of Skin Phenotype by Circulatory Pathogenic T Lymphocytes

B.J. Nickoloff

Introduction

Psoriasis is one of the most common skin diseases present throughout the worldwide population affecting about 2 % of individuals [1]. It has several different clinical appearances, but the most common phenotype consists of symmetrically distributed, persistent erythematous scaling plaques. Within these cutaneous lesions, there is infiltration of inflammatory cells, prominent keratinocyte hyperplasia with altered differentiation, neovascularization of the dermis, and activation of immunocompetent cells–T cells and dendritic antigen-presenting cells [2]. One of the most difficult problems for investigators studying this disease is to be able to determine with certainty which cellular and molecular events are of primary importance and which changes are secondary. The confederacy of cell types participating in this disorder, together with the panoply of cytokines and the rapidity of evolution and disappearance of skin lesions, has confounded even the most astute clinicians and bench researchers for the past century. Perhaps the greatest obstacle has been the lack of an appropriate and relevant animal model that recapitulates all of the important and characteristic cutaneous changes present in human psoriatic plaques.

Psoriasis is a disease in which the signs and symptoms are predominantly confined to the skin, although joints may be affected [3]. Because of its immediate accessibility and the obvious detection of lesions by the naked eye, most research activity has centered on the skin, with less regard for potential contributing factors present at nonskin sites such as the peripheral lymph nodes, systemic circulation, or bone marrow. The literature contains thousands of reports characterizing innumerable changes in the skin, beginning with the stratum corneum, moving down though all the layers of the epidermis, and into the dermis and subcutaneous tissues. Rather than reviewing the psoriasis literature from the perspective of the keratinocyte [2], this chapter will highlight the pathogenic role of immunocompetent cells such as T lymphocytes and dendritic antigen-presenting cells (collectively referred to as immunocytes).

Overview of Literature

One of the first issues to tackle when dealing with recruited cells that enter lesional skin sites from the blood is to distinguish inflammatory reactions from immunological activation. While these processes have some overlapping features, this chapter will deal primarily with the mechanistic aspects that lead to a specific immune response, and not with nonspecific inflammatory components of psoriatic plaques [4]. The key distinguishing feature of an immune response is the activation of a specific clone or group of

T cells that have responded to either a conventional (nominal) antigen or to a superantigen and that have bound to the surface of an antigen-presenting cell. In the skin, there are both nonprofessional (i.e., keratinocytes)and professional antigen-presenting cells (i.e., epidermal and dermal dendritic cells) that can mediate the activation of T cells [5–9]. Over the past two decades, considerable circumstantial evidence has accumulated implicating the immune system in the pathogenesis of psoriasis. From an epidemiological perspective, a role for the immune system in psoriasis first emerged with the recognition that there is an increased frequency of certain HLA alleles that have also been observed in other diseases linked to autoimmune reactions [10–12]. Next came the clinical observation that relatively low doses of methotrexate given systemically could induce remission of psoriatic skin lesions [13]. While the early interpretation of the mechanism of action for methotrexate highlighted its potential antimitotic activity on the proliferating psoriatic keratinocytes, more recent views indicate that this drug has previously unrecognized, potent immunomodulatory activity.

The serendipitous observation that the immunosuppressive agent cyclosporin A could not only prevent renal allograft rejection, but also improve psoriasis [14] provided further support for a cell-mediated immunological basis for psoriasis. Juxtaposed to these pharmacologically based human clinical observations highlighting immunocytes in psoriasis, other investigators were grafting skin onto nude mice, but concluded that there was an intrinsic defect in the skin and that psoriasis could be produced independent of circulating cellular and/or humoral factors [15–17]. We will return to the use of animal models at the end of this chapter, but suffice it to note at this point that the pendulum thus began to swing between the recruited T cell from the circulation and the indigenous epidermal keratinocytes as the key cellular determinant of the psoriasis phenotype. It has been the recent utilization of more sophisticated immunological techniques, additional pharmacological clinical trials, and new animal model-based experimental protocols that have caused the pendulum currently to swing in favor of a primary role for T lymphocytes in psoriasis.

Using various staining protocols, the initial psoriatic lesions examined reveal early infiltration of the skin by dendritic cells and T lymphocytes [18–20]. Follow-up studies revealed more definitive evidence for a role of specific T cell subsets in causing psoriasis [21, 22]. Investigators in the early 1990s began using molecular analysis of the T cell receptor (TCR) rearrangement to determine whether characteristic T cell activation pathways and collections of nonrandom subsets of lymphocytes were present at sites of presumptive immunologically mediated tissue reactions [23]. When investigative skin biologists began probing normal and psoriatic skin, several interesting results were observed. We designate healthy skin from a normal volunteer with no evidence of any skin disease or family history of psoriasis as NN skin; symptom-free or lesion-free skin from a patient with psoriasis elsewhere or with a family history of psoriasis is designated as PN skin; and untreated psoriatic plaque-derived skin is referred to as PP skin. Within normal human skin, T cells expressing certain Vβ genes was documented [24]. In various forms of psoriasis, including guttate and plaque-stage disease, nonrandom patterns of Vβ gene expression have also been observed by several groups [25–29]. As can be seen in Table 1, different laboratories have detected various T cell subsets in both normal and diseased skin specimens. Moreover, there are also differences in the type of T cell subset found between guttate and plaque-stage disease. Of particular interest is

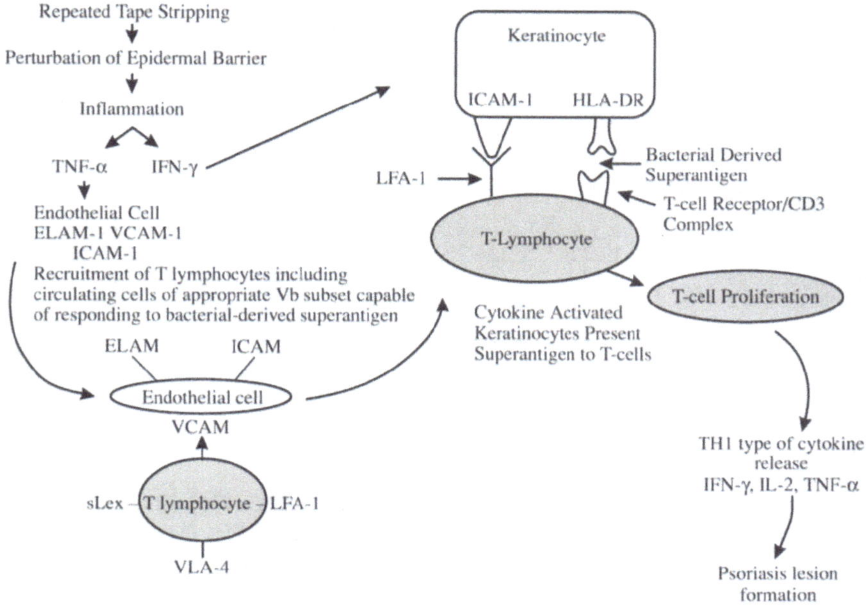

Fig. 1. Overview of proposed pathophysiological basis for psoriasis highlighting the role of T cells. In this scenario, inflammatory-induced changes in the skin induce endothelial cell leukocyte adhesion molecule (*ELAM*) expression, facilitating binding of T cells – positive for sialyl Lewis antigen, sLex), lymphocyte function-associated antigen (*LFA*)-1, and very late activation antigen (*VLA*)-4 – and entry into the skin. These recruited T cells include a subset capable of responding to external or intrinsically derived superantigen. The T cell activation leads to production of T-helper (*TH1*)-type cytokines with a net effect on keratinocytes that causes secondary hyperproliferation and altered differentiation of the epidermal cells, thereby leading to psoriasis lesion formation. *TNF*, tumor necrosis factor; *IFN*, interferon; *VCAM*, vascular cell adhesion molecule; *ICAM*, intercellular adhesion molecule

the facg that some groups found a clonal population of T cells, while others have documented nonclonal collections of T cells.

One possible explanation for the aforementioned differences between guttate and plaque-stage disease may relate to the involvement of bacterially derived superantigens. As a group, patients with guttate lesions are frequently associated with streptococcal throat infections [30]. The production of bacterially derived superantigens which could circulate from the pharynx and localize to skin sites, with subsequent activation of T cells, may be one mechanism to link the extracutaneous site of infection to the development of skin lesions [31–33]. A theoretical pathophysiological pathway for psoriatic plaque formation is portrayed in Fig. 1. Because bacterially derived superantigens are different from nominal or conventional antigens in that they stimulate several types (rather than a single clone) of Vβ-bearing T cells, the presence of several different VβT cell subsides in guttate lesions actively supports a role for superantigens in guttate psoriasis [20]. With respect to the more common form of plaque-stage disease, it is more likely that a nominal antigen is involved, although definitive evidence for such an antigen is currently lacking, and one group failed to detect any Vβ-selective (bacterial

Table 1. Evidence of specific immune responses in human skin

Type of skin	Pattern of TCR rearrangements Vβ profile	Junctional region	Reference
NN	1, 7, 14, 16	ND	[24]
NN	2, 6	Nonclonal	[26]
PP (guttate and plaque)	2, 5.1	ND	[25]
PP (guttate)	2	Nonclonal	[29]
PP (plaque stage)	2, 3, 6, 13.1	Oligoclonal	[26]
PP (plaque stage)	19, 22	-	[28]
PP (plaque stage)	3, 13.1	Clonal	[28]
PP (plaque stage)	No dominant T cell subset identified	-	[30]

ND, not done; NN, healthy skin from a normal volunteer with no evidence of any skin disease or family history of psoriasis; PP, untreated psoriatic plaque-derived skin

superantigen-related) T cell infiltration of psoriatic plaques [34]. Much more work obviously remains to be completed in this area, but it is clear that there is currently no consensus as to the prevalence of any specific type of T cell bearing a characteristic or unique Vβ in either normal or psoriatic lesional skin.

Returning to clinical trials, several pharmacological studies beyond methotrexate and cyclosporin A provide compelling (although indirect) evidence to support a role for T cells in psoriasis. These trials include antibodies against CD3 [35] and CD4 [36, 37], with the most recent and perhaps most definitive study using a fusion protein containing diphtheria toxin linked to interleukin (IL)-2 [38]. This latter agent should only destroy T cells bearing high-affinity IL-2 receptors. Indeed, when given systemically, remarkable clearance of psoriatic plaques was achieved with a good correlation between the reduction in intraepidermal $CD8^+$ T cells and epidermal thickness. However, it is not known whether the primary target for any of these regents is the pathogenic T cell, a regulatory T cell subset, or both. This same concern also applies to the TCR data in Table 1, i.e., in chronic lesions, are investigators really looking at a population predominantly made up of pathogenic T cells or regulatory T cells? Such a distinction is critically important, because the disease-initiating T cell may actually be a $CD4^+$ T cell, whereas the regulatory T cells may belong to the $CD8^+$ population. This dilemma in establishing cause–effect relationships highlights the main limitation in using pharmacological studies to determine mechanistic pathophysiological details. Obviously, what is required is an appropriate animal model that will permit definitive conclusions to be drawn from experimental protocols.

There have been many putative animal models suggested to be relevant to the study of psoriasis (for a review, see [39]). Beyond the early grafting studies using nude mice [15–17], other transgenic animal models in rodents have been described, including transgenic mice overexpressing BNF-1 oncogene [40], HLA-B27 transgenic rats [41], flaky skin mutant mice [42], murine epidermis–human dermis severe combined immunodeficient (SCID) mouse model [43], transgenic mice overexpressing β_1-integrins [44], and CD18-deficient polygenic mice [45]. Another two recent reports in which there was epidermal thickening included trangenic mice in which cyclin D1 was overexpressed [46] or IκBa deficiency was induced [47]. When each of these animal models is examined critically, it is clear that – despite having some erythema and scaling of the skin and even some increased epidermal thickness – none contains all of the changes present in human psoriatic plaques. A human psoriatic plaque contains a constellation of cellular and molecular changes in a very specific histological pattern, and simply finding a rodent that has erythematous scaling skin does not permit a diagnosis of psoriasis to be made. Given this void in the literature, we began several years ago to transplant relatively large pieces of human skin containing both epidermis and dermis onto SCID mice. Because human skin has very distinctive properties [48], we felt the best animal model would be to transplant full-thickness skin in its native anatomical configuration. The initial experiments were designed to examine the stability of the phenotype of skins from various donors after engraftment and revascularization in the SCID mouse [49].

By studying a member of parameters, it became clear that NN, PN, and PP skin retained a stable phenotype when comparing skin before and after engraftment. The cellular organization and basic pathological features were retained with a high degree of fidelity in this model system [49]. Initial experiments revealed that PP skin could be effectively treated and converted to PN skin by using cyclosporin A (T. Wrone-Smith and B.J. Nickoloff, unpublished observation). The next question was whether PN skin could be converted to PP skin.

As we contemplated the design of experiments to create psoriatic plaques, we were mindful of three reports that indicated the presence of circulatory pathogenic immunocytes in human subjects [50–52]. When we injected immunocytes derived from the peripheral blood of psoriatic patients into their transplanted PN skin, within 2–4 weeks the lesion-free skin developed into a full-fledged psoriatic plaque [53]. Thus the skin thickened with scale formation and underlying dermal neovascularization (i.e., angiogenesis). This phenotypic conversion of PN to PP skin was accompanied by prominent nonrandom trafficking of T cells from the injected dermis into the epidermal compartment. For most autologous combinations of skin and immunocytes, the T cells required a preactivation step with a cocktail of bacterially derived superantigens and IL-2. The injection of NN skin with autologous blood-derived immunocytes did not produce any psoriasiform changes, nor did we observe complete phenotypic conversion of PN skin to PP skin using various soluble mediators/cytokines [53]. Taken together, these results clearly indicate that psoriasis is caused by a subset of T cells that are present in the circulation. While it is not possible to exclude a contributory role for psoriatic keratinocytes, the current data provide the most definitive evidence to date that psoriasis can be transferred by immunocompetent cells. Work is currently underway to identify the precise phenotypic and genotypic characteristics of the unique T cells that are responsible for infiltrating into the epidermis and inducing massive epidermal hyperplasia.

Conclusion

As the pendulum of the psoriatic paradigm has oscillated between the primary role for keratinocytes and for T cells, recent data indicates it has swung predominantly in favor of the T cell [53]. Moreover, the pathogenic T cell is present in the general circulation and not confined to the skin. This conclusion, based on the SCID–human skin chimeric animal model, is supported by another recent study revealing the proliferation/activation of peripheral blood-derived T lymphotes and psoriasis [54]. The presence of pathogenic T cells in the blood, which can hence be distributed everywhere, may explain why psoriasis is a disease that can affect the entire skin surface [3]. Of course, it is unclear at the moment how the circulatory T cells enter the skin and what the inciting antigen is that is responsible for their activation. Furthermore, it is unclear why the disease is not present at other sites of epithelial lining beyond the skin, such as the gastrointestinal tract, and what all of the immunological reactions are that ultimately generate highly specific and consistent T-helper (Th)1-type cytokine networks [55].

Many more questions need to be resolved before all of the pieces of this perplexing puzzle can be put together to provide a clear view of psoriasis. However, it should not be underappreciated how far this field of dermatology has progressed in the last 5 years. Intervention at the immunological and molecular level can be more rationally considered with more highly targeted immunosuppressive agents designed with fewer side effects than corticosteroids, cyclosporin A, or methotrexate. Once the identity of the pathogenic T cell has been determined, I suspect that we will rapidly unravel the genetic basis for this common and chronic cutaneous eruption. By continuing to use the SCID mouse model and applying sophisticated immunological and molecular-based technologies, this disease will finally be understood, and better treatments and perhaps even cures with complete prevention of psoriasis can be envisioned during the early part of the next century.

Summary

During the past decade, the paradigm for psoriasis research has changed dramatically. This common skin disease, which features prominent thickening of the skin, was previously believed to be a result of a primary defect in the keratinocyte. However, a growing body of evidence points to a fundamental defect in the immune system, with the recognition that the massive epidermal hyperplasia is secondary to the influx into the skin of critically important disease-producing T lymphocytes. Thus psoriasis is not really primarily a skin disease, but rather a disease of the immune system in which the phenotype is manifested clinically by characteristic skin lesions. This chapter reviews the experimental and clinical discoveries that have shifted the paradigm away from the keratinocyte and towards the T cell in psoriasis. Hopefully, by continuing to follow this new investigative pathway, the specific type of T cell in the circulation responsible for causing psoriasis will be identified, and the molecular and genetic basis for this enigmatic disease resolved.

References

1. Krueger GG, Bergstresser PR, Lowe NJ, Voorhees JJ, Weinstein GD (1984) Psoriasis. J Am Acad Dermatol 11:937–947
2. Nickoloff BJ (1991) The cytokine network in psoriasis. Arch Dermatol 127:871–884
3. Farber E, Nall ML, Strefling A (1985) Psoriasis: a disease of the total skin. J Am Acad Dermatol 12:150–156
4. Christophers E, Mrowietz U (1995) The inflammatory infiltrate in psoriasis. Clin Dermatol 13:131–135
5. Valdimarsson H, Baker BS, Jonsdottir I, Fry L. (1986) Psoriasis: a disease of abnormal keratinocyte proliferation induced by T lymphocytes. Immunol Today 7:256–259
6. Gottlieb AB (1988) Immunologic mechanisms in psoriasis. J Am Acad Dermatol 18:1376–1380
7. Baadsgaard O, Fisher GJ, Voorhees JJ, Cooper KD (1990) The role of the immune system in the pathogenesis of psoriasis. J Invest Dermatol 95:32s–34s

8. Nickoloff BJ, Mitra RS, Green J, Zheng XG, Shimizu Y, Thompson C, Turka LA (1993) Accessory cell function of keratinocytes for superantigens: dependence on lymphocyte function-associated antigen-1/intercellular adhesion molecule-1 interaction. J Immunol 150:2148–2159
9. Nestle F, Turka LA, Nickoloff BJ (1994) Characterization of dermal dendritic cells in psoriasis: autostimulation of T lymphocytes and induction of Th1 type cytokines. J Clin Invest 94:202–209
10. Russell TJ, Schultes LM, Kuban DJ (1972) Histocompatibility (HL-A) antigens associated with psoriasis. N Engl J Med 287:738–740
11. White SH., Newcomer VD, Mickey MR, Terasaki PI (1972) Disturbance of HL-A antigen frequency in psoriasis. N Engl J Med 287:740–743
12. Henseler T, Christophers E (1985) Psoriasis of early and late onset: characterization of two types of psoriasis vulgaris. J Am Acad Dermatol 13:450–456
13. Van Scott R, Auerbach, Weinstein GD (1964) Parenteral methotrexate in psoriasis. Arch Dermatol 89:550–556
14. Mueller W, Herrmann B (1979) Cyclosporin A for psoriasis. N Engl J Med 301:555
15. Krueger GG, Manning DD, Malouf J, Ogden B (1975) Long-term maintenance of psoriatic human skin on congenitally athymic (nude) mice. J Invest Dermatol 64:307–312
16. Haftek M, Ortonne JP, Staquet MJ, Viac J, Thivolet J (1981) Normal and psoriatic human skin grafts on "nude" mice: morphological and immunochemical studies. J Invest Dermatol 76:48–52
17. Fraki JE, Briggaman RA, Lazarus GS (1982) Uninvolved skin from psoriatic patients develops signs of involved psoriatic skin after being grafted onto nude mice. Science 215:685–687
18. Burg G, Braun-Falco O (1970) Das entzündliche Infiltrat bei Psoriasis vulgaris. Arch Clin Exp Dermatol 236:297–314
19. Baker BS, Swain AF, Valdimarsson H, Fry L (1984) T-cell subpopulations in the blood and skin of patients with psoriasis. Br J Dermatol 110:37–44
20. Onuma S (1994) Immunohistochemical studies of infiltrating cells in early and chronic lesions of psoriasis. J Dermatol 21:223–232
21. Krueger JG, Krane JF, Carter MD, Gottlieb AB (1990) Role of growth factors, cytokines, and their receptors in the pathogenesis of psoriasis. J Invest Dermatol 94:135S–140S
22. Prens ER, Debets, Hegmans J (1995) T lymphocytes in psoriasis. Clin Dermatol 13:115–129
23. Marguerie CC, Lunardi C So A (1992) PCR-based analysis of the TCR repertoire in human autoimmune diseases. Immunol Today 13:336–338
24. Dunn DA, Gadenne AS, Simha S, Lerner EA, Bigby M, Bleicher PA (1993) T-cell receptor V beta expression in normal human skin. Proc Natl Acad Sci USA 90:1267–1271
25. Lewis HM, Baker BS, Bokth S, Powles AJ, Garioch JJ, Valdimarsson, Fry L (1993) Restricted T-cell receptor V beta gene usage in the skin of patients with guttate and chronic plaque psoriasis. Br J Dermatol 129:514–520
26. Menssen A, Trommler P, Vollmer S, Schendel D, Albert E, Gurtler L, Riethmuller G, Prinz JC (1995) Evidence for an antigen-specific cellular immune response in skin lesions of patients with psoriasis vulgaris. J Immunol 155:4078–4083
27. Boehncke WH., Kuenzlen C, Zollner TM, Mielke V, Sterry W (1994) Predominant usage of distinct T-cell receptor V beta regions by epidermotropic T cells in psoriasis. Exp Dermatol 3:161–163
28. Chang JC, Smith LR, Froning KJ, Schwabe BJ, Laxer JA, Caralli LL, Kurland HH, Karasek MA, Wilkinson DI, Brustoff SW (1994) CD8+ T cells in psoriatic lesions preferentially use T-cell receptor V beta 3 and/or V beta 13.1 genes. Proc Natl Acad Sci USA 91:9282–9286
29. Leung DY, Travers JB, Giorno R, Norris DA, Skinner R, Aelion J, Kazemi LV, Kim MH, Trumble AE, Kotb M, Schlievert PM (1995) Evidence for a streptococcal superantigen-driven process in acute guttate psoriasis. J Clin Invest 96:2106–2112
30. Wyyte JH, Baughman RD (1964) Acute guttate psoriasis and streptococcal infection. Arch Dermatol 89:350–356
31. Kotzin BL, Leung DY, Kappler J, Marrack P (1993) Superantigens and their potential role in human disease. Adv Immunol 54:99–166

32. Nickoloff BJ, Mitra RS, Green J, Shimizu Y, Thompson C, Turka LA (1993) Activated keratinocytes present bacterial-derived superantigens to T lymphocytes: relevance to psoriasis. J Derm Sci 6:127–133
33. Leung DY, Walsh P, Giorno R, Norris DA (1993) A potential role for superantigens in the pathogenesis of psoriasis. J Invest Dermatol 100:225–228
34. Boehncke WJ, Dressel D, Manfras B, Zollner TM, Wettstein A, Bohm OB, Sterry W (1995) T-cell-receptor repertoire in chronic plaque-stage psoriasis is restricted and lacks enrichment of superantigen-associated V beta regions. J Invest Dermatol 104:725–728
35. Weinshenker BG, Bass BH, Ebers GC, Rice GP (1989) Remission of psoriatic lesions with muromonab-CD3 (orthoclone OKT3) treatment. J Am Acad Dermatol 20:1132–1133
36. Morel P, Revillard JP, Nicolas JF, Wijdenes J, Rizova H, Thivolet J (1992) Anti-CD4 monoclonal antibody therapy in severe psoriasis. J Autoimmun 5:465–477
37. Rizova H, Nicolas JF, Morel P, Kanitakis J, Demidem A, Revillard JP, Wijdenes J, Thivolet J, Schmitt S (1994) The effect of anti-CD4 monoclonal antibody treatment on immunopathological changes in psoriatic skin. J Derm Sci 7:1-13
38. Gottlieb SL, Gilleaudeau P, Johnson R, Estes L, Woodworth TG (1996) Response of psoriasis to a lymphocyte-selective toxin (DAB-IL-2) suggest a primary immune, but not keratinocyte, pathogenic basis. Nat Med 1:442–447
39. Sundberg JP, Beamer WG, Shultz LD, Dunstan DW (1990) Inherited mouse mutations as models of human adnexal, cornification, and papulosquamous dermatoses. J Invest Dermatol 95:62S–63S
40. Wilson JB, Weinberg W, Johnson R, Yuspa S, Levine AJ (1990) Expression of the BNLF-1 oncogene of Epstein-Barr virus in the skin of transgenic mice induces hyperplasia and aberrant expression of keratin 6. Cell 61:1315–1327
41. Breban M, Hammer RE, Richardson JA, Taurog JD (1993) Transfer of the inflammatory disease of HLA-B27 transgenic rats by bone marrow engraftment. J Exp Med 178:1607–1616
42. Sundberg JP, Boggess D, Sundberg BA, Beamer WG, Shultz LD (1993) Epidermal dendritic cell populations in the flaky skin mutant mouse. Immunol Invest 22:389–401
43. Boehncke WH., Sterry W, Hainzl A, Scheffold W, Kaufmann R (1994) Psoriasiform architecture of murine epidermis overlying human psoriatic dermis transplanted onto SCID mice. Arch Dermatol Res 286:325–330
44. Carroll JM, Romero MR, Watt FM (1995) Suprabasal integrin expression in the epidermis of transgenic mice results in developmental defects and a phenotype resembling psoriasis. Cell 83:957–968
45. Bullard DC, Scharffetter-Kocharek K, McArthur MJ, Chosay JG, McBride MA, Montgomery CM, Beaudet AL (1996) A polygenic mouse model of psoriasiform skin disease in CD18-deficient mice. Proc Natl Acad Sci USA 93:2116–2121
46. Robles AJ, Larcher F, Whalin RB, Murillas R, Richie E, Gimenez-Conti IB, Jorcano JL, Conti (1996) Expression of cyclin D1 in epithelial tissues of transgenic mice results in epidermal hyperproliferation and severe thymic hyperplasia. Proc Natl Acad Sci USA 93:7634–7638
47. Klement JF, Rice NR, Car BD, Abbondanzo SJ, Powers GD, Bhatt H, Chen CH, Rosen CA, Stewart CL (1996) IκBβ deficiency results in a sustained NF-κB response and severe widespread dermatitis in mice. Mol Cell Biol 16:2341–2349
48. Montagna W (1971) Cutaneous comparative biology. Arch Dermatol 104:577–591
49. Nickoloff BJ, Kunkel SL, Burdick M, Strieter RM (1995) Severe combined immunodeficiency mouse and human psoriatic skin chimeras. Validation of a new animal model. Am J Pathol 146:580–588
50. Gardembas-Pain M, Ifrah N, Foussard C, Boasson M, Saint Andre JP, Verret JL (1990) Psoriasis after allogeneic bone marrow transplantation. Arch Dermatol 126:1523
51. Eedy DJ, Burrows D, Bridges JM, Jones FG (1990) Clearance of severe psoriasis after allogenic bone marrow transplantation. BMJ 300:908
52. Jowitt SN, Yin JA (1990) Psoriasis and bone marrow transplantation. BMJ 300:1398–1399
53. Wrone-Smith T, Nickoloff BJ (1996) Dermal injection of immunocytes induces psoriasis. J Clin Invest 98:1878–1887

54. Jeffes EW, Lee GC, Said S, Sabahi M, McCullough JL, Herrod R, Alzona CP, Linden KG, Soundararajan D, Edwards S et al (1995) Elevated numbers of proliferating mononuclear cells in the peripheral blood of psoriatic patients correlate with disease severity. J Invest Dermatol 105:733–738
55. Uyemura K, Yamamura M, Fivenson DF, Modlin RL, Nickoloff BJ (1993) The cytokine network in psoriasis is characterized by a T-helper type 1 cell mediated response. J Invest Dermatol 101:701–705

Vasculitis Allergica

B. Zelger

Introduction

The Department of Dermatology, University of Innsbruck, Austria, serves a population of about one million inhabitants as the only primary health care institution for dermatologic problems. Within the last decade, we consistently had approximately 40 inpatients per year suffering from vasculitis allergica (VA). Considering those cases seen in consultation on other wards and in peripheral hospitals, the incidence is at least five to six patients per 100 000 people annually. Thus VA is by far the most frequent problem of vasculitic disorders in dermatology.

VA was first distinguished from panarteritis nodosa as hypersensitivity angiitis by Zeek et al. [36]. Since then, a steadily increasing number of modern techniques has drastically broadened our knowledge of vascular disorders in general, and of VA in particular. It became evident that in the vast majority of cases (95 %) VA is an immune complex-mediated type III Arthus reaction [19], limited to capillaries and/or small postcapillary venules of the skin as well as a variety of other organs. However, in a minority additional pathogenetic mechanisms become effective, such as monoclonal/polyclonal immunoglobulins, cryoglobulins, and antinuclear (ANA), antineutrophil cytoplasmic (ANCA), or antiendothelial cell antibodies. VA may precede, accompany, or occur during a wide variety of other vasculitic and systemic disorders characterized by involvement of larger vessels and/or extravascular disease as part of a complex process, the exact classification and pathogenesis of which remains largely obscure.

The present article describes recent developments in diagnosis, pathogenesis, and therapy in this interesting field of dermatology.

State of the Art

Definition

VA, which is also called leukocytoclastic vasculitis, (cutaneous) necrotizing vasculitis, (cutaneous) necrotizing venulitis, and hypersensitivity angiitis, is a vasculitis of capillaries to postcapillary venules. It is clinically characterized by palpable purpura and histologically by fibrin, leukocytes, and nuclear debris within the (lumen and) wall of affected vessels.

Clinicopathologic Presentation

The clinical hallmark of VA is palpable purpura (Fig. 1). It is characterized by acute onset of hemorrhagic papules to nodules affecting areas of high venous pressure, usually the lower legs in mobile patients or dorsal body parts in bed-ridden patients. According to the acuity, recurrence, and extent of the underlying disease (see below), the clinical appearance may show considerable variations: peracute onset of extensive disease may lead to confluent hemorrhages of large parts of the extremities, often with bulla formation and necrosis imitating bullous and/or necrotizing erysipelas. In contrast, the smoldering, wheal-like infiltration of urticarial vasculitis [28] shows no or only minimal hemorrhage. Erythrocyte extravasation can often only be appreciated by slight hyperpigmentation after clearing of the lesions. In addition, the prolonged persistance of urticarial lesions (> 24 h) argues against ordinary urticaria. In some of these cases, VA may show anular configurations, which, when recurrent episodes of a vasculitic process occur, constitutes erythema gyratum repens (Fig. 2).

In all these cases, skin biopsies (Fig. 3) reveal capillaries to postcapillary venules characterized by fibrin, leukocytes, and nuclear debris within the lumen, wall, and surrounding connective tissue of affected vessels (leukocytoclastic vasculitis or venulitis). According to the extent of disease, this process may show considerable variation, with only minimal admixture of erythrocyte extravasation in urticarial vasculitis to extensive tissue necrosis in hemorrhagic–necrotic variants.

Clinical presentation obviously varies according to the extent of organ involvement: on the one hand, the gastrointestinal tract, synovia, and kidneys are frequently involved, e.g., in Henoch-Schönlein purpura. Apart from common constitutional symptoms such as fever, weight loss, weakness, fatigue, and malaise, organ-specific symptoms include abdominal cramps, diarrhea, melena, arthralgia, myalgia, and hematuria. On the other hand, VA may be limited to one organ, most commonly the skin. In rare cases, this organ may be the lung [25], the gut [5], or the kidneys, as discussed for patients with immune complex-mediated forms of isolated glomerulonephritis [13].

Additional complexity results in patients where VA accompanies various systemic disorders, such as rheumatoid arthritis (rheumatoid vasculitis [31]), hepatitis C (cryoglobulinemic vasculitis [11]), plasmocytoma, or lupus erythematosus (hypergammaglobulinemic vasculitis). Connective tissue disease occasionally begins as urticarial vasculitis or erythema gyratum repens [1].

In approximately 25% of patients with systemic (large vessel) vasculitis [2], the condition may also be complicated by or even begin with VA. Such patients may develop or present with additional dermatologic features, including persistent papules, nodules, and plaques.

In Wegener's granulomatosis, these lesions prefer the extensor surface of the upper extremities or trunk, in particular the hands, elbows, and buttocks. The vascular variant, which is histologically characterized by necrotizing vasculitis, is known as erythema elevatum et diutinum. In the early phase, extravascular variants look like folliculitis or Sweet syndrome, i.e., histologically, they have a neutrophil-rich, diffuse dermal infiltrate in common [18]. The longer these lesions persist, the more prominent a histiocytic component becomes. Clinically, this results in granuloma anulare-like to papulonecrotic lesions or even ulcers; histologically, it results in extravascular granulomas with or without central basophilic necrosis surrounded by a histiocytic palisading process

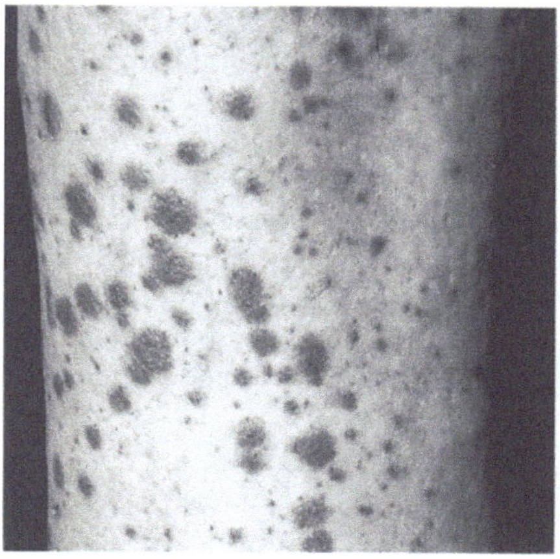

Fig. 1. Vasculitis allergica („palpable purpura")

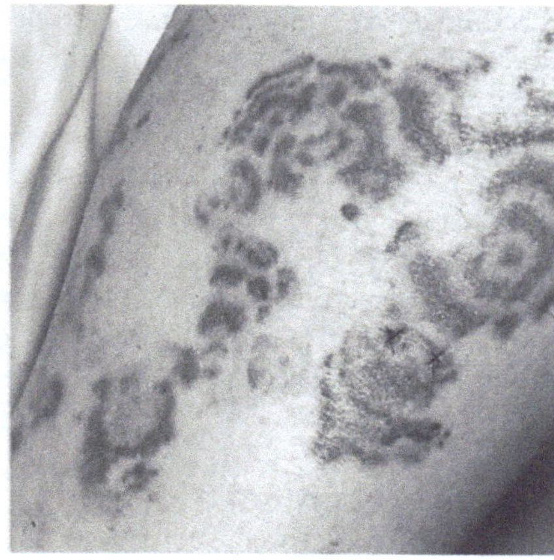

Fig. 2. Erythema gyratum repens

interspersed by neutrophils known as palisaded neutrophilic and granulomatous dermatitis [8].

Identical lesions may be seen in other systemic disorders, such as lupus erythematosus, dermatomyositis, or rheumatoid arthritis [8].

Lesions rich in eosinophils and eosinophilic debris are characteristic of Churg-Strauss granuloma. Such lesions usually affect the head of adults with a previous or concomitant history of allergic rhinitis or bronchial asthma; blood examinations reveal hypereosinophilia (> 1500 per ml).

Painful nodules often aligned along preexisting vessels are characteristic of microscopic panarteritis nodosa [35]. This entity has recently been distinguished from classic panarteritis nodosa, which affects the aorta and large arterial branches only; patients with the latter characteristically suffer from complications due to thrombembolism

Fig. 3. Necrotizing vasculitis

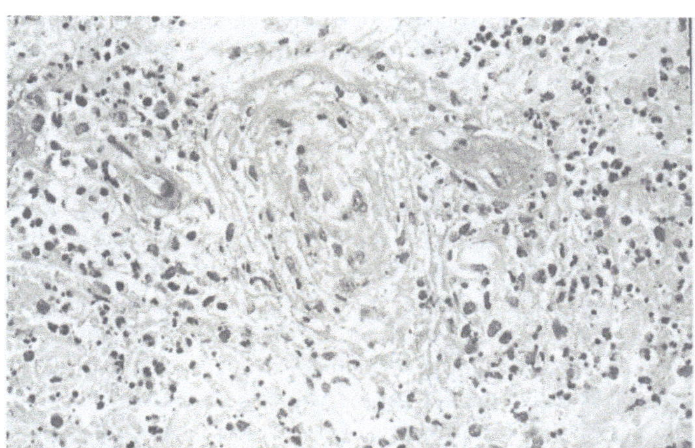

and/or aneurysms, but show no involvement of smaller arteries or even VA [22]. In contrast, microscopic panarteritis nodosa affects small to medium-sized arteries in a variety of organs, in particular kidneys, gut, and heart. Its skin-limited form [9] has previously been called cutaneous panarteritis nodosa [10].

Finally, one facultative clinical feature may give clues about pathogenetic mechanisms, namely livedo patterning [37]. When the underlying disease process mostly causes rheologic disturbances as in cryoglobulinemic or hypergammaglobulinemic vasculitis, a regular net-like livedo reticularis may occur; histologically, these cases are dominated by fibrin thrombi instead of leukocytoclasia. In the case of a localized inflammatory process of vessel walls, as in microscopic panarteritis nodosa, irregular bizarre livedo racemosa may be seen.

Diagnostic Approach

In addition to clinical presentation, previous history, serologic parameters, and histology are necessary for exact classification.

On the one hand, a precise short-term history of the patient's actual situation often reveals preceding or accompanying infectious disorders. Streptococcal infections, in particular angina tonsillaris, are typical, but any other infection might also be a trigger. We have seen VA complicating or following erysipelas, triggered by gastrointestinal infections or incarcerated hernias, or following various viral infections, in particular hepatitis B and C. A wide variety of pharmaceutical and alimentary agents may also occasionally trigger VA, sulfonamides [30] and polyvitamins [3] being the best established associations. On the other hand, a detailed long-term history for underlying diseases may reveal systemic disorders, such as lupus erythematosus, rheumatoid arthritis, or malignancies, which may be complicated by VA.

Serologically, there are three options:

1. Serologic and/or other laboratory parameters reveal *subclinical involvement of internal organs*, e.g., increased liver function parameters, increased muscle enzymes, a positive Hemoccult (modified guaiac test) or hematuria, increased daily urinary protein excretion, and decreased creatinine clearance. To further evaluate this process, various imaging and apparatus methods such as X-ray, sonography, computed tomography, magnetic resonance imaging, and endoscopy are necessary. Moreover, such methods may also reveal previously unsuspected disease, such as sinusoidal swellings or hemorrhagic lung infiltrates in Wegener's disease; still other methods, such as nerve conduction velocity or electromyography, confirm the clinical finding of mononeuritis multiplex, a characteristic presenting sign of many vasculitic disorders, or muscle involvement, respectively.
2. Laboratory investigations may detect or confirm *etiologically relevant factors*, such as elevated antistreptolysin and antistaphylosin titers or mixed cryoglobulinemia associated with hepatitis C; similarly, detection of cold agglutinins, cryoglobulins, lupus anticoagulans, anticardiolipin antibodies, or hypergammaglobulinemia necessitates an intensive search for underlying infectious, systemic, or neoplastic disorders, such as lupus erythematosus or plasmocytoma.
3. Serology helps to illuminate the *pathogenetic* mechanism. Thus circulating immune complexes are characteristic of classic VA [27], but are not always detectable; more frequently, complement consumption is recognized by decreased levels of comple-

ment factors 3 and 4, CH50, or CH100 [32]. A positive ANA titer detected by indirect immunofluorescence suggests the possibility of a underlying connective tissue disorder, and extractable nuclear antigens (ENA) or ANA subsets might be helpful for subtyping by enzyme-linked immunosorbent assay (ELISA). Similarly, positive antineutrophil cytoplasmic antibodies (ANCA) routinely screened by indirect immunofluorescence indicate a systemic vasculitis, and again subtyping may be helpful. Thus cytoplasmic ANCA (cANCA), characterized by diffuse cytoplasmic reactivity in indirect immunofluorescence and antibodies against proteinase 3 by ELISA, mostly occur in Wegener's granulomatosis [34], while perinuclear ANCA (pANCA), characterized by perinuclear accentuated cytoplasmic reactivity and antibodies against myeloperoxidase, most often show association with microscopic panarteritis nodosa [4].

The value of skin biopsies is also threefold:

1. Biopsies may exclude simulants of VA. Thus stasis bleedings show erythrocyte extravasation without vasculitis, but are often accompanied by stasis dermatitis. Multiple insect bites show a wedge-shaped infiltrate of lymphohistiocytes and eosinophils. Septic vasculitis, which mostly occurs in severely ill patients with bizarre acral bleedings, histologically shows fibrin thrombi. Similarly, early petechial bleedings of livedo vasculitis also show fibrin thrombi without significant inflammatory infiltrate.
2. Biopsies help to subclassify the vasculitic process, e.g., by detection of immunglobulin A deposits in direct immunofluorescence of patients with Henoch-Schönlein purpura or prominent fibrin thrombi indicative of cryoglobulinemia or hypergammaglobulinemia. Biopsies may confirm or detect clinically suspected or unsuspected large-vessel vasculitis.
3. Skin biopsies may sometimes make more invasive and risky biopsy techniques of affected internal organs unnecessary, e.g., when classic Churg-Strauss granulomas are detected or a dense, neutrophil-rich infiltrate with features of folliculitis, Sweet syndrome, or VA associated with cANCA is seen in the characteristic clinical setting of Wegener's granulomatosis, i.e., upper and lower respiratory tract lesions and glomerulonephritis.

Therapeutic Approach

The clinical course and natural history of VA are frequently self-limited, and the prognosis is usually good. Thus therapy should be based on a cause- and intensity-related stepwise approach.

In addition to bed rest, antibiotics are the first monotherapy to be effective in approximately 50 % of patients with VA. Thus penicillins, for example, are helpful when streptococci-induced angina is the trigger, and tetracyclines when mostly gram-negative gastrointestinal infections precede VA.

When VA is extensive with massive skin and additional extracutaneous involvement, in particular renal, or when antibiotics cannot stop recurrent episodes of palpable purpura within a couple of days, corticosteroids are indicated. Starting with approximately 1 mg methylprednisolone/kg per day, gradual tapering over 2–4 weeks will successfully heal VA in more than 90 % of cases. However, it is important not only to evaluate the effects on skin and joints, which are the most relevant signs for the patient, but also to carefully manage internal functions, in particular renal ones (urine analysis, blood pressure control). It is well established that renal function may deteriorate over a period of weeks, despite normalization of other organ functions.

The further therapy in these patients follows regimens which would similarily be applied to systemic vasculitis ab initio. Such regimens have proven enormously successful, e.g., in Wegener's granulomatosis, lowering the mortality rate of 80% within 2 years without therapy to less than 20% after 5 years with a combination of corticosteroids and cytotoxic agents [14]. There is some controversy in the literature about whether a continuous daily regimen with 2 mg cyclophosphamide/kg per os or a monthly pulse therapy with 1000 mg as a single-shot intravenous therapy is preferable. Pulsed regimens seem to be less toxic, but generally not as effective as daily medications [21]. If remission occurs, a gradual tapering of the glucocorticoid dose starting 1 month after initiation and continuation of cyclophosphamide therapy for at least 1 year beyond induction of remission is indicated. If complete remission is maintained within this year, the cyclophosphamide dose is then gradually reduced to zero within the next 6 months.

In the case of hemorrhagic cystitis or bone marrow cytotoxicity (the main complications of these cyclophosphamide regimens), 100-150 mg azathioprine per day [7] or 7.5 mg methotrexate split in three doses over 24 h once a week [23] are alternative treatments. Inadequate success, which occurs in less than 1% of all patients presenting with VA, may be managed by additional plasmapheresis (three sessions per week on alternate days for 3 weeks [20]) or more recently developed alternative immunosuppressive agents such as cyclosporin A (4–5 mg/kg per day orally [6]) or immunoglobulin therapy (2 g/kg split in equal doses over 5 days every month intravenously [16]).

There are anecdotal reports that other oral agents, such as dapsone (100–150 mg/ day) and colchicine (0.6 mg one to four times per day), are effective [33], but their use has been limited mainly to early lesions of Wegener's granulomatosis, such as erythema elevatum et diutinum or palisaded neutrophilic and granulomatous vasculitis. Similarly, indomethacin (150 mg/day) is of limited value in the early management of urticarial vasculitis [29]. Interferon-α (3 million units applied three times a week subcutaneously [24]) may be helpful in hepatitis C-associated cryoglobulinemic vasculitis. Moreover, rheologically influenced disorders might benefit from daily subcutaneous application of 5000 U high molecular weight heparin similar to the effect in livedo and septic vasculitis [15].

Two further facts are of therapeutic importance. First, long-term follow-up is mandatory for early recognition of relapses in patients where VA is the expression of systemic vasculitis or other systemic disorders [17]. Second, patients on long-term immunosuppressive therapy must be carefully managed to avoid and/or to recognize early therapeutic side effects, which are a great problem in approximately 20% of patients [6].

Discussion

Classification of vasculitis has always been a matter of great discussion and concern. Classification criteria followed the size of the affected vessels, the kind and number of organs affected, the histologic appearance, and, most recently, serologic parameters. In a literature research over the last 5 years, more than 85% of papers deal with ANCA, which drastically outlines the recent concentration of vasculitis research on these serologic phenomena. Various authors have tried to correlate clinical entities with serologic parameters, e.g., immune complexes with VA, cANCA with Wegener's granulomatosis, and pANCA with microscopic panarteritis nodosa. While these combinations are certainly valuable for classification and understanding of many cases, others fall outside these guidelines.

To overcome these problems, a number of reputed clinicians and scientists in the field of vasculitic disorders have tried to form a consensus classification [22] which primarily follows clinicopathological criteria, in particular the size of the affected vessel. Takayasu arteritis, giant cell arteritis, Winiwarter Bürger disease, classic panarteritis nodosa, and Kawasaki disease mainly affect the aorta or their main branches; microscopic panarteritis nodosa, Wegener's granulomatosis, and Churg-Strauss syndrome mainly affect medium to small-sized arteries, and VA small capillaries and postcapillary venules. Alongside additional histologic criteria, e.g., extravascular granulomas, and serologic criteria further help to differentiate between these entities.

In this classification, VA in the vast majority of cases (> 95 %) is an immune complex-mediated vasculitis of capillaries to postcapillary venules without large-vessel involvement. Pathogenetically, immune complexes result from a combination of various antigens with their respective immunglobulin M, and occasionally G, antibodies, which are usually removed by macrophages. When a disease process is overwhelming or the scavenger system of macrophages is temporarily ineffective, circulating immune complexes adhere via Fc receptors to capillaries and postcapillary venules; the slow blood flow in this part of the vascular system certainly favors adhesion of immune complexes. Next, the complement cascade is activated, and strongly chemotactic factors such as C3a and C5a become effective. Immigrant mast cells, neutrophils, and macrophages are then responsible for further chemotaxis and tissue degradation characterized by characteristic leukocytoclastic histology [19].

When no immune complexes are detectable, investigations for additional pathomechanisms may detect rheologic parameters such as hypergammaglobulinemia, cryoprecipitable proteins, and lupus anticoagulans factor or indirect parameters thereof, such as a prolonged partial thromboplastin time, ANA, and anticardiolipin antibodies. The resulting hypercoagulability slows down the blood flow in postcapillary venules. This is particularly the case when cryoglobulins, cryofibrinogen, or cold agglutinins are present. Clinically, these cases may show moderate livedo reticularis; histologically, fibrin thrombi dominate over the vasculitic process [37].

Finally, a third pathomechanism becomes evident in the case of ANCA [12]. These antibodies are usually directed against epitopes within intracytoplasmic granules of granulocytes and early macrophages, such as proteinase 3 or myeloperoxidase, and are thus ineffective. However, when granulocytes and macrophages become activated, e.g., by interleukin-1 or tumor necrosis factor-α during infections, these antigens become expressed on the cell surface, where the respective antibodies then can be fixed. ANCA-activated neutrophils and monocytes then adhere via Fc receptors to intra- and extravascular targets, i.e., endothelial cells, macrophages, or fibroblasts. As neutrophils and monocytes are metabolically active and thus mobile cells, this process is not dominated by rheologic phenomena, as in immune complex or cryoglobulinemic vasculitis, which may at least partially explain why this process is seen more frequently in larger arteries or even extravascularly. Perpetuation of the process leads to a granulomatous reaction. A similar process might occur with antiendothelial cell antibodies, which may be seen for example in large-vessel disorders such as Kawasaki disease [26].

Summary

Vasculitis allergica is a common vasculitic problem of capillaries and postcapillary venules with an incidence of six patients per 100 000 people annually. Palpable purpura and leukocytoclastic vasculitis are the characteristic clinical and histological findings of this polyetiologic (infections, drugs, alimentary ingredients, connective tissue disorders, neoplasms) immune complex-mediated disease. Unusual clinical presentations include urticarial vasculitis and erythema gyratum repens. Histologic pecularities include the immunglobulin A-positive Henoch-Schönlein purpura and the fibrin thrombi-rich variants of cryoglobulinemic vasculitis (hepatitis C) and hypergammaglobulinemic vasculitis (plasmocytoma, connective tissue disorders). Moreover, in rare cases (< 5%), vasculitis allergica can occur in patients with more serious systemic arteritis such as Wegener's granulomatosis (cANCA). Corticosteroids are an effective curative therapy in more than 90% of patients. Adverse outcome is mostly due to long-term renal problems.

References

1. Asherson RA, D'Cruz D, Stephens CJ, McKee PH, Hughes GR (1991) Urticarial vasculitis in a connective tissue disease clinic: patterns, presentations and treatment. Semin Arthritis Rheum 20:285–296
2. Barksdale SK, Hallahan CW, Kerr GS, Fauci AS, Stern JB, Travis WD (1995) Cutaneous pathology in Wegener's granulomatosis. A clinicopathologic study of 75 biopsies in 46 patients. Am J Surg Pathol 19:161–172
3. Bear RA, Lang PA, Garvey MB (1982) Vasculitis and vitamin abuse. Arch Pathol Lab Med 106:48
4. Bosch X, Font J, Mirapeix E, Revert L, Urbano-Marquez A, Ingelmo M (1993) Anti-neutrophil cytoplasmic autoantibodies (ANCA): antigenic specificities and clinical associations. Adv Exp Med Biol 336: 281–286
5. Burke AP, Sobin LH, Virmani R (1995) Localized vasculitis of the gastrointestinal tract. Am J Surg Pathol 19:338–349
6. Calabrese LH, Hoffman GS, Guillevin L (1995) Therapy of resistant systemic necrotizing vasculitis. Polyarteritis, Churg-Strauss syndrome, Wegener's granulomatosis, and hypersensitivity vasculitis group disorders. Rheum Dis Clin North Am 21:41–57
7. Callen JP, Spencer LV, Burruss JB, Holtman J (1991) Azathioprine. An effective, corticosteroid-sparing therapy for patients with recalcitrant cutaneous lupus erythematosus or with recalcitrant cutaneous leukocytoclastic vasculitis. Arch Dermatol 127:515–522
8. Chu P, Connolly MK, LeBoit PE (1994) The histopathologic spectrum of palisaded neutrophilic and granulomatous dermatitis in patients with collagen vascular disease. Arch Dermatol 130:1278–1283
9. Dewar CL, Bellamy N (1992) Necrotizing mesenteric vasculitis after longstanding cutaneous polyarteritis nodosa. J Rheumatol 19:1308–1311
10. Diaz-Perez JL, Winkelmann RK (1974) Cutaneous periarteritis nodosa. Arch Pathol 110: 407–414
11. Durand JM, Lefevre P, Harle JR, Boucrat J, Vitviski L, Soubeyrand J (1991) Cutaneous vasculitis and cryoglobulinemia type II associated with hepatitis C virus infection. Lancet 337:499–500
12. Ewert BH, Jennette JC, Falk RJ (1992) Anti-myeloperoxidase antibodies stimulate neutrophils to damage human endothelial cells. Kidney Int 41:375–383
13. Falk RJ, Jennette JC (1993) A nephrological view of the classification of vasculitis. In: Gross WL (ed) ANCA-associated vasculitides: immunological and clinical aspects. Plenum, New York, pp 197–208
14. Fauci AS, Haynes BF, Katz B, Wolff SM (1983) Wegener's granulomatosis: prospective clinical therapeutic experience with 85 patients for 21 years. Ann Intern Med 98:76–85
15. Fritsch PO, Zelger B (1995) Livedo-Vasculitis. Hautarzt 46:214–224

16. Gedalia A, Correa H, Kaiser M, Sorensen R (1995) Case report: steroid sparing effect of intravenous gammaglobulin in a child with necrotizing vasculitis. Am J Med Sci 309:226–228
17. Gordon M, Luqmani RA, Adu D, Greaves I, Richards N, Michael J, Emery P, Howie AJ, Bacon PA (1993) Relapses in patients with a systemic vasculitis. Q J Med 86:779–789
18. Goulart RA, Mark EJ, Rosen S (1995) Tumefactions as an extravascular manifestation of Wegener's granulomatosis. Am J Surg Pathol 19:145–153
19. Gower RG, Sams WM Jr, Thorne EG, Kohler PF, Claman HN (1977) Leukocytoclastic vasculitis-sequential appearance of immunoreactants and cellular changes in serial biopsies. J Invest Dermatol 69:477–484
20. Guillevin L, Fain O, Lhote F, Jarrousse B, Huong DLT, Bussel A, Leon A (1992) Lack of superiority of steroids plus plasma exchange to steroids alone in the treatment of polyarteritis nodosa and Churg-Strauss syndrome: a prospective randomized trial in 78 patients. Arthritis Rheum 35:208–215
21. Hoffmann GS, Leavitt RJ, Fleisher TA, Minor TA, Fauci AS (1990) Treatment of Wegener's granulomatosis with intermittent high-dose intravenous cyclophosphamid. Am J Med 89: 403–410
22. Jennette JC, Falk RJ, Andrassy K, Bacon PA, Churg J, Gross WL, Hagen EC, Hoffman GS, Hunder GG, Kallenberg CG, McCluskey RT, Sinico RA, Rees AJ, von Es LA, Waldherr R, Wiik A (1994) Nomenclature of systemic vasculitides. Proposal of an international consensus conference. Arthritis Rheum 37:187–192
23. Jorizzo JL, White LW, Wise CM, Zanolli MD, Sherertz EF (1991) Low dose weekly methotrexate for unusual neutrophilic vascular reactions: cutaneous polyarteritis nodosa and Behcet's disease. J Am Acad Dermatol 24:973–978
24. Karlsberg PL, Lee WM, Casey DL, Cockerell CJ, Cruz PD Jr (1995) Cutaneous vasculitis and rheumatoid factor positivity as presenting signs of hepatitis C virus induced mixed cryoglobulinemia. Arch Dermatol 131:1119–1123
25. Katzenstein AL, Locke WK (1995) Solitary lung lesions in Wegener's granulomatosis. Pathologic findings and clinical significance in 25 cases. Am J Surg Pathol 19:545–552
26. Leung DYM, Collins T, Lapierre LA, Geha RS, Pober JS (1986) Immunglobulin M antibodies present in the acute phase of Kawasaki syndrome lyse cultured vascular endothelial cells stimulated by gamma interferon. J Clin Invest 77:1428–1435
27. Mackel SE, Tappeiner G, Brumfield H, Jordon RE (1979) Circulating immune complexes in cutaneous vasculitis: detection with C1q and monoclonal rheumatoid factor. J Clin Invest 64:1652–1660
28. Mehregan DR, Hall MJ, Gibson LE (1992) Urticarial vasculitis: a histopathologic and clinical review of 72 cases. J Am Acad Dermatol 26:441–448
29. Millns JL, Randle HW, Solley GO, Dicken CH (1980) The therapeutic response of urticarial vasculitis to indomethacin. J Am Acad Dermatol 3:349–355
30. Mullick FG, McAllister HA, Wagner BM, Fendoglio JJ (1979) Drug related vasculitis. Hum Pathol 10:313–325
31. Scott DGI, Bacon PA, Tribe CR (1981) Systemic rheumatoid vasculitis: a clinical and laboratory study of 50 cases. Medicine 60:288–297
32. Soter NA, Mihm MC, Gigli I, Dvorak HF, Austen KF (1976) Two distinct cellular patterns in cutaneous necrotizing angiitis. J Invest Dermatol 66:344–350
33. Swerlick RA, Lawley TJ (1991) Small vessel vasculitis and cutaneous vasculitis. In: Churg A, Churg J (eds) Systemic vasculitis. Igaku-Shoin, New York, pp 193–201
34. Van der Woude FJ, Rasmussen N, Lobatto S, Wiik A, Permin H, van Es LA, van der Giessen M, van der Hem GK, The TH (1985) Autoantibodies against neutrophils and monocytes: tool for diagnosis and marker of disease activity in Wegener's granulomatosis. Lancet i:425–429
35. Waldherr R (1993) Classification of systemic vasculitis. In: Gross WL (ed) ANCA-associated vasculitides: immunological and clinical aspects. Plenum, New York, pp 165–172
36. Zeek PM, Smith CC, Wector JC (1948) Studies on periarteritis nodosa. III. The differentiation between the vascular lesions of periarteritis nodosa and of hypersensitivity. Am J Pathol 24:889–917
37. Zelger B, Plörer A, Sepp N, Fritsch PO (1995) Differentialdiagnose der Livedosyndrome. Hautarzt 46:369–379

Contact Dermatitis

A. H. Enk and J. Knop

Introduction

Chemicals that induce contact sensitivity (CS), called haptens, exhibit several common features that define them as allergens. They are of relatively low molecular weight and are chemically reactive and lipid soluble. In most cases, chemical reactivity leads to the formation of nonreversible chemical bonds between haptens and the cell surface and/or extracellular matrix proteins. This modification of self-proteins has been given several names, such as derivatization, haptenization, and conjugation. By binding to formerly nonimmunologic self-proteins, haptens convert them into immunogenically altered self-proteins recognized by antigen-specific T cells. Conjugates of protein and hapten become the target structures against which contact hypersensitivity (CH) responses are directed. The lipid solubility and small molecular weight allow these chemicals to easily enter the skin through the stratum corneum. Whereas some haptens induce sensitization in humans or animals, others, although of very similar structure, cause irritation or even tolerance induction. In contrast to haptens, substances such as sodium lauryl sulfate or sodium dodecyl sulfate cause rather nonspecific dermatitis and are called irritants. The mechanism by which allergic and irritant contact dermatitis are induced and the differences between these two immune reactions have been of long-standing interest for scientists. As early as 1942, Landsteiner and Chase [1] successfully showed that cutaneous reactivity against allergens could be conferred on immunologically naive guinea pigs by the adoptive transfer of peritoneal exudate from sensitized donors. These experiments for the first time established the transferability of CH with cells.

An important subsequent observation was made in 1957 by Frey and Wenk [2], who found that the destruction of afferent lymphatics draining sites of skin treated with allergens prevented effective sensitization, thus providing evidence for the requirement of lymphatic drainage for the induction of CH.

In 1969, Macher and Chase [3] conducted a series of studies that provided important insights into the balance between unresponsiveness and hypersensitivity. They immunized guinea pigs with an injection of hapten (picrylchloride, TNCB) into ear skin and excised the injected ears at various time points. When they excised the ear after 12 h, only one of 28 guinea pigs developed sensitivity. When the ears were left undisturbed, 16 of 20 animals were sensitized. It was concluded that hapten injection sites need to remain intact for at least 2 days to achieve maximal sensitization. In a second set of experiments, TNCB was injected into the remaining ears of guinea pigs whose ears were excised 12 h after the first treatment. Surprisingly, only a few animals developed sensitivity; a large percentage had become immunologically unresponsive to TNCB. Furthermore, Macher and Chase observed that, by using radioactively labeled TNCB, large portions of TNCB injected into the skin left the injection sites through venous outflow within minutes. Additionally, an intravenous injection of similar amounts of haptens before immunization led to unresponsiveness. It was concluded that the sensitizing depot was hapten that remained in the ear after early outflow. If the sensitizing depot is removed, a state of unresponsiveness is induced.

In the early 1970s, Silberberg showed that Langerhans' cells (LC) are involved in contact allergic reactions to a variety of allergens in humans [4] and in contact allergic reactions to 2,4-dinitro-1-chlorobenzene in guinea pigs [5, 6]. The observations that mononuclear cells, probably lymphocytes, were found in apposition to LC in the epidermis and dermis and that LC appeared in dermal lymphatics and in draining lymph nodes suggested the possibility that LC constitute a circulating population of cells that participate in contact allergy reactions. To investigate the possibility that LC can acquire an antigen, Silberberg-Sinakin et al. [7] conducted studies with the antigen ferritin. Their findings indicate that LC may appropriate an antigen in the skin and from there circulate to draining lymph nodes, thus performing functions analogous to those of macrophages. These studies suggested that LC may thereby present antigens to lymphocytes in skin and lymph nodes.

Toews et al. [8] provided evidence that LC are essential for the induction of CH. These investigators used the tail skin of mice, which is relatively deficient in LC, and compared it with normal body wall skin and abdominal wall skin that was depleted of LC by a short course of ultraviolet (UV) light irradiation to evaluate their capacity to sustain sensitization. Normal body wall skin supported the induction of sensitization, whereas tail skin or UV-treated skin (skin deficient in LC) induced a state of unresponsiveness.

These studies were complemented by Streilein and Bergstresser [9], who studied the relationship between the distribution and function of LC within the epidermis of inbred Syrian hamsters and the capacity of cutaneous surfaces to promote the induction of CH to dinitrofluorobenzene (DNFB). Similar to previous findings, Streilein and Bergstresser observed that cutaneous surfaces deficient in normally functioning LC were inefficient at promoting DNFB sensitization. Instead, an allergen applied to these skin regions induced a state of antigen-specific unresponsiveness.

In 1985, Knight et al. [10] showed that the transfer of small numbers of dendritic cells (DC) from mice skin painted with TNCB and oxazalone induced CS in recipient mice. Experiments reported by Macatonia et al. [11] extended these earlier observations by showing that lymph node cells taken 24 h after skin painting with fluorescein isothiocyanate (FITC) are capable of inducing delayed-type hypersensitivity (DTH) reactions in recipient mice. Skin painting increased the number of DC in the draining lymph nodes, and the antigen was preferentially located on DC. These DC were found to induce proliferative responses of syngeneic lymph node cells. DC were therefore proposed to be the prime cells for the induction of CS. In a further study, Macatonia et al. [12] examined changes in the number and properties of cells isolated from lymph nodes from 30 min to 6 days after skin painting with FITC. They showed that, during a 3-day period after skin painting, the antigen is located preferentially on DC in draining lymph nodes and that these cells are able to stimulate T cell proliferation in vitro.

In a continuing study [13], the cells involved in the development of DTH were studied. In an early stage in the immune response, DTH could be transferred by antigen-bearing DC, initiating a DTH response. This early stage was distinguished from a later stage in which T cells transferred sensitization.

In 1990, Kripke et al. [14] showed that Ia^+, $F4/80^+$ cutaneous cells, some of which were LC, leave the skin after epicutaneous sensitization with FITC and participate in the induction of CS in the regional lymph nodes. Nude BALB/c mice were sensitized with FITC at the site of an allogeneic skin graft. It was observed that the antigen-bearing DC subsequently found within draining lymph nodes were of graft donor origin.

All these data conveyed convincing evidence that LC were activated in situ by haptens. It was our goal to better define the factors responsible for this activation and to characterize differences between irritant and allergic contact reactions.

Differential Induction of Cytokines by Allergens and Irritants

In addition to LC, the epidermis contains cells of different lineages such as keratinocytes, melanocytes, dendritic epidermal T cells in mice, and some Merkel cells. In inflammatory conditions, macrophages, T cells, and mast cells infiltrate the epidermis. All of these cells are capable of exerting autocrine, paracrine, and endocrine influences by secreting soluble protein factors termed cytokines. In fact, keratinocytes, which comprise the vast majority of epidermal cells in both human and mouse skin, are a rich source of cytokines. Keratinocytes have been shown to produce interleukin (IL)-1 [15, 16], IL-7 [17], IL-3, IL-6, IL-8, IL-10 [18], IL-12 [19], tumor necrosis factor (TNF)-α, and interferon (IFN)-induced protein-10 (IP-10) [18]. Most of these cytokines are not constitutively produced in vivo, but can be induced by a variety of stimuli, including inflammatory agents, UV irradiation, tumor-promoting agents, and several types of injury. According to Barker et al. [20], keratinocytes thereby "prepare" the skin for specific immunological activity.

Because cytokines can nonspecifically be induced by many stimuli, one of the remaining key questions was whether there is a difference in cytokine expression between CS and irritant dermatitis. Early evidence for a distinct regulation of LC activation by irritants and allergens was provided by studies carried out by Aiba and Katz [21], who investigated phenotypic and functional changes of in vivo-activated LC. The investigators harvested LC from the ear skin of naive mice painted with various haptens and primary irritants at various time points. After 24 h, staining of epidermal sheets from allergen-treated mice using anti-I-A antibodies showed an increase in LC size and a more intense staining for major histocompatibility complex (MHC) class II antigens. Microfluorimetric analysis revealed a two- to threefold increase in I-A and I-E expression in 22%–55% of all LC. Forty-eight to 72 h after hapten painting, the peak of enhanced class II-expressing cells decreased. This phenotypic change was only observed with haptens that served as allergens. Application of irritants or vehicle controls did not induce these changes. Functionally, LC obtained from allergen-treated mice induced a two- to fivefold increase in proliferation by allogeneic or syngeneic T cells [21]. Thus the observed changes in vivo correlated with the changes occurring in the in vitro culture described by Schuler and Steinman [22]. From these results, it was concluded that epicutaneous treatment of the skin with haptens results in an in vivo activation of LC. This activation therefore represents an essential step in hapten-specific sensitization. Interestingly, the application of a panel of irritants (10–20% phenol, 10–30% sodium lauryl sulfate, ethanol, 50–75% methyl-salicylate, or 10–20% benzalkonium) did not induce activation.

As a critical question, the factor or factors responsible for the hapten-induced changes still remained to be identified. Haptens could either directly affect LC by an as yet unknown mechanism or induce the expression of mediators or growth factors by one of the several types of epidermal cells. A study by Enk and Katz [23] addressed the early events that occur after hapten painting of the skin in nonsensitized mice to identify cytokine alterations that may be critical in the induction of CS. Because epidermal cells have the capacity to produce a wide variety of cytokines that are known to modulate LC function and induce inflammation, they determined the changes in epidermis-derived cytokine mRNA levels after hapten painting in murine epidermis. These data indicate that haptens that are capable of inducing allergic CS cause profound selective changes in the signal strength of the mRNA of several cytokines. It was found that only contact sensitizers such as TNCB, DNFB, or dinitrochlorobenzene (DNCB) upregulated IL-1β, IL-1α, macrophage inflammatory protein (MIP)-2, IP-10, and I-Aα mRNA. The earliest of the observed changes was an increase in signal strength of the mRNA signal of IL-1. This upregulation occurred as early as 15 min after hapten painting. Cell depletion assays showed that the IL-1 mRNA signal was almost entirely derived from epidermal LC. Upregulation of I-A mRNA, reaching strength peak at 18 h, was consistent with the previous findings of Aiba and Katz, who reported an upregulation of MHC class II signals at the protein level within 24 h of hapten application [21]. Our findings also showed an allergen-specific induction of the two polypeptides IP-10 and MIP-2. IP-10 has been reported to be produced by keratinocytes in DTH reactions [24] and to have chemotactic and mitogenic functions associated with inflammation and cell proliferation. Although there was no constitutive mRNA signal for IP-10 in the murine epidermis, signals were detectable 1 h after hapten painting and reached peak strength at 4 h after hapten application. MIP-2 has been shown to elicit a localized inflammatory response in mice and to have chemotactic activity [25–27]. Until then, only lipopolysaccharide-stimulated macrophages had been shown to produce MIP-2 [28]. Allergen-specific induction of MIP-2 reached peak strength 4 h after hapten treatment. Importantly, the application of vehicle, irritant, or tolerogen did not induce the cytokine mRNA upregulations described. A rather nonspecific pattern of upregulation was observed for the mRNA of TNF-α and INF-γ, because these cytokines were induced by allergens and irritants or tolerogens. Taken together, it was proven that a complex array of signals, not a single cytokine, characterized the induction phase of allergic contact dermatitis and that cytokines might serve as differentiating markers for allergic and irritant reactions.

Because the increase in IL-1β mRNA preceded the increases of IL-1β, IL-10, MIP-2, or IP-10 mRNA signals, we conducted further studies to determine whether IL-1β production might be causally linked to epicutaneous sensitization [29]. IL-1 was injected intradermally into the ears of mice, and total mRNA was extracted 4 h later. A quantitative reverse-transcriptase polymerase chain reaction (RT-PCR) technique was used to compare the changes in IL-1β, IL-1α, MIP-2, TNF-α, I-Aα, and IL-10 mRNA signals that were caused by intradermally injected IL-1β to the changes caused by intradermal TNF-α or IL-1α and topical application of allergen. Injection of IL-1β, but not IL-1α, caused changes in the epidermal cytokine pattern almost identical to those resulting from epicutaneous application of contact sensitizers. IL-1β injection even enhanced its own message, providing evidence for an autocrine activation of LC. Furthermore, injection of IL-1β resulted in a dramatic increase in MHC class II molecules on the surface of LC, a change in their morphology, and a decreased number of resident LC in the epidermis, suggesting a possible effect on LC migration in vivo.

In vitro treatment of LC-depleted epidermal cells with IL-1 almost exactly mimicked the changes induced by in vivo application of allergen, with the exception of missing LC-derived IL-1β and MHC class II I-Aα signals. Most interestingly, stimulation of keratinocyte monolayers with water-soluble allergen in the absence of LC (i.e., in the absence of IL-1) failed to induce the characteristic cytokine cascade of CS.

Functionally, LC derived from IL-1β-injected skin showed increased accessory capacity in -CD3 proliferation assays compared with LC derived from control-injected skin, thus demonstrating the functional activation of the cells by IL-1β in situ [30]. Until recently, CS was thought to be a mainly T-helper (Th)1-mediated immune response. In several recent reports, however, a role for $CD8^+$ T cells and MHC class I-mediated antigen presentation was shown, adding complexity to the system. Indeed, IFN-γ-producing $CD8^+$ T cells seem to be among the major mediators of CS, at least in the murine system.

Counterregulatory Cytokines in Contact Sensitivity

Thus far, only the proinflammatory effects of cytokines in contact dermatitis have been discussed. However, there is no immune reaction in the human body that does not need to be terminated to prevent harmful effects for the human body. Indeed, early indications in our initial studies suggested that there were counterregulatory mechanisms in allergic contact dermatitis as well. Our initial time-course experiments of the induction phase of CS indicated that certain cytokines (e.g., IFN-γ or IP-10) were rapidly induced by allergens (within 1.5–2 h after allergen application). However, it was also observed that this rapid induction was followed by an early downregulation (within 4–6 h of hapten painting) of IFN-γ and IP-10, although the inflammatory process was still ongoing. Therefore, it was tempting to speculate that counterregulatory cytokines such as IL-10 might be involved in this process. IL-10, the "cytokine synthesis inhibitory factor," was initially characterized by its ability to inhibit Th1 cytokine production, especially IFN-γ production [31, 32]. To achieve this effect, the presence of functional antigen-presenting cells such as macrophages or DC is needed [33].

These findings and earlier reports [34, 35], which show the preferential generation of Th2 (rather than Th1) hapten-specific $CD4^+$ T cells after stimulation of nonprimed T cells with hapten-modified LC, led us [18] to study the role of IL-10 in the induction of CS. Various chemicals were applied to murine skin, and signals for IL-10 were sought by quantitative RT-PCR at various time points. Although IL-10 mRNA signals were occasionally identified in untreated normal epidermis, they were reproducibly enhanced 4 h after hapten application and were maximal after 12 h. Again, the induction of IL-10 mRNA signals proved to be an allergen-specific event, because irritants or tolerogens did not induce IL-10 mRNA. Cellular depletion assays showed that keratinocytes were the main source of IL-10 mRNA. IL-10 protein was detected by immunoprecipitation with an anti-IL-10 monoclonal antibody of supernatants obtained 16 h after hapten coupling of epidermal cells. The finding that murine keratinocytes are able to produce enhanced amounts of IL-10 after hapten stimulation might be relevant for the final development of Th cells toward a Th2 phenotype. Thus IL-10 might somehow interfere with LC by altering their antigen-presenting functions, e.g., by blocking costimulatory signals, in a manner that favors the development of Th2 cells. It may also be that, through inhibition of IFN-γ, which is usually necessary for the development of Th1 cells, IL-10 inhibits Th1 cell development.

To answer these questions, we determined whether antigen-presenting functions of LC could be influenced by IL-10 [36]. Initial studies failed to show effects of IL-10 on MHC class II expression by LC or anti-CD3 monoclonal antibody- or alloantigen-induced, LC-dependent T cell proliferation. When the peptide-specific T cell clones AE7 (Th1) and D10.G4 (Th2) were substituted for unprimed T cells, differential effects of IL-10 on T cell proliferation were observed. Untreated and IL-10-pretreated LC supported Th2 cell proliferation equally well, and IL-10-pretreated LC were unable to induce Th1 cell proliferation. The inhibitory influence of IL-10 was observed when fresh or 1-day-cultured LC were used, and LC cultured for 2 or 3 days were influenced to a much lesser extent. These findings made it likely that the induction of some costimulatory molecule already expressed by cultured, but not by fresh LC was inhibited by IL-10. However, intact antigen presentation in the context of lacking costimulation should lead to T cell anergy. To test our hypothesis that IL-10-treated LC induce immunologic tolerance, classical tolerance experiments were performed. These experiments showed that IL-10-treated LC did indeed induce immunologic tolerance in Th1 cell clones. Thus IL-10 is capable of converting LC from potent inducers of T cell proliferation to tolerogenic antigen-presenting cells.

The finding that IL-10 is produced by cells within the epidermis on hapten stimulation and that IL-10 exerts significant influences on LC may have important implications. LC leaving the skin at early time points after hapten painting (i.e., when IL-1 is produced) might mature into very potent immunostimulatory cells and induce proliferation of Th1 cells in the regional lymph node. On the other hand, because IL-10 is induced relatively late in the hapten-specific cytokine cascade, LC that leave the skin at later time points might be converted to specifically tolerizing cells by IL-10. These cells may induce either T cell anergy in Th1 cells or induce proliferation of the "wrong" Th2 cells, thus limiting the number of specifically sensitized T cells. Furthermore, by abrogating IFN- and IL-2 production of Th1 cells, IL-10 might promote the outgrowth of Th2 cells, thus downregulating DTH reactions. To investigate whether IL-10 also serves the function of a tolerizing agent in vivo, mice were injected intradermally with recombinant murine IL-10 8 h before epicutaneous application of contact allergen (TNCB). As a control, mice were injected with IL-10 in the presence of neutralizing amounts of anti-IL-10 monoclonal antibody. Whereas control-treated mice showed a normal ear swelling response to epicutaneous challenge, the ear swelling response of IL-10-treated animals was significantly inhibited. Coinjection of the neutralizing α-IL-10 monoclonal antibody completely abrogated this effect. Resensitization of IL-10-pretreated mice after 14 days of rest and subsequent challenge 1 day later revealed a minimal response towards application of allergen. This induction of anergy was proved to be antigen specific. In an attempt to show the induction of antigen-specific tolerance in these mice in vitro, regional lymph nodes of mice initially treated with TNCB plus IL-10 and control-treated mice were prepared and restimulated in vitro with trinitrobenzene sulfonic acid (TNBS; a water-soluble analogue of TNCB) or control to measure antigen-specific proliferation. Lymph node cells from animals treated with TNCB plus IL-10 showed a significantly reduced proliferation toward TNBS compared with controls. To elucidate the mechanisms of action of IL-10, the epidermal cytokine pattern was analyzed on the mRNA level after the injection of IL-10 or control and application of allergen. Injection of IL-10, but not control, significantly impeded the induction of proinflammatory cytokines IL-1β, TNF-α, and IL-1α [37]. In aggregate, these data show that IL-10 also exerts tolerizing functions in vivo.

In addition to the above-mentioned reports on the immunoinhibitory effects of IL-10 during the induction of CS responses, recent reports have also dealt with the tolerizing effect of low doses of hapten. It was recently shown by Steinbrink and Macher that doses of allergen that were insufficient to cause sensitization resulted in the induction of specific unresponsiveness to a certain hapten. Obviously, these low allergen doses bypass sensitization by essentially being ignored by the skin immune system. This means that no measurable activation of epidermal LC or epidermal cytokines occurs. In contrast, the haptens seem to be drained to more central immunological compartments such as lymph nodes or spleen, where they induce T suppressor cells. These $CD8^+$ T_S cells are characterized by a Th2-type cytokine pattern (IL-4) [5, 10] and are therefore called T_S2 cells. This works demonstrates that low, epidermally applied doses of hapten exert tolerance-inducing capacities. This might reflect a mechanism that prevents sensitization in people that are frequently exposed to low doses of allergen, thereby avoiding easy sensitization.

Discussion

The experimental progress and the better understanding of the pathogenesis of CS reactions has led to a number of new diagnostic and therapeutic strategies.

In terms of diagnosis, the fact that LC specifically release IL-1β following the application of an allergen can be used as a screening assay for contact allergens. Thus far, the preparation of human LC has been extremely tedious and time-consuming and the number of cells generated usually too low to be used for test purposes. Fortunately, rather recently, culture systems for DC from human peripheral blood have been developed that allow for the generation of large numbers of DC [38]. These DC can now be exposed to potential contact allergens in culture. Afterwards, mRNA signals for IL-1β production can be determined as a marker for sensitization. This system might provide an easy test assay for contact allergens that would allow for the predictive testing of potential contact allergens.

The other novelty arising from the experiments outlined is a therapeutic one. Over the last 30 years, CS has mainly been treated with topical or systemic corticosteroids. However, the fact that DC and LC are important in the generation of allergic contact dermatitis, and the fact that their function can be modified with cytokines such as IL-10, opens up their use as therapeutic tools. As already mentioned, large numbers of DC can now be grown in an autologous system from the blood of patients. The DC grown from patients sensitized to a known hapten could then be exposed to IL-10, a cytokine known to inhibit the accessory functions of these cells. Furthermore, these "tolerizing" autologous DC would be pulsed with the respective hapten and reinfused into the patient. As DC are highly migratory, these "tolerizing" antigen-presenting cells would reach the appropriate T cell compartments easily. As they would attach to the hapten-specific T cells without being able to fully activate them due to their lack of costimulatory molecules, these DC might switch off an ongoing, hapten-specific immune response. Thus this therapy might serve as a hapten-specific hyposensitization strategy for type IV allergens. The possibility of using DC with this aim is currently being tested in our laboratory.

Summary

Allergic contact dermatitis is a frequent dermatological disorder with a high socioeconomic impact. Incidence rates in the general population range from 5% to 15%. As allergic contact dermatitis has subserved the function of a model for a primary immune response for a number of years now, the pathogenesis of the disease is comparatively well understood. It is known that contact allergens are usually reactive chemical structures called haptens that need to be coupled to protein structures in order to function as allergens and to be recognized by the immune system. These haptens bind to epidermal structures in a random fashion, thereby activating the immune cells of the epidermis, the antigen-presenting LC. These cells become activated, start to migrate to the regional lymph node, and induce hapten-specific T cells. These T cells then recirculate via blood and lymph to skin-associated tissues. Specifically sensitized T cells then induce the inflammatory infiltrate when the sensitizing hapten is again applied to the skin.

While new details concerning the pathogenesis of allergic contact dermatitis have been explored, the therapeutic principles have remained unchanged for the last 30 years. Corticosteroids either applied topically or given systemically are still the primary treatment option for allergic contact dermatitis. However, recent breakthroughs in the culture of DC and the understanding of ways to modify them functionally might soon introduce new therapeutic concepts in this field.

References

1. Landsteiner K, Chase M (1942) Experiments on transfer of cutaneous sensitivity to simple compounds. Proc Soc Exp Biol Med 49:688–690
2. Frey J, Wenk P (1957) Experimental studies on the pathogenesis of contact eczema in guinea pigs. Arch Allergy Appl Immunol 11:81–100
3. Macher E, Chase MW (1969) Studies on the sensitization of animals with simple chemical compounds. XII. The influence of excision of allergenic depots on onset of delayed hypersensitivity and tolerance. J Exp Med 129: 103–121
4. Silberberg I (1973) Apposition of mononuclear cells to Langerhans cells in contact allergic reactions. An ultrastructural study. Acta Derma Venereol (Stockh) 53:1–12
5. Silberberg I, Baer RL, Rosenthal SA et al (1975) Dermal and intravascular Langerhans cells at sites of passively induced allergic contact sensitivity. Cell Immunol 18:435–453
6. Silberberg I, Baer RL, Rosenthal SA (1974) The role of langerhans cells contact allergy. I. An ultrastructural study in actively induced contact dermatitis in guinea pigs. Acta Derm Venereol (Stockh) 54:321–331
7. Silberberg-Sinakin I, Thorbecke GJ, Baer RL et al (1976) Antigen-bearing Langerhans cells in skin, dermal lymphatics and in lymph nodes. Cell Immunol 25:137–151
8. Toews GB, Bergstresser PR, Streilein JW (1980) Epidermal Langerhans cells density determines whether contact hypersensitivity or unresponsiveness follows skin painting with DNFB. J Immunol 124:445–453
9. Streilein JW, Bergstresser PR (1981) Langerhans cell function dictates induction of contact hypersensitivity or unresponsiveness to DNFB in Syrian hamsters. J Invest Dermatol 77:272–277
10. Knight SC, Krejci J, Malkovsky M et al (1985) The role of dendritic cells in the initiation of immune responses to contact sensitizers. I. In vivo exposure to antigen. Cell Immunol 94:427–434
11. Macatonia SE, Edwards AJ, Knight SC (1986) Dendritic cells and the initiation of contact sensitivity to fluorescein isothiocyanate. Immunology 59:509–514
12. Macatonia SE, Knight SC, Edwards AJ et al (1987) Localization of antigen on lymph node dendritic cells after exposure to the contact sensitizer fluorescein isothiocyanate. Functional and morphological studies. J Exp Med 166:1654–1667

13. Macatonia S, Knight S (1989) Dendritic cells and T cells transfer sensitization for delayed-type hypersensitivity after skin painting with contact sensitizer. Immunology 66:96–99
14. Kripke ML, Munn CG, Jeevan A et al (1990) Evidence that cutaneous antigen-presenting cells migrate to regional lymph nodes during contact sensitization. J Immunol 145:2833–2838
15. Luger TA, Stadler BM, Katz SI et al (1981) Epidermal cell (keratinocyte)-derived thymocyte-activating factor (ETAF). J Immunol 127:1493–1498
16. Luger TA, Stadler BM, Luger BM et al (1983) Characteristics of an epidermal cell thymocyte-activating factor (ETAF) produced by human epidermal cells and a human squamous cell carcinoma cell line. J Invest Dermatol 81:187–193
17. Heufler C, Topar G, Grasseger A et al (1993) Interleukin 7 is produced by murine and human keratinocytes. J Exp Med 178:1109–1114
18. Enk AH, Katz SI (1992) Identification and induction of keratinocyte-derived IL-10. J Immunol 149:92–95
19. Müller G, Saloga J, Germann T et al (1994) Identification and induction of keratinocyte-derived IL-12. J Clin Invest 94:1799–1805
20. Barker JN, Mitra RS, Griffiths CE et al (1991) Keratinocytes as initiators of inflammation. Lancet 337:211–214
21. Aiba S, Katz SI (1990) Phenotypic and functional characteristics of in vivo-activated Langerhans cells. J Immunol 145:2791–2796
22. Schuler G, Steinman R (1984) Murine epidermal Langerhans cells mature into potent immunostimulatory dendritic cells in vitro. J Exp Med 161:526–546
23. Enk AH, Katz SI (1992) Early molecular events in the induction phase of contact sensitivity. Proc Natl Acad Sci USA 89:1398–1402
24. Kaplan G, Luster AD, Hancock G et al (1987) The expression of a gamma inteferon-induced protein (IP-10) in delayed immune responses in human skin. J Exp Med 166:1098–1108
25. Wolpe SD, Cerami A (1989) Macrophage inflammatory proteins 1 and 2: members of a novel superfamily of cytokines. FASEB J 3:2565–2573
26. Tekamp Olson P, Gallegos C, Bauer D et al (1990) Cloning and characterization of cDNAs for murine macrophage inflammatory protein 2 and its human homologues. J Exp Med 172: 911–919
27. Sherry B, Cerami A (1991) Small cytokine superfamily. Curr Opin Immunol 3:56–60
28. Wolpe SD, Sherry B, Juers D et al (1989) Identification and characterization of macrophage inflammatory protein 2. Proc Natl Acad Sci USA 86:612–616
29. Enk AH, Angeloni VL, Udey MC et al (1993) An essential role for Langerhans cell-derived IL-1 beta in the initiation of primary immune response in skin. J Immunol 150:3698–2704
30. Zubiaga AM, Munoz E, Huber BT (1991) Production of IL-1 alpha by activated Th type 2 cells. Its role as an autocrine growth factor. J Immunol 146:3849–3856
31. Fiorentino DF, Bond MW, Mosmann TR (1989) Two types of mouse T helper cell. IV. Th2 clones secrete a factor that inhibits cytokine production by Th1 clones. J Exp Med 170:2081–2095
32. Fernandez Botran R, Sanders VM, Mosmann TR et al (1988) Lymphokine-mediated regulation of the proliferative response of clones of T helper 1 and T helper 2 cells. J Exp Med 168:543–558
33. Fiorentino DF, Zlotnik A, Vieira P et al (1991) IL-10 acts on the antigen-presenting cell to inhibit cytokine production by Th1 cells. J Immunol 146:3444–3451
34. Hauser C, Katz SI (1988) Activation and expansion of hapten- and protein-specific T helper cells from nonsensitized mice. Proc Natl Acad Sci USA 85:5625–5628
35. Hauser C, Yokoyama WM, Katz SI (1989) Characterization of primary T helper cell activation and T helper cell lines stimulated by hapten-modified, cultured Langerhans cells. J Invest Dermatol 93:649–655
36. Enk AH, Angeloni VL, Udey MC et al (1993) Inhibition of Langerhans cell antigen-presenting function by IL-10. A role for IL-10 in induction of tolerance. J Immunol 151:2390–2398
37. Enk AH, Saloga, J, Becker D et al (1994) Induction of hapten-specific tolerance by IL-10 in vivo. J Exp Med 179:1397–1402
38. Romani N, Gruner S, Brang D et al (1994) Proliferating dendritic cell progenitors in human blood. J Exp Med 180:83–88

Pyoderma Gangrenosum

P. Schmid-Grendelmeier

Introduction

Pyoderma gangrenosum (PG) is a relatively rare, chronic, ulcerative skin condition, sometimes idiopathic, but often associated with underlying systemic disease. First described by Brunsting et al. 60 years ago [1], this ulcerating skin disease was called "pyoderma gangraenosum," because the authors thought that streptococcal infection was the main component leading to secondary cutaneous gangrene. Later, this was shown to be not relevant, although the cause of PG remains obscure in many cases. Many other associated conditions have been reported, e.g., inflammatory bowel disease (IBD; particularly colitis ulcerosa), arthritis, paraproteinemias, and myeloproliferative disorders. Clinical and histological overlap with other neutrophilic skin diseases such as Sweet's syndrome, subcorneal pustular dermatosis Sneddon-Wilkinson disease, and erythema elevatum have been described [2].

PG is now divided into four different variants: ulcerative, pustular, bullous, and vegetative type [3]. These types differ not only in their clinical and histological appearance, but also in diseases that are often associated with them. Ulcerative PG is the most frequent and most aggressive type and seems often to be associated with chronic IBD, arthritis, and monoclonal gammopathy. Pustular PG is more frequently seen with acute IBD and can progress to the ulcerative form. Bullous PG is often associated with myeloproliferative disorders. Vegetative PG is a less aggressive, superficial variant, frequently without associated systemic disease.

Diagnosis is based primarily on clinical features, because there are no specific histopathological findings. Nevertheless, a skin biopsy should be performed in suspected PG to provide additional support for the diagnosis and to exclude other clinically similar ulcerative diseases, such as granulomatous, infectious, or vascular ulcers.

The pathogenesis of PG has not yet been fully elucidated. There is no doubt that an inflammatory process takes place, but the causative agents are unclear. Skin hyperreactivity to external or internal agents as well as a local or systemic defective immune system have been suggested [3]. The use of therapeutic agents is therefore sometimes based on their antimicrobial activity, but even more so on their immunosuppressive and anti-inflammatory properties. Thus PG is open to many different forms of immunosuppressive or immunomodulative intervention as treatment. This chapter summarizes the variety of approaches in PG treatment, with special emphasis on established methods and preliminary immunointervention.

Management

The management of PG is based on general measures, both topical and systemic therapy, the latter being necessary in most cases. In this chapter, emphasis is placed on systemic therapy, in which immunosuppressive intervention has an important role. Nevertheless, general measures and topical treatment are also discussed briefly, because only by considering these measures as well can optimal treatment of patients with PG be achieved.

General Measures and Investigations

A correct diagnosis of PG is critical, as other similar diseases such as venous ulcers or infectious diseases need completely different therapy. PG is often associated with underlying systemic disease; therefore, an appropriate general approach and search for internal diseases should be performed. Most patients with severe PG require hospitalization to establish the diagnosis, perform the necessary investigations, and initiate appropriate therapy.

A skin biopsy should always be obtained, combined with different stains and cultures for different infectious agents. The necessity of establishing a correct diagnosis outweighs the risk of precipitating new lesions as a pathergic reaction to the trauma.

Laboratory investigations, including serum protein electrophoresis, immunoelectrophoresis, and screening for syphilis, human immunodeficiency virus (HIV), hepatitis, and antiphospholipid antibodies should be performed. In addition, chest radiography and an appropriate investigation of the gastrointestinal tract should be carried out in the case of suspected IBD [3–5].

Local Therapy

Most patients with PG require systemic immunosuppressive treatment, but in some uncomplicated or early cases, local therapy may be sufficient. In other patients, local therapy can help to relieve pain or to allow doses of systemic agents to be reduced.

Nonspecific local measures can be used to treat and prevent secondary bacterial infection and to accelerate wound healing. Thus measures used in other ulcers such as daily cleaning with antiseptic solutions and the use of wet compresses or hydrocolloid dressings are also worthwhile in PG.

Skin grafting in PG is often unsuccessful and can provoke new PG lesions at the donor site. Long et al. [6] recommend skin grafting only with concomitant use of immunosuppressive agents and when PG activity is low. Furthermore, the use of subcutaneous sutures should be used to avoid puncture of the skin surface. Following these precautions, we were able to perform skin grafting successfully in a 73-year-old woman with two large PG on the lower limbs; we administered 30 mg prednisolone and 100 mg cyclosporine A (CyA; 3 mg/kg body weight per day), and the patient did not develop any new lesions either at the recipient or at the donor site for over 2 years.

Specific topical treatments for PG include the use of topical or intralesional corticosteroids and sodium cromoglycate. Only a few reports about effective therapy with topical corticosteroids exist [7]. However, intralesional use seems to be more successful, as described in some earlier reports [8, 9], at least as an adjunctive therapy [10]. Others only obtained similarly good results using intralesional steroids in mild cases [3]. For successful treatment, repeated injections at multiple sites at the border of the lesion have to be given at regular intervals of a few days to up to several weeks.

Another interesting topical treatment consists in application of sodium cromoglycate in a 1% or 2% solution, especially with occlusive dressing [11]. Tamir et al. [12] described five patients with PG (four of which also received systemic steroids, 60 mg/day); an initial improvement 3–7 days after sodium cromoglycate application and complete healing of the ulcers between 5 and 8 weeks occurred. The authors conclude that topical sodium cromoglycate can be effective as adjunctive or sole treatment in PG. The mode of action of sodium cromoglycate in PG remains unclear. Theories range from inhibition of mast cell degranulation or response to platelet-activating factor and decreased inflammatory response mediated by suppression of chemotaxis to neutrophils and eosinophils. As sodium cromoglycate has also been described as being helpful in chronic, uncomplicated leg ulcers, there might also be a nonspecific wound-healing effect.

Only isolated reports exist about the use of other topical agents, such as amino salicylic acid, nitrogen mustard, and more recently CyA [13].

Another topical, though not pharmacological therapy approach in PG is the use of hyperbaric oxygen. Its effectiveness has been described by several authors [14, 15]. The main benefit of hyperbaric oxygen consists in rapid relief of pain, beginning almost immediately after administration [14].

Systemic Therapy

Systemic therapy is the most commonly used treatment in PG patients. It can be a single drug or, in many cases, a combination of various drugs. Most of these drugs have an immunomodulatory or even immunosuppressive action. Among the most important are systemic corticosteroids and immunosuppressives such as azathioprine, chlorambucil, and cyclophosphamide. In recent years, CyA has shown very promising results. Diaminophenylsulfone (DDS, dapsone) and clofazimine have an antibacterial effect, but also their mode of action in PG seems to be largely related to their effect on inflammatory cells rather than to their antibacterial activity. Other modalities have been tried in several cases, such as plasmapheresis [4], intravenous immunoglobulins [16], and interferons [17].

Another aspect of treatment of PG is the adequate management of an underlying systemic disease. Controlling this systemic disease can lead to healing of the secondary PG and can improve the success of the treatment for PG with all other agents used.

Corticosteroids

Corticosteroids such as prednisone are considered to be consistently successful agents in the treatment of PG. In patients resistant to local therapy, they are particularly effective in treating the acute, rapidly progressive form of the disease. Multiple reports attest their efficacy [3–5, 18–22]. The beneficial effects of corticosteroids are not entirely clear. Immunosuppressive, anti-inflammatory, and other mechanisms are being discussed [20].

It is important to control the disease quickly; so substantial dosages (40–120 mg daily, approximately 1 mg/kg) at the initiation of therapy are preferable. Gradual increases or smaller doses do not fully control the eruption of disease. Absence of pain, reduction of erythema, and reduction of granulation at the base of the ulcer indicate disease control. If the disease is controlled, the dose of the corticosteroids can be reduced slowly. Too rapid a decrease (> 10 mg/week) may result in severe recurrence, and prolonged low-dose maintenance therapy is therefore sometimes required [3]. Adding another agent such as sulfapyridine or dapsone when the steroid is withdrawn can maintain the improvement and reduce the complications of prolonged steroid therapy [18].

Intravenous "high-dose pulse steroid therapy" can produce rapid improvement in lesions previously unresponsive to oral corticosteroids. Such a treatment normally consists of 1000 mg methylprednisolone in 150 ml of 5% dextrose given once daily for 1–5 days. A rapid decrease in pain and inflammation with fewer side effects than oral therapy can be observed [21, 22]. However, pulse therapy must always be administered in a hospital with cardiac monitoring during and 24 h after infusions in order to prevent serious complications due to electrolyte shifts with subsequent cardiac arrhythmia.

Cyclosporine

CyA has shown the most promise in the management of PG. In 1985, Curely et al [23] described the patient with idiopathic PG who responded to CyA therapy. The initial dose was 10 mg/kg per day, and the ulcers started to heal 3 weeks later. A relapse was observed with a dosage below 3 mg/kg, but went into remission again with 4 mg/day. Since then, many other authors have described the use of CyA to treat PG, mostly in combination with oral corticosteroids [23–27]. Chow and Ho [4] summarized results of over 40 patients treated with CyA reported so far. CyA is effective in treating severe and or refractory PG, regardless of the associated disease. Only four of the reported 41 patients showed no response to CyA. Almost all of these cases had been chronic and refractory to high doses of corticosteroids, and in many of them to other drugs such as dapsone, azathioprine, minocycline, pulse methylprednisolone, and cyclophosphamide.

An initial dose of 4.5–7.5 mg/kg per day is usually recommend. Recent studies use doses lower than 6 mg/kg per day without a significant loss of efficacy compared to the higher doses in earlier studies. Response typically starts within 1–3 weeks, with complete healing within 1–7 months. In the maintenance period, CyA can be reduced to as low as 1.5–3 mg/kg after successful initiation of response. Healing can be observed up to 12–36 months after the end of CyA therapy, and relapses reported after successful CyA therapy are rare. In the case of PG relapse, there was usually a good response to CyA when started again. The combination with CyA allows reduction of oral corticosteroids at daily doses of lower than 10 mg/day. This can minimize the side effects of long-term corticosteroids significantly.

CyA influences the early events in antigenic activation by blocking the synthesis and or release of interleukin (IL)-1 from monocytes and IL-2 from activated T-helper (Th) cells [28]. CyA does not cause significant myelosuppression [29]. Nevertheless, CyA also has potentially serious side effects. These include nephrotoxicity, hypertension, electrolyte changes, and increased risk of malignancy, hepatotoxicity, neurotoxicity, and minor-risk hypertrichosis and hyperplasia of the gingiva [30]. However, because the majority of patients achieve remission with low doses of CyA (< 5 mg/kg per day), side effects of CyA in PG patients are usually mild and transient.

Because of concomitant systemic diseases requiring potent systemic drugs, it is of great importance to know about possible interactions of these drugs with CyA. Thus the efficacy of CyA is increased by imidazoles, macrolide antibiotics, tetracyclines, oral contraceptives, and antihistaminics and reduced by anticonvulsants, tuberculostatics, and sulfonamides. Furthermore, the parallel use of potentially nephrotoxic drugs such as aminoglycosides, nonsteroidal anti-inflammatory drugs (NSAID), acyclovir, or sulfonamide has to be handled with caution.

FK 506 (Tacrolimus)

FK 506 is a novel macrolide antibiotic that has immunosuppressive properties similar to CyA but is more potent [28,29]. Nine patients with PG have been treated with FK 506 with very encouraging results [31]. FK 506 was given twice daily (0.15 mg/kg), and steroid therapy was tapered or discontinued. Except for one (noncompliant) patient, all had complete and durable responses. The adverse effects of FK 506 in long-term use are nephrotoxicity, neurotoxicity, and diabetes mellitus, but these may be reduced by short-term therapy as necessary in PG [32]. To our knowledge, two other drugs with similar activities, rapamycin and leflunomide, have not been described so far for treatment of PG.

Immunosuppressants

Immunosuppressants can be used in patients with PG when systemic corticosteroids are unsuccessful or have intolerable side effects. Because of their severe adverse effects, especially bone marrow suppression, these agents should be reserved for severe or refractory cases.

Azathioprine/Mercaptopurine

Azathioprine, a purine analogue, is the most frequently used immunosuppressive drug for treating PG. The use of azathioprine for the treatment of PG has produced controversial results, as it is effective only in some of the cases reported by Chow and Ho [4]. It is normally used at a dosage of 100–150 mg per day, alone or in combination with systemic corticosteroids. Azathioprine is a slow-acting drug, and a therapeutic or steroid-sparing effect cannot be expected before 6–8 or even 12 weeks [33].

The most severe adverse effect is dose-related, and sometimes delayed, bone marrow suppression leading to leukopenia and thrombocytopenia. Other complications include opportunistic infections, hepatotoxicity, and an increased risk of neoplasias. Mercaptopurine, the active metabolite of azathioprine, has also been reported to be effective in PG patients, but side effects are more frequent.

Alkylating Agents

Some reports exist about the use of alkylating agents in patients with PG. All the used drugs (cyclophsophamide, mephalan, and chlorambucil) are effective by blocking DNA replication, and all have a predictable myelosuppressive effect, which is the dose-limiting side-effect [33].

Cyclophosphamide, one of the most cytotoxic and immunosuppresssive agents, was reported to be effective in a few cases, but failure of treatment has also been documented [4]. In the cases of successful treatment, cyclophosphamide was used at dosages of between 100 and 150 mg/day for 3–5 months in combination with corticosteroids after failures with other treatments (e.g., dapsone, plasma exchange). In these cases, the drugs were finally withdrawn without relapses. Zonana-Nacach et al. recently reported two PG patients treated with several high-dose pulses of cyclophosphamide (500 mg/m^2) with oral prednisone over a few weeks [34]. Both patients showed rapid healing and no relapses for 24 and 36 months, respectively.

Although these results are good, the serious adverse effects of cyclophosphamide [33] have to be considered: myelosuppression with leukopenia after 10–14 days after beginning therapy, severe hemorrhagic cystitis, risk of malignancy, and other risks such as hepatotoxicity, cardiotoxicity, and aphthous ulcers.

Chlorambucil and mephalan have also been reported in a few patients [35, 36]. Here, too, the main adverse effect is myelosuppression with neutropenia, which can make cessation of treatment necessary.

Antimicrobial Agents

Antimicrobial agents are widely used to treat PG, mostly in combination with corticosteroids or other immunosuppressive agents. As their efficacy in PG is mostly due to an immunosuppressive than an antimicrobial effect, they are also summarized here.

Diaminodiphenylsulfone (Dapsone)

Dapsone is of considerable benefit in PG. It is usually used in combination with oral or intravenous pulse steroids in dosages of 100–200 mg daily [37]. Its mechanism of action is not fully understood, but it is thought that it exerts its effect via modulation of the inflammatory response rather than by an antibacterial effect. Sulfones inhibit the myeloperoxidase-H_2O_2-mediated cytotoxic system in polymorphonuclear leukocytes and are also effective in many other disorders characterized by intense neutrophilic infiltration. The main side effects are hemolysis, particularly in patients with glucose-6-phosphate dehydrogenase deficiency and other hematological disorders.

Clofazimine

Clofazimine, a phendimetrazine tartarate, is used mainly in the treatment of leprosy and other mycobacterial diseases. It has also been used successfully in PG and was first described by Michaelssson et al. [38]. These authors treated eight patients with 300 or 400 mg/day and noted improvement within 1–2 weeks and healing in 1–4 months. Ryan [5] recommends the use of 200–400 mg/day to control the disease. Other authors observed no response or only short improvement with clofazimine [39].

The mode of action of clofazimine is also thought to be associated more with its effect on inflammatory cells than with its antibacterial activity. Side effects are rare and include possible exacerbation of an underlying Crohn's disease and discoloration of the skin (orange-red) and bowel (orange-black).

Minocycline

Other antimicrobacterial agents such as vancomycin, meclocillin [3, 4], and especially tetracyclines have also been reported to be effective in the treatment of PG . Most experience exists with minocycline, usually given in a dose of 200–300 mg. In the literature, favorable reports about 15 patients treated with minocycline exist. The effects seem to be due to the anti-inflammatory activity of the tetracyclines [4]. Minocycline is reported to be especially useful in subacute or uncomplicated cases [40]. Although partial or complete healing can be observed, relapses are frequent when minocycline is reduced or discontinued.

Discussion

The treatment of PG remains a challenge. As the origin and pathogenesis of PG is not yet fully understood, a specific therapeutic agent is still lacking. The diversity of therapeutic modalities with different modes of actions reflects the lack of a specific, highly effective therapeutic agent. Except for the treatment of PG with corticosteroids, only reports of isolated cases can be found. Despite the many reports, no randomized controlled studies in the treatment of PG exist to compare the different described and suggested modalities. Nevertheless, some conclusions can be drawn from the various treatments of PG.

In an initial step, other diagnoses should always be excluded. A biopsy, although not specific for PG, should support the clinical picture of PG. It is of the greatest importance to discover any underlying disease, which, if present, should be treated, which can help to heal the associated PG. Therefore, careful evaluation of skin and internal conditions before diagnosis and treatment is critical.

For mild or early cases, topical treatment can be sufficient. However, in most cases systemic therapy is required. Nevertheless, topical treatment can help to induce pain relief, prevent bacterial infection, or allow doses of systemic drugs to be reduced.

Nonspecific ulcer treatment is worthwile in all PG patients. Of the different specific topical treatments, intralesional corticosteroids and the application of topical sodium cromoglycate have been reported to be effective in a number of cases. Treatment with topical sodium cromoglycate entails no severe adverse effects and is therefore a worthwhile topical treatment in addition to systemic therapy. Hyperbaric oxygen in PG seems to be especially helpful to induce pain relief.

The cornerstone of treatment of any severe and refractory PG remains systemic therapy. Systemic corticosteroids are the mainstay in all patients resistant to local therapy or with aggressive disease. With a few exceptions, corticosteroids form part of the treatment regimen in most of the cases reported – used as a single drug or in combination with various other agents. To obtain rapid control of the disease, initiation of therapy with high dosages (about 1 mg/kg) is necessary. In addition, high-dose pulse therapy with corticosteroids can shorten the course of PG. After the ulcer has improved, corticosteroids can be tapered, but in most cases maintenance therapy at lower doses for some months is required.

If corticosteroids alone are not effective or have unacceptable side effects, various additional drugs such as dapsone, clofazimine, minocycline, alkylating agents, and other immunosuppressive substances can be used, as has been reported.

Of all these agents, CyA and, as preliminary data show, FK 506 seem to be the most promising. These drugs permit substantial reduction of the corticosteroid dose required. Furthermore, short-term treatment with these drugs can induce long-term remission. Other similar drugs, such as leflunomide or rapamycin, with less adverse effects than CyA but a comparable mechanism of action could also play a role in treating PG in the future. Other immunosuppressants, such as azathioprine, are effective only after prolonged use; others, such as the alkylating substances, have severe and sometimes life-threatening and hence limiting adverse effects. These drugs should be used only in cases of very recalcitrant PG or pronounced adverse effects due to corticosteroids. As additional drugs, dapsone, clofazimine, and minocycline have been reported to be quite effective at doses causing very few adverse effects. Plasma exchange or hyperbaric oxygen may also be useful in some cases.

Thus treatment of PG remains a dermatological challenge. Diagnosis and treatment of potential underlying systemic diseases is critical and requires an interdisciplinary medical approach. The mainstay of therapy consists in systemic corticosteroids in sufficiently high doses and long-term treatment periods. Various other drugs can be added to reduce corticosteroid doses; of these, especially immunosuppressants such as CyA and its recently developed derivatives seem to be very promising, as prolonged remission can be achieved.

Summary

PG is a chronic, ulcerative skin condition often associated with underlying systemic disease. The pathogenesis has not yet been fully elucidated, and treatment of PG remains a challenge.

This chapter summarizes the variety of therapeutic approaches in PG. General measures and local and systemic therapy are reviewed. Special emphasis is placed on treatment with immunosuppressive agents such as corticosteroids, CyA, and alkylating drugs. Mode of action, recommended doses, and adverse effects of these drugs in the treatment of PG are listed and discussed to permit the appropriate choice of agent.

References

1. Brunsting LA, Goeckerman WH, O'Leary PA (1930) Pyoderma gangraenosum: clinical and experimental observations in five cases occurring in adults. Arch Dermatol 22:655–680
2. Vignon-Pnenamen MD, Walch D (1991) Cutaneous manifestations of neutrophilic disease: a study of seven cases. Dermatologica 183:255–264
3. Powell FC, Su WPD, Perry HO (1996) Pyoderma gangrenosum: classificiation and management. J Am Acad Dermatol 34:395–409
4. Chow RKP, Ho VC (1996) Treatment of pyoderma gangrenosum. J Am Acad Dermatol 34: 1047–1060
5. Ryan TJ (1992) Pyoderma gangrensosum. In: Rook, Wikinson, Elbling (eds) Textbook of dermatology, 5th edn. Blackwell Scientific, Oxford
6. Long CC, Jessop J, Young M (1992) Minimizing the risk of post-operative pyoderma gangrenosum. Br J Dermatol 127:45–48

7. Ko CB, Walton S, Wyatt EH (1992) Pyoderma gangrenosum: associations revisited. Int J Dermatol 31:574–577
8. Gardener LW, Acker DW (1972) Triamcinolone and pyoderma gangrenosum. Arch Dermatol 106:559–560
9. Jennings JL (1983) Pyoderma gangrenosum: successful treatment with intralesional steroids. J Am Acad Dermatol 9:575–578
10. Duffill MB (1994) Cyclosporine, azathioprine and local therapy for pyoderma gangrenosum. Aust J Dermatol 35:15–18
11. Smith KC, Su WPD, Leiferman KU (1987) Cromolyn sodium in 2% aqueous solution under an occlusive hydrocolloid dressing may be effective adjunctive treatment in management of pyoderma gangrensoum. J Am Acad Dermatol 17:509–511
12. Tamir A, Landau M, Brenner S (1996) Topical treatment with 1% sodium cromo-glycate in pyoderma gangrenosum. Dermatology 192:252–254
13. Mrowietz U, Chrsitophers E (1990) Clearing of pyoderma gangrenosum by intralesional cyclosporine A. Br J Dermatol 123:389–393
14. Davis JC, Landeen JM, Levine RA (1987) Pyoderma gangrenosum: skin grafting after preparation with hyperbaric oxygen. Plast Reconst Surg 79:200–206
15. Wasserteil V, Bruce S, Sessoms SL et al (1992) Pyoderma gangrenosum treated with hyperbaric oxygen therapy. Int J Dermatol 31:594–596
16. Gupta AK, Shear NH, Sauder DN (1995) Efficacy of human intraevenous immune globulin in pyoderma gangrenosum. J Am Acad Dermatol 32:140–142
17. Smith JB, Shenefelt PD, Soto O et al (1996) Pyoderma gangrenosum in a patient with cryoglobulinemia and hepatitis C successfully treated with interferon alfa. J Am Acad Dermatol 34:901–903
18. Perry HO (1982) Pyoderma gangrenosum. Aust J Dermatol 23:53–61
19. Lebbé C, Moulonguet-Michau I, Perrin P et al (1992) Steroid-responsive pyoderma gangrenosum with vulvar and pulmonary involvement. J Am Acad Dermatol 27:623–625
20. Norris DA, Weston WL, Thorne EG et al (1978) Pyoderma gangrenosum: abnormal monocyte function corrected in vitro with hydrocortisone. Arch Dermatol 114:906–911
21. Johnson RB, Lazarus GS (1982) Pulse therapy: therapeutic efficacy in the treatment of pyoderma gangrenosum. Arch Dermatol 118:76–84
22. Pinto GM, Cabecas MA, Riscado M et al (1991) Pyoderma gangrenosum associated with systemic lupus erythematosus: response to pulse steroid therapy. J Am Acad Dermatol 24:818–821
23. Curley RK, MacFarlane AW, Vickers CFH (1985) Pyoderma gangrenosum treated with cyclosporine A. Br J Dermatol 113:601–604
24. Shelley ED, Shelley WB (1988) Cyclosporine therapy for pyoderma gangrenosum associated with sclerosing cholangitis and ulcerative colitis. J Am Acad Dermatol 18:1084–1088
25. Elgart G, Stover P. Larson K et al (1991) Treatment of pyoderma gangrenosum with cyclosporine: results in seven patients. J Am Acad Dermatol 24:83–86
26. Matis J (1992) Cyclosporine A and pyoderma gangrenosums. Arch Dermatol 128:1060–1066
27. Zumdick M, Schuppe HC, Goerz G (1993) Cyclosporine A therapy in pyoderma gangrenosum. Hautarzt 44:306–308
28. Schreiber SL, Crabtree GR (1992) The mechanism of action of cyclosporine A and FK 506. Immunol Today 13:136–142
29. Johansson A, Moller E (1990) Evidence that the immunosupressive effects of FK 506 and cyclosporine are identical. Transplantation 50:1001–1007
30. Fradin MS, Ellis CN, Voorhees JJ (1990) Managment of patients and side effects during cyclosporine therapy for cutaneous disorders. J Am Acad Dermatol 23:1265–1275
31. Abu-Elmagel K, Van Thiel DH, Jegasothy BV et al (1993) Resolution of severe pyoderma gangrenosum in a patient with streaking leokocyte factor disease after treatment with tacrolimus (FK 506). Ann Intern Med 119:595–598
32. Fung JJ, Alessiani M, Abu-Elmagd K et al (1991) Adverse effects associated with the use of FK 506. Transplant Proc 23:3105–3108
33. Rapini RP (1991) Cytotoxic drugs in the treatment of skin diseases. Int J Dermatol 30:313–322

34. Zonana-Nacach A, Jimenez-Balderas FJ et al (1994) Intravenous cyclo-phosphamides pulses in the treatment of pyoderma gangrenosum associated with rheumatoid arthritis: report of 2 cases and review of the literature. J Rheumatol 21:1352–1356
35. Resnik BI, Rendon M, Kerdel FA (1992) Successful treatment of aggressive pyoderma gangrenosum with pulse steroids and chlorambucil. J Am Acad Dermatol 27:635–636
36. Jones RR, Black AK, Donaghy M et al (1983) Defective monocyte function in pyoderma gangrenosum with IgG kappa paraproteinemia. Clin Exp Immunol 52:685–692
37. Galun E, Flugelman MY, Rachmilewitz D (1986) Pyoderma gangrenosum complicating ulcerative colitis: successful treatment with methylprednisolone pulse therapy and dapsone. Am J Gastroenterol 81:988–989
38. Michaelsssson G, Molin L, Oehman S et al (1976) Clofazimine: a new agent for the treatment of pyoderma. Arch Dermatol 112:344–349
39. Kaplan B, Trau H, Sofer E et al (1992) Treatment of pyoderma gangrenosum with clofazimine. Int J Dermatol 31:591–593
40. Berth-Jones, Tan SV, Graham RAC et al (1989) The successful use of minocycline in pyoderma gangrenosum in a report of seven cases and a review of the literature. J Dermatol 1:23–25

Viral Infections: Human Papillomavirus Infections Treated with Immunostimulatory Drugs and Vaccination Therapies

G. Gross

Introduction

During the last decade, herpesviruses have become effectively treated using acyclovir and its prodrug valaciclovir as well as penciclovir and its prodrug famciclovir. Similarly, antiretroviral drugs which inhibit the viral RNA-directed DNA polymerase and reverse transcriptase, such as zidovudine and dideoxyinosine, have recently been developed.

Development of antiviral compounds against human papillomaviruses (HPV), however, is extremely difficult, because only few enzymes are encoded by HPV and none of them are kinases, polymerases, or proteases which could act as targets for already established antiviral substances [1]. Because papillomaviruses are highly dependent on normal cellular enzymes to complete the virus life-cycle, there is a potential risk for a substantial host cell toxicity from agents active against HPV DNA replication and expression.

Available therapies for symptomatic HPV disease are directed toward destruction or excision of the infected tissue. Such methods comprise cytodestructive and cytotoxic substances such as podophyllin, podophyllotoxin, 5-fluorouracil, and trichloroacetic acid, as well as surgical methods including cryotherapy, electrosurgery, and laser surgery. Some of these methods are either expensive or painful, and all are associated with an extremely high recurrence rate of up to 80% [2–4]. No effective antiviral chemotherapeutic agent is currently available for HPV infections.

Unlike infection with other human pathogenic viruses such as human immunodeficiency virus (HIV), cytomegalovirus, and hepatitis B and C virus, infection with HPV is usually focal and develops on more or less accessible cutaneous or mucosal surfaces. Infection may occur through a small break in the epidermis. It can take months before a wart develops, and up to 90% of HPV infections have no clinically visible manifestation but remain subclinical or even latent [5]. In the latter case, the viral DNA persists silently in the basal or germinative layer cells of the epidermis, probably at an extrachromosomal level. No concise information exists on the trigger mechanisms that finally induce wart formation.

Skin warts tend to regress spontaneously. In about 70% of subjects with cutaneous warts, the warts disappear without therapy within 2 years [6]. Sometimes warts persist for decades. Mechanisms of persistence and of spontaneous regression are poorly understood. In many instances, however, warts regress simultaneously at multiple sites, suggesting a systemic immune response [7]. Many lines of evidence suggest that cellular rather than humoral immune mechanisms are of primary importance for regression of papillomavirus-induced lesions. The substantial increase in the incidence of warts and squamous cell carcinoma noted in immunosuppressed patients such as renal transplant recipients and HIV-infected patients is also indicative of a cell-mediated immune mechanism involved in wart regression [8]. Furthermore, patients with established warts have a depressed cellular immune system [9]. Patients suffering from epidermodysplasia verruciformis (EV), a rare syndrome with a congenital deficiency of the cellular immune system, have a life-long increased incidence of disseminated warts and flat, wart-like lesions [10]. It is well understood that mechanisms that account for tumor rejection and immune surveillance are impaired in these populations, leading to an enhanced susceptibility to disseminated benign wart disease and a higher probability for progression to malignancy [11]. The presence of HPV-16 or HPV-18 in cervical intraepithelial neoplasia (CIN) correlates with a decreased number of Langerhans cells [12]. HPV infections are found nine times more often among renal transplant recipients than in the general population [13], and these patients also have an increased incidence of CIN lesions [11]. Decreased numbers of $CD4^+$ cells are observed in CIN lesions [14], and patients with HPV carrying CIN or cervical cancer have decreased natural killer (NK) cell activity [15]. Cervical cancer is associated with certain major histocompatibility complex (MHC) class II alleles [16]. Complete loss of MHC class I expression is found in about 15% of tumors, and a further 20% of tumors exhibit a partial loss of class I alleles [17]. Under normal circumstances, infected subjects have effective mechanisms for the immunologic elimination of virus-infected cells. If spontaneous regression of viral warts occurs, acute inflammation is often prominent, with infiltration of T cells and macrophages promoting local cytodestruction of infected keratinocytes [7]. Identification of the viral antigens which participate in immune rejection might lead to the developement of clinically useful, epitope-specific immunostimulatory therapies to promote systemic rejection of infected tissue. Some evidence suggests that persistent papillomavirus-induced lesions are deficient for antigen presentation, partly because of a reduced number of Langerhans cells [12] or downregulation of MHC expression [17–21]. Alternatively, immunologic unresponsiveness may be due to presentation of viral antigens in tolerogenic form on infected keratinocytes or to the induction of a focal T cell suppression [22].

Immunotherapies

Stimulation of the immune system has long been an appealing therapeutic approach for cutaneous and mucosal warts. Reagents such as autogenous vaccines, levamisole, dinitrochlorobenzene (DNCB), and bacillus Calmette-Guérin (BCG) have been used, but with very limited success.

In contrast to most of the established therapies which are defined only by the method used to most effectively eliminate the infected tissue rather than by biologic or pharmacologic inhibition of virus replication, immunomodulatory compounds such as interferons (IFN), retinoids, inosine pranobex, cimetidine, and most recently a cytokine inducer (imiquimod) have come into broader use in HPV infections, especially of those located in the genitoanal tract [23–26].

Interferons

The various properties of IFN have led to a variety of strategies for treating HPV-induced lesions [3, 24–26]. It is well accepted that antiviral and antiproliferative properties are seen at high IFN doses (> 5 million IU/day), whereas immunomodulating activities are prevalent at lower IFN doses (< 5 million IU/day) and decrease with increasing dosage [3, 24, 25].

IFN can be used as single treatment in cutaneous warts and HPV-associated genital warts, either topically as a gel, by intralesional injection, or parenterally in the form of intramuscular or subcutaneous injections. Furthermore, IFN can be combined with surgical methods such as electrosurgery, cryotherapy, or laser therapy or with cytotoxic agents such as podophyllin and podophyllotoxin [24].

In cutaneous warts, treatment is rarely indicated. In patients suffering from disseminated warts or from EV, however, parenteral IFN can be used with some success combined with retinoids. In large tumors, intralesional IFN injection may help to reduce the tumor size and the virus load, leading to improved removal using ablative therapies [25, 26].

Facial flat warts have been treated sucessfully with IFN-β gel. This is an alternative approach to local vitamin A acid therapy or superficial cryotherapy in this difficult issue. Current indications for single IFN therapy in anogenital HPV infections include recalcitrant anogenital warts refractory to any other treatment and extensive disease in which conventional therapy is not fully practicable [26]. Unusual conditions associated with HPV infections, such as Buschke-Löwenstein tumors [27], vulvodynia, and and vestibulitis [28], and HPV infection in children, particularly juvenile laryngeal papillomatosis and anogenital warts, have profited to some extent from the use of IFN therapy [25].

Single Interferon Therapy

Despite a number of optimistic open studies using IFN-α and IFN-β gel [29–34], no beneficial effects have been consistently demonstrated with single topical gel application compared with locally applied placebo or 0.5% podophyllotoxin [35]. This is especially true in keratotic lesions of the outer genitalia. Probably this is due to the fact that the available preparations do not deliver adequate quantities of IFN to infected basal cells which act as target cells for HPV infection [24]. Intralesional administration of IFN was long favored as a promising approach, despite a number of disadvantages. More recent studies have demonstrated, however, that only limited beneficial effects occur in lesions that are not treated by intralesional IFN injection and located elsewhere [25, 26, 36]. In general, intralesional IFN treatment requires frequent visits and causes repetitive local pain, as multiple injections are required. Furthermore, the effect of intralesional IFN therapy is far lower or even absent in immunocompromised patients, as shown for HIV-positive individuals [37]. In contrast to traditional ablative methods, however, intralesional IFN therapy does not lead to ulceration and scarring. It is of interest that, some years ago, intralesionally administered recombinant IFN-α_{2b} was licensed in the United States by the Food and Drug Administration (FDA) for treatment of genital warts.

Single parenteral IFN therapy of anogenital warts has not achieved general acceptance, although some favorable results were obtained in clinical trials [24–26]. This is mainly due to the delayed therapeutic effect and to variable patient outcomes, and less to patients discomfort and side effects, which are absent or tolerable with low-dose treatment. A number of studies have clearly shown that low doses of IFN-α or IFN-γ are

Table 1. Influence of adjuvant interferon (IFN) on the recurrence rate of recalcitrant condylomata acuminata (randomized controlled studies)

Ablative therapy	Recurrence rate (%) No IFN	IFN	IFN type	Dose (million IU)	Route	Reference
Co_2 laser	38	19	α_{2b}	1.0–5.0	Perilesional	[41]
Co_2 laser	45	21	α_{2b}	10.0	Perilesional	[42]
Podophyllin 25%	65	67	α_{2b}	1.5	Intralesional	[43]
Co_2 laser	75	54	β	0.1/1g	Gel	[4]
Cryotherapy	60	71	α_{2a}	3.0	s.c. continouus	[44]
Cryotherapy	73	69	α_{2a}	3.0	s.c. continuous	[45]
Co_2 laser	81	42	α_{2b}	1.0	s.c. cyclic	[46][a]
Co_2 laser	77	48	α_{2b}	3.0	s.c. continuous	[47]
Co_2 laser	61	68	α_{2a}	3.0	s.c. continuous	[48]
Co_2 laser	32	38	α_{2a}	3.0	s.c. continuous	
Co_2 laser	63	41	α_{2a}	1.5	s.c. cyclic	[50]
Podophyllin 25%	74	64	α_{2a}	3.0	s.c. continuous	[51]
Co_2 laser	51	52	α_{2a}	1.0		[52]
Cryotherapy		49	α_{2a}	3.0		
Electrocautery						
[a] Diathermy loop						

more effective than high doses if given subcutaneously [24,38]. Furthermore, cyclic IFN treatment (5–7 days of therapy, followed by a 3- to 4-week interval, repeated for up to three cycles) appears to be superior to continuous IFN treatment application (three times weekly for 4–6 weeks) [39]. The main disadvantage of parenteral IFN therapy, however, is that, similar to intralesional IFN therapy, efficacy is widely reduced or even absent in immunocompromised patients such as HIV-positive patients and drug addicts [37,40].

Adjuvant Interferon Therapy

A very favorable approach is the use of IFN as an adjuvant to surgical procedures [24, 25] (Table 1). Application of IFN-β hydrogel after destruction of the epithelial barrier by either CO_2 laser, electrocauter, or cryotherapy has led to a lower recurrence rate of condylomata acuminata as compared with a gel containing placebo (54% vs. 75%) [4]. Controlled studies have shown that the combination of intralesional IFN with CO_2 laser is a beneficial approach to reduce the recurrence of visible HPV infections in the anogenital tract [41, 42]. Although somewhat controversial (Table 1), it is obvious that recurrence rates of condylomata acuminata tend to decrease if adjuvant systemic IFN therapy is used together with ablative methods. Data from a recently published placebo-controlled, double-blind study suggest that the outcome of patients with genital warts treated by parenteral adjuvant IFN-α_{2a} therapy depends on the therapy regimen [50]. Patients with refractory condylomata acuminata received daily subcutaneous injections of 1 million IU recombinant IFN (rIFN)-α_{2a} given cyclically in three cycles consisting of 5 days of therapy with a 4-week interval between each cycle (total dose, 15 million IU IFN-α_{2a}; Table 1). In addition to the significantly lower recurrence rate in the IFN-treated patient group compared to the group that received placebo, the tolerability of cyclically administred rIFN-α_{2a} at a low dose (1 million IU per day injection) was

Table 2. Concept of adjuvant immunotherapy for severre and recalcitrant condylomata acuminata

Type of disease	Involved area (cm^2)	Adjuvant treatment	Dosage
Circumscribed	< 10	IFN-β gel	1 million IU/g gel, 5×daily, 4 weeks
Severe	> 10	Subcutaneous IFN-α	1.5 million IU IFN-α_{2a} or 1.5 million IU IFN-α_{2b} daily, 7 days, 3-week interval[a]

Adjuvant therapy after surgery, CO2 laser, Nd-yttrium-aluminium garnet (YAG) laser, cryotherapy, or electrocautery.
IFN, interferon
[a] Maximum of three cycles

excellent and did not differ significantly from that in placebo-treated patients [50]. Cyclic treatment with rIFN-α_{2a} was much more effective than continuous treatment in previous treatments [44, 45, 48, 49, 51, 52]. Accordingly, in problem cases it is recommended that surgery is followed by adjuvant IFN administration (low-dose and cyclic or local IFN gel therapy) in order to break the vicious cycle of recalcitrance (Table 2). For direct, definitive comparion of the clinical benefits of the cyclic and continuous regimen, a comparative trial is now warranted.

It is understood that both parenteral and local adjuvant IFN gel therapy, which is useful in circumscribed cases of condylomata acuminata (affected area, < 10 cm^2), require a high degree of motivation and compliance from the patients (Table 2).

Safety and Precautions

Side effects are clearly dose dependent. Influenza-like symptoms, the most common side effects, are noted in most of the patients a few hours after parenteral IFN administration. Leukopenia, thrombocytopenia, and temporary elevation of liver function tests may transiently occur in patients receiving high doses of parenteral IFN (5 million IU IFN per day). The same is true for fever, chills, myalgias, headache, myalgia, and nausea. The latter symptoms are self-limited, lasting only for the first 2–3 days of treatment [53]. More dangerous side effects include autoimmune diseases (e.g., thrombocytopenic purpura, autoimmune thyroiditis), which may be triggered by IFN therapy and which usually improve after therapy suspension. Testing for absence of autoimmune antibodies before and during treatment is recommended.

Development of higher levels of neutralizing antibodies has been shown preferentially directed against rIFN-α_{2a}, but to a lesser degree also against rIFN-α_{2b} and natural IFN-α [25]. In a recent study, however, treatment-induced IFN-α antibodies did not impair the beneficial effect of low-dose cyclic rIFN-α_{2a} treatment [54].

Absolute contraindications against IFN therapy are autoimmune diseases, concurrent heparin therapy, severe general diseases such as cardiovascular disease, renal dysfunction, history of attacks or psychosis, pregnancy, immunosuppression (endogenous and exogenous), active psoriasis, and low levels of thrombocytes (< 70000 per μl) [53]. Local IFN gel apparently is also active if given after debulking skin or mucosal warts in immunodeficient patients [27, 55]. This is in contrast to both intralesional and systemic IFN application in immunocompromised individuals [37, 40]. A similar effect was recently obtained in acquired immunodeficiency syndrome (AIDS) patients suffering from giant mollusca contagiosa which have been refractory to other common therapies [56]. As recurrence of such lesions can be prevented, there is a great impact on the psychological state of these patients.

Retinoids

Studies on the role of vitamin A and retinoids have been performed particularly in patients with cervical cancer. This was based on the fact that one of the risk factors for cervical neoplasia is likely to be deficiency of dietary vitamin A. It has been suggested that vitamin A may be protective against cervical cancer, which was shown in some studies [57, 58]. Thus the possibility exists that vitamin A or related retinoids could be administered therapeutically early in the neoplastic process (either systemically or locally) to inhibit progression of the disease. It has also been suggested that combining the antiproliferative effect of retinoids with the oncogene-inhibitory effect and the antiproliferative, immunostimulatory, and immunopotentiating activities of IFN-α may provide an enhanced beneficial effect with regard to reduction of cervical tumor size. It is very likely that each of these agents inhibits cervical cell proliferation by distinct pathways.

Imiquimod

Imiquimod is an immunomodulator which upregulates cell-mediated immune responses, presumably by inducing cytokines, especially IFN-α. Thus imiquimod, a imidazoquinolinamine derivative (1-(2-methylpropyl)-1H-imidazo[4,5-C]quinolin-4-amine), has the potential to act against genital warts. This substance is currently being tested in genital HPV-associated lesions in immunocompetent and immunodeficient patients [59], and good overall results have been obtained both in clearing warts and in preventing recurrence of warts. In the future, it may well be used in all human sites infected by HPV, even the skin, either as single treatment or after surgical removal of the lesions for prevention of recurrence.

Cimetidine

Cimetidine is a H_2 receptor antagonist which has been in use for years in the treatment of peptic ulcer disease. Because of its immunomodulatory activities if given at a high dose, cimetidine has also been used to treat patients with different conditions, such as mucocutaneous candidiasis [60], common variable immunodeficiency [61], shingles, and herpes simplex. Cimetidine has been shown to enhance a variety of immunologic functions. It has inhibitory effects on suppressor T cell function [62, 63] and augments delayed-type hypersensitivity responses [64]. The results of some trials have suggested that cimetidine may also be useful for the treatment of viral warts [65–67]. A double-blind study, recently performed by Yilmaz et al. [68], however, was unable to confirm this hypothesis. Cimetedine has been shown to be no more effective than placebo in the treatment of patients with common warts.

In addition, a controlled trial performed in children suffering from warts had to be terminated early after enrolling because of the lack of any distinct advantage of cimetidine compared with standard treatment [69]. In summary, the performed studies suggest that, at present, cimetidine might be helpful as adjuvant therapy for warts, but is unlikely to be effective by itself.

Inosine Pranobex

Inosine pranobex has been used for several years for treating common warts, although placebo-controlled trials have not been performed to show its efficacy in this indication. Combination of inosine pranobex with hot water treatment and keratolysis using salicylic acid plaster or tincture is most useful in periungal, subungual, and plantar warts if given orally at a dosage of 1 mg per kg body weight three times daily for up to 6 weeks (personal observation). Inosine pranobex has been shown to increase the success rate in the treatment of HPV-induced condylomata acuminata combined with conventional therapy [70]. Its clinical role in the primary treatment of HPV disease, however, warrants further investigation. Recently, the efficacy of inosine pranobex was assessed in a double-blind, placebo-controlled trial in the treatment of persistent subclinical HPV infection of the vulva [71]. Inosine pranobex induced significant regression of disease in nearly two thirds of the treated women and reduced the severity of pruritus in more than half of the patients. It is advantageous that inosine pranobex is administered orally and that adverse drug reactions are rarely noted and are mild.

Vaccines

HPV-induced tumors can progress to squamous cell carcinoma, e.g., HPV-16-associated cervical carcinoma [72]. Current epidemiological studies suggest that the prevalence of HPV infection in developed countries may be increasing dramatically, and, if these trends continue, a proportional increase in the prevalence of cervicovaginal carcinoma can be expected in the future. Cervical carcinoma is actually the second leading cause of cancer death in developing countries. Further increase also with regard to the squamous cell carcinoma of the skin, the outer genitalia, the anus, and the upper respiratory tract has to be expected in the next few years in immunodeficient and iatrogenically immunosuppressed patients. Thus there is a requirement for prophylactic and therapeutic vaccines which could both protect against infection and accelerate rejection of established tumors. Two HPV-specific oncogenic proteins, E6 and E7, are important in the induction and maintenance of cellular transformation and are coexpressed in the majority of HPV-containing carcinomas. Therefore, vaccines targeted to these proteins may provide an opportunity to prevent and treat HPV-associated malignancies.

With regard to the cervix uteri, which is currently of primary concern for vaccine strategies, immunological control could be envisaged at three stages of HPV infection:

1. *Before onset of sexual contact.* A population-based vaccination program should start in young teenage girls in order to induce neutralizing antibodies against HPV- 16 at the cervix. This would imply induction of antibodies against the HPV-16 viral capsid proteins L1 and L2.

2. *During viral persistence in the cervical tissue.* This is calculated to be on average two decades until cervical cancer occurs (peak incidence at about 43 years of age) [73]. In this period, HPV infection can be subclinical or can manifest itself as visible condyloma or CIN. Furthermore, in this period regression of lesions and even clearance of HPV infection may happen.
3. *When cancer of the cervix uteri has become established.* A future immunotherapeutic approach could lead to stimulatuation of a cytotoxic T cell response against E6 and E7 proteins and consequently induce tumor involution.

In contrast to large parts of the viral genome which have been integrated into the host cell genome, the transforming genes E 6 and E 7 are generally expressed and may be targets for immunotherapy [72]. Of all three stages of cervical HPV infection, the viral-persistence phase is currently the most attractive phase for immunotherapeutic intervention protocols.

In view of the long list of high-risk or intermediate-risk HPV types involved in cervical dysplasia, it must be taken into account that immunotherapy effective against all HPV types will probably not be achievable. However, as HPV-16 alone is associated with at least 60% of high-grade CIN lesions and with about 50% of cervical cancers [74], reduction of the prevalence of HPV-16 carriers would result in a significant decrease in the incidence of anogenital neoplasias.

Prophylactic Vaccination

Virus-like particles (VLP) are most likely to fulfill the requirements of efficacy and safety. A series of studies have shown that VLP contain the conformationally sensitive neutralizing epitopes of the intact virions [75–77] and that immunization with VLP induces equally high titers of neutralizing antibodies as immunization with native virions [78]. Before clinical trials of VLP vaccines can start, however, some important questions have to be considered.

Route of Immunization

It is not yet clear whether immunization favoring IgA production, such as the oral route or even the vaginal route, might result in better protective efficacy than intradermal immunization.

Candidates for Vaccination

Vaccine trials should be targeted at teenage girls seeking contraceptive advice. This is based on longitudinal cohort studies indicating that no teenage girls who had had no or only one partner had antibodies against HPV-16 or HPV-33, whereas 54% of teenage girls who had had more than five sexual partners had seroconverted against either of these viruses [79].

Viral Types To Include in the Vaccine

In a recent worldwide survey of HPV types, 93% of over 1000 cervical cancers were HPV positive [80]. HPV-16 was found in 50%, and the four most common types (HPV-16, HPV-18, HPV-31, and HPV-45) were detected in 77% of cancers. In order to decide whether additional HPV types apart from HPV-16 should be included in a vaccine, it will be most important to obtain data on the degree of cross-protection between the oncogenic HPV types.

There is a still growing list of alternative preventive and therapeutic vaccines that are currently under investigation. Prophylactic vaccines include VLP, DNA vaccines, live virus expression vector-based vaccines, subunit vaccines, and synthetic peptide-based vaccines. Therapeutic vaccines consist in synthetic CTL epitope vaccination. Advantages of some of these approaches, such as low cost and/or stability, are opposed by certain long-term risks, such as integration of HPV DNA into host cell DNA (DNA vaccines) and vaccinia viral disease in immunocompromised patients receiving live virus expression vectors.

Therapeutic Vaccination

A series of strategies exist for eliciting cytotoxic T cell (CTL)-mediated immunity. One of the most straightforward vaccination approaches stimulating CTL response using peptides is to mimic endogenously degraded HPV E6 and E7 peptides with MHC class I-binding ability that also constitute CTL epitopes [81]. Preliminary results from initial clinical trials of therapeutic peptide vaccination have, however, been disappointing so far. Thus future work should also comprise optimization of immunization protocols for synthetic peptide CTL epitope vaccination.

Summary

A number of immunomodulatory drugs have been in use for viral infections over a long period of time with only limited success. In contrast to herpesvirus infections, which have currently become very effectively treated by the development of the nucleoside analogue acyclovir and its successors valaciclovir, penciclovir, and famciclovir, no antiviral compounds exist so far for HPV infections. In visible HPV infections and HPV-associated intraepithelial neoplasia, IFN have a role to play when given combined with ablative methods such as CO_2 laser or electrocautery. Further compounds used to some extent together with ablative methods or combined with IFN are retinoids, inosine pranobex, and the H_2 receptor antagonist cimetidine.

Cytokine induction by locally active imidazaquinolinamines, i.e., imiquimod, is a straightforward development which is most likely to turn out to be efficicacious as primary therapy of anogenital and cutaneous warts in both immunocompetent and immunodeficient patients. The advantage of this approach is that visible lesions are cleared with a very low rate of recurrence.

Vaccines targeted at the oncogenic HPV E6 and E7 proteins, which are coexpressed in the majority of HPV-containing carcinomas, may provide an opportunity to both prevent and specifically treat HPV-associated squamous cell malignancies, particularly of the cervix. It is assumed that immunotherapy using therapeutic vaccines is most attractive during the period of viral persistence, when HPV infection is either subclinical or manifest as visible condyloma or cervical intraepithelial neoplasia (CIN).

References

1. Phelps WC, Alexander KA (1995) Antiviral therapy for human papillomaviruses: rationale and prospects. Ann Intern Med 123:368–382
2. Kraus SJ, Stone KM (1990) Management of genital infection caused by human papilomavirus. Rev Infect Dis12 [Suppl]: S620–632
3. Gross G (1996) Interferons. In: Elsner P, Eichmann A (eds) Sexually transmitted diseases. Advances in diagnosis and treatment. Basel, Karger, pp 233–246 (Current problems in dermatology, vol 24)
4. Gross G, Rogozinski T, Schöfer H et al (1994) Recombinant interferon beta gel as an adjuvant in the treatment of recurrent genital warts: results of a placebo-controlled double-blind study in 120 patients. J Interferon Res 14 [Suppl 1]:151
5. Schneider A (1994) Natural history of genital papillomavirus infections. Intervirology 37: 201–214
6. Messing AM, Epstein WL (1963) Natural history of warts. Arch Dermatol 87:306–310
7. Tagami H, Ogino A, Tagigawa M et al (1974) Regression of plane warts following spontaneous inflammation. A histopathological study. Br J Dermatol 90:147–154
8. Benton C, Shahidullah H, Hunter J (1992) Human papillomavirus in the immunosuppressed. Papillomavirus Rep 3:23–26
9. Morison WL (1975) Viral warts, herpes simplex and herpes zoster in patients with secondary immune deficiencies and neoplasms. Br J Dermatol 92:625–630
10. Jablonska S, Orth G (1985) Epidermodysplasia verruciformis. Clin Dermatol 3:83–96
11. Aloub MI, Barr BB, McLaren KM et al (1989) Human papillomavirus infection and cervical intraepithelial neoplasia in women with renal allografts. BR Med J 298:153–156
12. Hawthorn RJ, Murdoch JB, MacLean, Mackie RM (1988) Langerhans'cells and subtypes of human papillomavirus in cervical intraepithelial neoplasia. Br Med 297:643–646
13. Halpert R, Frachter RG, Sedlis A et al (1986) Human papillomavirus and lower genital tract neoplasia in renal transplant patients. Obstet Gynecol 68:251–258
14. Tay SK, Jenkins D, Maddox P et al (1987) Tissue macrophage response in human papillomavirus infection and cervical intraepithelial neoplasia. Br J Obstet Gynecol 94:104–107
15. Malejczik J, Majewskii S, Jablonska S et al (1989) Abrogated NK-cell lyysis of human papillomavirus (HPV)16 bearing keratinocytes in patients with precanceroous and cancerous HPV-induced anogenital lesions. Int J Cancer 43:209–214
16. Wank R, Thomssen C (1991) High risk of squamous cell carcinoma of the cervix for women with HLA-DQW3. Nature 352:723–725
17. Connor ME, Stern PL (1990) Loss of MHC Class I expression in cervical carcinoma. Int J Cancer 46:1029–1031
18. Hughes RG, Norval M, Howie SE (1988) Expression of major histocompatibility class II antigens by Langerhans' cells in cervical intraepithelial neoplasia. J Clin Pathol 41:253–259
19. Viac J, Soler C, Chardonnet Y et al (1993) Expression of immune associated surface antigens of keratinocytes in human papillomavirus-derived lesions. Immunobiology 188:393–396
20. Jochmus I, Dürst M, Reid R et al (1994) Major histocompatibility complex and human papillomavirus type 16 E7 expression in high-grade vulvar lesions. Hum Pathol 24:519–523
21. Glew SS, Duggan-Keen M, Cabrera T, Stern PL (1992) HLA class II antigen expression in human papillomavirus-associated cervical cancer. Cancer Res 52:4009–4016
22. Cooper KD, Androphy EJ, Lowy D, Katz SI (1990) Antigen presentation and T-cell activation in epidermodysplasia verruciformis. J Invest Dermatol 94:769–776
23. Beutner K, Spruance S, Douglas J et al (1994) Double-blind, vehicle-controlled, randomized multicenter trial of 5% imiquimod cream for the treatment of genital and perianal warts. 2nd Int Congress Papillomaviruses Hum Pathol, Paris (abstr)
24. Gross G (1990) Interferons in genital HPV disease. In: Gross G, Jablonska S, Pfister H, Stegner HE (eds) Genital papillomavirus infections. Springer, Berlin Heidelberg New York, pp 393–412
25. Rockley PF, Tyring SK (1995) Interferons alpha, beta and gamma therapy of anogenital human papillomavirus infections. Pharmacol Ther 65:265–287

26. Gross G (1995) Treatment of human papillomavirus infection. In: Mindel A (ed) Genital warts. Human papillomavirus infection. Arnold, London, pp 198–236
27. Gross G, Roussaki A, Pfister H (1989) Recurrent vulvar Buschke-Löwenstein tumor-like condylomata acuminata and Hodgkin's disease effectively treated with recombinant interferon alpha-2c gel as adjuvant to electrosurgery. Curr Probl Dermatol 18:178–184
28. Bornstein J, Pascal B, Abramovici H (1991) Treatment of a patient with vulvar vestibulitis by intramuscular interferon beta; a case report. Eur J Obstet Gynecol Reprod Biol 42:237–239
29. Ikic D, Bosnic N, Smerdel S (1975) Double-blind clinical study with human leukocyte interferon in the therapy of condylomata acuminata. Proc Symp Clin Use Interferon, Zagreb, pp 167–177
30. Möller BR, Johannesen P, Osther K et al (1983) Treatment of dysplasia of the cervical epithelium with an interferon gel. J Obstet Gynecol 62:625–629
31. Marcovici R, Peretz BA, Paldi E (1983) Human fibroblast interferon therapy in patients with condylomata acuminata. Isr J Med Sci 19:104
32. Vesterinen E, Meyer B, Cantell K et al (1984) Topical treatment of flat vaginal condyloma with human leukocyte interferon. Obstet Gynecol 64:535–538
33. De Virgilis C, Crippa L, Leopardi O et al (1987) The role of beta-interferon in the therapy of female genital viral diseases. Int J Immunol 3:147–150
34. Schneider A, Papendick U, Gissmann L (1987) Interferon treatment of human genital papillomavirus infections: importance of viral type. Int J Cancer 3:147–150
35. Syed TA, Cheema KM, Ahmad SA et al (1995) Human leukocyte interferon-alpha versus podophyllotoxin in cream for the treatment of genital warts in males. Dermatology 191: 129–132
36. Eron LJ, Judson F, Tucker S et al (1986) Interferon therapy for condylomata acuminata. N Engl J Med 315:1059–1069
37. Douglas JM, Rogers U, Judson FN (1986) The effect of asymptomatic infection with HTLV-3 on the response of anogenital warts to intralesional treatment with recombinant alpha-2-interferon. J Infect Dis 154:331–334
38. Gross G, Degen KW, Fierlbeck G et al (1991) Recombinant interferon gamma in anogenital warts: results of a multicentre placebo-controlled clinical trial. J Interferon Res 11 [Suppl 1]:76
39. Gross G, Ikenberg H, Roussaki A (1986) Systemic treatment of condylomata acuminata with recombinant interferon alpha-2a: low dose superior to high-dose regimen. Chemotherapy 32:537–541
40. Gross G, Roussaki A, Ikenberg H, Drees N (1991) Genital warts do not respond to systemic recombinant interferon alpha-2a treatment during cannabis consumption. Dermatologica 183:203–207
41. Vance JC, Davis D (1990) Interferon alpha-2b injections used as an adjuvant therapy to carbon dioxide laser vaporization of recalcitrant anogenital condylomata acuminata. J Invest Dermatol 995:146–148
42. Davis BE, Noble MJ (1992) Initial experience with combined interferon alpha and carbon dioxide laser for the treatment of condylomata acuminata. J Urol 197:627–629
43. Douglas JM Jr, Eron LJ, Judson FN et al (1990) A randomized trial of combination therapy with intralesional interferon alpha-2b and podophyllin versus podophyllin alone for the therapy of anogenital warts. J Infect Dis 162:52–59
44. Handley JM, Horner T, Maw RD et al (1991) Subcutaneous interferon alpha-2a combined with cryotherapy vs. cryotherapy alone in the treatment of primary anogenital warts: A randomised observer-blind placebo-controlled study. Genitour Med 67:297–307
45. Eron LJ, Alder MB, O'Rourke JM et al (1993) Recurrence of condylomata acuminata following cryotherapy is not prevented by systemically administered interferon. Genitourin Med 69: 91–93
46. Hohenleutner U, Landthaler M, Braun-Falco O (1990) Postoperative adjuvante Therapie mit Interferon-alpha-2b nach Laserchirurgie von Condylomata acuminata. Hautarzt 41:545–548
47. Petersen CS, Bjerring P, Larsen J, Blakkaer J (1991) Systemic interferon alpha-2b increases the cure rate in laser-treatment patients with multiple persistent genital warts: a placebo-controlled study. Genitourin Med 67:99–102

48. The Condylomata International Collaborative Study Group (1993) Randomized placebo-controlled double-blind combined therapy with laser surgery and systemic interferon-alpha-2a in the treatment of anogenital condylomata acuminata. J Infect Dis 167:824–829
49. Nieminen P, Aho M, Lehtinen M et al (1994) Treatment of genital HPV infection with carbon dioxide laser and systemic interferon alpha-2a. Sex Transm Dis 21:59–65
50. Gross G, Roussaki A, Baur S et al (1996) Systemically administered interferon alpha-2a prevents recurrence of condylomata acuminata following CO2-laser ablation. The influence of the cyclic low-dose therapy regimen. Results of a multicentre double-blind placebo-controlled clinical trial. Genitourin Med 72:71
51. Armstrong DKB, Maw RD, Dinsmore WW et al (1994) Randomised, double-blind, parallel group study to compare subcutaneous interferon alpha-2a plus podophyllin with placebo plus podophyllin in the treatment of primary condylomata acuminata. Genitourin Med 70: 389–393
52. Armstrong DKB, Maw RD, Dinsmore WW et al (1996) Combined therapy trial with interferon alpha-2a and ablative therapy in the treatment of anogenital warts. Genitourin Med 72: 103–107
53. Dianzani F (1992) Interferon treatments: how to use an endogenous system as a therapeutic agent. J Interferon Res (special issue), pp 109–118
54. Prümmer O, Gross G, Baur S, Herrmann F The beneficial effect of low-dose interferon alpha-2a treatment in patients with condylomata acuminata is not impaired by interferon-alpha antibodies. J Interferon Cytokine Res (in press)
55. Gross G, Roussaki A, Brzoska J (1990) Topical interferon beta gel as adjuvant therapy in immunocompromised patients with recurrent genital warts. J Interferon Res 10 [Suppl 1]:112
56. Gross G, Roussaki A Recalcitrant giant molluscum contagiosum in a patient with AIDS successfully treated by a combination of CO2 laser Swift LaseTM and interferon beta gel. J Am Acad Dermatol submitted for publication
57. Lippmann SM, Kavanagh JJ (1992) Paredes-Espinoza M, 13-cis-retinoic acid plus interferon-alpha-2a: highly active systemic therapy for squamous cell carcinoma of the cervix. J Natl Cancer Inst 84:241–245
58. Bollag W (1991) Retinoids and interferon: a new promising combination? Br J Haematol 79 [Suppl 1]:87–91
59. Beutner K, Spruance S, Douglas J et al (1994) Double-blind, vehicle-controlled, randomized multicenter trial of 5% imiquimod cream for the treatment of genital and perianal warts. 2nd Int Congress Papillomaviruses Hum Pathol, Paris (abstr)
60. Jorizzo JL, Sams WM, Jegasothy BV et al (1980) Cimetidine as an immunomodulator: chronic mucocutaneous candidiasis as a model. Ann Intern Med 92:192–195
61. White WB, Ballow M (1985) Modulation of suppressive-cell activity by cimetidine in patients with common variable hypoglobulinemia. N Engl J Med 312:198–202
62. Jin Z, Kumar A, Cleveland RP et al (1986) Inhibition of suppressor cell function by cimetidine in a murine model. Clin Immunol Immunopathol 38:350–356
63. Strejcek J, Suhajowa E, Jira M et al (1984) Further evidence of immunomodulatory effects of cimetidine. Allerg Immunol (Leipz) 30:117–122
64. Avella J, Madsen JE, Binder HJ et al (1978) Effect of histamine-receptor antagonists on delayed hypersensitivity. Lancet 1:624–626
65. Orlow SJ, Paller A (1993) Cimetidine therapy for multiple viral warts in children. J Am Acad Dermatol 28:794–796
66. Choi YS, Hann SK, Park YK (1993) The effect of cimetidine on verruea plana juvenilis: clinical trials in six patients. J Dermatol (Tokyo) 20:497–500
67. Glass AT, Solomon BA (1996) Cimetidine therapy for recalcitrant warts in adults. Arch Dermatol 132:680–682
68. Yilmaz E, Alpsoy E, Basaran E (1986) Cimetidine therapy for warts: a placebo-controlled, double-blind study. J Am Acad Dermatol 34:1005–1007
69. Bauman C, Francis JS, Vanderhooft S, Sybert VP (1996) Cimetidine therapy for multiple viral warts in children. J Am Acad Dermatol 35:271–272

70. Davidson-Parker J, Dinsmore W, Khan MH et al (1988) Immunotherapy of genital warts with inosine pranobex and conventional treatment: double blind placebo-controlled study. Genitourin Med 64:383–386
71. Tay SK (1996) Efficacy of inosine pranobex oral therapy in subclinical human papillomavirus infection of the vulva: a randomized double-blinded placebo controlled study. Intern J STD AIDS 7:276–280
72. Zur Hausen H (1991) Human papillomaviruses in the pathogenesis of anogenital cancer. Virology 184:9–13
73. Gustafsson L, Adami HO (1989) Natural history of cervical neoplasia: consistent results obtained by an identification technique. Br J Cancer 60:132–135
74. Lorincz AT, Reid R, Jenson AB et al (1992) Human papillomavirus infection of the cervix: relative risk associations of 15 common anogenital types. Obstet Gynecol 79:328–337
75. Christensen ND, Kirnbauer R, Schiller JT et al (1994) Human papillomavirus types 6 and 11 have antigenically distinct strongly immunogenic conformationally dependent neutralizing epitopes. Virology 205:329–332
76. Rose RC, Reichmann RC, Bonnez W (1994) Human papillomavirus type 11 recombinant virus-like particles induce the formation of neutralizing antibodies and detect HPV-specific antibodies in human sera. J Gen Virol 75:2075–2078
77. Breitburd F, Kirnbauer R, Hubbert NL et al (1995) Immunization with virus-like particles from cottontail rabbit papillomavirus (CRPV) can protect against experimental CRPV infection. J Virol 69:3959–3962
78. Kirnbauer R, Booy F, Cheng N et al (1992) Papillomavirus L1 major capsid protein self-assembles into virus-like particles that are highly immunogenic. Proc Natl Acad Sci USA 12: 180–184
79. Andersson-Ellström A, Dillner J, Haagmar B et al (1996) Comparison of development of serum antibodies to HPV 16 and HPV 33 and acquisition of cervical HPV DNA among sexually experienced and virgin young girls. A longitudinal cohort study. Sex Transm Dis 23(3): 234–238
80. Bosch FX, Manos MM, Munoz N et al (1995) Prevalence of human papillomavirus in cervical cancer: a worldwide perspective. J Natl Cancer Inst 87:796–799
81. Wu TC (1994) Immunology of the human papilloma virus in relation to cancer. Curr Opinions Immunol 6:746–754

Immunostimulation and Vaccination Therapy of Human Immunodeficiency Virus Infection

N. S. Penneys

If any infectious disease seems to be a candidate for therapy via immunostimulation, human immunodeficiency virus (HIV) is the one. HIV has a devastating and profound impact on the immune system. This retrovirus causes a progressive destruction and misfunction of $CD4^+$ lymphocytes after selectively binding to a surface receptor on their membranes [1]. Since $CD4^+$ lymphocytes are pivotal in the immune response to infections, their loss leads to a cascade of secondary immune dysfunction [2–4] and an increased risk of infection, frequently to exotic pathogens. In addition, HIV-induced autoimmune phenomena, inappropriate mechanisms of T cell death, and dysregulation of other normal homeostatic mechanisms of the immune system play a role in the pathogenesis of the disease [5].

The dermatologic manifestations of HIV infection are legion and have been extensively described [6–8]. A lack of immune response leads to perpetuation of skin lesions associated with common infections such as human papillomavirus, molluscum contagiosum, herpesvirus group infections, and superficial fungal disease. Other less specific manifestations of HIV infection in the skin may be a consequence of dysregulation of the immune system. For example, persistent insect bite reactions have been described in this site associated with increased circulating antibody titers to mosquito salivary gland antigens [9]. The chronic pruritic eruption of acquired immunodeficiency syndrome (AIDS) (eosinophilic folliculitis, chronic papular eruption) may represent an immune dysfunction related to an unknown eliciting antigen.

Conventional therapy for HIV infection includes a variety of approaches and combinations. Antiretroviral medications are generally directed at inhibiting specific metabolic sequences necessary for viral replication. One significant drawback of antiretroviral therapies has been the rapid emergence of drug-resistant isolates during therapy [10, 11]. The high rate of mutability of the virus may ultimately limit all antiretroviral therapies [12]. On the other hand, immune-based therapies are designed to modulate or reconstitute the immune system. These therapies do not target the retrovirus directly, but may affect viral propagation indirectly by improving or enhancing the immune system. Theoretically, immune-based therapies would be less susceptible to escape mutations. Immune-based therapies directed at suppression of HIV infection include those which affect (either suppress or stimulate) cytokine release and those that promote immune system reconstitution.

Cytokine Alteration

HIV virus production is affected by host-related factors. These include physical factors as well as agents that influence the differentiation of bone marrow-derived precursor cells. Cytokines represent the major factors involved in the communication between T cells, macrophages, and other immune cells in the course of an immune response to antigens and infectious agents. These substances coordinate immune responses, communicate and mediate between antagonistic functions of different cell types, generate inflammatory responses, and maintain general homeostasis. Furthermore, different cellular activities are associated with different cytokine profiles [13]. Although many cytokine functions have been described, this is a dynamic field in which new effectors and new functions for recognized cytokines are still being described. Well-known cytokines include tumor necrosis factor (TNF)-α, interferons, and the interleukins. Many of these substances also have profound effects on cutaneous homeostasis [14].

Cytokine function in individuals infected by HIV may be significantly altered. Many cytokines appear to drive HIV infection. TNF-α is such a cytokine. Serum from patients with AIDS and secondary infections have abnormally elevated levels of TNF-α [15], and there is evidence that TNF-α levels correlate with disease state. Furthermore, in some in vitro systems, TNF-α [16] increases the expression of HIV. Pentoxifylline, a substance that inhibits TNF expression, may modestly inhibit HIV-1 propagation [17]. IL-4, a cytokine expressed by a subset of activated T cells and cells of the basophil/mast cell lineage, is another cytokine that upregulates production of HIV RNA [18]. Therefore, strategies that inhibit these cytokines might be clinically beneficial.

Stimulation of cytokines that are not deleterious and possibly beneficial could result in clinical improvement. The cytokine interleukin (IL)-2 is such a candidate. Patients with AIDS have abnormally low production of IL-2. IL-2 in vitro stimulates T lymphocytes, increases the release of cytokines, and is a potent T lymphocyte growth factor. In vivo, IL-2 restores T lymphocyte responsiveness in athymic mice, enhances the primary immune response of animals, and generates natural killer (NK) cell activity [19]. The addition of IL-2 to cells from HIV-1-infected patients can correct a number of their immunological abnormalities, and the administration of low-dose polyethylene glycol IL-2 in patients with HIV disease has resulted in sustained immune enhancement in the absence of toxicity [20]. Unfortunately, the use of IL-2 in patients with AIDS resulted only in transient increase in immunity. A more recent study using a longer-acting derivative of IL-2 coupled with the simultaneous administration of antiretroviral therapy has produced some elevation of CD4 counts [21]. Cytokines elaborated by $CD8^+$ T lymphocytes such as RANTES, macrophage inflammatory protein (MIP)-1a, and MIP-1b suppress HIV [22]; administration of these cytokines may also eventually have roles in suppression of HIV infection.

Cytokines that have limited and specific biologic effects are more likely to be clinically useful. Such an example might be interferon (INF)-α, which has activity that is restricted to antiviral activity and has been efficacious against a variety of chronic viral infections. Stimulatory effects of cytokines may be limited by their pharmacokinetics. Short-lived cytokines may not be feasible clinical therapeutic agents.

Lastly, some cytokines either induce or suppress virus replication in vitro as a function of the model system; this observation suggests that hidden pitfalls may surface during clinical trials of cytokines and means that claims of clinical benefit that have been made prior to trials may be premature.

Immune Reconstitution

Immune reconstitution represents a broad category of potential therapies. Any and all abnormalities can be addressed. Therapeutic avenues can be broad (e.g., the use of vaccination therapies) or focused (e.g., attempting to correct a specific biochemical abnormality). Broad approaches such as immune reconstitution involving transfer of lymphoid or precursor cell populations are just beginning, but remain a hopeful alternative. As an example of a focused abnormality, decreased concentrations of glutathione in the serum [23] and lymphocytes [24] have been described in the context of HIV, and replacement of glutathione can inhibit HIV replication in vitro [25]. Clinical trials of agents that replenish glutathione would represent a focused attempt to correct a specific immune abnormality.

In several viral diseases, neutralizing antibodies are thought to be an important component of a protective immune response [26]. Initial HIV-1 vaccine studies demonstrated that antisera elicited by immunization with HIV-1 envelope glycoproteins gp120 or gp160 or by peptides derived from the third variable region of gp120 could neutralize HIV-1 in vitro [27]. Furthermore, chimpanzees vaccinated with recombinant envelope glycoprotein products were protected from infection when challenged with HIV-1 [28]. These results have focused current vaccine efforts on envelope subunit vaccines and on their ability to induce neutralizing antibodies. A large number of vaccines have been tested in human volunteers, including purified recombinant envelope glycoproteins and vectors expressing HIV-1 envelope glycoprotein; these vaccines have successfully induced neutralizing antibody to heterologous laboratory strains of HIV-1. However, it appears that envelope subunit vaccine products are not efficient in inducing neutralizing antibodies against primary isolates of HIV-1 [29]. A recent study seems to confirm that vaccines that appear to be efficacious in vitro may fail in vivo; a 5-year test of a genetically engineered version of gp160 involving 608 HIV-infected people revealed disease progression in the vaccinated group at the same rate as the placebo group [30].

Summary

The usefulness of immunostimulatory therapies is unproven. Broad application of these approaches must await the results of controlled studies demonstrating efficacy.

References

1. McDougal JS, Kennedy MS, Sligh JM et al (1986) Binding of HTLV-III/LAV to T4+ T cells by a complex of the 110 K viral protein and the T4 molecule. Science 231:382–385
2. Pahwa S, Pahwa R, Good RA et al (1986) Stimulatory and inhibitory influences of human immunodeficiency virus on normal B lymphocytes. Proc Natl Acad Sci USA 83:9124–9128
3. Lane HC, Masur H, Edgar LC et al (1983) Abnormalities of B-cell activation and immunoregulation in patients with the acquired immunodeficiency syndrome. New Engl J Med 309: 453–458
4. Gartner S, Markovits P, Markovitz DM et al (1986) The role of mononuclear phagocytes in HTLV-III/LAV infection. Science 233:215–219
5. Fauci AS (1993) Multifactorial nature of human immunodeficiency virus disease: implications for therapy. Science 262:1011–1018
6. Penneys NS (1995) Skin manifestations of AIDS, 2nd edn. Dunitz, London
7. Kaplan MH, Sadick N, McNutt NS et al (1987) Dermatologic findings and manifestations of acquired immunodeficiency syndrome (AIDS). J Am Acad Dermatol 16:485–506

8. Goodman D, Teplitz ED, Wishner A et al (1987) Prevalence of cutaneous disease in patients with acquired immunodeficiency syndrome (AIDS) or AIDS-related complex. J Am Acad Dermatol 17:210–220
9. Penneys NS, Nayar JK, Bernstein H et al (1989) A chronic pruritic eruption in 5 patients with AIDS associated with increased antibody titers to mosquito salivary gland antigens. J Am Acad Dermatol 21:421–425
10. Larder BA, Kemp SD (1989) Multiple mutations in HIV-1 reverse transcriptase confer high-level resistance to zidovudine (AZT). Science 246:1155–1158
11. Saag MS, Hahn BH, Gibbons J, Li Y, Parks ES, Parks WP et al. (1988) Extensive variation of human immunodeficiency virus type-1 in vivo. Nature 334:440–444
12. Lederman MM (1995) Host-directed and immune-based therapies for human immunodeficiency virus infection. Ann Int Med 122:218–222
13. Belardelli F (1995) Role of interferons and other cytokines in the regulation of the immune response. APMIS 103:161–179
14. Schroder JM (1995) Cytokine networks in the skin. J Invest Dermatol 105:20S–24S
15. Nunez E, Christeff N (1994) Steroid hormone, cytokine, lipid and metabolic distrubances in HIV infection. In: Clinical endocrinology and metabolism. Tindall, London, pp 803–824
16. Kalebic T (1996) Human fetal glial cells constitutively produce HIV-inducing cytokines. Exp Cell Res 223:452–458
17. Luke DR, McCreedy BJ, Sarnoski TP, Bookout JB, Johnston AM, Lell JE (1993) Phase I/II study of pentoxifylline with zidovudine on HIV-1 growth in AIDS patients. Int J Clin Pharmacol Ther Toxicol 31:343–350
18. Naif H, Ho-Shon M, Chang J, Cunningham AL (1994) Molecular mechanisms of IL-4 effect on HIV expression in promonocytic cell lines and primary human monocytes. J Leukoc Biol 56:335–339
19. Malkovsky M, Sondel PM, Strober W (1988) The interleukins in acquired disease. Clin Exp Immunol 74:151–161
20. Teppler H, Kaplan G, Smith KA, Montana AL, Meyn P, Cohn ZA (1993) Prolonged immunostimulatory effect of low-dose polyethylene glycol interleukin 2 in patients with human immunodeficiency virus type 1 infection. J Exp Med 177:483–492
21. Clark AG, Holondiy M, Schwartz DH (1992) Decrease in HIV provirus in peripheral blood mononuclear cells during zidovudine and human rIL-2 administration. J Acq Immun Defic Syndr 5:52–59
22. Cocchi F, DeVico AL, Garzino-Demo A, Arya SK, Gallo RC, Lusso P (1995) Identification of RANTES, MIP-1 alpha, and MIP-1 beta as the major HIV-suppressive factors produced by CD8+ cells. Science 270:1811–1815
23. Skurnick JH, Bogden JD, Baker H, Kemp FW, Sheffet A, Quattrone G, Louria DB (1996) Micronutrient profiles in HIV-1-infected heterosexual adults. J Acquir Immun Defic Syndr Human Retrovirol 12:75–83
24. Buhl R, Jaffe HA, Holroyd KJ, Wells FB, Mastrangeli A, Saltini C, et a. (1989) Systematic glutathione deficiency in symptom-free HIV-seropositive individuals. Lancet 2:1294–1298
25. Kalebic T, Kinter A, Poli G, Anderson ME, Meister A, Fauci AS (1991) Suppression of human immunodeficiency virus expression in chronically infected monocytic cells by glutathione, glutathione ester, and N-acetylcysteine. Proc Natl Acad Sci USA 88:986–990
26. Suss J, Sinnecker H (1991) Immune reactions against rabies viruses – infection and vaccination. Exp Pathol 42:1–9
27. Steimer KS, Haigwood NL (1992) Immunization of primates with native, recombinant HIV-SF2 gp 120 generates broadly effective neutralizing antibodies directed to conformational epitopes. AIDS Res Hum Retroviruses 8:1391
28. Berman PW, Gregory TJ, Riddle L et al (1990) Protection of chimpanzees from infection by HIV-1 after vaccination with recombinant glycoprotein gp120 but not gp160. Nature 345:622–625
29. Mascola JR, Snyder SW, Weislow OS, Belay SM,Belshe RB, Schwartz DH, Clements ML, Dolin R, Graham BS, Gorse GJ, Keefer MC, McElrath MJ, Walker MC, Wagner KF, McNeil JG, McCutchan FE, Burke DS (1996) Immunization with envelope subunit vaccine products elicits neutralizing antibodies against laboratory-adapted but not primary isolates of human immunodeficiency virus type 1. J Infect Dis 173:340–348
30. Kaiser J (1996) AIDS vaccine trial disappointing. Science 272:341

Cytokine Therapy and Vaccination in Tropical Diseases (Leishmaniasis and Leprosy)

G. Kolde and C. Sunderkötter

Introduction

The rationale for the immunotherapy applied in leishmaniasis and leprosy derives from the recent knowledge which has been gained from the pathophysiology of experimental leishmaniasis, i.e., from experiments with inbred mouse strains which are either resistant (e.g., C3He, C57BL/6) or susceptible (e.g., BALB/c) to infection with *Leishmania major*. These studies have shown that the outcome of the disease depends on the development of leishmania-specific CD4 cells into T-helper type-1 (Th1) cells in resistant mice or into T-helper type-2 (Th2) cells in susceptible mice (for a review, see [32]). The decisive factor is the cytokine profile released by these cells. Th2 cells release interleukin (IL)-4, IL-5, and IL-10, for example, which mediate progression of disease. Th1 cells, in contrast, release exclusively IL-2 and interferon (IFN)-γ, by which the infection is successfully combated. IFN-γ, in particular, has potent effects, as it supports the further propagation of Th1 cells and activates macrophages to kill the intracellular parasites. Macrophages are about the only cells which phagocytose the obligate intracellular leishmania. They therefore present the effector cells which, according to whether they are stimulated by Th1 or Th2 cytokines, either eliminate the intracellular pathogen or allow its propagation. Consequently, the application of IFN-γ has been found to have beneficial effects in experimental leishmaniasis [32].

In humans, infections with *L. major* also have different courses, but are not confined to the two genetically determined extremes encountered in mice. However, humans do show a genetically determined spectrum of diseases with two polar ends when infected with *Mycobacterium leprae*. Similar to experimental leishmaniasis, the immune response in human leprosy is tightly linked to a Th1/Th2 response. The tuberculoid forms are characterized by (a) the development of organized granulomas which contain marked levels of mRNA for IL-2 and IFN-γ [45] and (b) *M. leprae*-reactive Th1 cells in the cirulation [16]. The selective lack of cellular immunity to *M. leprae* in lepromatous leprosy has been correlated with (a) high levels of mRNA of Th2 cytokines in the diffuse inflammatory infiltrate [45], (b) more $CD4^+$ T cells that produce IL-4 than IFN-γ [33], and (c) $CD8^+$ cells that suppress the proliferative response of specific $CD4^+$ cells [33]. Macrophages again serve as antigen-presenting and decisive effector cells because, in addition to Schwann cells, they harbor the mycobacteriae and either kill them or facilitate their propagation.

With this knowledge about the immunological events in leishmaniasis and leprosy, it was conceivable that the application of Th1 cytokines might present a promising form of immunotherapy in human infection. Insights into the development of cellular immunity have also revived interest in the vaccination strategies used in these diseases. In this

Table 1. Forms of human leishmaniasis

Clinical form	Species	Subgenus
Cutaneous leishmaniasis	*L. major, L. tropica, L. aethiopica, L. mexicana* complex	*L. saf'janova*
Visceral leishmaniasis (including post-kala-azar dermal leishmaniasis)	*L. donovani, (L. infantum)*	*L. saf'janova*
Mucocutaneous leishmaniasis	*L. braziliensis* complex	*L.* viannia

chapter, we report on the currently available cytokine therapy and vaccination in leishmaniasis and leprosy and compare their efficacy with conventional treatment regimens.

State of the Art

Leishmaniasis

Human leishmaniasis has been divided into three major forms, as outlined in Table 1. In this chapter, we will concentrate on cutaneous leishmaniasis, but will also mention immunotherapy of the other forms.

Cutaneous Leishmaniasis

Cutaneous leishmaniasis can have different clinical courses, which are partially dependent on the species of the leishmania, but mostly on the leishmania-specific immune status of the infected patient (for a review, see [15]). A papule usually develops at the side of inoculation; this papule grows, ulcerates, and finally heals within 2 years leaving a scar (acute cutaneous leishmaniasis). In some cases, healing takes longer (chronic cutaneous leishmaniasis). In about 3–5 % of patients, papulous lesion recurs after initial healing, although the patients present with a positive cellular immune response to leishmania antigen (recurrent cutaneous leishmaniasis). Especially after infection with *L. aethiopica* and *L. mexicana amazonensis*, cutaneous lesions may disseminate and do not heal; these patients have a selective anergy towards leishmania antigens (disseminated/diffuse cutaneous leishmaniasis). Cutaneous erythematous papules or hypopigmented macules also occur in patients recovering from visceral leishmaniasis caused by *L. donovani* (post-kala-azar dermal leishmaniasis). Recently, a new form was described after infection with *L. tropica* without apparent involvement of the skin, but involving visceral organs (viscerotropic leishmaniasis).

Most forms of cutaneous leishmaniasis are self-limited. Therefore, uncomplicated courses of acute cutaneous leishmaniasis do not require immunotherapy. Conventional treatment has recently been proposed to be applied in the following order of preference (for a review, see [25]):

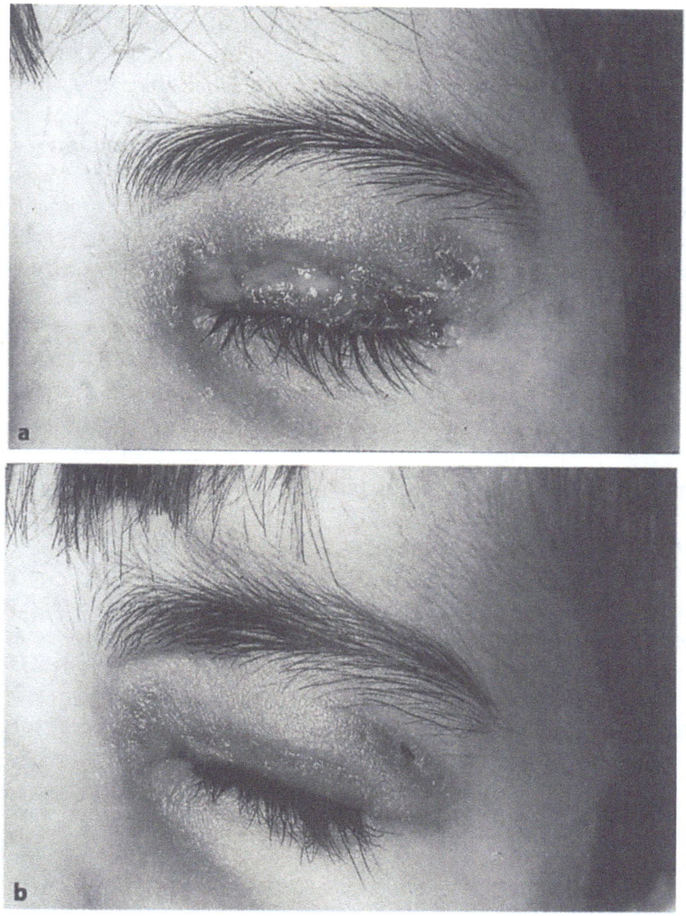

Fig. 1a,b. Lesion of cutaneous leishmaniasis on the upper eyelid **a** before and **b** 28 days after systemic monotherapy with interferon (IFN)-γ. (From [26], with permission)

- *First line:* cryosurgery or thermotherapy
- *Second line:* surgical excision of small lesions or intralesional antimonial therapy (except for antimony-resistant *L. aethiopica*)
- *Third line:* oral itraconazol or ketoconazol for at least 2 months

Cytokine Therapy. Although conventional treatment is sufficient for most patients, there are cases in which it fails or cannot be applied. For example, a young boy was admitted to our hospital whose upper eyelid was endangered by acute leishmaniasis (Fig. 1a). Although the disease could have eventually been self-limited, rapid treatment was necessary in order to prevent a disfiguring scar and functional impairment of the eyelid. As surgical therapy was not possible, we treated him with systemic IFN-γ (100 mg/m^2 per day), which was well-tolerated and led to rapid healing with a functionally and cosmetically excellent result (Fig. 1b) [26]. Administration of IFN-γ was associated with a decline of less mature macrophages in the infiltrate, as also observed in healing lesions of IFN-γ producing resistant mice [26, 39]. Thus, in contrast to surgical measures or chemotherapeutic treatment, which interferes with the metabolism of leishmania, IFN-γ initiates a rather physiological immune response against intracellular parasites. In other reports, IFN-γ (25 mg) was injected intradermally (perilesionally) in 13 patients with *L. tropica*, leading to complete resolution of lesions and histological features of cell-mediated immune responses in nine of the patients [17]. However, in a subsequent report, the same group reported that weekly perilesional injection of methylglucamine antimonate was superior to weekly perilesional injection of 25 μg IFN-γ [18]. It it possible that daily, and not necessarily perilesional injections of IFN-γ are more efficacious. Daily administration of IFN-γ (100 mg/m^2) has been successfully combined with methylglucamine antimonate in a patient suffering from cutaneous leishmaniasis refractory to methylglucamine antimonate alone [27]. In disseminated cutaneous leishmaniasis, daily injections of IFN-γ with pentavalent antimony may also evolve as a promising therapy [5]. The application of recombinant IL-2 is another immunotherapeutic attempt in this form of leishmaniasis [1].

Visceral and Mucocutaneous Leishmaniasis

In contrast to cutaneous leishmaniasis, all patients with visceral and mucocutaneous leishmaniasis require treatment. With regard to mucocutaneous leishmaniasis, this means that all patients with cutaneous infection in areas endemic for species of the *L. braziliensis* complex and therefore in danger of mucosal spread, need to be treated efficiently and monitored carefully. Again, there are several forms of conventional treatment with a certain order of preference [15]:

- *First line:* stibogluconate
- *Second line:* pentamidine or amphotericin B
- *Third line:* ketoconazol or allopurinol

Because of the severity of disease and the often toxic side effects of most of these drugs, the decision for immunotherapy could be made more readily. However, also because of the severity of infection, except for in one uncontrolled pilot trial [38], IFN-γ has been used in addtion to and in combination with approved conventional regimens instead of being applied as a monotherapeutic agent. Combinations of IFN-γ and antimony were effective in several patients with visceral leishmaniasis [4, 5, 19, 37] and mucocutaneous leishmaniasis [6, 12].

Vaccination

There is still no effective and safe vaccination for use in patients with human leishmaniasis. Deliberate infection with viable leishmania species tried in some endemic areas has been shown to induce T cell-mediated protective immunization, but this "leishmanization" can become as troublesome as naturally acquired disease [28]. In 1987, Convit et al. [10] reported on successful vaccination against American cutaneous leishmaniasis using killed leishmania amastigotes and live bacille Calmette-Guérin (BCG) as adjuvant. Current knowledge suggests that this immunization may be mediated by the adjuvant-induced release of IL-12 from macrophages [3] and thus represents a combination of immunostimulation and vaccination. It is not yet clear whether the alternative administration of recombinant IL-12 is more efficacious than BCG. A partly purified fraction of *L. braziliensis braziliensis* injected without adjuvant was effective as an immunoprophylactic agent in a preliminary trial in Brazil [29]. For evaluation of this strategy regarding the degree and duration of protection, a longer follow-up is necessary. It also has to be determined whether the effective, safe, and successful vaccination strategies recently developed in experimental leishmaniasis are suitable for use in humans. These methods include avirulent vaccine from mutant leishmania [42], induction of low-zone immunization by repeated administration of a few viable leishmania [7], and very recently DNA vaccination with the leishmania surface protein gp63 [43].

Leprosy

Infections with *M. leprae*, an intracellular bacterium of macrophages and peripheral nerve Schwann cells, usually begins as indeterminate leprosy that may spontaneously resolve. Otherwise, the disease progresses to a wide spectrum of clinical and histopathologic manifestations, with Th1 cell-associated tuberculoid leprosy (TT) at the one end, and Th2 cell-associated progressive lepromatous leprosy (LL) at the other. These polar forms frame the borderline types – borderline tuberculoid (BT), borderline borderline (BB), and borderline lepromatous (BL) – with corresponding modifications of the immune response (for a review, see [2]).

The multidrug therapy (MDT) for leprosy recommended by the WHO [44] consists of rifampicin and dapsone in the paucibacillary TT and BT types, and rifampicin, dapsone, and clofazimine in the multibacillary BB, BL, and LL types. These chemotherapeutic regimens are administered for at least 6 months and 2 years, respectively. Several studies have shown that the MDT is highly effective, with relapse rates of about one per 1000 paucibacillary cases and 0.2 per 1000 multibacillary cases. The treatment regimens are usually well tolerated, but may have serious side effects, such as rifampicin-induced hepatic failure, dapsone-induced agranulocytosis, and the occasionally fatal "sulfone syndrome."

Cytokine Therapy

Leprosy was one of the first bacterial diseases treated successfully with IFN-γ to activate the infected macrophages. In 1986, Nathan et al. [30] reported that the local application of IFN-γ into a single cutaneous lesion of LL resulted in migration of $CD4^+$ and $CD8^+$ cells as well as monocytes into the dermis, and formation of granulomas similar to those in BT. Half of the patients showed an approximately tenfold decrease in acid-fast bacilli due to activation of the infected macrophages. Further studies suggested that IFN-γ may also have beneficial systemic effects when injected intramuscularly at higher multiple doses [31]. No toxic effects of IFN-γ therapy were observed. However, there is some evidence that this therapy produces more adverse immune complex-mediated type-2 leprosy reactions than MDT, with manifestation of erythema nodosum leprosum in a substantial number of patients [22, 34]. This form of vasculitis can be successfully controlled by administration of thalidomide and pentoxifylline, which reduce the high serum levels of tumor necrosis factor (TNF)-γ in affected patients [22,41]. Nevertheless, there is as yet no controlled trial demonstrating that costly monotherapy with IFN-γ is superior to MDT.

Intradermal injections of recombinant IL-2 have more recently been shown to be effective in LL [8, 23]. In general, this Th1 cell-derived cytokine is crucial in vitro for the blastogenesis and differentiation of specific $CD4^+$ cells and the release of IFN-γ. IL-2 treatment of anergic leprosy could mimic the immune response to *M. leprae* observed in TT and BT patients and induces both T cell-mediated and humoral immune response, in contrast to IFN-γ [22]. When using a combination of IL-2 and MDT, the bacterial clearance was more pronounced than with the combined application of MDT and IFN-γ. The difference is thought to result from both an increased immigration of specific $CD8^+$ cells into the lesions and an increased release of IFN-γ and macrophage activation [22]. Remarkably, no adverse leprae reactions were reported in the various studies using IL-2 therapy. Furthermore, there was no severe toxicity of the treatment, except for a transient erythematous and edematous response similar to capillary leak syndrome, as observed by Kaplan [22] during the first days of administration. Thus immunotherapy using IL-2 seems to be more efficacious and less toxic than with IFN-γ.

Vaccination

Vaccination is used both for induction of protective immunity and for immunotherapeutic treatment of already infected patients. BCG, an attenuated strain of *M. bovis*, is the most widely used vaccine to induce protective immunization against *M. leprae* due to its cross-protective capacity against various strains of mycobacteriae. The efficacy of BCG vaccination against leprosy, however, ranges from 80% in Uganda to less than 20% in some other countries [13]. This variability of efficacy is thought to result from different antigenic determinants of the leprosy bacillus endemic in the different parts of the world and the use of different strains of BCG for immunization. However, immunoprophylaxis was not significantly improved by a vaccine consisting of BCG plus killed *M. leprae* [11]. Interestingly, a recent study investigated whether BCG vaccination is indeed able to induce protective immunization against leprosy antigens [14]. This study suggests that BCG rather functions as a nonspecific adjuvant that helps to acquire protective immunity resulting from the natural exposure to *M. leprae* in the endemic parts of the world.

The first immunotherapeutic vaccination strategy for patients already suffering from multibacillary leprosy was developed was by Convit et al. [9], using killed *M. leprae* and BCG. After therapy, numerous patients with active and inactive LL and BL showed development of specific T cell-mediated immunity with formation of tuberculoid granulomas, conversion of the lepromin test, and clinical improvement. Recovery from disease was found to be increased when vaccination was combined with chemotherapeutic MDT. In the last few years, chemotherapy has mostly been used in combination with *Mycobacterium w* vaccine [24, 46]. *Mycobacterium w* is a nonpathogenic, rapidly growing strain of an atypical mycobacterium that shares a number of B and T cell epitopes with *M. leprae* and induces propagation of Th1 cells and release of IL-2 and IFN-γ in experimental leprosy of mice [36]. Patients receiving combined MDT and *Mycobacterium w* vaccine therapy showed rapid formation of tuberculoid granulomas and enhanced bacterial clearance [46]. The accelerated onset of these effects may explain why some of the treated patients developed adverse type-1 leprosy reactions characterized by sudden generation of cell-mediated immunity that can result in a loss of function of the infected nerves.

Discussion

All available studies indicate that immunotherapy with the Th1 cytokines IL-2 and IFN-γ can be effective in the treatment of human leishmaniasis and leprosy. IFN-γ, in particular, has already been proven to induce appropriate activation of the infected macrophages, thereby leading to killing of the intracellular microbes and to resolution of the disease. As macrophages function as both effector cells and antigen-presenting cells in several infections with intracellularly residing microbes, their cytokine activation also seems to be an efficacious and physiologic therapeutic approach in other cutaneous and systemic diseases, such as tuberculosis. However, it should be mentioned that the application of recombinant IFN-γ and IL-2, which is usually well tolerated, is much more expensive than conventional therapy. Furthermore, there are as yet only few, if any clinical trials on the most effective dosage and application route (lesional versus systemic) of these cytokines and on their efficacy when combined with chemotherapy or surgical measures.

Although IFN-γ and IL-2 are effective in leprosy, their administration is evidently not able to reverse the infection-specific anergy in leprosy patients [22]. Both cytokines are rather distant mediators in the cytokine network which mediate the immunological control of the infectious agents, but at least in leishmaniasis they play a less decisive role in the differentiation of CD4 cells into Th1 cells [32], in contrast to IL-12 [35]. This cytokine is mainly released from cells of the monocyte/macrophage series and is one of the most powerful inducers of IFN-γ production in other cells. The application of IL-12 has indeed recently been shown to reverse the anergy of susceptible mice by inducing curative cellular immune response against leishmania [20, 40]. There is substantial evidence that the efficacy of vaccines and in particular vaccine adjuvants is also directly related to their ability to induce IL-12 production [3]. Macrophages and accessory dendritic cells expressing costimulatory molecules are equally known to be crucial for the development of a Th1 response (for a review, see [21]). Thus the injection of activated dendritic cells pulsed with antigenic proteins from infectious agents may become another approach for immunotherapy.

Before these experimental approaches are suitable for use in humans, we suggest the following cytokine treatment and vaccination:

- *In leishmaniasis*, the monotherapeutic subcutaneous application of IFN-γ (100 mg/m^2 per day) presents an effective treatment for cutaneous disease that should be applied in complicated courses of acute disease, in chronic cutaneous leishmaniasis when conventional therapy has failed, and in disseminated cutaneous leishmaniasis. In mucocutaneous and visceral leishmaniasis, IFN-γ or IL-2 may be added to chemotherapeutic regimens to enhance their efficacy. For prophylactic immunization against cutaneous leishmaniasis, final studies with purified protein vaccines from different leishmania species should be awaited. For prophylactic immunization against the more severe mucocutaneous and visceral disease, people living in endemic areas could already be subjected to vaccination strategies that have appeared to be safe and promising in preliminary trials.

- *In multibacillary leprosy*, immunotherapy with IFN-γ and IL-2 had marked local effects mimicking a physiological cell-mediated immune response. However, the systemic effects of such monotherapy seem too weak to combat the systemic distribution of *M. leprae* [23]. In contrast, the combination of IFN-γ or IL-2 with MDT is worthwhile in treating otherwise intractable LL and BL. Immunization with *Mycobacterium w* vaccine, in particular, has also been proven to enhance the efficacy of MDT. As long as the efficacy of this vaccine in prophylactic immunization is not clear, well-established BCG vaccination should continue to be performed in areas endemic for leprosy.

In conclusion, the currently available cytokine therapy and vaccination have markedly improved the treatment of leishmaniasis and leprosy. It is reasonable to assume that immunotherapeutic strategies will soon become the most important tool for both the prevention and treatment of these infections. Both leishmaniasis and leprosy are definitely still endemic in many parts of the world; they are increasingly being imported into northern Europe and North America, and they now often affect immunocompromised patients due to HIV infection.

Summary

Healing of leishmaniasis and leprosy requires microbicidal activation of macrophages which harbor the obligate intracellular pathogens. In experimental leishmaniasis of mice, macrophage activation is known to be mediated by the cytokines IL-2 and IFN-γ released by pathogen-specific Th1 cells. IFN-γ, the most potent cytokine for macrophage activation, has recently been shown to be a very successful immunotherapeutic agent for cutaneous leishmaniasis, particularly in complicated cases. Its use was also effective in mucocutaneous and visceral leishmaniasis. In anergic leprosy, therapy with IFN-γ or IL-2 induced a local reaction resembling that seen in cell-mediated immunity. Vaccination is another form of immunotherapy which is efficacious in leprosy in both the prevention and treatment of disease. In leishmaniasis, an effective and safe vaccine is still lacking. but there are some promising new experimental strategies which will soon become suitable for use in human disease.

References

1. Akuffo H, Kaplan G, Kiessling R et al (1990) Administration of recombinant interleukin-2 reduces the local parasite load of patients with disseminated cutaneous leishmaniasis. J Infect Dis 161:775–780
2. All India Institute of Medical Sciences (1995) Leprosy. Lancet 345:697–703
3. Alfonso LCC, Scharton TM, Vieira LQ et al (1994) The adjuvant effect of interleukin-12 in a vaccine against Leishmania major. Science 263:235–237
4. Badaro R, Falcoff E, Badaro FS et al (1990) Treatment of visceral leishmaniasis with pentavalent antimony and interferon gamma. N Engl J Med 322:16–22
5. Badaro R, Johnson WD (1993) The role of interferon-γ in the treatment of visceral and diffuse cutaneous leishmaniasis. J Infect Dis 167:S13–17
6. Botasso O, Cabrini J, Falcoff R (1992) Successful treatment of an antimony-resistant American mucocutaneous leishmaniasis: a case report. Arch Dermatol 128:996–997
7. Bretscher PA, Wie G, Menon JN, Bielefeldt-Ohmann H et al (1992) Establishment of stable, cell-mediated immunity that makes "susceptible" mice resistant to Leishmania major. Science 257:539–542

8. Converse P, Ottenhoff THM, Teklemariam SW et al (1990) Intradermal recombinant interleukin-2 enhances peripheral blood T cell responses to mitogen and antigens in lepromatous leprosy. Scand J Immunol 32:83–91
9. Convit J, Aranzazu N, Ulrich M et al (1982) Immunotherapy with a mixture of Mycobacterium leprae and BCG in different forms of leprosy and in Mitsuda negative contacts. Int J Lepr 50:415–424
10. Convit J, Castellanos PL, Rondon A et al (1987) Immunotherapy versus chemotherapy in localised cutaneous leishmaniasis. Lancet i:401–404
11. Convit J, Sampson C, Zuniga M et al (1992) Immunoprophylactic trial with combined Mycobacterium leprae/BCG vaccine against leprosy: preliminary results. Lancet 339: 446–450
12. Falcoff E, Taranto NJ, Remondegui CE et al (1994) Clinical healing of antimony-resistant cutaneous or mucocutaneous leishmaniasis following the combined administration of interferon-gamma and pentavalent antimonial compounds. Trans R Soc Trop Med Hyg 88:95–97
13. Fine PEM (1988) BCG vaccination against tuberculosis and leprosy. Br Med Bull 44:691–703
14. Fine PEM, Sterne JA, Ponnighaus JM, Rees RJ (1994) Delayed-type hypersensitivity, mycobacterial vaccines and protective immunity. Lancet 344:1245–1249
15. Grevelink SA, Lerner EA (1996) Leishmaniasis. J Am Acad Dermatol 34:257–272
16. Haanen JB, de Waal Malefijt R, Res PC et al (1991) Selection of human T helper type 1-like T cell subset by mycobacteria. J Exp Med 174:583–592
17. Harms G, Zwingenberger K, Chéhadé AK et al (1989) Effects of intradermal gamma-interferon in cutaneous leishmaniasis. Lancet i:1287–1292
18. Harms G, Chéhadé AK, Dooba M et al (1991) A randomized trial comparing a pentavalent antimonial drug and recombinant interferon gamma in the local treatment of cutaneous leishmaniasis. Trans R Soc Trop Med Hyg 85:214–216
19. Harms G, Zwingenberger K, Sandkamp B et al (1993) Immunochemotherapy of visceral leishmaniasis: a pilot trial of sequential treatment with recombinant interferon-gamma and pentavalent antimony. J Interferon Res 13:39–41
20. Heinzel FP, Schoenhaut DS, Rerko RM et al (1993) Recombinant interleukin 12 cures mice infected with Leishmania major. J Exp Med 177:1505–1512
21. Jenkins MK, Johnson JG (1993) Molecules involved in T-cell costimulation. Curr Opinion Immunol 5:361–367
22. Kaplan G (1993) Recent advances in cytokine therapy in leprosy. J Infect Dis 167:S18–S22
23. Kaplan G, Britton WJ, Hancock GE et al (1991) The systemic influence of recombinant interleukin-2 on the manifestation of lepromatous leprosy. J Exp Med 173:993–1006
24. Katoch K, Katoch VM, Natrajan M et al (1995) Treatment of bacilliferous BL/LL cases with combined chemotherapy and immunotherapy. Int J Lepr Other Mycobact Dis 63:202–212
25. Koff AB, Rosen T (1994) Treatment of cutaneous leishmaniasis. J Am Acad Dermatol 31:693–708
26. Kolde G, Luger T, Sorg C, Sunderkötter C (1996) Successful treatment of cutaneous leishmaniasis using systemic interferon-gamma. Dermatology 192:56–60
27. Kürkcüoglu N, Tandogda R (1990) Interferon gamma therapy for cutaneous leishmaniasis. Arch Dermatol 126:831–832
28. Modabber F (1989) Experiences with vaccines against cutaneous leishmaniasis of mice and men. Parasitology 98:S49–S60
29. Monjour L, Silva OA, Vouldoukis I et al (1992) Immunoprophylaxis in cutaneous leishmaniasis. Lancet 340:1098–1099
30. Nathan CF, Kaplan G, Levis WR et al (1986) Local and systemic effects of intradermal recombinant interferon-γ in patients with lepromatous lepra. N Engl J Med 315:6–15
31. Nathan C, Squires K, Griffo W et al (1990) Widespread intradermal accumulation of mononuclear leukocytes in lepromatous leprosy patients treated systemically with recombinant interferon gamma. J Exp Med 172:1509–1512
32. Reiner Sl, Locksley RM (1995) The regulation of immunity to Leishmania major. Annu Rev Immunol 13:151–177
33. Salgame G, Abrams JS, Clayberger C et al (1991) Differing lymphokine profiles of functional subsets of human CD4 and CD8 T cell clones. Science 254:279–282

34. Sampaio EP, Moreira AL, Sarno EN et al (1992) Prolonged treatment with recombinant interferon-γ induces erythema nodosum leprosum in lepromatous leprosy patients. J Exp Med 175:1729–1737
35. Scott P (1993) IL-12: initiation cytokine for cell-mediated immunity. Science 260:496–497
36. Singh IG, Mukherjee R, Talwar GP, Kaufmann SH (1992) In vitro characteristics of T cells from Mycobacterium w vaccinated mice. Infect Immunol 60:257–263
37. Squires KE, Rosenkaimer F, Sherwood JA et al (1993) Immunochemotherapy for visceral leishmaniasis: a controlled pilot trial of antimony versus antimony plus interferon-gamma. Am J Trop Med Hyg 48:666–669
38. Sundar S, Rosenkaimer F, Lesser ML, Murray HW(1995) Immunochemotherapy for a systemic intracellular infection: accelerated response using interferon-gamma in visceral leishmaniasis. J Infect Dis 171:992–996
39. Sunderkötter C, Kunz M, Steinbrink K et al (1993) Resistance of mice to experimental leishmaniasis is associated with more rapid appearance of mature macrophages in vitro and in vivo. J Immunol 151:4891–4901
40. Sypek JP, Chung CL, Mayor SE et al (1993) Resolution of cutaneous leishmaniasis: interleukin 12 initiates a protective T helper type 1 immune response. J Exp Med 177:1797–1802
41. Talhari S, Orsi AT, Talhari AC et al (1995) Pentoxifylline may be useful in the treatment of type 2 leprosy reactions. Lepr Rev 66:261–263
42. Titus RG, Gueiros-Filho FJ, de Freitas LA, Beverley SM (1995) Development of a safe live leishmania vaccine line by gene replacement. Proc Natl Acad Sci USA 92:10267–10271
43. Walker PS, Scharton-Kersten TM, Hengge U et al (1996) Direct targeting of skin and muscle for genetic immunization in a murine model of leishmaniasis. J Invest Dermatol 106:810 (abstract)
44. World Health Organisation (1982) Chemotherapy of leprosy for control programmes. World Health Organ Tech Rep Ser 675:21–24
45. Yamamura M (1992) Defining protective responses to pathogens: cytokine profile in leprosy lesions. Science 255:12
46. Zaheer SA, Mukherjee R, Ramkumar B et al (1993) Combined multidrug and Mycobacterium w vaccine therapy in patients with multibacillary leprosy. J Infect Dis 167:401–410

Cutaneous Lymphomas

G. Burg, R. Dummer, and F. Nestle

Introduction

The skin is an immunoregulatory organ that hosts various types of immunoregulatory cells, both professional ones (such as lymphocytes and dendritic cells) and nonprofessional ones (such as keratinocytes, endothelial cells, and others), which may become actively involved under certain pathophysiologic circumstances in immunoregulatory events. These cells are either resting in or traveling through the skin depending on a network of chemotactic, adhesion, promoting, or blocking factors in a permanently interactive feedback context.

Cutaneous lymphomas like nodal lymphomas are tumors arising from the immunocompetent cell system. In cutaneous B cell lymphomas (CBCL), as in cutaneous T cell lymphomas (CTCL), the primary event may be antigenic stimulation through the help of dendritic cells and T cells. Formation of follicular structures corresponding to secondary follicles in the lymph node is seen in the skin following *Borrelia burgdorferi* infection by a tick bite. Transformation into CBCL has been reported [6, 32], paralleling the situation in mucosa-associated lymphoid tissue (MALT) lymphomas of the gastrointestinal tract associated with *Helicobacter pylori* infection.

In CTCL, the first step may be chronic antigenic stimulation, attracting T-helper (Th) memory cells from the dermal microvasculature into the dermis and into the epidermis by specific ligand–adhesion receptor interactions: lymphocyte function-associated antigen (LFA)-1/intercellular adhesion molecule (ICAM)-1; very late activation antigen (VLA)-4/vascular cell adhesion molecule (VCAM)-1; cutaneous lymphocyte antigen (CLA)/E selectin [51].

Keratinocytes are potential providers of a battery of cytokines, including interleukin (IL)-1, IL-3, IL-6, IL-7, IL-8, IL-10, tumor necrosis factor (TNF)-α, granulocyte-macrophage colony-stimulating factor (GM-CSF), transforming growth factor (TGF), and others [21].

IL-1 costimulates thymocytes and T and B cells, as well as hematopoietic stem cells, which in autocrine stimulatory loops and probably due to the lack of natural regulatory blocking mechanisms, such as apoptosis or senescence of the cells, may lead to unlimited cell proliferation with the potential risk of accumulation of gene mutations, finally leading to tumor formation.

IL-7 and IL-15 may be important factors for the proliferation of lymphoid cells in CTCL [14]. It has been shown that peripheral blood mononuclear cells from patients with Sézary syndrome, the leukemic form of CTCL, have a Th2 cell cytokine (IL-4, IL-5, and IL-10) production pattern. Peripheral blood mononuclear cells in nonleukemic CTCL patients also show preferential secretion of a Th2-like cytokine pattern upon stimulation [20]. The presence of a Th2 cytokine pattern correlates with a malignant T cell clone in different stages of cutaneous involvement among patients with CTCL. In all stages of cutaneous involvement of CTCL, IL-4 and IL-5 mRNA is variably detectable [77]. However, rare forms of CTCL exist in which tumor cells secrete high amounts of interferon (INF)-γ [9].

Moreover, occurrence of depigmentation, development of squamous cell carcinomas, and susceptibility to infections provide additional clinical evidence for alteration of the immune system in cutaneous lymphoma (CL).

Taken together, CL seem to be ideal target diseases for immunointerventional therapy. This approach should be used early during disease progression rather than in advanced stages of the diseases [23].

Immunomodulatory Agents and Their Application in the Treatment of Cutaneous Lymphoma

Interferons

IFN consist of at least three different gene products with different subtypes, binding to different receptors, the number of which is different on various cell types. They show pleiotropic effects, including antiviral and antineoplastic effects in vitro and in vivo. The antitumor effect is due to enhanced expression of cell surface antigens. IFN activates macrophages, T cells, and natural killer (NK) cells and modulates antibody production. Moreover, modulation of various enzymes involved in cell proliferation takes place. Nevertheless, the response depends on the type of IFN used. IFN-α increases class I molecules on lymphocytes, whereas IFN-γ induces class I and II histocompatibility molecules. IFN-α, particularly pertinent to the treatment of CTCL, induces a shift from a Th2 cytokine profile to a Th1 profile, reducing IL-4 and IL-5 production by T cells. IFN receptor expression on the cell surface depends on cell activity and may be significantly higher on lymphoma cells than on normal lymphocytes. IFN have been extensively used for the treatment of CTCL, either as monotherapy or in combination with other immunomodulating substances. The different designs and dosages used prevent detailed comparison of the various trials. Early stages seem to benefit better from immunomodulatory treatment modalities than advanced stages of CTCL.

Interferon-α

Most studies conducted so far have been done with IFN-α. In the beginning, high doses (50 MU/m^2) were used [7] in a phase II study, resulting in a 45% response rate. Responses developed gradually over a period of weeks to months. An overview of the literature shows that lower doses (3–9 MU/m^2) are as effective, but are less toxic [8, 52]. The studies clearly show that IFN are active agents that produce responses nearly as often as single-agent chemotherapy, but with less toxicity when low doses are used.

Different tumors have different threshold levels of sensitivity for IFN. For example, hairy cell leukemia is sensitive to much lower doses of IFN-α than CTCL [52]. The lowest dose to begin with is 3 MU/m^2 every second day. Patients on low-dose IFN-α who do not achieve complete response can have a remission induced with dose escalation [52].

It has not yet been evaluated whether administration every second day or three times a week is superior to daily administration.

Published studies on interferon in CTCL show an average of 15–20 % complete remissions and of 30–40 % partial remission; thus approximately 50–60 % of the patients benefit objectively from this type of treatment.

The lengths of treatment of CTCL with recombinant IFN should be at least 6 months, followed by a maintenance dose for up to 2 years.

There are almost no limitations for recruiting CTCL patients for treatment with IFN. As with any other treatment, early stages of the disease do better than advanced stages with high tumor burden.

The major side effects associated with IFN-α treatment are influenza-like symptoms such as fever, chills, myalgias, and malaise during the initial exposure to the drug. These are easily controlled with nonsteroidal anti-inflammatory drugs (NSAID). Other side effects include gastrointestinal complaints, anorexia, leukopenia, decrease in blood platelet count or elevation of liver function tests, telogen effluvium, and fatigue. As with other immunomodulatory drugs, concommitant autoimmune thyroiditis or vitiligo may occur.

Possible dissemination in a patient with CTCL involving visceral organs under treatment with recombinant IFN-α_2 has been reported [73]. Intermittent high-dose recombinant IFN-α_{2a} was used in advanced mycosis fungoides (MF) and Sézary syndrome (SS) refractory to one or more standard therapies in order to reduce side effects. Patients received 10 MU IFN-α/m^2 i.m. on day 1 followed by 50 MU/m^2 i.m. on days 2–5 every 3 weeks; after the first four cycles, stable and partially responding patients underwent dose escalation to twice the starting dose. One complete and six partial responses were observed (response rate, 29 % and 95 %, respectively), lasting 4–19 months. No improvement in objective response was seen in the eight patients who received dose escalation [41].

Intralesional IFN may be given safely and has a beneficial effect, both locally and systemically [74, 79].

One major problem may be the development of IFN antibodies [57], comprising both binding antibodies and neutralizing antibodies. Both may be relevant in affecting the efficacy of IFN treatment. Incidences reported so far with IFN-α are within a broad range of 3 % to over 30 % neutralizing antibodies developing in patients treated with recombinant IFN-α. This broad spectrum indicates that the type of IFN used, dose, frequency, and form of application may have a great impact on the incidence of antibody formation. The presence of IFN antibodies (binding and neutralizing) may have impact on the outcome of CTCL treatment with IFN-α therapies [57].

Interferon-β

IFN-β is produced mainly by fibroblasts and some epithelial cells. It binds to the same receptor as IFN-α. However, in contrast to IFN-α, IFN-β is strictly species specific. It is involved in the regulation of nonspecific humoral immune responses, it increases the expression of HLA class I antigens, and it blocks the expression of HLA class II antigens, which are stimulated by IFN-γ. IFN-β also stimulates NK cells and suppressor cells. It shows antiproliferative activity against tumor cells.

In dermatology, IFN-β has mostly been used in the topical treatment of condylomata acuminata. There are only very few reports on the use of IFN-β for CTCL [37, 84]; these reports indicate one partial response among seven patients treated with low-dose IFN-β intramuscularly [84], whereas excellent results have been reported on local application of IFN-β in CTCL [37]. In summary, experience with IFN-β is very limited so far and seems not to be superior to that known from other IFN.

Interferon-γ

IFN-γ, also referred to as immune IFN or formerly as macrophage-activating factor (MAF), is produced mainly by T cells and NK cells activated by antigens or by IL-2 and is part of the Th1 cytokine pattern. The expression of the IFN-γ receptor on human peripheral blood monocytes is significantly increased by GM-CSF. In addition to its antiviral and antiparasitic activities, IFN-γ inhibits the proliferation of a number of normal and transformed cells. The growth-inhibitory activities of IFN-γ are more pronounced than those of the other IFN. Its synthesis in Th cells is induced by IL-2; it acts synergistically with IL-1 and IL-2 and seems to be required for the expression of IL-2 receptors on the cell surface of T lymphocytes. It modulates T cell growth and functional differentiation and is a growth-promoting factor for T lymphocytes. Blocking of the IL-2 receptor also inhibits the synthesis of IFN-γ. Differentiation of human promyelocytic leukemia cells into monocytes can be induced by IFN-γ. IFN-γ stimulates major histocompatibility complex (MHC) class II gene expression and the expression of CD4 in Th cells. It stimulates keratinocytes and is chemotactic for $CD4^+$ lymphocytes through inducible protein (IP)-10. This protein seems to be overexpressed in suprabasal keratinocytes in CTCL lesions [63].

Consequently, it was proposed that production of IFN-γ by the lymphoid infiltrate in CTCL induces the epidermal keratinocytes to secret IP-10, which due to its chemotactic effect on CTCL cells accounts for their epidermotropism [63]. On the other hand, lack of epidermotropism and subcutaneous localization of the infiltrate was the predominant feature in a case of lipotropic CTCL with IFN-γ production by the tumor cells [9].

Among the many indications for clinical use, IFN-γ has also been used in the treatment of CL alone or in combination with other substances [38, 39, 50, 63, 81].

Early reports came from Japan [38, 50] using IFN-γ intravenously or intralesionally. IFN-γ may also be effective in CTCL patients refractory to recombinant IFN (rIFN)-α and results in long-lasting (up to 32 months) partial responses [39]. More recent reports [81] have recommended the use of intralesional rIFN-γ applied to residual tumors following systemic chemotherapy [81].

The toxicities seen with IFN-γ were similar to those observed with rIFN-α, but were perhaps more frequent and more severe [52], including reversible dose-limiting neutropenia and nephrotic syndrome.

In summary, the objective response rate (complete and partial responses) in patients receiving systemic IFN-γ, as obvious from the few studies done, is about 50%, with a complete response rate of less than 10%.

Interleukin-2

IL-2 has many alternative names, including lymphocyte proliferation factor, T cell growth factor (TCGF), thymocyte-stimulating factor, and many others. Under physological conditions, IL-2 is produced mainly by $CD4^+$ T cells following activation by mitogens or allergens. Production is suppressed by dexamethasone or cyclosporin A.

The biological activities of IL-2 are mediated by a membrane receptor that is expressed almost exclusively on activated, but not on resting T cells. The expression of the IL-2 receptor is modulated by several interleukins (IL-5, IL-6, IL-12). At least three subunits of the IL-2 receptor (low, intermediate, and high affinity) can be differentiated. Activated lymphocytes and leukemia cells may secrete fragments of the Tac antigen and other chains, which circulate in the serum as soluble IL-2 receptor (sIL2R), the concentration of which in cutaneous lymphomas is closely related to the tumor burden. There is evidence that elevated sIL2R levels account for diminished NK activity by neutralizing IL-2 in CTCL patients [19, 24].

IL-2, IL-7, and IL-15 are known to be potential autocrine or paracrine growth factors in CTCL, stimulating cell proliferation. On the other hand, it was demonstrated that sIL-2R inhibit IL-2-dependent proliferation and cytotoxicity, explaining diminished NK cell activity in CTCL [19]. Almost 10 years ago, rIL-2 was successfully used for local treatment in a case of CTCL [49]. After six injections of rIL-2, four out of five nodules disappeared and the remaining large nodule was diminished in size. The histology showed mostly cells reactive for histiocytic markers.

In a recent series, seven patients (three MF, three Sézary syndromes, and one nonepidermotropic large cell CTCL) were treated with high-dose rIL-2 (20×10^6 IU/m^2 per day) [33, 45]. There were three complete responses lasting 6, 28, and 33 months and two partial responses. The sequential immunophenotypic studies showed an increase in $CD1^+$ cells in the dermal infiltrates without significant modification of NK cells or cytotoxic T lymphocytes (CTL). After six injections of rIL-2, four out of five nodules in a patient with large-cell CTCL disappeared, and the remaining large nodule was diminished in size for a period of 13 months [49]. These studies and our own experiences in four cases of advanced CTCL indicate that high-dose rIL-2 may be an alternative treatment approach in patients in whom other therapies, including aggressive chemotherapy, have failed.

The rationale for using IL-2 in a T cell lymphoproliferative disease might come from the observation that malignant cells do not depend on IL-2, since they seem to be Th2 cells that block reactive T lymphocytes by sIL-2R or IL-10 [25].

IL-2 supports the proliferation and clonal expansion of T cells that specifically attack certain tumor types by generating lymphokine-activated killer (LAK) cells and tumor-infiltrating lymphocytes (TIL). In a CTCL-derived cell line (SeAx), IL-2 inhibits ICAM-1 release [21].

Most experience was gained in the use of IL-2 for treatment of nonlymphoid neoplasias.

Intravenous administration of IL-2 alone or in combination with other immunomodulatory substances or with cytostatics was performed in various neoplasias, including malignant melanoma [22]. Only 30–40% of patients responded favorably to IL-2 therapy. High-dose IL-2 stimulates nonspecific LAK cell activity through low-affinity IL-2 receptors without leading to systemic immunity. Low-dose IL-2 exhibits immunomodulatory activities by inducing secretion of other soluble mediators, such as TNF-α, TNF-β, and IFN-γ. Intratumoral low doses of IL-2 can be highly effective with low toxic side effects. However, stimulation of lymphoid cell proliferation by IL-2 could be detrimental in patients with CTCL. Future aspects include construction of IL-2–toxin protein chimeras or vaccination with IL-2-transduced tumor cells.

Cyclosporin A

Cyclosporine (CSA) is a polypeptide which inhibits transcription of IL-2 and several other cytokines, most notably in Th lymphocytes. Th cells are preferentially inhibited, whereas suppressor T cell activity is not affected. Due to its immunosuppressive properties, it has been used in a wide range of dermatoses in which immunoregulatory dysfunction is a suspected etiological factor. Considering the stimulatory effect of IL-2 on T lymphocytes, therapeutic use of CSA for blocking this mediator theoretically seems to be appropriate.

CSA has been reported to exhibit cytostatic and cytolytic effects against selected T lymphoblastic leukemic cell lines [69]. Several reports on treatment of CTCL with CSA, initiated after the failure of conventional therapy, have been reported in the literature [58, 65, 70]. Post-treatment tissue biopsy specimens from patients with Sézary syndrome have demonstrated an overall decrease in tumor cell masses in the skin and lymph nodes. The marked clinical improvement with dramatic improvement of pruritus correlated with the expression of T cell activation "markers" [70]. Most patients had widespread disease, some with lymph node involvement. Side effects include hypertrichosis, gingival hyperplasia, and neurological and gastrointestinal effects. These are usually of mild or moderate severity and resolve after dosage reduction. Serious, irreversible damage of renal function may occur after long-term treatment and deserves regular laboratory monitoring.

Two of 11 patients with CTCL responded to treatment with CSA in a phase II study; however, rapid recurrence occurred, suggesting that CSA was cytostatic rather than cytocidal or that the clinical remissions were mediated by the anti-inflammatory effects of the drug [13]. In a patient with MF that was refractory to cytotoxic combination chemotherapy, CSA showed immediate improvement of subjective symptoms accompanied by a decrease in skin infiltration noted on physical examination and microscopically. Despite continued administration of CSA, symptoms recurred after 3½ months of therapy [44].

Dissemination of the disease into extracutaneous organs in a patient with MF treated with CSA (5 mg/kg body weight) for 5 weeks [67] and transformation of Sézary syndrome to high-grade T cell lymphoma has been reported [10].

From a series of three patients with MF and two patients with Sézary syndrome [65], it was concluded that CSA alone is not sufficient therapy in CTCL. As with other tumors, it is hard to predict which patients will benefit from treatment with CSA and which may deteriorate.

Monoclonal Antibodies

Monoclonal antibodies (mAb) seem to be ideal substances to target antigens expressed on the surface of the tumor cells. The proliferating cells in CTCL, however, tend to show loss rather than presentation of tumor cell-specific antigens. The generation of human anti-mouse antibodies constitutes an additional obstacle in using mAb in vivo.

An early pilot study with T-101, a murine antibody directed against CD5, was conducted in 1984 [15]. Four CTCL patients were treated with mAb to human T cells (T101) as infusion therapy. Immunofluorescence confirmed that circulating cells bound the antibody in vivo and were subsequently removed from the circulation. There are limitations of effector cell-mediated cytotoxicity at the tissue level. Moreover, production of anti-mouse antibodies may result in the production of neutralizing antibodies, possibly depending on the underlying immune status of the patient or the amount of mouse protein to which immunocompetent cells are exposed.

Radiolabeled murine monoclonal antibody (T101) was used for imaging and therapy of six CTCL patients [62]. Two patients showed regression of skin lesions, peripheral adenopathy, and resolution of pruritus. Duration of responses ranged from 3 weeks to 3 months. Signs of acute toxicity included myelosuppression as a major side effect, which limits the use of labeled mAb for therapy. Several other studies have been performed (for a review, see [8]).

The relative specificity and efficacy of mAb therapy is encouraging, but the limited clinical benefit and problems with anti-mouse antibody production underscore the need for continued research.

Autologous Bone Marrow Transplantation

There are only a few reports available on the effect of autologous bone marrow transplantation (ABMT) in patients with advanced CTCL. Early reports date back 10 years [12]. In one trial involving six patients treated with ABMT, only two were alive with no sign of diesease 1 year after treatment [5].

In four patients with high- and intermediate-grade cutaneous nonepidermotropic lymphoma, high-dose chemotherapy (cyclophosphamide, carmustine, and etoposide) and total body irradiation (12 Gy) in combination with AMBT resulted in complete remission lasting 22–51 months [47].

Fusion Toxins

Fusion toxins (FT), generated by fusion of a plant or bacterial toxin to a receptor ligand, have been constructed in order to specifically target a cellular antigen. Fusion of the IL-2 gene with the diphtheria toxin A chain gene resulted in a IL-2 fusion protein which contained 486 amino acids from the diphtheria toxin protein (DAB 486 IL-2) and was the first fusion toxin to enter phase I clinical trials. DAB 486 IL-2 binds to the high-affinity IL-2 receptor, is internalized by receptor-mediated endocytosis, and subsequently inhibits protein synthesis of neoplastic lymphocytes bearing the high-affinity IL-2 receptor by diphtheria toxin.

The biologic activity and toxicity of DAB 486 IL-2 was tested in 20 patients with hematologic malignancies, especially MF. Biologic activity was noted in patients with

MF showing clearing of skin lesions and relief of pruritus. However, there were also considerable dose-dependent signs of toxicity [43]. Significant toxicity observed in the phase I clinical trials with this recombinant protein could be reduced by a second-generation molecule, characterized by a deletion of 97 amino acids, resulting in DAB 389 IL-2, a second-generation molecule of this type with a more favorable pharmacological profile.

Three of five CTCL patients treated with DAB 486 IL-2 attained a complete response, which lasted more than 33 months without any interval treatment. The two other patients achieved partial remission. Treatment was well tolerated, except for a transient increase in hepatic transaminases in all patients [35].

In a phase II study, the correlation of the activity of chimeric fusion protein toxin DAB 486 IL-2 in advanced MF and the Sézary syndrome with IL-2 receptor expression was studied [28]. None of the 14 patients with CTCL enrolled achieved complete remission. There was one partial response, whereas most patients did not significantly benefit from the treatment. From this study, it was concluded that FT has valuable activity in patients with CTCL and that expression of the IL-2 receptor may be necessary, but not sufficient to predict response [29].

Studies with DAB 389 IL-2, the second-generation IL-2 FT, in which MF and Sézary syndrome patients with tumor cells expressing the IL-2 receptor were enrolled, have shown encouraging results in 38% of patients [31]. Toxicities have been mild and reversible.

Considering the fact that IL-7 binding to the respective receptor on CTCL cells is a potent stimulus for the proliferation of neoplastic lymphoid cells, appropriate constructs could be designed, targeting lymphoid cells expressing IL-7 receptor [14, 29]. Another target could be the IFN-γ receptor, since it is overexpressed in Sézary cells [25].

Thymopentin

Thymopentin (TP-5) is a synthetic pentapeptide corresponding to the active site of human thymopoietin. It has been used in patients with MF and Sézary syndrome intraveneously or subcutaneously, with minor improvement in some patients [56]. An overall response of 75% was achieved in patients with Sézary syndrome receiving TP-5 at a dose of 50 mg intravenously three times a week. Responses were more likely to occur in patients with Sézary counts below 2600/mm^3 [3]. Mostly minor responses were seen in a study recently reported by the National Cancer Institute (NCI) [31].

Miscellaneous

Changes in the IL-1 and IL-8 functional activities seen in the epidermis of CTCL lesions may also be targets for future immunomodulatory treatment modalities [34, 72, 78].

Expression of MY7 (CD13) antigen, normally found in normal basal cell keratinocytes but not in CTCL basal cell keratinocytes, can be induced by IFN-α_{2a} [11, 17].

Increased TNF production as a result of extracorporeal photopheresis may have important implications for the immunomodulatory effect in CTCL, mediating numerous antitumor effects [76].

Considering the fact that neoplastic lymphocytes in CTCL preferentially express a Th2 cytokine profile, which is responsibe for an array of clinical and hematological disturbances, IL-12 would seem to be an excellent candidate for shifting the profile back to a Th1 pattern [20, 77]. However, there has not been any clinical testing so far in CTCL patients.

Retinoids are known to modulate the growth and differentiation effects of TNF. They have been used in the treatment of CTCL alone or in combination treatment regimens.

With isotretinoin, complete remission was obtained in 21% of patients with MF or Sézary syndrome and partial remission in 38 %; with etretinate, complete remission was achieved in 21% and partial remission in 46%. The first sign of remission occurred within 2–4 weeks. During continued treatment, remissions could not always be maintained. Isotretinoin and etretinate were considered to be of equal potency in the treatment of MF [46].

Seven patients with CTCL were treated with low-dose IFN-α_{2b} (2 million units, three times per week) in combination with oral 13-*cis* retinoic acid (1 mg/kg per day). The combination therapy resulted in two complete and two partial remissions. Responses were maintained by continuous therapy for up to 15 months even after dose reduction of both agents by 50 % [40].

Combination Therapy

IFN-α has been used in combination with several other treatment modalities, including fludarabine [30], etretinate [1, 18, 68], photochemotherapy [48, 60, 64], and pentostatin [27]. In early studies [66, 82], high dosages of IFN-α (up to 36 million units daily for 3 months) in combination with etretinate (0.7 mg/kg) were given.

In a series of 45 patients [16], an objective response was achieved in 62 % of patients receiving combination therapy of IFN-α and etretinate. Similar reports have been published by other groups [1, 40]. We have seen significant remission of clinical symptoms in a patient with tumor-stage MF receiving low-dose IFN-α in combination with acitretin after chemotherapy had failed [2].

The response rate among 102 patients in seven studies using a combination of IFN with retinoids, including 13-*cis* retinoic acid and etretinate, was 60 %, and the complete response rate was 11% (for a review, see [8]). The combination of IFN-α with photochemotherapy seems to be more effective, resulting in an overall objective response rate of more than 90 % [42, 48, 53, 59, 64]. There is no clear information about the optimal dose of IFN and duration of psoralen ultraviolet A (PUVA) therapy to be used in order to maintain treatment results.

Extracorporeal photochemotherapy (EPC) and low-dose IFN-α are well tolerated. Combined therapy may result in a long-term disappearance of the malignant clone from the blood in patients with Sézary syndrome [61], although this therapy does not appear to be effective in patients with advanced Sézary syndrome [75]. The combination of IFN with pentostatin may be an active regimen in patients with advanced stages of MF without visceral involvement [27]. Local hypothermia in combination with recombinant IFN-γ has shown to be very effective in one patient with advanced tumor stage of adult T cell lymphoma [50].

Vaccination Therapy

Considering the fact that one or a few clones of neoplastic T cells bearing clone-specific T cell receptors are involved in CTCL, vaccination techniques could be an appropriate concept for the treatment of CTCL (see "Rapamycin," this volume). This approach aims at inducing an effective immune response to individually characterized pathogenic lymphocytes by administering dendritic cells previously pulsed with the idiotype protein of interest in the specific patient [4, 36]. The following steps had to be performed in this endeavour: (a) identification of the clonal population of malignant T cells in the individual patient; (b) sequencing of the specific T cell receptor for identification of the idiotypic region; (c) production of synthetic peptides containing the unique sequence for the individual Vb idiotypic region [54]; (d) combining the synthetic peptide with cocultured autologous blood-derived dendritic cells; and (e) vaccination of the patient with dendritic cells bearing the immunogenic peptide. Addition of adjuvants and of cytokines (IL-2, GM-CSF, TNF-α, IL-12) might be of additional benefit.

The dendritic cell antigen presentation system induces activation and expansion of large numbers of antigen-specific T cells for use in adoptive cellular immunotherapy against cancer, using antigen-pulsed dendritic cells as a vaccine and/or immunotherapeutic agent to accelerate an individual's immunopotential to an antigenic epitope specific for a distinct tumor cell clone.

Specific Indications

Most immunomodulatory treatment modalities in CL rely on cutaneous T cell lymphomas, especially MF and Sézary syndrome (SS). However, there have also been attempts at treating lymphomatoid papulosis [55, 80], non-MF/-SS CTCL, and follicular cell-derived lymphomas [26, 71, 83].

Conclusion

As in nonhematologic neoplasias and in extracutaneous proliferative diseases of the hematopoietic system, malignant lymphomas primarily occurring in the skin are prone to immunomodulatory treatment modalities. Early stages of the diseases exhibit a more favorable ratio between tumor cells and cytotoxic T cells and are thus the best candidates for an immunotherapeutic approach. Further detection of significant pathogenetic events and factors associated with the stepwise transformation of a normal lymphocyte into a neoplastic cell, through stages of genetic instability and sequential accumulation of mutations, possibly affecting oncogenes, suppressor genes, DNA repair genes, or proteins influencing signal transduction, will open up future prospects for designing effective treatment schedules specifically tailored to target the individual tumor cell clone.

Summary

Cutaneous lymphomas (CL), like nodal lymphomas, are tumors arising from the immunocompetent cell system, possibly resulting from persistent antigenic stimulation with unlimited cell proliferation and accumulation of gene mutations according to the multistep pathogenesis of tumor formation.

Among the many immunomodulatory treatment approaches in CL, interferons (IFN), especially IFN-α, have proved to be effective in low doses in up to 50–60% of patients with cutaneous T-cell lymphoma (CTCL). Even if stimulation of lymphoid cell proliferation by IL-2 may be detrimental for patients with CTCL, this cytokine has been beneficial in patients resistent to other treatment modalities when used in high doses. Cyclosporin A (CSA) has been effective in some patients with CTCL, and ineffective or even detrimental in others. Relatively few reports with less encouraging results exist on the use of monoclonal antibodies, thymopentin (TP), or autologous bone marrow transplantation (ABMT) in CL. Preliminary reports on the use of IL-2 fusion toxin (FT) for more specific targenting of IL-2-positive tumor cells have been promising. The use of peptide-pulsed dendritic cells for vaccination strategies will hopefully open up new dimensions in the treatment of malignant lymphomas, provided that tumor-specific antigens can be identified on clonal cell populations.

References

1. Altomare GF, Capella GL, Pigatto PD, Finzi AF (1993) Intramuscular low dose alpha-2B interferon and etretinate for treatment of mycosis fungoides. Int J Dermatol 32:138–141
2. Bauch B, Barraud-Klenovsek M, Burg G, Dummer R (1995) Eindrucksvolle Remission einer Mycosis fungoides im Tumorstadium unter low-dose Interferon alpha und Acitretin nach erfolgloser Chemotherapie. Z H G 70:200–202
3. Bernengo MG, Doveil GC, Meregalli M et al (1988) Immunomodulation and Sezary syndrome: experience with thymopentin (TP-5). Br J Dermatol 119:207–221
4. Bhardwaj N, Bender A, Gonzalez N et al (1995) Stimulation of human anti-viral CD8+ cytolytic T lymphocytes by dendritic cells. Adv Exp Med Biol 378:375–379
5. Bigler RD, Crilley P, Micaily B et al (1991) Autologous bone marrow transplantation for advanced stage mycosis fungoides. Bone Marrow Transplant 7:133–137
6. Braun-Falco O, Guggenberger K, Burg G et al (1978) Immunozytom unter dem Bild einer Acrodermatitis chronica atrophicans. Hautarzt 29:644–647
7. Bunn PJ, Foon KA, Ihde DC et al (1984) Recombinant leukocyte A interferon: an active agent in advanced cutaneous T-cell lymphomas. Ann Intern Med 101:484–487
8. Bunn PJ, Hoffman SJ, Norris D et al (1994) Systemic therapy of cutaneous T-cell lymphomas (mycosis fungoides and the Sezary syndrome). Ann Intern Med 121:592–602
9. Burg G, Dummer R, Wilhelm M et al (1991) A subcutaneous delta positive T-cell lymphoma that produces interferon gamma. N Engl J Med 325:1078–1081
10. Catterall MD, Addis BJ, Smith JL et al (1983) Sezary syndrome: transformation to a high grade T-cell lymphoma after treatment with cyclosporin A. Clin Exp Dermatol 8:159–169
11. Celerier P, Fleischmann M, Basset SN et al (1993) In vitro induction of basal keratinocyte MY7 antigen expression in cutaneous T-cell lymphoma is associated with response to interferon-alfa therapy. Arch Dermatol 129:1136–1140
12. Chen YC, Wang CH, Huang SC et al (1968)Autologous bone marrow transplantation after supralethal dose of total body irradiation in a case of mycosis fungoides. Taiwan I Hsueh Hui Tsa Chih 85:304–314
13. Cooper DL, Braverman IM, Sarris A et al (1993) Cyclosporine treatment of refractory T-cell lymphomas. Cancer 71:2335–2341
14. Dalloul A, Laroche L, Bagot M et al (1992) Interleukin-7 is a growth factor for Sezary lymphoma cells. J Clin Invest 90:1054–1060
15. Dillman RO, Shawler DL, Dillman JB et al (1984) Therapy of chronic lymphocytic leukemia and cutaneous T-cell lymphoma with T101 monoclonal antibody. J Clin Oncol 2:881–891
16. Dreno B, Claudy A, Meynadier J et al (1991) The treatment of 45 patients with cutaneous T-cell lymphoma with low doses of interferon-alpha 2a and etretinate. Br J Dermatol 125:456–459

17. Dreno B, Fleischmann M, Valard S et al (1992) Induction of myelo-monocytic My7 antigen (CD13) expression by interferon-alpha in basal cells of cutaneous T-cell lymphomas. Br J Dermatol 126:320–323
18. Dreno B (1993) Roferon-A (interferon alpha 2a) combined with Tigason (etretinate) for treatment of cutaneous T cell lymphomas. Stem Cells Dayt 11:269–275
19. Dummer R, Posseckert G, Nestle F et al (1992) Soluble interleukin-2 receptors inhibit interleukin 2-dependent proliferation and cytotoxicity: explanation for diminished natural killer cell activity in cutaneous T-cell lymphomas in vivo? J Invest Dermatol 98:50–54
20. Dummer R, Kohl O, Gillessen J et al (1993) Peripheral blood mononuclear cells in patients with nonleukemic cutaneous T-cell lymphoma. Reduced proliferation and preferential secretion of a T helper-2-like cytokine pattern on stimulation. Arch Dermatol 129:433–436
21. Dummer R, Sigg ZS, Kalthof K et al (1994) Various cytokines modulate ICAM-1 shedding on melanoma- and CTCL-derived cell lines: inverse regulation of ICAM-1 shedding in a Sezary cell line by interferon-gamma. Dermatology 189:120–124
22. Dummer R, Gore ME, Hancock BW et al (1995) A multicenter phase II clinical trial using dacarbazine and continuous infusion interleukin-2 for metastatic melanoma. Clinical data and immunomonitoring. Cancer 75:1038–1044
23. Dummer R, Heald P, Nestle F et al (1996) Sézary syndrome T-cell clones display T-helper 2 cytokines and express the accessory factor-1 (interferon-γ receptor β-chain). Blood 88:1383–1389
24. Dummer R, Posseckert G, Sugamura K et al (1996) Circulating interleukin-2 receptors are a group of multimeric proteins with immunoreactivity for interleukin-2 receptor α, β and γ chains. J Interferon Cytokine Res 16:315–320
25. Dummer R, Häffner A, Hess M et al (1996) A rational approach to the therapy of cutaneous T-cell lymphomas. Onkologie 19:226–230
26. Foon KA, Roth MS, Bunn PJ (1986) Alpha interferon treatment of low-grade B-cell non-Hodgkin's lymphomas, cutaneous T-cell lymphomas, and chronic lymphocytic leukemia. Semin Oncol 13:35–42
27. Foss FM, Ihde DC, Breneman DL et al (1992) Phase II study of pentostatin and intermittent high-dose recombinant interferon alfa-2a in advanced mycosis fungoides/Sézary syndrome. J Clin Oncol 10:1907–1913
28. Foss FM, Borkowski TA, Gilliom M et al (1994) Chimeric fusion protein toxin DAB486IL-2 in advanced mycosis fungoides and the Sezary syndrome: correlation of activity and interleukin-2 receptor expression in a phase II study. Blood 84:1765–1774
29. Foss FM, Koc Y, Stetler SM et al (1994) Costimulation of cutaneous T-cell lymphoma cells by interleukin-7 and interleukin-2: potential autocrine or paracrine effectors in the Sezary syndrome. J Clin Oncol 12:326–335
30. Foss FM, Ihde DC, Linnoila IR et al (1994) Phase II trial of fludarabine phosphate and interferon alfa-2a in advanced mycosis fungoides/Sezary syndrome. J Clin Oncol 12:2051–9
31. Foss FM, Kuzel TM (1995) Experimental therapies in the treatment of cutaneous T-cell lymphoma. Hematol Oncol Clin North Am 9:1127–1137
32. Garbe C, Stein H, Dienemann D et al (1991) Borrelia burgdorferi-associated cutaneous B cell lymphoma: clinical and immunohistologic characterization of four cases. J Am Acad Dermatol 24:584–590
33. Gisselbrecht C, Maraninchi D, Pco JL et al (1994) Interleukin-2 treatment in lymphoma: a phase II multicenter study. Blood 83:2081–2085
34. Hansen ER, Vejlsgaard GL, Lisby S et al (1991) Epidermal interleukin 1 alpha functional activity and interleukin 8 immunoreactivity are increased in patients with cutaneous T-cell lymphoma (see comments). J Invest Dermatol 97:818–823
35. Hesketh P, Caguioa P, Koh H et al (1993) Clinical activity of a cytotoxic fusion protein in the treatment of cutaneous T-cell lymphoma. J Clin Oncol 11:1682–90
36. Hsu FJ, Benike C, Fagnoni F et al (1996) Vaccination of patients with B-cell lymphoma using autologous antigen-pulsed dendritic cells. Nat Med 2:52–58
37. Ito Y, Jimbow K, Miura S et al (1984) Local application of interferon beta to skin lesions of malignant melanoma and malignant lymphoma-clinical and histopathological analysis. Gan To Kagaku Ryoho 11:1263–1268

38. Jimbow K, Yamana K, Ishida O et al (1987) Evaluation of rIFN-gamma in the treatment of lymphoma and melanoma of the skin by systemic and intralesional administration. Gan To Kagaku Ryoho 14:152–158
39. Kaplan EH, Rosen ST, Norris DB et al (1990) Phase II study of recombinant human interferon gamma for treatment of cutaneous T-cell lymphoma. J Natl Cancer Inst 82:208–212
40. Knobler RM, Trautinger F, Radaszkiewicz T et al (1991) Treatment of cutaneous T cell lymphoma with a combination of low-dose interferon alfa-2b and retinoids. J Am Acad Dermatol 24:247–252
41. Kohn EC, Steis RG, Sausville EA et al (1990) Phase II trial of intermittent high-dose recombinant interferon alfa-2a in mycosis fungoides and the Sézary syndrome. J Clin Oncol 8:155–160
42. Kuzel TM, Gilyon K, Springer E et al (1990) Interferon alfa-2a combined with phototherapy in the treatment of cutaneous T-cell lymphoma. J Natl Cancer Inst 82:203–207
43. Kuzel TM, Rosen ST, Gordon LI et al (1993) Phase I trial of the diphtheria toxin/interleukin-2 fusion protein DAB486IL-2: efficacy in mycosis fungoides and other non-Hodgkin's lymphomas. Leuk Lymph 11:369–377
44. Maddox AM, Kahan BD, Tucker S et al (1985) Remission in skin infiltrate of a patient with mycosis fungoides treated with cyclosporine. J Am Acad Dermatol 12:952–956
45. Marolleau JP, Baccard M, Flageul B et al (1995) High-dose recombinant interleukin-2 in advanced cutaneous T-cell lymphoma (see comments). Arch Dermatol 131:574- 579
46. Molin L, Thomsen K, Volden G et al (1987) Oral retinoids in mycosis fungoides and Sézary syndrome: a comparison of isotretinoin and etretinate. A study from the Scandinavian Mycosis Fungoides Group. Acta Derm Venereol (Stockh) 67:232–236
47. Moreau P, LeTortorec S, Mahe MA et al (1994) Autologous bone marrow transplantation using TBI and CBV for disseminated high/intermediate grade cutaneous non-epidermotropic non-Hodgkin's lymphoma. Bone Marrow Transplant 14:775–778
48. Mostow EN, Neckel SL, Oberhelman L et al (1993) Complete remissions in psoralen and UV-A (PUVA)-refractory mycosis fungoides-type cutaneous T-cell lymphoma with combined interferon alfa and PUVA (see comments). Arch Dermatol 129:747–752
49. Nagatani T, Kin ST, Baba N et al (1988) A case of cutaneous T cell lymphoma treated with recombinant interleukin 2 (rIL-2) Acta Derm Venereol (Stockh) 68:504–508
50. Nakayama J, Yamada A, Hori Y et al (1989) Cutaneous lesion of adult T-cell lymphoma treated successfully with local hyperthermia in combination with intravenous administration of rINF-gamma. Nippon Hifuka Gakkai Zasshi 99:907–914
51. Nestle FO, Nickoloff BJ (1994) Role of dendritic cells in benign and malignant lymphocytic infiltrates of the skin. Dermatol Clin 12:271–282
52. Olsen EA, Bunn PA (1995) Interferon in the treatment of cutaneous T-cell lymphoma. Hematol Oncol Clin North Am 9:1089–107
53. Otte HG, Herges A, Stadler R (1992) Combination therapy with interferon alfa 2a and PUVA in cutaneous T-cell lymphoma. Hautarzt 43:695–699
54. Potoczna N, Boehncke W, Nestle F et al (1996) T-cell receptor beta variable region (Vbeta) usage in cutaneous T-cell lymphomas (CTCL) in comparison to normal and eczematous skin. J Cutan Pathol 23:298–305
55. Proctor SJ, Jackson GH, Lennard AL et al (1992) Lymphomatoid papulosis: response to treatment with recombinant interferon alfa-2b (letter). J Clin Oncol 10:170
56. Przybilla B, Burg G, Schmoeckel C et al (1983) Treatment of cutaneous T-cell lymphomas with TP-5. Evaluation of the clinical effect in 8 patients. Acta Derm Venereol (Stockh) 63:524–529
57. Rajan GP, Seifert B, Pruemmer O et al (1996) Incidence and in-vivo relevance of anti-interferon antibodies during treatment of low-grade cutaneous T-cell lymphomas with interferon alpha-2a combined with acitretin or PUVA. Arch Dermatol Res 288:543–548
58. Ramon D, Betlloch I, Jimenez A et al (1986) Remission of Sezary's syndrome with cyclosporin A. Mild capillary leak syndrome as an unusual side effect. Acta Derm Venereol (Stockh) 66:80–82
59. Roenigk HJ, Kuzel TM, Skoutelis AP et al (1990) Photochemotherapy alone or combined with interferon alpha-2a in the treatment of cutaneous T-cell lymphoma. J Invest Dermatol 95:198–205

60. Roenigk HH, Kuzel T, Rosen S (1993) Interferons for cutaneous T-cell lymphoma monotherapy or combination with PUVA. Aust J Dermatol 34:13–15
61. Rook AH, Prystowsky MB, Cassin M et al (1991) Combined therapy for Sezary syndrome with extracorporeal photochemotherapy and low-dose interferon alfa therapy. Clinical, molecular, and immunologic observations. Arch Dermatol 127:1535–1540
62. Rosen ST, Zimmer AM, Goldman LR et al (1987) Radioimmunodetection andradioimmunotherapy of cutaneous T cell lymphomas using an 131I-labeled monoclonal antibody: an Illinois Cancer Council Study. J Clin Oncol 5:562–573
63. Sarris AH, Esgleyes RT, Crow M et al (1995) Cytokine loops involving interferon-gamma and IP-10, a cytokine chemotactic for CD4+ lymphocytes: an explanation for the epidermotropism of cutaneous T-cell lymphoma? Blood 86:651–658
64. Stadler R, Otte HG (1995) Combination therapy of cutaneous T cell lymphoma with interferon alpha-2a and photochemotherapy. In: Herfarth C, Senn H-J (eds) Recent results in cancer research, vol 139. Springer, Berlin Heidelberg New York, pp 391–401
65. Street TH, Muller Sm Pittelkow M (1990) Cyclosporine in the treatment of cutaneous T cell lymphoma. J Am Acad Dermatol 23:1084–1089
66. Thestrup PK, Hammer R, Kaltoft K et al (1988) Treatment of mycosis fungoides with recombinant interferon-alpha 2a2 alone and in combination with etretinate. Br J Dermatol 118: 811–818
67. Thomsen K, Wantzin GL (1987) Extracutaneous spreading with fatal outcome of mycosis fungoides in a patient treated with ciclosporin A: a word of caution. Dermatologica 174: 236–238
68. Torii H, Kaneko T, Matsuyama T et al (1994) Interferon-alpha (INF-alpha) and etretinate in the treatment of mycosis fungoides. J Dermatol 21:767–770
69. Totterman TH, Danersund A, Nilsson K et al (1982) Cyclosporin-A is selectively cytotoxic to human leukemic T cells in vitro. Blood 59:1103–1107
70. Totterman TH, Scheynius A, Killander A et al (1985) Treatment of therapy-resistant Sezary syndrome with cyclosporin-A: suppression of pruritus, leukaemic T cell activation markers and tumour mass. Scand J Haematol 34:196–203
71. Tourani JM, Leaute JB, Lessana LM et al (1989) Complete remission following recombinant interferon alpha-2a in a patient with diffuse large B cell cutaneous lymphoma. Nouv Rev Fr Hematol 31:315–316
72. Tron VA, Rosenthal D, Sauder DN (1988) Epidermal interleukin-1 is increased in cutaneous T-cell lymphoma. J Invest Dermatol 90:378–381
73. Tulli A, Biele MM, Capizzi R (1988) A possible visceralization in a case of cutaneous T cell lymphoma under treatment with recombinant interferon alfa 2 (letter). G Ital Dermatol Venereol 123:262
74. Vonderheid EC, Thompson R, Smiles KA et al (1987) Recombinant interferon alfa-2b in plaque- phase mycosis fungoides. Intralesional and low-dose intramuscular therapy. Arch Dermatol 123:757–763
75. Vonderheid EC, Bigler RD, Greenberg AS et al (1994) Extracorporeal photopheresis and recombinant interferon alfa 2b in Sezary syndrome. Use of dual marker labeling to monitor therapeutic response. Am J Clin Oncol 17:255–263
76. Vowels BR, Cassin M, Boufal MH et al (1992) Extracorporeal photochemotherapy induces the production of tumor necrosis factor-alpha by monocytes: implications for the treatment of cutaneous T-cell lymphoma and systemic sclerosis. J Invest Dermatol 98:686–692
77. Vowels BR, Lessin SR, Cassin M et al (1994) Th2 cytokine mRNA expression in skin in cutaneous T-cell lymphoma. J Invest Dermatol 103:669–673
78. Wismer JM, McKenzie RC; Sauder DN et al (1994) Interleukin-8 immunoreactivity in epidermis of cutaneous T-cell lymphoma patients. Lymphokine Cytokine Res 13:21–27
79. Wolff JM, Zitelli JA, Rabin BS et al (1985) Intralesional interferon in the treatment of early mycosis fungoides. J Am Acad Dermatol 13:604–612
80. Wyss M, Dummer R, Dommann SN et al (1995) Lymphomatoid papulosis-treatment with recombinant interferon alfa-2a and etretinate. Dermatology 190:288–291

81. Yamamoto T, Sasaki G, Sato T et al (1995) Cytokine profile of tumor cells in mycosis fungoides: successful treatment with intra-lesional interferon-gamma combined with chemotherapy. J Dermatol 22:650–654
82. Zachariae H, Thestrup PK (1990) Interferon alpha and etretinate combination treatment of cutaneous T-cell lymphoma. J Invest Dermatol 95:206–208
83. Zenone T, Catimel G, Barbet N et al (1994) Complete remission of a primary cutaneous B cell lymphoma treated with intralesional recombinant interferon alpha-2a (letter). Eur J Cancer 30A:246–247
84. Zinzani PL, Mazza P, Gherlinzoni F (1988) Beta interferon in the treatment of mycosis fungoides (letter). Haematologica 73:547–548

Non-melanoma Skin Cancer

S. A. Buechner

Introduction

Non-melanoma skin cancers (NMSC) comprised of basal cell carcinoma (BCC) and squamous cell carcinoma (SCC) are the most common human cancers [14, 24, 25]. The annual incidence of NMSC is rapidly increasing, with an average increase between 3% and 6% per year in most populations, and has been reported to be almost 1000 per 100000 people in Australia [1, 14, 24]. An estimated 2750000 new cases of NMSC occurred worldwide in 1985. It is also estimated that there were 1200000 cases of BCC in the United States in 1995 [1, 15]. BCC is by far the most common skin malignancy throughout the world, accounting for about 75% of NMSC [15, 24]. Given that the incidence of NMSC continues to increase yearly, the dermatologist will diagnose and treat an increasing number of patients with skin cancer. The majority of BCC begin as small lesions typically less than 1 cm in diameter that can be successfully treated in a variety of ways [15, 26]. Treatment goals focus on complete tumor removal and minimization of cosmetic and functional defects. Effective methods of treatment include excisional surgery, curettage and electrodesiccation, cryosurgery, radiotherapy, and Mohs' micrographic surgery [15]. However, many BCC may present considerable therapeutic difficulties because of the location of the tumor, its size, and the age of the patient. Large and recurrent tumors, in particular, usually require extensive resection with rotation of tissue or free or composite grafts. Recently, results from several clinical trials have shown that intralesional interferon (IFN) is an effective treatment modality for BCC [4, 8, 9, 11, 22]. IFN, a group of glycoproteins, have a broad spectrum of biologic activities, including the control of cell growth and differentiation, regulation of cell surface antigen expression, and modulation of humoral and cellular immune responses [31]. With the advent of recombinant DNA technology, large quantities of IFN have become available for clinical studies. This chapter reviews the growing data from human studies employing intralesional IFN to treat NMSC and discusses the indications, effectiveness for cure, side effects, and cosmetic results.

Basal Cell Carcinoma

Clinical Studies

The successful introduction and the use of IFN for several malignancies, including renal cell carcinoma, cutaneous T cell lymphoma, and Kaposi's sarcoma, was the main stimulus for recent interest in the therapeutic use of IFN in BCC. Clinical trials have used several different dosages, intervals, and duration of treatment. Various dosing

Table 1. Studies using intralesional interferon for basal cell carcinoma

Reference	Interferon	Evaluable patients (*n*)	Dose per injection (IU)	Schedule	Duration of treatment (weeks)	Complete remission (*n*)	Complete remission (%)[c]	Histologic cure rate (*n*)	Histologic cure rate (%)[c]	Follow-up (months)
[16]	IFN-α_2	8	1.5×10^6	3x/week	3	8	100	8	100	2
[18]	IFN-α_{2a}	7[a]	$1.5–6.0\times10^6$	3x/week	5–11	8	100	8	100	3–8
[37]	IFN-α_2	11	0.9×10^6	3x/week	3	0	0	0	0	3
[34]	IFN-γ	7	2×10^5	2x/week	4	0	0	0	0	2
[9]	IFN-α_{2b}	120	1.5×10^6	3x/week	3	103	86	96[d]	81	12
[11]	IFN-α_{2b}	33 30	10×10^6 10×10^6	1x/week 1x/week	1 3	17 24	52 80	17 24	52 80	4 4
[35]	IFN-α_{2b}	10	1.5×10^6	3x/week	3	6	60	–	–	3–21
[12]	IFN-γ	15 14	20×10^3 100×10^3	3x/week 3x/week	3 3	1 7	7 50	1 7	7 50	3 3
[22]	HNLI	72	$0.4–1.2\times10^6$	5x/week	3–6	52	72	52	72	–
[4]	IFN-α_{2b}	19	1.5×10^6	3x/week	3	8	42	8	42	6
[20]	IFN-α_{2b}	10	1.5×10^6	3x/week	3	6	55	6	55	12–26
[2]	IFN-α_{2b}	27	1.5×10^6	3x/week	3	14	52	14	52	2–12
[8]	IFN-α_{2b}	140	1.5×10^6	3x/week	4–8	94	67	–	–	12–54
[6]	IFN-α_{2b}	43[b]	$1.5–3.0\times10^6$	3x/week	3	43	88	43	88	12–36

HNLI, human natural leukocytic interferon
[a] Eight tumors
[b] 49 tumors
[c] Percentage of evaluated tumors
[d] 96 out of 118 tumors

schedules have been compared in order to determine the optimum dose and to assess side effects and long-term results. Data from these studies are summarized in Table 1.

Greenway et al. [16] first reported that eight out of eight BCC treated intralesionally three times a week for 3 weeks with 1.5×10^6 IU IFN-α_{2b} per injection were clinically and histologically cured 2 months after completion of therapy. There were three nodular BCC and five superficial BCC, ranging in size from 7×6 mm to 14×12 mm. In another study, eight BCC with surface area ranging from 2 cm to 35 cm were treated by intralesional injection of IFN-a_{2a} [18]. Most of these lesions were located in esthetically important areas, including the eyelids, the canthi, and the cheek. The dose per injection varied from 1.5×10^6 to 6.0×10^6 IU, according to the size of the lesions. Injections were given three times a week. After 6–11 weeks of treatment using a total dose of IFN-α_{2a} varying from 24×10^6 to 156×10^6 IU, all patients underwent complete clinical and histologic remission. Ten patients with BCC were treated with sublesional injections of IFN-α_{2b} three times a week for 3 weeks [35]. Eight patients received 1.5×10^6 IU per injection, whereas two patients with larger lesions were treated with 3.0×10^6 IU and 6.0×10^6 IU per injection, respectively. Six treated lesions measuring less than 19×19 mm cleared completely. Two of the nonresponders had large BCC with tumor diameters greater than 25 mm. Eleven BCC injected intralesionally three times weekly for 3 weeks with a low dose (0.9×10^6 IU) of IFN-α_2 failed to respond to the treatment [37]. In a subsequent study, 65 BCC were treated with intralesional sustained-release protamine zinc chelate 10×10^6 IU IFN-α_{2b} per injection [11]. Only lesions ranging in size from 0.5 to 1.5 cm for nodular tumors or 2 cm for superficial lesions at their largest diameter were included. Patients were randomized to receive IFN-α_{2b} either in a single dose of 10×10^6 IU or in one dose of 10×10^6 IU per week for 3 consecutive weeks. At study week 16, the entire test lesion was excised. Histologic examination of excisional biopsies confirmed elimination of tumor in 17 (52%) out of 33 patients treated with single injection of 10×10^6 IU, whereas 24 (80%) out of 30 patients treated with three weekly injections were histologically cured. The efficacy of intralesional IFN-α in BCC was further evaluated in another study using a treatment regimen of 1.5–3.0×10^6 IU three times a week for 4–8 weeks. A complete remission was observed in 94 (67%) of the 140 patients with BCC. Partial response was achieved in 33 (24%) patients. No recurrences have been observed in patients with complete clinical remission during a follow-up period of 12–54 months [8].

In our study of 43 patients with 49 biopsy-established BCC, patients were treated with three injections of 1.5–3.0×10^6 IU per week for 3 weeks and 43 (88%) of the tumors were clinically and histologically cured. Twelve patients observed for 2–3 years showed no recurrence [6]. Effectiveness of IFN-α in the treatment of BCC was also confirmed by a multicenter placebo-controlled trial. A total of 172 patients with biopsy-proven noduloulcerative or superficial BCC were given IFN-α_{2b} or placebo three times weekly for 3 weeks with a cumulative dosage of 13.5×10^6 IU [9]. Recurrent tumors and large tumors penetrating to deep tissue were not treated. At study weeks 16 and 20,86% of IFN-treated patients and 29% of placebo-treated patients had negative biopsy specimens. Of the 103 biopsy-negative, IFN-treated patients at weeks 16 and 20, 101 had an excisional biopsy of the test lesions at month 12. Ninety-six (95%) of these patients remained tumor free 1 year after initiation of treatment. Recently, the efficacy of intralesional IFN-α_{2b} in the treatment of primary morpheaform and recurrent tumors was evaluated. Fifteen patients received 1.5×10^6 IU IFN-α_{2b} injected intralesionally

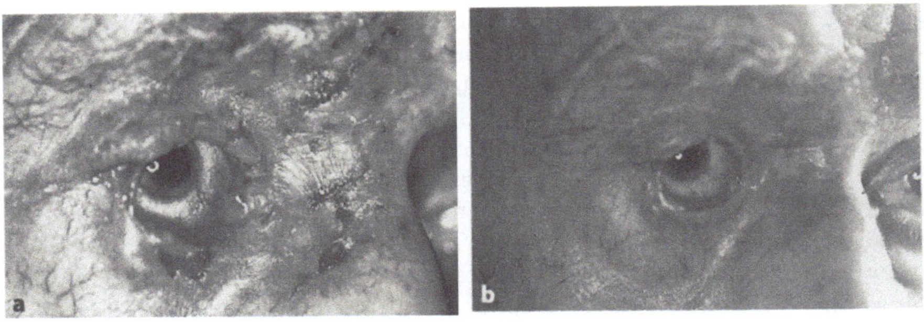

Fig. 1. **a** Superficial multifocal basal cell carcinoma of the periorbital region before treatment with intralesional interferon-α_{2b}. **b** Clinical appearance of skin cancer site 16 weeks after therapy. No evidence of residual tumor

three times a week for 3 weeks. About 2 months after completion of treatment, all tumors were excised using Mohs' micrographic surgery. In four (27 %) of the 15 patients, no residual tumor was found at surgery. A tumor reduction of 75 % was observed in five (33 %) of these patients [33]. For small, uncomplicated tumors measuring less than 2 cm in diameter, the treatment regimen of 1.5×10^6 IU three times a week for 3 weeks appears to be the most effective. Larger BCC may require a total dose greater than 13.5×10^6 IU. If lesions respond, they begin to regress 4–6 weeks after completion of therapy. However, maximum responses usually require 8–12 weeks. A case of invasive BCC has been reported which involved intraorbital structures and the frontal bone of the skull. Despite various treatments, including radiation, excision, cryosurgery, and two Mohs' surgical procedures, the tumor continued to grow. Regional injections into the intraorbital tumor three times per week for 6 weeks with 2×10^6 IU IFN-α_{2b} resulted in a dramatic, complete tumor regression. Tumor overlying the frontal bone responded to 4×10^6 IU IFN-a_{2b} intralesionally in the same dosage schedule. There was no evidence of residual tumor 16 months after therapy [10]. Recently, we have treated a patient who presented with an extremely large, recurrent, multifocal BCC involving the entire periorbital region (Fig. 1a). A remarkable response to intralesional treatment with IFN-α_{2b} using 3.0×10^6 IU per injection with a cumulative dose of 40×10^6 IU was observed 3 months after completion of therapy (Fig. 1b). In a pilot clinical trial, intralesional low-dose recombinant IFN-γ failed to show any effectiveness in seven patients with nodular BCC [34]. In another study, the efficacy of two different doses of IFN-γ was evaluated in 29 patients with BCC [12]. Fifteen patients treated with 0.01 mg IFN-γ, injected intralesionally three times a week for 3 weeks, were compared with a group of 14 patients receiving 0.05 mg intralesionally. Twelve weeks after therapy, excision of biopsy specimens revealed no tumor in seven of 14 patients treated with the higher dose, although only one of 15 patients treated with low-dose IFN-γ was cured according to histologic criteria. However, further controlled studies are needed in order to evaluate the efficacy of IFN-γ in the treatment of BCC.

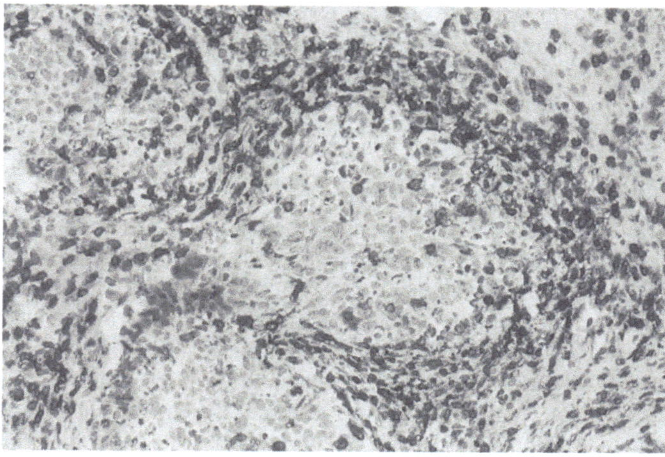

Fig. 2. $CD3^+$ T cells surrounding and infiltrating nests of basal cell carcinoma during treatment with intralesional interferon-α_{2b}

Histologic and Immunohistochemical Studies

Skin biopsy specimens taken from the sites of previous BCC after the completion of intralesional treatment with IFN show a papillary and mid-dermal perivascular inflammatory infiltrate that consists of lymphocytes and histiocytes. There may be a focal exocytosis of lymphocytes into the epidermis, accompanied by mild spongiosis. Numerous ectatic blood vessels are usually present in the dermis. Benign epidermoid cysts and residual fibrosis can be frequently observed after treatment [5, 6, 16]. The majority of cells in the infiltrate are $CD3^+$, $CD4^+$ T cells (Fig. 2). Among these T cells, the number of $CD4^+$ T cells outnumber $CD8^+$ T cells in a ratio ranging from 2:1 to 3:1. A small number of $CD20^+$ B cells are observed within the infiltrate. When compared with the peritumoral infiltrate before therapy, there is a considerable increase in the number of $CD4^+$ cells in the infiltrate after intralesional injections of IFN-α_{2b} [5, 27]. The inflammatory infiltrate strongly expressed lymphocyte function-associated antigen (LFA)-1, and the expression of interleukin (IL)-2 receptor (CD25) is also increased. There is no expression of HLA-DR antigen on tumor cells of IFN-α-treated BCC at subsequent stages of regression. Endothelial cells within blood vessels surrounding the tumors strongly express intercellular adhesion molecule (ICAM)-1, but this molecule is not expressed by tumor cells during treatment with IFN-α, except for isolated tumor cells located at the borders of BCC nests.

Squamous Cell Carcinoma

Limited data are available on the intralesional use of IFN in the treatment of SCC. In an early study, three patients with SCC were treated successfully with 0.9×10^6 IU intralesional IFN-α_2 [37]. Thirty-four SCC ranging in size from 0.5 to 2.0 cm were treated with 1.5×10^6 IU IFN-α_{2b} injected intralesionally three times per week for 3 weeks. Eighteen weeks after therapy, 33 (97%) of 34 evaluable lesions were cured histologically on follow-up excision [13]. This study demonstrated that IFN-α applied intralesionally is successful in small, primary SCC. More recently, encouraging results were obtained with

SCC using three weekly injections of $1.5–3.0 \times 10^6$ IU IFN-α_{2a} for periods of 4–8 weeks [7]. The lesions ranged from 1.5 to 4 cm in diameter. A complete response was achieved in 25 (69.5%) of 36 patients, and a partial response was noted in seven (19.5%). No recurrences were noted during a follow-up period of 12–48 months.

Side Effects

Adverse reactions to IFN are, for the most part, limited to influenza-like symptoms and consist of mild fever, chills, headache, arthralgias, and myalgias. The severity of adverse reactions is directly related to the dosage of IFN. The symptoms start 2–4 h post-injection and may last for 4–8 h. They usually occur at doses over $1.0–2.0 \times 10^6$ IU per day and decrease with repeated doses. Thus treatment can be given late in the day, and the vast majority of the side effects occur during the evening and night hours. These symptoms respond to acetaminophen or paracetamol, which should be given orally at the time of injection. Among the patients treated with intralesional injections of IFN-a, adverse effects of any degree of severity were noted in 30–70% of patients [8, 9]. About 15% of the patients receiving IFN-α at a dosage of 1.5×10^6 IU per injection showed decreases in the total white blood cell count [9]. Local reactions at the injection site are minimal and consist of occasional pruritus and burning sensation.

Discussion

The rationale for the use of IFN for BCC and SCC is based primarily on their ability to control cell growth and differentiation. In addition, IFN have been shown to have immunomodulatory properties, including the regulation of cell surface antigen expression and modulation of humoral and cellular immune responses [17, 23]. Consequently, the IFN have been evaluated as potential anticancer agents in various human malignancies in a relatively large number of studies. The effectiveness of intralesional IFN therapy in BCC has been established in a number of clinical trials. However, the duration and dosing of IFN-α for BCC is still controversial. There is evidence to suggest that the cure rate decreases if lower doses of IFN and fewer injections are used [11, 37]. Most frequently, dosages of $1.5–3.0 \times 10^6$ IU of IFN-α have been injected intralesionally three times a week for 3 weeks. Using this treatment, regimen cure rates of 42–100% have been reported (Table 1). The reasons for the various responses may include different histologic types of lesions, anatomic site, size of tumors, tumor weight variability, and inadequate distribution of IFN within the lesion. However, recent studies suggested that there is no significant difference between the cure rates of nodular and superficial BCC, regardless of the dosing schedule used [8, 9, 11, 12]. Cornell et al. [9] found in their study of 120 BCC that large tumors (200 mm^2) were cured in 88% of cases, and a similar cure rate of 79–94% was documented in the smaller lesions. However, only lesions with their largest diameter less than 1.5 cm for noduloulcerative BCC and between 0.5 and 2.0 cm for superficial BCC were included in this study. Therefore, the differences in terms of lesion cure found in other studies utilizing a regimen of 1.5×10^6 IU IFN-α injected intralesionally three times a week for 3 weeks may be explained by the large size of the tumors of more than 2 cm at their largest diameter. In our opinion, to increase efficacy large BCC require a total dose greater than 13.5×10^6 IU. Patients receiving high-dose IFN treatment may experience more severe adverse reactions. This should be taken into consideration, particularly in elderly patients. More importantly, BCC treated with intralesional IFN need to be followed up for at least 3 months after completion of therapy, because response to treatment may be delayed. Trials that allow longer follow-up before post-treatment biopsy of the injected lesion would be necessary in order to confirm the regression of the tumor. In most studies, primary surgical resection of BCC is associated with a 95 % cure rate [15]. With the use of cryosurgery for primary BCC, 5-year cure rates ranging from 94 % to 99 % have been reported. Although intralesional therapy does not offer cure rates as high as the more conventional treatments, it is a promising new treatment modality for BCC and may find a role particularly for patients desiring a more favorable cosmetic result and the avoidance of a surgical procedure. Adjuvant intralesional IFN therapy may be indicated for large or recurrent tumors in anatomic areas in which it is difficult to obtain clear surgical margins without cosmetic or functional loss. The mechanisms of action by which IFN acts on BCC are only partially known. IFN-α inhibits growth and proliferation of normal and malignant cells by prolonging the length of the cell cycle [17,31]. Direct evidence was provided showing that IFN-α treatment of human cells downregulates epidermal growth factor receptor expression on these cells, reflected in a subsequent abrogation of cell proliferation. The IFN have also been shown to induce cellular differentiation [2]. The presence of epidermoid cysts at various stages of tumor regression suggests that IFN-α may be involved in the regression process by enhancing the terminal differentiation of tumor cells. There is also increasing body of evidence that IFN indirectly act on tumor cells by inducing a variety of immune effects [23]. Both IFN-α and IFN-γ can stimulate the activity of natural killer cells and macrophages. Enhancement of expression of tumor-associated antigens and receptors for tumor necrosis factor (TNF) may result in more efficient immune recognition and killing of tumor cells by cytotoxic leukocytes or antibody-dependent cell-mediated cytotoxicity. In fact, it has been shown by our and other studies that treatment of BCC with intralesional IFN-α is associated with an increase in $CD4^+$ T cells at the periphery and within the tumor nests [5,27]. Our studies showed that the relative number of $CD4^+$ cells surrounding and infiltrating the tumor nests during the intralesional IFN treatment correlated directly with regression of BCC. Recently, it has been reported that there are significantly more $CD4^+$ T cells in regressing BCC when compared with actively growing tumors [21]. In addition, intradermal injections of IFN-α_{2b} into normal human skin caused an increase in the numbers of dermal $CD3^+$, $CD4^+$, and HLA-DR^+ cells [36]. Both $CD4^+$ and $CD8^+$ T cell subsets can express cytolytic activity against a variety of target cells [19]. One of the mechanisms by which cytotoxic T cells kill target cells is by inducing apoptosis [38]. Recent evidence has demonstrated that $CD4^+$ cytotoxic T cells can induce apoptosis in their targets preferentially via engagement with the Fas antigen, a cell surface molecule belonging to the TNF family [28,32]. When Fas ligand binds to Fas, the target cell undergoes apoptosis. Prior studies have shown that Fas antigen is not expressed on tumor cells in BCC [29]. More recently, induction of apoptotic cell death in squamous cell carcinoma cell lines by IFN-α has been reported [30]. Therefore, it is possible that Fas-based cytotoxicity by $CD4^+$ T cells might be involved in the death of tumor cells during intralesional treatment with IFN-α.

In conclusion, the use of IFN in treatment of BCC and SCC is a fascinating and rapidly advancing area of research. Intralesional IFN-α has been shown to be an effective and safe modality in the treatment of BCC. One of the first priorities in terms of the future direction must be to clarify the role of currently available IFN in comparison with conventional methods of treatment. A second aim which should receive rapid attention is to document the additive antitumor effect, especially in treating recurrent, high-risk BCC by surgical excision. Furthermore, long-term follow-up is necessary to detect recurrences, even when the clinical appearance of the treated site does not show any visible evidence of residual tumor 12 months after therapy.

Summary

BCC and SCC are the most common skin cancers. Recent evidence has emerged that intralesional IFN-α and IFN-γ provide an effective treatment for BCC and SCC. Intralesional IFN are indicated for the treatment of BCC at critical anatomic sites where there is a need for preservation of function with more favorable cosmetic results. In addition, IFN will have to be considered as adjuvant therapy for advanced, high-risk BCC and SCC. Highly promising results indicate that IFN, either alone or in combination with standard therapies, will play an important role in the management of NMSC.

References

1. Armstrong BK, Kricker A (1995) Skin cancer. Dermatol Clin 13:583–594
2. Baron S, Tyring SK, Fleishmann WR (1991) The interferons: mechanism of action and clinical application. JAMA 266:1375–1383
3. Boneschi V, Brambilla L, Chiappino G, Mozzanica N, Finzi AF (1991) Intralesional alpha 2b recombinant interferon for basal cell carcinoma. Int J Dermatol 30:220–224
4. Bottomley WW, Keczkes K (1991) Treatment of basal cell carcinomas with intralesional recombinant interferon-alfa-2b. J Dermatol Treat 2:15–16
5. Buechner SA (1991) Intralesional interferon alfa-2b in the treatment of basal cell carcinoma. J Am Acad Dermatol 24:731–734
6. Buechner SA, Lautenschlager S, Schiller P, Itin P, Bigliardi P, Izakovic J, Yilmaz B, Müller D, Courvoisier S (1995) Treatment of basal cell carcinomas with intralesional interferon alfa-2b. Dermatology 191:173–174
7. Chimenti S, Cotellessa C, Peris K, Di Cristofaro S, Fargnoli MC, Torlone G (1995a) Use of recombinant interferon alpha-2a in the treatment of squamous cell carcinoma. J Dermatol Treat 6:163–166
8. Chimenti S, Peris K, Di Cristofaro S, Fargnoli MC, Torlone G (1995b) Use of recombinant interferon alfa-2b in the treatment of basal cell carcinoma. Dermatology 190:214–217
9. Cornell RC, Greenway HT, Tucker SB, Edwards L, Ashworth S, Vance JC, Tanner DJ, Taylor EL, Smiles KA, Peets EA (1990) Intralesional interferon therapy for basal cell carcinoma. J Am Acad Dermatol 23:694–700
10. DiLorenzo PA, Goodman N, Lansville F, Markel W (1994) Regional and intralesional treatment of invasive basal cell carcinoma with interferon alfa-n2b. J Am Acad Dermatol 31:109–111
11. Edwards L, Tucker SB, Perednia D, Smiles KA, Taylor EL, Tanner DJ, Peets EA (1990a) The effect of an intralesional sustained-release formulation of interferon alfa-2b on basal cell carcinoma. Arch Dermatol 126:1029–1032
12. Edwards L, Whiting D, Rogers D, Luck K, Smiles KA (1990b) The effect of intralesional interferon gamma on basal cell carcinomas. J Am Acad Dermatol 22:496–500
13. Edwards L, Berman B, Rapini RP, Whiting DA, Tyring S, Greenway HT, Eyre SP, Tanner DJ, Taylor EL, Peets E, Smiles KA (1992) Treatment of cutaneous squamous cell carcinomas by intralesional interferon alfa-2b therapy. Arch Dermatol 128:1486–1489
14. Gloster HM, Brodland DG (1996) The epidemiology of skin cancer. Dermatol Surg 22:217–226
15. Goldberg LH (1996) Basal cell carcinoma. Lancet 347:663–667
16. Greenway HT, Cornell RC, Tanner DJ, Peets E, Bordin GM, Nagi C (1986) Treatment of basal cell carcinoma with intralesional interferon. J Am Acad Dermatol 15:437–443

17. Gresser I (1990) Biolologic effects of interferons. J Invest Dermatol 95:66S–71S
18. Grob JJ, Collet AM, Munoz MH, Bonerandi JJ (1988) Treatment of large basal cell carcinomas with intralesional interferon alpha-2a. Lancet 1:878–879
19. Hahn S, Gehri R, Erb P (1995) Mechanism and biological significance of CD4-mediated cytotoxicity. Immunol Rev 146:57–79
20. Healsmith MF, Berth-Jones J, Fletcher A, Graham-Brown RAC (1991) Treatment of basal cell carcinoma with intralesinal interferon alpha-2b. J R Soc Med 84:524–526
21. Hunt MJ, Halliday GM, Weedon D, Cooke BE, Barnetson RS (1994) Regression in basal cell carcinoma: an immunohistochemical analysis. Br J Dermatol 130:1–8
22. Ikic D, Padovan I, Pipic N, Knezevic M, Djakovic N, Rode B, Kosutic I, Belicza M (1991) Basal cell carcinoma treated with interferon. Int J Dermatol 30:734–737
23. Knop J (1990) Immunologic effects of interferon. J Invest Dermatol 95:72s–74s
24. Marks R (1995a) The epidemiology of non-melanoma skin cancer: who why and what can we do about it. J Dermatol 22:853–857
25. Marks R (1995b) An overview of skin cancers. Incidence and causation. Cancer 75:607–612
26. Motley RJ (1995) The treatment of basal cell carcinoma. J Dermatol Treat 6:121–125
27. Mozzanica N, Cattaneo A, Boneschi V, Brambilla L, Melotti E, Finzi AF (1990) Immunohistological evaluation of basal cell carcinoma immunoinfiltrate during intralesional treatment with alpha-2-interferon. Arch Dermatol Res 282:311–317
28. Nagata S, Golstein P (1995) The Fas death factor. Science 267:1449–1456
29. Oishi M, Maeda K, Sugiyama S (1994) Distribution of apoptosis-mediating Fas antigen in human skin and effects of anti-Fas monoclonal antibody on human epidermal keratinocyte and squamous cell carcinoma cell lines. Arch Dermatol Res 286:396–407
30. Rodriguez-Villanueva J, McDonnell TJ (1995) Induction of apoptotic cell death in non-melanoma skin cancer by interferon-a. Int J Cancer 61:110–114
31. Stadler R, Ruszczak Z (1993) Interferons. New additions and indications for use. Dermatol Clin 11:187–199
32. Stalder T, Hahn S, Erb P (1994) Fas antigen is the major target molecule for CD4+ T cell-mediated cytotoxicity. J Immunol 152:1127–1133
33. Stenquist B, Wennberg AM, Gisslen H, Larko O (1992) Treatment of aggressive basal cell carcinoma with intralesional interferon: evaluation of efficacy by Mohs surgery. J Am Acad Dermatol 27:65–69
34. Tank B, Habets JMW, Naafs B, Damsma O, Stolz E, van Joost T (1989) Intralesional treatment of basal cell carcinoma with low-dose recombinant interferon gamma. J Am Acad Dermatol 21:734–735
35. Thestrup-Pedersen K, Jacobsen IE, Frentz G (1990) Intralesional Interferon-a 2b treatment of basal cell carcinoma. Acta Derm Venereol (Stockh) 70:512–514
36. Tong Y, Tucker SB (1993) Normal human skin lymphocytic and Langerhans' cell responses to intradermal interferon a-2b injections. Am J Med Sci 306:23–27
37. Wickramasinghe L, Hindson TC, Wacks H (1989) Treatment of neoplastic skin lesions with intralesional interferon. J Am Acad Dermatol 20:71–74
38. Williams GT (1994) Apoptosis in the immune system. J Pathol 173:1–4

Therapy of Kaposi's Sarcoma

W. Kempf

Clinical Aspects and Pathogenesis

Kaposi's sarcoma (KS), described in 1872 as "idiopathic multiple pigmented sarcoma of the skin" by M. Kaposi [1], occurs in four different epidemiological forms, which have been described in detail in recent review articles [2, 3].

The *classic-sporadic type* of KS affects predominantly elderly men (male to female ratio of 10–15:1), aged 50–70 years, particularly those of the Mediterranean region or Jews from Eastern Europe. Patients present with brown–violet nodules on the lower legs, sometimes accompanied by a lymphedema, and the disease shows a slowly progressive course with an overall good prognosis.

The *African endemic type* of KS is found primarly in young men, aged 25–40 years, and children in Central Africa and represents 3–18 % of all malignant neoplasms in the black population in these areas. This KS type usually shows a rapidly fatal course.

The *iatrogenic or immunosuppression-related KS type* is a rare complication of immunosuppressive medication in organ transplant recipients and patients receiving long-term corticosteroid therapy or chemotherapy, occurring 10–22 months after initiation of immunosuppressive medication. In most cases, a regression of the tumor can be observed after discontinuation of the immunosuppressive medication, but lesions tend to reappear during subsequent phases of immunosuppressive therapy.

Since the onset of the acquired immunodeficiency syndrome (AIDS) epidemic, *AIDS-asssociated or epidemic KS* is one of the most common neoplasms in AIDS patients, despite its decreasing prevalence over the past few years. Particularly homosexual or bisexual men, accounting for up to 90 % of all patients with epidemic KS, develop this KS type, whereas other human immunodeficiency virus (HIV) risk groups are rarely affected by KS. Similarly to the other epidemiological forms of KS, there is a male predominance, with a male to female ratio of 100:1 in epidemic KS. The KS lesions are often multiple and typically localized in the oral cavity and on the acral localizations, such as the penis and the top of the nose; they usually appear after $CD4^+$ cell counts begin to decrease to under 200 $CD4^+$ cells/mm^3. In contrast to the classic-sporadic KS type, the clinical course ranges from a chronic disease with recurrent single lesions at varying localizations to a highly aggressive disease with a very poor prognosis and quality of life. Autopsy studies demonstrated that up to half of the patients have an involvement of internal organs, especially of the lungs and the gastrointestinal tract. KS is the cause of death in about 12 % of affected patients, mainly due to severe hemorrhages by gastrointestinal or pulmonal involvement, but the majority of the patients with epidemic KS die from opportunistic infections or other malignancies as complications of the HIV infection [4].

Histology and Histogenesis

Three characteristic stages (patch, plaque, and nodular stage) in KS lesions can be differentiated, composed of three cellular components occurring in varying proportion: (1) a proliferation of dilated, irregularly shaped, and thin-walled vessels (patch stage), which become slit-like during tumor progression; (2) a predominating population of spindle cells in the plaque and nodular stage; (3) and an inflammatory mixed infiltrate consisting of lymphocytes, plasma cells, and macrophages, which can be found in all stages [5].

Endothelial cells, either of lymphatic origin or deriving from blood vessels, are thought to be the actual tumor cell, but the exact nature of the KS progenitor cells remains to be determined.

Pathogenesis

Epidemiological studies indicated that KS, at least in its AIDS-associated form, can be regarded as a sexually transmitted disease caused by a viral agent whose transmission is linked to particular sexual practices [6, 7]. Several viruses, particularly cytomegalovirus and human papillomaviruses, have been proposed as causal "KS agents," but could not be confirmed to be involved in the etiology of KS (for a review, see [8]). Recently, DNA sequences of a new human herpesvirus (HHV) detectable in more than 90% of AIDS-associated KS have been identified [9]. Subsequent studies demonstrated that this new herpesvirus, called KS-associated herpesvirus (KSHV) or HHV-8, can be detected in all epidemiological forms of KS, indicating a causal role of HHV-8 in the development of KS [10].

Based on studies on long-term cultures of KS cells, several growth factors have been identified to be involved in the propagation and maintenance of KS growth (for reviews, see [11, 12]). Interleukin (IL)-1, tumor necrosis factor (TNF)-α, and oncostatin M, a potent mitogenic growth factor, have been shown to stimulate the proliferation of endothelial cells and KS spindle cells. The KS spindle cells themselves secrete basic fibroblast growth factor (bFGF), which is an important growth factor for KS in vivo and in vitro. These cytokines stimulate the proliferation and migration of endothelial cells and promote self-preservation of activated cells and recruitment of normal surrounding cells in an autocrine and paracrine stimulation. In addition to the cellular angiogenic factors, HIV tat protein has been shown to be a potent angiogenic peptide stimulating KS growth [13].

These findings led to the following pathogenetical concept. The infection with HHV-8 and other viral cofactors results in a growth stimulaton of KS progenitor cells, either by direct transformation or indirectly by inducing a cytokine cascade which maintains and propagates the growth of KS cells via an autocrine and paracrine stimulation. In addition, HIV promotes tumor growth directly by expression of HIV tat protein which has angiogenic properties. Therefore, KS has been regarded by some authors as a potentially reversible hyperproliferative reactive process in the initial stages [14], which becomes a true neoplastic process in the later stages. The clinical course of KS varying between the individual patients and different epidemiological forms may be determined by the pattern of other involved infectious agents (e.g., Epstein-Barr virus), genetic predisposition, hormonal influence, and immunological factors.

Principles of Therapy

Considering the pathogenetical steps in the development of KS, various sites of actions for therapeutical interventions exist, as listed in Table 1. Local therapy is usually applied in limited disease, while systemic therapy is required in disseminated KS. In addition, local therapy is effective in the management of complications such as lymphedema and pain accompanying localized lesions and to achieve a cosmetic improvement of residual cutaneous lesions after a systemic therapy for disseminated KS.

Treatment depends on the extent of disease and has to take into account the epidemiological type of KS. A staging classification for AIDS-associated KS including the clinical extent of KS, immunological status, and HIV-related systemic diseases has been developed by the AIDS Clinical Trial Group (ACTG) (Table 2) [15]. The immunological status has been found to be the most important prognostic factor in prediciting survival.

In the classic-sporadic KS, patients generally respond well to local therapies, whereas patients with African endemic KS – with exception of the lymphadenopathic subtype – respond favorably to systemic chemotherapy. In patients with iatrogenic KS, regression of KS can be effectively achieved by discontinuation or reduction of immunosuppressive therapy.

Despite the spectrum of possible therapeutical approaches, no curative therapy for AIDS-associated KS exists up so far, and neither local nor systemic therapies have been found to prolong the survival of patients with AIDS-associated KS [2]. However, therapy of AIDS-associated KS can provide palliation of symptoms and improve quality of life. In the following section, various therapeutical approaches for KS will be reviewed with emphasis on immunomodulatory strategies in the treatment of the AIDS-associated KS.

Local Therapy

Radiotherapy and Cryotherapy

Radiotherapy and cryotherapy are regarded as the mainstay of local therapy in various KS forms, with clinical response rates up to 85%. The lesions treated with cryosurgery tend to recur after weeks or months probably due to persistent KS in the deep portion of reticular dermis not reached by cryotherapy [2, 16]. Surgical excision is useful for the rapid treatment of socially stigmatizing and isolated lesions at selected localizations such as the face, oral cavity, and genitalia. Laser therapy (argon, pulsed dye, and CO_2 laser) can be used for cutaneous macular lesions, but recurrence is usually observed within 3 months. In addition, sclerotherapy and photodynamic therapy have been described as successful approaches to treat oral mucosal lesions [2, 16, 17].

Immunomodulatory Approaches

Interferon (INF)-α showed a complete (CR) or partial remission (PR) rate of 20% and 70%, respectively, in ten patients with classic-sporadic KS treated with intralesionally injected INF-α (three million U) three times per week for 1 month and variable doses for an additional month [18]. Dupuy et al. reported a CR or PR in 85% of the lesions in 14 patients with AIDS-associated KS receiving additional systemic therapy with azidothymidine (AZT), using intralesionally administered IFN-α (one million U) three

Table 1. Therapeutical approaches for Kaposi's sarcoma

Local	Systematic
Physical methods	Chemotherapy (CT)
Radiotherapy	Single-agent/multiagent CT[a]
Cryosurgery	+ AZT
Surgical excision	+ AZT + IFN-α
Laser therapy	+ AZT + IFN-α + GM-CSF
Infrared coagulation	
Photodynamic therapy	
Sclerotherapy	
Intralesional chemotherapy	
Vinblastine/vincristine	
Intralesional immunomodulatory drugs	Immunomodulatory drugs
IFN-α	IFN-α
TNF-α	IFN-α + AZT
GM-CSF	IFN-α + AZT + GM-CSF
	Intravenous immunoglobulin therapy
	Autologous, activated $CD8^{+}$T cytotoxic cells + IL-2
Antiangiogenic substances	Antiangiogenetic substances
Topical tretinoin	Retinoids
	Platelet factor 4, Fumagillol
	βHCG

IFN, interferon; TNF, tumor necrosis factor; GM-CSF, granulocyte-macrophage colony-stimulating factor; AZT, azidothymidine; IL, interleukin; HCG, human chorionic gonatropin.
[a] Includes: vinblastine, vincristine, etoposide, bleomycin, liposomal dauno- or doxorubicin, paclitaxel.

Table 2. Staging classification of AIDS-associated Kaposi's sarcoma (KS) (from Krown et al. 1989)

	Good risk (0) (all of the following)	Poor risk (1) (any of the following)
Tumor (T)	Confined to skin and/or lymph nodes and/or minimal oral disease	Tumor-associated edema or ulceration
Immune system (I)	CD4 cell > 200 µl	CD4 cells < 200 µl
Systemic illness (S)	No history of oppurtunistic infection or thrush No "B" symptoms[b] Performance status > 70 (Karnofsky)	History of opportunistic infection and/or "B" symptomsb Performance status < 70 (Karnofsky) Other HIV-related illness (e.g., neurologic disease, lymphoma)

HIV, human immunodeficiency virus.
[a] Minimal oral disease is non-nodular KS confined to the palate.
[b] Unexplained fever, night sweats, > 10 % involuntary weight loss, or diarrhea persisting more than 2 weeks

times per week for 6 weeks, but this approach failed to demonstrate superior efficacy over placebo in this study [19].

Intralesional TNF-α, which has antiangiogenic properties, resulted in a clinical response in 15 of 16 patients with AIDS-associated KS, but was accompanied by relatively severe side effects such as fever, rigors, chills, pain, nausea, and vomiting, which limits its use [20].

Granulocyte-monocyte colony-stimulating factor (GM-CSF) has been reported to resolve bothersome lesions within days after local perilesional injection, without adverse or systemic effects [21].

Topical tretinoin, inhibiting KS cell growth in vitro [22], has been shown to induce partial remissions in seven of eight (87%) patients with AIDS-associated KS [23].

Up to now, intralesionally applied immunomodulatory substances such as IFN-α and TNF-α have been found to be similarly effective as cryotherapy and intralesional chemotherapeutics. Two major disadvantages limit their use: (1) they are more expensive than the other approaches, and (2) side effects are more severe compared to conventional therapies; they are therefore not suitable as a first-line approach.

Intralesional Chemotherapy

Intralesionally injected vinblastine and vincristine have been reported to result in CR or PR rates of 60–88% in AIDS-associated and other forms of KS. Recurrences may occur in 40% of patients within 4–6 months [24]. Intralesional chemotherapy is particularly indicated for the treatment of oral lesions and nodular lesions larger than 1 cm in diameter. Side effects include postinflammatory hyperpigmentation, which limit its use in exposed body areas, pain for 1–2 days after injection, and transient mononeuropathy when injected near nerves [2, 16].

Systemic Therapy

Considering the growth maintenance and stimulation of KS cells by various cytokines, treatment with immunomodulatory and antiangiogenic factors is of particular interest as a therapeutic strategy. Whereas in local treatment of KS the value of immunomodulating drugs remains to be defined, systemic therapeutic immunointervention is an important part of the treatment of KS.

Chemotherapy

Whereas patients with disseminated classic-sporadic and African endemic KS respond well to chemotherapy with vinca alkaloids, bleomycin, etoposide, and cisplatin [25], single-agent chemotherapy with these cytotoxic drugs resulted in a response rate of 40–80% in patients with AIDS-associated KS [26]. Because an increased toxicity of cytotoxic drugs in AIDS patients was observed, multiagent chemotherapy regimens were investigated in an attempt to reduce toxicity, but no particular combination has been demonstrated to be superior. Cytotoxic chemotherapy is indicated particularly to reduce tumor burden in patients with extended visceral KS lesions or generalized cutaneous KS. Dose-related neutropenia and opportunistic infections are the most important side effects of cytotoxic chemotherapy, but at least the myelotoxic effect of cytotoxic drugs can be reduced by additional therapy with hematopoietic growth factors such as GM-CSF or erythropoietin.

Liposomal formulations of daunorubicin and doxorubicin, which are thought to be taken up selectively by KS tumor tissue, have been reported to induce CR of short duration in up to 8 % and PR in up to 85 % of patients, even in those with extensive AIDS-associated KS [27, 28].

Systemic chemotherapy has been used in combination with the antiviral agent AZT and has been proven to be a safe and effective regimen, but patients have to be carefully monitored [29]. AZT may retard KS growth by improving the immune dysfunction of the patients and by reducing the viral load of HIV and HIV tat protein, a potent angiogenic stimulus for KS tumor cells.

Immunotherapy

IFN-a is now the most important immunomodulating drug in the treatment of AIDS-associated KS based upon its antiproliferative, antiangiogenic, antiviral, and cytokine-regulating effects, thereby increasing the activity of natural killer cell, T cell-mediated cytotoxicity, and macrophage function [30]. Comparing various dosage regimens, IFN-α as a single agent shows a mean response rate of approximately 30 %, when a dose greater than 20 million U/m^2 body surface area is used in a three times per week or alternate-week schedule, whereas lower doses revealed response rates less than 10 % [31, 32]. A dose dependency of response rates and of the onset of response has been noted, while maximal responses can usually be observed after 6 months or more [33]. The duration of the response remains uncertain. Best response rates can be achieved in patients with CD4$^+$ T cell counts of more than 400 cells/mm^3 and low levels of endogenous INF, β2-microglobulin, and neopterin. In contrast, patients with CD4$^+$ T cell of counts less than 200 cells/mm^3, prior opportunistic infections and "B" symptoms, including weight loss, fever, and night sweats exhibit a poor response to systemic IFN-a therapy [30, 34]. The response rates do not depend on whether IFN-α is administrated subcutaneously, intramuscularly, or intravenously. Common side effects of IFN-α treatment include hematologic alterations such as neutropenia and thrombocytopenia, elevations of hepatic enzymes (chemical hepatitis), and a flu-like syndrome with malaise, high fevers, chills, myalgia, and anorexia, which are reversible after discontinuation of IFN [30]. These side effects can be reduced by low doses of IFN-α at initiation of therapy, followed by gradual dosage escalation or dosage attenuation during treatment [30].

In analogy to the combination of cytotoxic agents with antiviral drugs, systemic IFN-a therapy in combination with AZT has also been studied. Response rates ranged from 30 % to 60 % [35–37]. Maximal doses of 18 millions U IFN-α per day and 100 mg AZT every 4 h have been recommended [35]. The most impressive benefit with response rates up to 30 % was noted in patients with CD4$^+$ T cell counts of less than 100–200 cells/mm^3, in whom IFN-α therapy alone is not effective. The combination of IFN-α and AZT is limited by neutropenia, anemia, thrombocytopenia, and hepatopathia occurring in approximately 50 % of patients. These side effects can be alleviated by the additional use of GM-CSF, without reducing the response rates [38].

Because IFN-α therapy is associated with various side effects and high treatment costs, this therapy modality has been considered as useful particularly for patients with CD4$^+$ cell counts greater than 400 cells/mm^3, no prior opportunistic infections, and generalized, preferentially cutaneoeus lesions [2]. In patients with severly impaired immune function (i.e., $CD4^+$ cell counts of less than 100–200 cells/mm^3), combination with AZT and in some cases GM-CSF is indicated.

Retinoids are known to possess antiproliferative and antiangiogenic properties. 13-*cis*-Retinoic acid has been shown to inhibit growth of KS cells in vitro and to induce programmed cell death (apoptosis) in high concentrations [22, 39]. Conflicting results about the effect of all-*trans*-retinoic acid in the treatment of epidemic KS exist. Whereas in a phase II pilot trial, partial (mostly minor) responses or stabilization of KS could be noted in 14 out of 24 patients with disease progression after 16–22 weeks [40], another study could not demonstrate a benefit, neither of a monotherapy with retinoids nor of retinoids in combination with IFN-α [41].

Intravenous immunoglobulin therapy has recently been demonstrated to have a beneficial effect in one patient with a immunosuppression-related KS and polymyositis who had not shown an improvement of KS after reduction of immunosuppressive therapy [42].

Lymphokine-activated killer (LAK) cells cytotoxic to AIDS-associated KS cells and LAK receptors on KS cells have been identified in vitro, suggesting that KS cells could be killed by the use of LAK cells in vivo [43]. Regression of KS in seven of eight patients with epidemic KS has been observed after treatment with interleukin (IL)-2 and autologous, activated $CD8^+$ cytotoxic T cells directed against HIV-infected cells, suppressing replication of HIV-infected cells leading to a decrease in HIV-induced growth factors [44].

Antiangiogenic Drugs

A range of various angiogenic growth factors are involved in the development of KS. These factors are targets to block the cytokine cascade as a crucial element maintaining and propagating KS tumor growth. Recombinant platelet factor 4 (rPF4), inhibiting angiogenesis in vitro, was reported to be effective as local treatment when injected intralesionally in six out of 12 (50%) patients with AIDS-associated KS [45]. The fumagillin analog TNP-470 decreases the proliferation of KS spindle cells by inhibiting bFGF and has been demonstrated to be active against KS spindle cells in vitro [46].

Antiangiogenic Hormones

Men are up to a hundredfold more frequently affected by KS than women, regardless of the epidemiological form of KS, suggesting an influence of steroidal sex hormones on KS growth. Recent studies on metastasizing KS-like tumors in nude mice demonstrated that tumor growth and metatstasis can be blocked by the human β-chorionic gonadotropin (βHCG) [47]. Despite these convincing observations, there are controversial reports on the therapeutic benefit of βHCG [48].

Antiviral Drugs

Considering the potential causal role of HHV-8, therapeutic interventions to block the viral infection should be able to modify the clinical course of KS. Recent reports concerning the influence of antiherpetic medications on the occurrence and progression of KS gave inconsistent results. In one study, only foscarnet was associated with a significant reduction in the risk for KS, whereas acyclovir and gancyclovir minimally affected the risk for KS in AIDS patients [49] . Other investigators did not find a benefit of antiherpetics [50], but it should be kept in mind that HHV-8 may be insensitive to classical antiherpetic agents such as acyclovir and gancyclovir.

Additionally, HIV tat protein supporting the angiogenic process in KS may be blocked by a benzodiazepine tat antagonist [51]. Similar effects may be expected by gene therapy targeting HIV replication by antisense oligonucleotide or other techniques resulting in a reduction of HIV viral load.

Summary

Epidemic KS is one of the most common neoplasms in patients with AIDS. Recent studies demonstrate that several growth factors and angiogenic factors are involved in the maintenance and propagation of KS tumor growth. In addition, a new human herpesvirus (HHV-8) has been considered to be etiologically involved in the pathogenesis of various epidemiological forms of KS. In this review, several therapeutic approaches for local and systemic treatment of KS are discussed, with an emphasis on immunomodulating and antiangiogenic substances. The recently described and experimental strategies directed against factors involved in the pathogenesis of KS are compared with standard modalities of treatment.

References

1. Kaposi M (1872) Idiopathisches multiples Pigmentsarkom der Haut. Arch Dermatol Syphil 4:742–749
2. Tappero JW, Conant MA, Wolfe SF, Berger TG (1993) Kaposi's sarcoma. Epidemiology, pathogenesis, histology, clinical spectrum, staging criteria and therapy. J Am Acad Dermatol 28:371–395
3. Friedman-Kien AE, Saltzman BR (1990) Clinical manifestations of classical, endemic African, and epidemic AIDS-associated Kaposi's sarcoma. J Am Acad Dermatol 22:1237–1250
4. Mitsuyasu RT (1993) Clinical aspects of AIDS-related Kaposi's sarcoma. Curr Opin Oncol 5:835–844
5. Ackerman AB and Gottlieb GJ (eds) (1988) Kaposi's sarcoma: a text and atlas. Atlas of the gross and microscopic features. Lea and Febiger, Philadelphia, pp 29–33
6. Beral V, Peterman TA, Berkelman RL et al (1990) Kaposi's sarcoma among persons with AIDS: a sexually transmitted infection? Lancet 335:123–128
7. Beral V, Bull D, Darby S et al (1992) Risk of Kaposi's sarcoma and sexual practices associated with faecal contact in homosexual or bisexual men with AIDS. Lancet 339:632–635
8. Kempf W, Adams V (1996) Viruses in the pathogenesis of Kaposi's sarcoma – a review. Biochem Mol Med 58:1–12
9. Chang Y, Cesarman E, Pessin MS et al (1994) Identification of herpesvirus-like DNA sequences in AIDS-associated Kaposi's sarcoma. Science 266:1865–1869
10. Moore PS, Chang Y (1995) Detection of herpesvirus-like DNA sequences in Kaposi's sarcoma in patients with and without HIV infection. N Engl J Med 332:1181–1185
11. Stürzl M, Brandstetter H, Roth WK (1992) Kaposi's sarcoma: a review of gene expression and ultrastructure of KS spindle cells in vivo. AIDS Res Hum Retroviruses 8:1753–1763
12. Miles SA (1994) Pathogenesis of HIV-related Kaposi's sarcoma. Curr Opin Oncol 6:497–502
13. Ensoli B, Barillari G, Salahuddin SZ et al (1990) Tat protein of HIV-1 stimulates growth of cells derived from Kaposi's sarcoma lesions of AIDS patients. Nature 345:84–86
14. Brooks JJ (1986) Kaposi's sarcoma: a reversible hyperplasia. Lancet ii:1309–1311

15. Krown SE, Metroka C, Wernz JC (1989) Kaposi's sarcoma in the acquired immunodeficiency syndrome: a proposal for uniform evaluation, response, and staging criteria. J Clin Oncol 7:1201–1207
16. Zalla MJ (1996) Kaposi's sarcoma. An update. Dermatol Surg 22:274–287
17. Webster GF (1995) Local therapy for mucocutaneous Kaposi's sarcoma in patients with acquired immunodeficiency syndrome. Dermatol Surg 21:205–208
18. Trattner A, Reizis Z, David M et al (1993) The therapeutic effect of intralesional interferon in classical Kaposi's sarcoma. Br J Dermatol 129:590–593
19. Dupuy J, Price M, Lynch G et al (1993) Intralesional interferon and zidovudine in epidemic Kaposi's sarcoma. J Am Acad Dermatol 28:966–972
20. Kahn J, Kaplan L, Volberding P et al (1989) Intralesional tumor necrosis factor-a for AIDS-associated Kaposi's sarcoma. J Acquir Immune Defic Syndr 2:217–223
21. Boente P, Sampaio C, Brandao MG et al (1993) local peri-lesional therapy with rhGM-CSF for Kaposi's sarcoma (letter). Lancet 341:1154
22. Corbeil J, Rapaport E, Richman DD et al (1994) Antiproliferative effect of retinoid compounds on Kaposi's sarcoma cells. J Clin Invest 93:1981–1986
23. Bonhomme L, Fredj G, Averous S et al (1991) Topical treatment of epidemic Kaposi's sarcoma with all-trans-retinoic acid. Ann Oncol 2:234
24. Boudreaux AA, Smith LL, Cosby CD et al (1993) Intralesional vinblastine for cutaneous Kaposi's sarcoma associated with acquired immunodeficiency syndrome. J Am Acad Dermatol 28:61–65
25. Klein E, Schwartz RA, Laor Y et al (1980) Treatment of Kaposi's sarcoma with vinblastine. Cancer 45:427–431
26. Volberding PA (1987) The role of chemotherapy for epidemic Kaposi's sarcoma. Semin Oncol 14 [Suppl 3]:23–26
27. Gill PS, Espina BM, Muggia F et al (1995) Phase I/II clinical and pharmacokinetic evaluation of liposomal daunorubicin. J Clin Oncol 13:996–1003
28. Harrison M, Tomlinson D, Stewart S (1995) Liposomal-entrapped doxorubicin: an active agent in AIDS-related Kaposi's sarcoma. J Clin Oncol 13:914–920
29. Brunt AM, Goodman AG, Philips RH et al (1989) The safety of intravenous chemotherapy and zidovudine when treating epidemic Kaposi's sarcoma. AIDS 3:457–460
30. Pluda JM, Parkinson DR, Feigal E et al (1993) Non-cytotoxic approaches to the treatment of HIV-associated Kaposi's sarcoma. Oncology 7:25–33
31. Real FX, Oettgen HF, Krown SE (1986) Kaposi's sarcoma and the acquired immunodeficiency syndrome: treatment with high dose and low doses of recombinant leukocyte A interferon. J Clin Oncol 4:544–551
32. Krown SE (1987) The role of interferon in the therapy of epidemic Kaposi's sarcoma. Semin Oncol 14 [2 Suppl 3]:27–33
33. Monfardini S, Tirelli V, Vaccher E (1994) Treatment of acquired-immunodeficiency syndrome (AIDS)-related cancer. Cancer Treatment Rev 20:149–172
34. Rosenbaum W, Gharakhanian S, Navarette MS et al (1990) Long-term follow-up of 120 patients with AIDS-related Kaposi's sarcoma treated with interferon alpha-2A. J Invest Dermatol 95:161S–165S
35. Krown SE, Gold JWM, Niedzwiecki D et al (1990) Interferon-a with zidovudine: safety, tolerance, and clinical and virologic effects in patients with Kaposi's sarcoma associated with the acquired immunodeficiency syndrome (AIDS). Ann Intern Med 112:812–821
36. Stadler R, Bratzke B, Schaart F et al (1990) Long-term combined rIFN-alph-2A and zidovudine therapy for HIV-associated Kaposi's sarcoma: clinical consequences and side effects. J Invest Dermatol 95:170S–175S
37. Baumann R, Tauber MG, Opravil M et al (1991) Combined treatment with zidovudine and lymphoblastoid interferon-alpha in patients with HIV-related Kaposi's sarcoma. Klin Wochenschr 69:360–367
38. Scadden DT, Bering HA, Levine JD et al (1991) Granulocyte-macrophage colony-stimulating factor mitigates the neutropenia of combined interferon alfa and zidovudine treatment of acquired immune deficiency syndrome-associated Kaposi's sarcoma. J Clin Oncol 9:802–808

39. Guo WX, Gill PS, Antakly T (1995) Inhibition of AIDS-Kaposi's sarcoma cell proliferation following retinoic acid receptor activation. Cancer Res 55:823–829
40. Gill PS, Espina BM, Moudgil T et al (1994) All-trans retinoic acid for the treatment of AIDS-related Kaposi's sarcoma: results of a pilot phase II study. Leukemia 8 [Suppl 3]:S26–S32
41. Bailey J, Pluda JM, Foli A et al (1995) Phase I/II study of intermittent all-trans-retinoic acid, alone and in combination with interferon alfa-2A, in patients with epidemic Kaposi's sarcoma. J Clin Oncol 13:1966–1974
42. Carmeli Y, Mevorach D, Kaminski N, Raz E (1994) Regression of Kaposi's sarcoma after intravenous immunoglobulin treatment for polymyositis. Cancer 73:2859–2861
43. Rahman MU, Mazumder A (1992) Recognition of heterogeneous lymphokine-activated killer (LAK) receptors on Kaposi's sarcoma cells, endothelial cells, and monocytes/macrophages: evidence of distinct LAK-cell antigen on Kaposi's sarcoma cells – potential for use of LAK cells for immunotherapy. J Clin Immunol 12:281–288
44. Klimas N, Flechter M, Walling J et al (1993) Response of Kaposi's sarcoma to autologous CD8 cells expanded and activated ex vivo and reinfused with rIL-2 (abstract WS-B15-2). IX Internat. Conf AIDS 1:58
45. Kahn J, Ruiz R, Kerschmann R et al (1993) A phase I/II study of recombinant platlet factor 4 (rPF4) in patients with AIDS-related Kaposi's sarcoma (abstract). Proc Am Soc Clin Oncol 12:50
46. Saville MW, Foli A, Broder S et al (1993) In vitro activity of TNP-470, a novel angiogenesis inhibitor in Kaposi's sarcoma (KS)- related spindle cells (abstract). J Cell Biochem [Suppl] 17E:22
47. Lunardi-Iskandar Y, Bryant JL, Zerman RA et al (1995) Tumorigenesis and metastasis of neoplastic Kaposi's sarcoma cell line in immunodeficient mice blocked by a human pregnancy hormone. Nature 375:64–68
48. Harris PJ (1995) Treatment of Kaposi's sarcoma and other manifestations of AIDS with human chorionic gonadotropin. Lancet 346:118–119
49. Jones J, Hanson DL, Chu SY et al (1995) AIDS-associated Kaposi's sarcoma. Science 267:1078–1079
50. Costagliola D, Mary-Krause M (1995) Can antiviral agents decrease the occurence of Kaposi's sarcoma? Lancet 346:578
51. Hsu M, Schutt AD, Holly M et al (1991) Inhibition of HIV replication in acute and chronic infections in vitro by Tat antagonist . Science 254:1799

Adjuvant Melanoma Therapy

A. Hauschild and E. Stockfleth

Introduction/Rationale

Although progress is being made in the prevention and diagnosis of malignant melanocytic skin diseases, approximately 20 % of patients suffering from malignant melanoma worldwide still die. Patients who have had malignant melanoma of a thickness (maximal vertical diameter of the tumor, according to Breslow) of less than 0.75 mm diagnosed early and surgically removed can usually be considered as cured. In contrast, patients with melanomas 1.5–4.0 mm in thickness (medium-risk group) carry a risk of up to 50 % of occult lymphogenic or hematogenic metastases (Table 1) [26].

The probability of developing subclinical hematogenic metastases is even greater in patients experiencing locoregional tumor cell seeding in transit or in lymph nodes (Table 1). In Germany, all patients with primary or metastasizing melanomas are usually subjected to a standard staging program, consisting in obligatory abdominal and lymph node sonography and chest X-ray examination, and optional brain computed tomography/magnetic resonance imaging (CT/MRT) and bone and lymph scintigraphy. Even if these examinations yield negative results, micrometastasis cannot be ruled out. As yet there is no established serological tumor marker for melanoma.

Therefore, the aim of an adjuvant ("supportive") therapy must be the destruction of existing micrometastasis and the prevention of recurrences. The concept of adjuvant therapeutic methods was developed 20 years ago using human tumors implanted into experimental animals [2].

Table 1. Stage-independent prognosis of melanoma

Tumor stage	5-year survival rate (%)
I Primary tumors	
tumor thickness (mm)	
< 0.75	96
0.75–1.5	85
> 1.5–4.0	70
> 4.0	50
II Locoregional metastases	
In transit	30
Lymph nodes	20
III Distant metastatses	
Nonvisceral	5
Visceral	0

The following has been shown [15]:

1. The success of the treatment was reciprocally proportional to the tumor mass.
2. Clinically inapparent micrometastases were more susceptible to treatment than larger primary tumors.
3. Substances that were effective against advanced tumors promised to be even more successful against small numbers of micrometastases.

The time interval between therapeutic surgery and subsequent adjuvant therapy should be as short as possible, i.e.. preferably not longer than 4–6 weeks [15, 29].

Clinical Studies of Adjuvant Therapy: Results

During the past 30 years, numerous prospective, randomized studies or comparisons with historical controls have been carried out (reviews by [1, 3, 16]). Here we discuss in detail the results of prospective randomized clinical studies that usually evaluate treatments in comparison with untreated controls.

Adjuvant Immunotherapy

The rationale of melanoma immunotherapy is based on the known immunogenicity of this tumor. Melanomas belong to the category of solid tumors most frequently showing spontaneous remissions in the primary tumor. So-called regression zones are histologically characterized by infiltrating activated T lymphocytes. The simultaneous occurrence of vitiligo in melanoma patients, especially those receiving immunotherapy, appears to be correlated with an improved prognosis. Another sign indicating the immunogenicity of malignant melanomas is the increased prevalence in immunosuppressed patients [28].

Nonspecific Immunostimulation

Early phase II studies on metastasizing melanomas indicated that intralesional or systemic therapy using nonspecific immunostimulants could induce the regression of metastases [25]. Patients in certain subgroups treated with *Calmette-Guérin bacillus (BCG)* or *Corynebacterium parvum* showed a prolongation of the disease-free interval in initial studies; however, this had no effect on the overall survival time [4, 13, 20]. In none of the prospective randomized BCG studies involving large numbers of patients with high-risk primary melanomas or surgically removed lymph node metastases was a statistically significant influence either on the disease-free interval or on overall survival time detected. Patient numbers varied between eight and 203, and the median follow-up time was between 1 and 10 years [3, 12]. This demonstrates that analyses of patient subgroups are meaningful only when large patient numbers are frequently quoted. Adjuvant therapy trials with BCG-treated or BCG plus dacarbazine (DTIC)-treated patients (World Health Organization Melanoma Group) did not find that treated patients had any advantage compared to untreated controls [32]. However, the analysis of patient subgroups indicated that BCG treatment resulted in longer survival times in patients whose BCG skin tests were negative prior to therapy [8].

The use of *C. parvum* for nonspecific immunostimulation does not provide an advantage over BCG, as shown in a large number of patients with advanced primary tumors or regional metastases with subcutaneous or intravenous therapy [22, 30].

Interferons/Interleukin-2

In contrast to nonspecific immunostimulants, interferons (IFN) and interleukin (IL)-2 are capable of activating tumor-specific immunocompetent cells.

IFN-γ enhances the expression of HLA class I and II molecules on the surface membrane of melanoma cells; it also activates macrophages [18]. The Southwestern Oncology Group (SWOG/USA) carried out an IFN-γ trial with stage I and II patients. The study was terminated when IFN-γ-treated patients had significantly more relapses than untreated patients [24]. No differences in recurrent diseases and survival rates between IFN-γ-treated patients and a control group was seen in a EORTC study (Kleeberg, personal communication). IFN-γ is no longer used in the systemic therapy of melanoma.

Recombinant INF-b (rINF-b) is currently being tested in intermediate- and high-risk melanoma patients (tumor thickness 1.5 mm) as part of a prospective randomized trial in Germany.

A comparison of *natural INF-β (nINF-β)*-treated patients with matched pairs from the central melanoma registry of the German Dermatological Society pointed to a potential beneficial effect of the treatment [5].

Recombinant $INF\text{-}\alpha_{2a}$ (Roferon A) and $INF\text{-}\alpha_{2b}$ (Intron A) were used to treat patients with distant melanoma metastases and proved to be effective by producing remission rates of approximatelly 15%. The mechanism of action is thought to be enhancement of expression of HLA class I molecules and of specific melanoma-associated proteins on the surface of the target cells. In addition, an antiproliferative effect on the melanoma cells – inhibition of protein synthesis – and the activation of natural killer cells may be important factors in the destruction of the tumor cells [6].

Several reports in recent years have claimed significant improvement in disease-free survival rates of patients following rIFN-α treatment; however, observation periods are still too short to allow a final judgement on this point. The most interesting study involving adjuvant IFN-α therapy was published by the Eastern Cooperative Oncology Group (ECOG, USA; EST 1984 trial). Patients carrying high-risk primary melanomas or clinically occult or detectable lymph node metastases were treated intravenously with high-dose $IFN\text{-}\alpha_{2b}$ (20 million IU/m^2 per day, 5 days a week over 4 weeks), followed by maintenance therapy with $IFN\text{-}\alpha_{2b}$ (10 million IU/m^2, three times a week) given subcutaneously for 11 months [19]. In comparison with untreated controls, it was demonstrated that not only the disease-free survival time was improved in IFN-α-treated patients (1.72 years vs. 0.98 years; 5-year disease-free interval, 37% vs. 26%), but also a prolonged median survival time (3.82 years vs. 2.78 years) and an increased 5-year survival rate (46% vs. 37%) were achieved [19]. This is the first study ever showing that significant improvement of survival can be obtained with an adjuvant therapy. It is important to note at this time that high-dose IFN therapy has significant side effects. Therefore, in 1990 the ECOG study group initiated a trial to compare the high-dose regimen (EST 1684) with low-dose therapy (3 million IU $IFN\text{-}\alpha_{2b}$ three times a week for 2 years). Preliminary results are not yet available.

Another low-dose IFN-a study (3 million IU IFN-α_{2a} three times a week) was presented by the WHO Melanoma Group (Trial 16 [9]). A preliminary evaluation showed that 46 % of 218 patients, who had lymph node metastases surgically removed and were subsequently treated with IFN-α_{2a}, remained disease-free after 2 years, compared with 27 % of patients in the control group. It appears, however, that the beneficial effect of this therapy (duration, 3 years) is diminished after termination of the treatment (Cascinelli, Milan, personal communication).

A third large, prospective adjuvant IFN-a therapy study was conducted with 497 French melanoma patients (tumor thickness > 1.5 mm). According to a preliminary evaluation, the treatment (3 million IU rIFN-α_{2a} three times a week for 18 months) resulted in a statistically significant prolongation of the disease-free survival time, which extended beyond the point of treatment termination (J.J. Grob, Marseille, personal communication).

The lowest treatment dose of rIFN-α (1 million IU every second day for 1 year) was used by the EORTC (Trial 18871) and failed to demonstrate beneficial effects. It can be assumed, therefore, that IFN treatment with these dose levels is ineffective (Kleeberg, Hamburg, personal communication).

The only trial using *interleukin (IL)-2 (Proleukin)* in the adjuvant therapy of malignant melanoma was conducted by a German–Swiss study group. Recombinant IL-2 combined with rIFN-α_{2b} was given subcutanously for 48 weeks. This randomized study involved 228 patients with malignant melanoma (tumor thickness > 1.5 mm) and untreated control patients. Immunological monitoring data showed that soluble IL-2 receptors in serum can be expressed even after several months of combined therapy. The clinical outcome of this study will become available in the near future.

Active Specific Immunization

In order to enhance immune reactivity against weak tumor-associated antigens, there have been attempts to treat patients with their own melanoma cells infected with nonpathogenic oncolytic viruses. Encouraging results were obtained in phase II studies when Newcastle disease virus [10] and vaccinia virus [21] recovered from lysed melanoma cells were used for vaccination. A single phase III study comparing active specific immunization (ASI) with untreated controls in a prospective, randomised manner was recently published by Wallack et al. [33]. This study with a vaccinia virus–melanoma oncolysate or placebo (vaccinia virus) involved 250 patients who had surgically removed lymph node metastases. A preliminary evaluation of the recurrence-free survival did not find any differences between treated and control patients. The observation period of 30 months is too short to assess the overall survival time. However, a significant difference between the immune reactivity of male and female patients was found [33]. At present, several phase III studies are being carried out worldwide to assess the potential benefits of adjuvant ASI therapy.

Adjuvant Chemotherapy

Systemic Application

During the past 30 years, many studies comparing melanoma patients receiving either adjuvant chemotherapy with dacarbazine or methyl-chloroethyl-nitrosourea (CCNU) with patients having standard excision procedures without further treatment have been conducted. All randomized investigations agreed that adjuvant chemotherapy did not provide reliable benefits (for a review, see [3]). One of the most comprehensive studies - by the Central Oncology Group (COG) in the United States - demonstrated remarkably poorer survival rates in the chemotherapy group than in untreated controls [17].

In another clinical study of patients with more than five histologically proven lymph node metastases, no success was recorded after autologous bone marrow transplantation and subsequent high-dose chemotherapy [23].

At the cellular level, a natural resistance against cytostatic drugs might explain the poor response of melanoma micrometastases to adjuvant chemotherapy in the majority of these adjuvant therapy studies.

Retsas et al. [27] recently published the results of a study with vindesine-treated patients after surgical removel of lymph node metastases compared with historical controls. Vindesine was given intravenously (3 mg/m^2 body surface) every second week during the first year, every third week for the following 6 months, and every fourth week during the last 6 months. After a median observation period of 8 years, vindesine-treated patients had a 5-year survival rate of 49 %, compared with 28 % in a simultaneously monitored group in which the patients had a similar tumor development but remained untreated [27].

Locoregional Application

Adjuvant locoregional chemotherapy results in higher concentrations of toxic drugs in the target tissue than systemic application. The North American Perfusion Group (NAPG), EORTC, and WHO conducted a large joint project to evaluate the effect of hyperthermic adjuvant extremity perfusion using melphalan. While it was possible to lower the rate of recurring in-transit metastases, the overall survival time of treated patients was not significantly altered (Eggermont, Rotterdam, personal communication). Because of the well-known toxicity problems, this form of therapy is discouraged as a routine measure subsequent to removal of a primary tumor.

Adjuvant Radiation Therapy

The X-ray sensitivity of melanomas is well established, as demonstrated by radiation therapy of the lentigo maligna melanoma and palliative treatment of brain, soft tissue, or bone metastases (for a review, see [31]). In the only randomized trial to study adjuvant radiation, the area of lymph node dissection was subsequently irradiated. Rates of local relapses and survival were not improved when radiation-treated patients were compared with untreated controls [11]. The Radiation Therapy Oncology Group (USA) is currently carrying out a new study of regional postoperative radiation therapy using 5×6 Gy on head and neck melanomas with lymph node metastases. The results of the study are not yet available.

Neoadjuvant Therapy

The term "neoadjuvant therapy" was introduced by Frei [14, 15] and refers to a primary systemic therapy to be applied before any surgical measures are taken. Frequently, neoadjuvant therapy reduces tumor size, which is almost a precondition for surgery for certain solid tumors, e.g., renal carcinoma.

Buzaid and coworkers of the M.D. Anderson Cancer Center in Houston/Texas carried out preoperative adjuvant polychemotherapy with cisplatin, vinblastine, and dacarbazine (CVD schedule). A total of 48% of the 52 melanoma patients with clinically detectable lymph node metastases showed either complete (10%) or partial (38%) remission. After 2 months of neoadjuvant therapy, all patients except the complete responders had a radical lymph node dissection. In this phase II study, postoperative treatment consisted of a continuation of polychemotherapy for all responding patients. After 5 years, 38% of the treated patients are still free of recurrent disease [7].

Summary and Future Perspectives

In spite of some progress and encouraging new findings, in particular with adjuvant INF treatment of malignant melanoma, further investigations are necessary in order to develop a meaningful approach for the therapy of high-risk melanomas. One important aspect of adjuvant therapy – as with any treatment – is the relationship between acceptable adverse reactions and the expected benefit. Adjuvant therapy on a routine basis can be applied only if the potential benefits to the patient are deemed significant, with the possible exception of patients with a very poor prognosis. Future investigations should not only focus on an increase in disease-free time, but in particular on prolongation of total survival time of treated patients. To answer these questions definitively, studies involving long follow-up periods for well-defined patient risk categories need to be carried out. Whereas unspecific immunostimulation, chemotherapy and radiation procedures have failed to demonstrate clinical value in terms of prolongation of survival in the adjuvant treatment of malignant melanoma, our current knowledge suggests that the most promising candidates for successful adjuvant therapy are interferons. At this time, there is also insufficient information on the usefulness of IL-2 in an adjuvant setting. Combination therapy with cytotoxic drugs and cytokines also warrants further study. It is to be expected that results of randomized studies on the use of ASI or genetically modified tumor cells (gene therapy) will become available in the next few years and that the clinical value of experimental approaches will be determined.

Acknowledgement. We thank Professor Dr. Dr. Aldinger and Mrs. Sandra Paul for careful preparation of the manuscript.

References

1. Balch CM, Hersey P (1988) Heutiger Stand der adjuvanten Therapie. In: Balch CM, Milton GW, Shaw HM, Seng-jaw Soong (eds) Hautmelanome. Springer, Berlin Heidelberg New York, pp 192–211
2. Balch CM, Maddox WA (1978) The logic of adjunctive therapy in surgical patients with resectable cancer. South Med J 71:951
3. Barth A, Morton DL (1995) The role of adjuvant therapy in melanoma management. Cancer 75(2):726–734
4. Bast RC Jr, Zbar B, Borsos T, Rapp HJ (1974) BCG and cancer. N Engl J Med 290:1413
5. Beiteke U, Ruppert P, Garbe C, Oxenfarth R, Kastl I, Türker T, Tronnier H, Frosch PJ (1993) Adjuvante Therapie des primären malignen Melanoms mit natürlichem humanen Interferon beta. Hautarzt 44:365–371
6. Bonnem EM (1991) Alpha interferon: the potential drug of adjuvant therapy: past achievements and future challenges. Eur J Cancer 27(4):S2–S6
7. Buzaid AC, Legha SS, Balch CM, Ross M, Ring S, Plager C, Papadopoulos NE, El-Naggar AK, Benjamin RS (1994) Pilot study of preoperative chemotherapy with cisplatin, vinblastine, and dacarbazine in patients with localregional recurrence of melanoma. Cancer 74:2476–2482
8. Cascinelli N, Rümke P, MacKie R, Morabito A, Bufalino R (1989) The significance of conversion of skin reactivity to efficacy of bacillus Calmette-Guérin (BCG) vaccinations given immediately after radical surgery in stage II melanoma patients. Cancer Immunol Immunother 28:282–286
9. Cascinelli N, Bufalino R, Morabito A, MacKie R (1994) Results of adjuvant interferon study in WHO melanoma programme. Lancet 343:913–914
10. Cassel WA, Murray DR, Phillips HS (1983) A phase II study on the postsurgical management of stage II malignant melanoma with a Newcastle disease virus oncolysate. Cancer 52:856
11. Creagan ET, Cupps RE, Ivins JC, Pritchard DJ, Sim FH, Soule EH et al (1978) Adjuvant radiation therapy for regional nodal metastases from malignant melanoma: a randomized, prospective study. Cancer 42:2206–2210
12. Czarnetzki BM, Macher E, Suciu S, Thomas D, Steerenberg PA, Rümke P (1993) Long-term adjuvant immunotherapy in stage I high risk malignant melanoma, comparing two BCG preparations versus non-treatment in a randomised multicentre study (EORTC Protocol 18781). Eur J Cancer 29A(9):1237–1242
13. Eilber FR, Townsend CM Jr, Morton DL (1976) Results of BCG adjuvant immunotherapy for melanoma of the head and neck. Am J Surg 132:476
14. Frei E III (1982) Clinical cancer research: an embattled species. Cancer 50:1979–1992
15. Goldie JH (1987) Scientific basis for adjuvant and primary (neoadjuvant) chemotherapy. Semin Oncol 14(1):1–7
16. Hauschild A, Sterry W (1992) Adjuvante Therapie des malignen Melanoms. DMW 117:303–306
17. Hill GJ, Moss SE, Golomb FM, Grage TB, Fletcher WS, Minton JP et al (1981) DTIC and combination therapy for melanoma, III: DTIC (NSC 45388) Surgical Adjuvant Study COG protocol 7040. Cancer 47:2556–2562
18. Kirkwood J, Agarwala S (1993) Systemic cytotoxic and biologic therapy of melanoma. Lippincott, Philadelphia (Principles and practice of oncology updates, vol 7)
19. Kirkwood JM, Strawderman MH, Ernstoff MS, Smith TJ, Borden EC, Blum RH (1996) Inteferon alfa-2b adjuvant therapy of high-risk resected cutaneous melanoma: the Eastern Cooperative Oncology Group Trial EST 1684. J Clin Oncol 14:7–17
20. Lamoureux G, Turcotte R, Portelance V (eds) (1976) BCG in Cancer Immunotherapy. Grune and Stratton, New York
21. Lindemann J, Klein PA (1967) Viral oncoloysis: increased immunogenicity of host cell antigen associated with influenza virus. J Exp Med 126:93

22. Lipton A, Harvey HA, Balch CM, Antle CE, Heckard R, Bartolucci AA (1991) Corynebacterium parvum versus bacille Calmette-Guérin adjuvant immunotherapy of stage II malignant melanoma. J Clin Oncol 9:1151–1156
23. Meisenberg BR, Ross M, Vredenburgh JJ, Jones R, Shpall EJ, Seigler HF et al (1993) Randomized trial of high-dose chemotherapy with autologous bone marrow support as adjuvant therapy for high-risk, multi-node-positive malignant melanoma. J Natl Cancer Inst 85:1080–1085
24. Meyskens FL, Kopecky K, Samson M, Hersh E, MacDonald J, Jaffe H et al (1990) Recombinant human interferon gamma: adverse effects in high-risk stage I and II cutaneous malignant melanoma. J Natl Cancer Inst 82:1071
25. Morton DL, Eilber FR, Malmgren RA, Wood WC (1970) Immunological factors which influence response to immunotherapy in malignant melanoma. Surgery 68:158–164
26. Morton DL, Davtyan DG, Wanek LA, Foshag LJ, Cochran AJ (1993) Multivariate analysis of the relationship between survival and the microstage of primary melanoma by Clark level and Breslow thickness. Cancer 71:3737–3743
27. Retsas S, Quigley M, Pectasides D, Macrae K, Henry K (1994) Clinical and histologic involvement of regional lymph nodes in malignant melanoma. Cancer 73(8): 2119–2130
28. Rhodes AR, Weinstock MA, Fitzpatrick TB, Mihm MC Jr, Sober AJ (1987) Risk factors for cutaneous melanoma: a practical method of recognizing predisposed individuals. JAMA 258:3146–3154
29. Schabel FM Jr (1995) Concepts for systemic treatment of micrometastases. Cancer 35:15
30. Thatcher N, Mene A, Banerjee SS, Craig P, Gleave N, Orton C (1986) Randomized study of corynebacterium parvum adjuvant therapy following surgery for (stage II) malignant melanoma (abstract). Br J Surg 73:111–115
31. Tilgen W (1995) Therapie des malignen Melanoms: Derzeitiger Stand und Perspektiven. In: Macher E, Kolde G, Bröcker EB (eds) Jahrbuch der Dermatologie. Biermann, Zülpich, pp 123–150
32. Veronesi U, Adamus J, Aubert C, Bajetta E, Beretta G, Bonadonna G et al (1982) A randomized trial of adjuvant chemotherapy and immunotherapy in cutaneous melanoma. N Engl J Med 307:913–916
33. Wallack MK, Sivanandham M, Balch CM, Urist MM, Bland KI, Murry D, Robinson WA, Flaherty LE, Richards JM, Bartolucci AA, Rosen L (1995) A phase III randomized, double-blind, multiinstitutional trial of vaccinia melanoma oncolysate-active specific immunotherapy for patients with stage II melanoma. Cancer 75(1):34–42

Cytokine-Based Treatments for Advanced Melanoma

U. Keilholz and C. Scheibenbogen

Introduction

Most patients with advanced metastatic melanoma who cannot be controlled by surgery experience rapid disease progression and die within 6–8 months. Many agents have been used for antitumor acitivity in melanoma, but there is no accepted standard therapy. Dacarbazine is the only single agent approved by the United States Food and Drug Administration for treating metastatic melanoma. It should be noted, however, that approval of dacarbazine today would not be very likely under the current, stringent Food and Drug Administration rules. The response rate achieved with dacarbazine as a single agent is 15–20 %, with a response duration of 4–6 months [1,2] and an uncertain survival benefit. Chemotherapy combinations of two or more drugs may increase the response rate to 40 % at the cost of considerable toxicity, but complete response rates do not exceed 10%, and survival rates are not improved [2, 3]. The 2-year survival rate for patients enrolled in chemotherapy phase II trials from the Mayo Clinic is 9% and the 5-year survival rate 2% [4]. These figures are identical to those in historical controls reported by Balch et al. [5].

The advent of cytokines resulted in a large number of phase II trials in metastastic melanoma. Interferon (IFN)-α alone has only little efficacy in the treatment of metastatic melanoma [6]. A number of responses have been reported from phase II trials; however, a summary of phase II trials from the Mayo Clinic resulted in a 9 % survival rate after 2 years and 2 % after 5 years [7], which, again, is identical to those in historical controls. The activity of interleukin (IL) 2 also has been extensively tested over the past decade in patients with advanced melanoma. The contribution of IL-2 has never been evaluated formally in any randomized phase III trial; however, encouraging results have been obtained in phase II studies [8]. This chapter focuses on IL-2 based treatment for metastatic melanoma.

Background

Mechanism of Action of IL-2

The mechanism of action and pharmacokinetics of the T cell growth factor IL-2 has been extensively reviewed elsewhere [8], this section summarizes the most important features. In high concentrations IL-2 stimulates the cytotoxicity of T lymphocytes, natural killer cells, and macrophages. In developing treatment strategies it must be recognized that different effector cells of the immune system are activated by varying concentrations of IL-2, based on differences in expression of IL-2 receptors. The IL-2 receptor consists of three chains: one low-affinity α-chain (CD25), a β-chain (P75) with intermediate affinity, and a γ-chain. The high-affinity IL-2 receptor is formed by assembly of all three chains. T lymphocytes, natural killer cells, and monocytes/macrophages constitutively express only the intermediate-affinity chain (β-chain) of the IL-2 receptor, requiring high concentration of IL-2 (100–300 ng/ml) for induction of a transmembrane signal. After contact with antigen T cells express the α-chain of the IL-2 receptor, leading to formation of a high-affinity receptor complex, and an IL-2 concentration in the range of 0.5 ng/ml is sufficient for maximal activation. The α-chain of the IL-2 receptor on T lymphocytes is induced not only by contact with antigen but also by incubation with IL-2 at a high concentration, leading to a positive feedback mechanism: after induction of the high-affinity IL-2 receptor low-dose IL-2 is sufficient to further stimulate T lymphocytes.

Pharmacokinetics

IL-2 is a glycoprotein with a molecular weight of 15 kDa, which is secreted by CD4 T lymphocytes after antigen recognition. The serum half-life of intravenously administered IL-2 is short, the α half-life (distribution half-life) is 6–7 min, and the β half-life (elimination half-life) is approximately 60 min. IL-2 is excreted by the kidneys. Intravenous bolus administration leads to a brief peak of IL-2 followed by rapid subsequent decline. Continuous intravenous infusion leads to constant serum levels after 4–6 h. The bioavailibility of subcutaneously administered IL-2 is very variable, leading to a wide variation in serum levels. The peak serum concentration is only 2% of the same dose administered intravenously. When kidney function is blocked experimentally in animal models, the half-life of IL-2 increases to 24 h, and hepatic metabolism is responsible for its elimination.

The biological pharmacokinetics are complex because IL-2 does not mediate immunological effects directly but acts by the activation of immunological effector cells. In addition, IL-2 induces secretion of a number of secondary cytokines (e.g., tumor necrosis factor α, IL-1, and IFN-γ) which are thought to be relevant for the clinical effects of IL-2 as well as for mediating most side effects. The therapeutic window of IL-2 is narrow. The maximal tolerable dose is approximately 2 mg when administered as rapid bolus every 8 h and approximately 1 mg per 24 h when administerd by continuous infusion. The dose-limiting toxicity varies from patient to patient.

Clinical Trials in Melanoma Patients Involving IL-2

IL-2 as a Single Agent

IL-2 as a single agent or in conjunction with adoptive transfer of immunological effector cells results in objective responses in up to 20% of patients with metastatic melanoma when IL-2 is administered in high-dose regimens [10–24] (Tables 1, 2). The addition of cellular treatments to intravenous infusion of IL-2 has not proven clearly beneficial [16, 19] and has not been further pursued in recent years. Some long-term survivors have been reported in most trials. These results led to subsequent studies combining IL-2 with IFN-α and/or cytotoxic agents.

Table 1. Adoptive immunotherapy

Treatment	No. of responders/ no. of patients	Reference
LAK cells + IL-2		
LAK + IL-2 b	4/7	Rosenberg et al. 1985 [10]
LAK + IL-2 civ	5/10	West et al. 1987 [11]
LAK + IL-2 b	10/48	Rosenberg et al. 1989 [12]
LAK + IL-2 b	6/32	Dutcher et al. 1989 [13]
LAK + IL-2 b + civ	7/40	Bar et al. 1990 [14]
LAK regional (liver) + IL-2 civ	3/9	Keilholz et al. 1994 [15]
Randomized study		Rosenberg et al. 1993 [16]
IL-2 b	6/22	
LAK + IL-2 b	6/27	
Total	47/195 (24 %)	
TIL + IL-2		
TIL + IL-2 b	11/20	Rosenberg et al. 1988 [17]
TIL + IL-2 civ	5/21a	Dillman et al. 1991 [18]

LAK, Lymphokine-activated killer cells; TIL, tumor-infiltrating lymphocytes; b, intravenous bolus; civ, continuous intravenous infusion.
[a] TIL cultures were initiated for 82 patients; however, 61 patients could not receive TIL because of slowly growing culture or rapid tumor progression. The data are on the 21 remaining patients only

Combinations of IFN-α and IL-2

The clinical activity of IL-2 and IFN-α has been shown in a number of phase II trials. The rationale of combining these two cytokines is based on in vitro observations in which IFN-α and IL-2 are synergistic. IFN-α can synergize with IL-2 in activating immunological effector cells, especially when IL-2 is used at suboptimal concentrations [25]. Furthermore, IFN-α upregulates the expression of HLA class I molecules and adhesion antigens on tumor cells, which is thought to be important for recognition of tumor cells by antigen-specific CD8 lymphocytes [26]. In larger phase II studies [27–34] (Table 2) the objective response rates of the combination treatment has been between 15 and 41%. However, the role of IFN-α in addition to IL-2 remains unconfirmed. The only randomized trial investigating IL-2 alone versus IL-2 plus IFN-α was terminated prematurely because of low response rates in both treatment arms [30]. The results of several very small trials suggest that subcutaneous administration of IL-2 does not lead to objective responses in metastatic melanoma. One trial of high-dose bolus IL-2 plus IFN-α showed that a 5-day regimen is significantly more active than a 3-day regimen, but the 5-day treatment was associated with considerable toxicity [33]. The administration of IL-2 in decreasing doses over 5 days (initial high-dose administration and subsequent tapering to a low maintenance dose) rather than a continuous dose infusion reduces the rate of side effects while the clinical efficacy is similar or higher [29].

The published data concerning duration of responses and survival are too limited and patient selection in phase II trials too heterogeneous to permit meaningful conclusions on the long-term effects of IFN-α/IL-2 combinations. However, most trials observe a proportion of patients with durable remissions. In one cohort of 65 patients 17% survived more than 3 years, and 11% more than 5 years, of whom 9% had no evidence of clinical disease at that time [35]. Similar results have been reported by other groups.

Table 2. Studies of IL-2-based melanoma treatments

Reference	IL-2 administration and concomitant treatment	*n*	Response rate (%)	Response duration (months)
IL-2 only				
Rosenberg et al. 1989 [12]	b	42	24	2–41
Thatcher et al. 1989 [20]	b	31	3	n.r.
Parkinson et al. 1990 [21]	b	46	22	4–20
Whitehead et al. 1991 [22]	b	42	10	n.r.
Dorval et al. 1992 [23]	civ	27	22	4–45
Legha et al. 1995 [24]	civ	33	22	n.r
Total		221	21	
IL-2 + IFN-α				
Rosenberg et al. 1989 [27]	b + IFNα	44	36	n.r.
Kruit et al. 1991 [28]	civ (reduced dose) + IFNα	54	20	n.r.
Keilholz et al. 1993 [29]	civ + IFNα	27	18	3–22
	Decrescendo + IFNα	27	41	3–36
Sparano et al [1993 [30]	b (reduced dose) + IFNα	41	10	2–15
Dillmann et al. 1993 [31]	civ + IFNa	66	11	n.r.
Marincola et al. 1995 [32]	b + IFNα	82	24	n.r.
Kruit et al. 1996 [33]	b + IFNα (5 days)	17	41	2–37
	b + IFNα (3 days)	25	20	4–10
EORTC MCG [34][a]	Decrescendo + IFNα	66	18	3–36
Total		449	22	
IL-2 + chemotherapy				
Stoter et al. 1989 [36]	civ + DTIC 850 mg/m^2	24	25	2–13
Dillmann et al. 1990 [37]	civ + LAK + DTIC 1.2 g/m^2	27	26	3–24
Flaherty et al. 1990 [38]	civ + DTIC 1 g/m^2	32	22	2–22
Demchak et al. 1991 [39]	b + CDDP 150 mg/m^2	27	37	1–30
Flaherty et al. 1993 [40]	s.c. + DDTP + DTIC	27	41	3–20
Atkins et al. 1994 [41]	b + Tam + CDDP + DTIC	38	42	2–20
Dummer et al. 1995 [42]	civ + DTIC 850 mg/m^2	57	25	n.r.
Total		232	31	
Il-2 + IFNα + chemotherapy				
Richards et al. 1992 [43]	b + IFNα + CDDP + DTIC + BCNU + Tam	74	57	5–10
Khayat et al. 1993 [44]	civ + IFNα + Tam + CDDP	39	54	3–21
Buzaid et al. 1994 [45]	b + IFNα + CDDP + DTIC	151	54	3–24
Proebstle et al. 1996 [46]	Decrescendo + IFNα + DTIC + CDDP ('poor risk' patients)	21	24	4–9
EORTC MCG [34][a]	Decrescendo + IFNα + CDDP	60	33	3–36
Total		375	45	

b, Intarvenous bolus; civ, continuous infusion; DTIC, dacarbazine; CDDP, cisplatin; BCNU, carmustine; LAK, lymphokine-activated killer cells; Tam, tamoxifen.

[a] Randomized study, interim analysis as of April 1996

Combination with Cytotoxic Agents: Chemo-immunotherapy

Response rates exceeding 50% have more recently been achieved in several phase II trials combining cytotoxic agents and IL-2 [36–45] (Table 2). It was of initial concern to determine whether the cytotoxic agents impair immune-mediated antitumor responses in vivo. However, dacarbazine and cisplatin do not reduce the induction neither of cytotoxic effector cells [47] nor of secondary cytokine secretion mediated by IL-2 [48]. The serum levels of neopterin are even significantly higher after administration of cisplatin than without previous chemotherapy. Because neopterin is a specific marker for activated macrophages, these observations suggest that cisplatin may even synergize with IL-2 in the activation of macrophages.

Comparing all published phase II trials shows that response rates exceed 50% with regimens containing the three drugs cisplatin, IFN-α, and IL-2 with or without further agents. However, data on response duration and survival are scarce, and the importance of any of the three drugs on survival of melanoma patients remains to be verified prospectively in phase III trials. The first comparative phase III trials were initiated in 1993. The Melanoma Group of the European Organization for Research and Treatment of Cancer (EORTC) performed a trial evaluating IFN-α (10 MU/m^2 on days 1–5) and IL-2 (decreasing intravenous infusions on days 4–9) with or without a single dose of cisplatin (100 mg/m^2 on day 1) [34]. The Karnofsky scores of 90% of patients were 90 or above. In contrast to previous phase II trials, where usually some 50% of patients had metastases confined to cutaneous, subcutaneous sites and lymph nodes and visceral involvement, 86% of the patients in the EORTC trial had visceral metastatic disease, indicating an advanced diseased stage in the majority of patients. The toxicity of the regimen was managable; dose adjustments were necessary in only 9% of cycles. The overall response rate was 18% among patients receiving IFN-a and IL-2, as expected for this advanced patient cohort, and increased to 35% with the addition of cisplatin. The series was stratified according to previously determined prognostic factors including serum LDH level and the presence of bulky metastatic disease (product of cross sectional diameter greater than 30 cm^2) [35]. More than 80% of patients with low tumor load and normal LDH levels also exhibited visceral disease. In these patients immunotherapy alone resulted in a response rate of 23%, which increased to 38% with the addition of cisplatin. In the remaining patients with high tumor load or elevated serum LDH levels the response rate was 13% with immunotherapy alone and 32% with the addition of cisplatin. Disease progression occurred on average after 53 days in patients treated with cytokines alone and after 92 days in those treated with chemotherapy. Overall survival was identical in the two treatment groups but was affected by stratification criteria for prognosis of disease. This trial shows that in patients with advanced melanoma with visceral disease the response rate can be increased from approximately 15 to 35% with the addition of just a single dose of cisplatin, and that progression-free survival can be doubled. However, the addition of cisplatin did not influence overall survival.

In 1995 the EORTC initiated a second trial (18951) which is evaluating a different dose of cisplatin (30 mg/m^2 for 3 days) plus dacarbazine (250 mg/m^2 for 3 days) and IFN-α (10 MU/m^2) for 5 days with or without the addition of IL-2 to determine whether IL-2 affects survival. Similar trials are being performed at the National Cancer Institute in Bethesda and by the Eastern Cooperative Oncology Group which will define the value of cytokine treatment for survival in patients with advanced melanoma.

Special Clinical Considerations: Combined Modality Treatment

Second-Line Surgery

The median duration of responses after cytokine treatment is usually between 5 and 9 months if no complete remission is achieved. The most frequent site of initial progression is from remaining tumor lesions. Therefore it seems logical to attempt surgical resection of residual tumor lesions in patients with partial response after IL-2 based treatments if this can be achieved with acceptable morbidity. One study observed long-term responses in melanoma patients after resection of residual lesions in partial and even in minor remission [49].

Brain Metastases

IL-2 treatment is not recommended in patients with symptomatic brain metastases because of the risk of increased perifocal edema and subsequent seizures. In small series of patients with cerebral metastases who were asymptomatic, concomitant chemo-immunotherapy and irradiation of the brain were administered without major toxicity [46], but the patient cohort was too small to draw definite conclusions concerning the efficacy of treatments.

Another recognized problem is the development of cerebral metastases after successful IL-2 treatment for systemic metastases. IL-2 crosses the blood-liquor barrier; however, as long as this barrier remains intact, lymphocytes do not reach brain metastases. IL-2-treatment is of limited value in the brain since lymphocytes are thought to mediate important therapeutic effects of IL-2. Stereotactic irradiation and/or whole-brain irradiation can be used in patients presenting with brain metastases after successful IL-2-treatment, especially in the absence of systemic disease (unpublished observations).

Immunological Mechanisms

Patients with hematogenous spread of melanoma have circulating melanoma cells in the peripheral blood, as shown by the extremely sensitive polymerase chain reaction assay for tyrosinase mRNA [50–53]. It is of interest that all patients tested in complete remssion after IL-2 based treatment show circulating melanoma cells for several years in the absence of clinical relapse [54]. It is unclear whether this state should be regarded as “tumor dormancy” or “immune surveillance.”

Three observations suggest that IL-2 mediated melanoma regression is mediated by T lymphocytes:

- A small proportion of patients responding to IL-2 based treatment develop HLA-associated autoimmune diseases [55], where T cells recognizing self-antigens are thought to play an important role.
- Vitiligo-like depigmentation of the skin has been observed in melanoma patients after IL-2 based treatment [43, 56] but not in renal cell cancer patients treated according to the same regimen.

- The response to IL-2 based treatment was associated with the presence of certain HLA class I molecules in one European study of a patient cohort with a rather homogeneous genetic background [57] but not in a second study performed in the United States in a genetically more heterogeneous population [58].

The relevance of tumor-specific lymphocytes can be demonstrated only in situ. As a first step, polymerase chain reaction analysis of the T cell receptor repertoire suggests a T cell response limited to a small number of Vb families in all patients with IL-2 mediated melanoma regression but not prior to immunotherapy or in progressing lesions [59], suggesting that the IL-2 mediated regression of melanoma is T cell mediated, or that T cells are at least important, and that the majority of the T cell response is directed against a limited number of targed epitopes.

Melanoma was the first tumor shown to be recognized by T lymphocytes specific for several distinct antigens, as reviewed elsewhere in this volume. The majority of the melanoma rejection antigens recognized by tumor-infiltrating lymphocytes are melanocyte lineage specific proteins (tyrosinase, Melan A/MART 1, gp 100), which are expressed by both normal melanocytes and melanoma cells. Current investigations are examining whether T lymphocytes mediating melanoma regression after IL-2 treatment are specific for these differentiation antigens [60], which would further elucidate the mechanism of immune-mediated melanoma regression and may also help to explain the interesting observation of the development of vitiligo in melanoma patients responding to IL-2 based treatment.

Summary

The treatment of patients with distant melanoma metastases is controversial and unsatisfactory. Cytotoxic chemotherapy and interferon-α alone have limited activity. The activity of Interleukin-2 (IL-2) has been tested during the past decade in numerous phase I and II trials. Encouraging results have been reported especially with combinations of IL-2 with IFN-α and cisplatinum-based chemotherapy. These treatments are currently being studied in larger randomized Phase III trials, evaluating the influence of intensive treatment regimens on survival and quality of life of patients with advanced melanoma.

References

1. Kirkwood JM (1994) Systemic therapy of melanoma. Curr Opin Oncol 6:204–211
2. Legha S (1989) Current therapy for malignant melanoma. Semin Oncol 16:34–44
3. Lakhani S, Selby P, Bliss JM, Perren TJ, Gore ME, McElwain TJ (1990) Chemotherapy for malignant melanoma: combinations and high doses produce more responses without survival benefit. Br J Cancer 61:330–334
4. Ahman DL, Creagan ET, Hahn RG, Edmonson JH, Bisel HF, Schaid DJ (1989) Complete responses and long-term survivals after systemic chemotherapy for patients with advanced malignant melanoma. Cancer 63:224–227
5. Balch CM, Soong SJ, Shaw HM, Milton GW (1985) An analysis of prognostic factors in 4000 patients with cutaneous melanoma. In: Balch CM, Milton GW (eds) Cutaneous melanoma. Lippincott, Philadelphia, pp 321–352
6. Kirkwood JM (1991) Studies of Interferons in the therapy of melanoma. Semin Oncol 18:83–90

7. Creagan ET, Schaid DJ, Ahmann DL, Frytak S (1990) Disseminated malignant melanoma and recombinant interferon: analysis of seven consecutive phase II investigations. J Invest Dermatol 95:188S–192S
8. Keilholz U (1995) Chemo-immunotherapy of melanoma: Is it time for phase III trials? Editorial. Cancer 75:905–907
9. Whittington R, Faulds D (1993) Interleukin-2. A review of its pharmacological properties and therapeutic use in patients with cancer. Drugs 46:446–514
10. Rosenberg SA, Lotze MT, Muul LM, Leitman S, Chang AE, Ettinghausen SE et al (1985) Observations on the systemic administration of autologous lymphokine-activated killer cells and recombinant interleukin-2 to patients with metastatic cancer. N Engl. J Med 313: 1485–1492
11. West WH, Tauer KW, Yanelli JR, Marshall GD, Orr DW, Thurman GB et al (1987) Constant infusion recombinant interleukin-2 in adoptive immunotherapy of advanced cancer. N Engl. J Med 316:898–905
12. Rosenberg SA, Lotze MT, Yang JC, Abersold JC, Linehan WM, Seipp C et al (1989) Experience with the use of high dose interleukin-2 in the treatment of 652 cancer patients. Ann Surg 210:474–485
13. Dutcher JP, Creekmore S, Weiss GR, Margolin K, Markowith AB, Roper M et al (1989) A phase II study of interleukin-2 and lymphokine-activated killer cells in patients with metastatic malignant melanoma. J Clin Oncol 7:477–485
14. Bar MH, Sznol M, Atkins MB, Ciobanu N, Mitocich KG, Boldt DH, Margolin KA, Aronson PR, Rayner AA, Hawkins MJ (1990) Metastatic malignant melanoma treated with a combined bolus and continuous infusion interleukin-2 and lymphokine-activated killer cells. J Clin Oncol 8:1138–1147
15. Keilholz U, Scheibenbogen C, Schlag P, Brado M, Kauffmann GW, Tilgen W, Hunstein W (1994) Regional adoptive immunotherapy with IL-2 and LAK cells for liver metastases of malignant melanoma. Eur J Cancer 30:103–105
16. Rosenberg SA, Lotze MT, Yang JC, Topalian SL, Chang AE et al (1993) Prospective randomized trial of high-dose interleukin-2 alone or in conjunction with lymphokine-activated killer cells for the treatment of patients with advanced cancer. J Nat Cancer Inst 85:622–632
17. Rosenberg SA, Packard BS, Aebersold BS, Solomon D, Topalian SL, Toy ST et al (1988) Special report. Use of tumor-infiltrating lymphocytes and interleukin-2 in the immunotherapy of patients with metastatic melanoma. N Engl J Med 319:1676–1680
18. Dillman RO, Oldham RK, Barth NM, Cohen RJ, Minor DR, Birch R, Yanelli JR, Maleckar JR, Sferruzza A, Arnold J, West WH (1991) Continuous interleukin-2 and tumor-infiltrating lymphocytes as treatment of advanced melanoma. Cancer 68:1–8
19. Dorval T, Mathiot C, Brandely M, Escande MC, Fridman WH et al (1991) Lack of effect of tumour infiltrating lymphocytes in patients with metastatic melanoma who failed to respond to interleukin 2. Correspondence. Eur J Cancer 27 [Suppl 2]:S99
20. Thatcher N, Dazzi H, Gosh A, Johnson RJ (1989) Recombinant IL-2 given intra-splenically and intravenously in advanced malignant melanoma: a phase I/II study. Cancer Treat Rev 16 [Suppl A]:49–52
21. Parkinson DR, Abrams JS, Wiernik PH, Rayner AA, Margolin KA et al (1990) Interleukin-2 therapy in patients with metastatic malignant melanoma: a phase II study. J Clin Oncol 8:1650–1656
22. Whitehead RP, Kopecky KJ, Samson MK, Constanzi JJ, Natale RB et al (1991) Phase II study of intravenous bolus recombinant interleukin-2 in advanced malignant melanoma: Southwest Oncology Group study. J Nat Cancer Inst 83:1250–1251
23. Legha SS, Gianan MA, Plager C, Eton OE, Papadopoulous NEJ (1996) Evaluation of interleukin-2 administered by continuous infusion in patients with metastatic melanoma. Cancer 77:89–96
24. Dorval T, Mathiot C, Brandely M, Escande MC, Fridman WH et al (1991) Lack of effect of tumour infiltrating lymphocytes in patients with metastatic melanoma who failed to respond to interleukin 2 (correspondence). Eur J Cancer 27 [Suppl 2]:S99

25. Cameron RB, McIntosh JK, Rosenberg SA (1988) Synergistic antitumor effects of combination immunotherapy with recombinant interleukin-2 and a recombinant hybrid alpha-interferon in the treatment of established murine hepatic metastases. Cancer Res 48:5810–5817
26. Giacomini P, Aguzzi A, Pestka S et al (1984) Modulation by recombinant DNA leukocyte (alpha) and fibroblast (beta) interferons of the expression and shedding of HLA and tumor-associated antigens by human melanoma cells. J Immunol 133:1649–1655
27. Rosenberg SA, Lotze MT, Yang JC, Linehan WM, Seipp C, Calabro S et al (1989) Combination therapy with interleukin-2 and alpha-interferon for the treatment of patients with advanced cancer. J Clin Oncol 7:1863–1874
28. Kruit WH, Goey SH, Monson JR, Stahel RA, Calabresi R et al (1991) Clinical experience with the combined use of recombinant interleukin-2 (IL-2) and interferon-alpha-2a (IFN alpha) in metastatic melanoma. Br J Haematol 79 [Suppl 1]:84–86
29. Keilholz U, Scheibenbogen C, Tilgen W, Bergmann L, Weidmann E, Seither E, Richter M, Brado B, Mitrou PS, Hunstein W (1993) Interferon-a and interleukin-2 in the treatment of malignant melanoma: a comparison of two phase II trials. Cancer 72:607–614
30. Sparano JA, Micetich KC, Sunderland M, Margolin K, Aronson F et al (1993) A randomized phase III trial of treatment with high-dose interleukin-2 (IL-2) either alone or in combination with interferon-a2A (IFN) in patients with advanced melanoma (abstract no 1332). Proc Am Soc Clin Oncol 12:390
31. Dillman RO, Church C, Oldham RK, West WH, Schwartzberg L et al (1993) Inpatient continuous-infusion interleukin-2 in 788 patients with cancer. The National Biotherapy Study Group experience. Cancer 71:2358–2370
32. Marincola FM, White DE, Wise AP, Rosenberg SA (1995) Combination therapy with interferon alpha-2a and interleukin-2 for the treatment of metastatic cancer. J Clin Oncol 5:1110–1122
33. Kruit WHJ, Punt CJA, Goey SH, de Mulder PHM, Gratama JW, Eggermont AMM, Bolhuis RLH, Stoter G (1996) Dose-efficacy study of two schedules of high-dose bolus administration of interleukin-2 and alpha-interferon in patients with metastatic melanoma. Br J Cancer 74:951–955
34. Keilholz U, Goey SH, Punt CJA et al (1996) IFNα/IL-2 with or without cisplatinum in metastatic melanoma: a randomized trial of the EORTC melanoma cooperative group, proceedings of the ASCO. J Clin Onc 15:436
35. Keilholz U, Scheibenbogen C, Sommer M, Pritsch M, Geueke AM (1996) Prognostic factors for response and survival in patients with metastatic melanoma receiving immunotherapy. Melanoma Res 6:173–178
36. Stoter G, Shiloni E, Aamdal S, Cleton FJ, Iacobelli S et al (1989) Sequential administration of recombinant human interleukin-2 and dacarbazine in metastatic melanoma. A multicentre phase II study. Eur J Cancer Clin Oncol 25[Suppl 3]:41–43
37. Dillman RO, Oldham RK, Barth NM, Birch R, Arnold J et al (1990) Recombinant interleukin-2 and adioptive immunotherapy alternated with dacarbazine therapy in melanoma: a National Biotherapy Study Group trial. J Nat Cancer Inst 82:1345–1349
38. Flaherty LE, Redman BG, Chabot GG, Martino S, Gualdoni SM et al (1990) A phase I-II study of dacarbazine in combination with outpatient interleukin-2 in metastatic malignant melanoma. Cancer 65:2471–2477
39. Demchak PA, Mier JW, Robert NJ, O'Brien K, Gould JA et al (1991) Interleukin-2 and high-dose cisplatin in patients with metastatic melanoma: a pilot study. J Clin Oncol 9:1821–1830
40. Flaherty LE, Robinson W, Redman BG, Gonzalez DR, Martino S, Kraut M, Valdivieso M, Rudolph AR (1993) A Phase II study of dacarbazine and cisplatin in combination with outpatient administered interleukin-2 in metastatic malignant melanoma. Cancer 71: 3520–3525
41. Atkins MB, KR O'Boyle, JA Sosman, GR Weiss, KA Margolin, ML Ernest et al (1994) Multiinstitutional phase II trial of intensive combination chemotherapy for metastatic melanoma. J Clin Oncol 12:1553–1560
42. Dummer R, ME Gore, BW Hancock, PJ Guillou, HC Grobben, JC Becker et al (1995) A multi-center phase II clinical trial using dacarbazine and continuous infusion of interleukin-2 in metastatic melanoma: clinical data and immunomonitoring. Cancer 75:945–948

43. Richards JM, Mehta N, Ramming K, Skosey P (1992) Sequential chemoimmunotherapy in the treatment of metastatic melanoma. J Clin Oncol 10:1338–1343
44. Khayat D, Borel C, Tourani JM, Benhammouda A, Antoine E, Rixe O, Vuillemin E, Bazex PA, Thill L, Franks R, Auclerc G, Soubrane C, Banzet P, Weil M (1993) Sequential chemoimmunotherapy with cisplatin, interleukin-2 and interferon alpha-2 for metastatic melanoma. J Clin Oncol 11:2173–2180
45. Buzaid AC, Legha SS (1994) Combination of chemotherapy with interleukin-2 and interferon-alpha for the treatment of advanced melanoma. Semin Oncol 6 [Suppl 14]:23–28
46. Proebstle TM, Keilholz U, Scheibenbogen C, Sterry W, Hunstein W (1996) A phase II study of DTIC, CDDP, a interferon, and high dose IL-2 in 'poor risk' melanoma. Eur J Cancer 32: 1530–1533
47. Redman BG, Flaherty L, Chou TH, Nakeff A, Pillote K, Kaplan J (1991) Sequential dacarbazine/cisplatin and interleukin-2 in metastatic melanoma: immunological effects of therapy. J Immunother 10:147–151
48. Keilholz U, Scheibenbogen C, Möhler T, Brossart P, Geueke AM, Jochim A, Hunstein W (1995) Addition of dacarbazine or cisplatin to IFNα/IL-2 in metastatic melanoma: toxicity and immunological effects. Melanoma Res 5:283–287
49. Keilholz U, Scheibenbogen C, Stoelben E, Saeger H, Hunstein W (1994) Immunotherapy of metastatic melanoma with IFNa and IL-2: Pattern of progression in responders and patients with stable disease without or with resection of residual lesions. Eur J Cancer 30A:955–958
50. Smith B, Selby P, Southgate J, Pittman K, Bradley C, Blair GE (1991) Detection of melanoma cells in peripheral blood by means of reverse transcriptase and polymerase chain reaction. Lancet 338:1227–1229
51. Brossart P, Schmier J, Krüger S, Willhauck M, Scheibenbogen C, Möhler T, Keilholz U (1995) A PCR-based semiquantitative assessment of malignant melanoma cells in peripheral blood. Cancer Res 55:4065–4068
52. Battayani Z, Grob JJ, Xerri L, Noe C, Zarour H, Houvaeneghel G, Delpero JR, Birmbaum D, Hassoun J, Bonerandi JJ (1995) Polymerase chain reaction detection of circulating melanocytes as a prognostic marker in patients with melanoma. Arch Dermatol 131:443–447
53. Mellado B, Colomer D, Castel T, Munoz M, Galan M, Vives Corrons J et al (1996) Detection of circulating neoplastic cells by reverse-transcriptase polymerase chain reaction (RT-PCR) correlates with stage and prognosis in malignant melanoma. Proceedings of ASCO, 433
54. Brossart P, Keilholz U, Scheibenbogen C, Möhler T, Willhauck M, Hunstein W (1994) Detection of residual tumor cells in patients with malignant melanoma responding to immunotherapy. J Immunother 15:38–41
55. Scheibenbogen C, Keilholz U, Pezzutto A, Hunstein W (1993) Rheumatic disease following immunotherapy. Ann Rheum Dis 52:165–68
56. Scheibenbogen C, Keilholz U (1994) Vitiligo-like lesions following immunotherapy with IFNa and IL-2 in melanoma patients. Eur J Cancer 30A:1209–1211
57. Scheibenbogen C, Keilholz U, Mytilineos J, Suciu S, Manasterski M, Hunstein W (1994) HLA class I alleles and responsiveness to immunotherapy with IFNa and IL-2. Melanoma Res 4:191–194
58. Marincola FM, Shamamian P, Rivoltini L, Salgaller M, Cormier J, Restifo NP, Simonis TB, Venzon D, White DE, Parkinson D (1996) HLA associations in the antitumor response against malignant melanoma. J Immunotherapy 18:242–252
59. Willhauck M, Möhler T, Scheibenbogen C, Pawlita M, Brossart P, Schmier J, Keilholz U (1996) T cell receptor b variable region diversity in melanoma metastases after IL-2-based immunotherapy. Clinical Cancer Res 2:767–772
60. Scheibenbogen C, Lee KH, Stevanovic S et al (1997) Analysis of the T cell response to tumor and viral peptide antigens by an IFN-γ-ELISPOT assay. Int J Cancer (in press)

Gene Therapy: A New Perspective for the Treatment of Malignant Melanoma

D. Schadendorf and R. Dummer

Introduction

Definition and Overview

Over the last 15 years various methods for delivering genes into mammalian cells have been developed. A great number of possible therapeutic applications have been envisaged. Medical specialists and the public have followed these recent developments with great interest. It is generally admitted that no attempts to introduce germline genetic alterations should be made. Therefore, this paper will focus on somatic gene therapy, in which genetic modifications are applied to somatic cells of an individual patient. The expected clinical benefit from genetic modification of somatic cells needs to be assessed carefully, and its potential risks have to be taken in consideration. Regardless of the technological strategy chosen by the scientist/physician, nonpropagating and nontransmissive gene transfer delivery systems are mandatory at the present time.

In principle, gene transfer consists of the insertion of a foreign sequence of nucleic acid into the nucleus of a (deficient) target cell. This transfer is mediated by a (virus-derived or macromolecular) vector system carrying the nucleic acid sequence. Current approaches use mainly modified or attenuated viruses as vectors to carry the genetic material into the cell (reviewed in [6, 21, 40]). Clinical protocols commonly use defective retroviruses or defective adenoviruses. Alternative gene therapy products include other delivery methods: DNA–liposome mixtures for direct tumor injection, naked DNA, and DNA combined with a targeted receptor-mediated delivery system (reviewed in [29]).

Melanoma is an antigenic tumor [4, 37]. Several proteins specific for melanocytic cells have been identified that are presented as peptides in the groove of the HLA class I complex and are recognized by cytotoxic T cells (CTL). These proteins include members of the MAGE family, gp100, tyrosinase, or MART-1 (melanoma antigen recognized by T cells)/Melan A (reviewed in [31]). Lymphokine-activated killer cells [14, 15] and tumor-infiltrating lymphocytes are capable of becoming enriched in melanoma metastases [41]. This infiltration of tumor sites by reactive lymphocytes seems to be the mechanism of interleukin (IL)-2-induced tumor regression [13]. Gene therapy, particularly cytokine gene transfer, is thought to be a potent tool to modify the interaction between melanoma cells and the immune system.

Table 1. Methode for delivering genes into mammlian cells and likely applications in gene therapy

Method	Application in gene therapy Ex vivo	In vivo	Transient (T) or stable (S) expression
Viral			
Retrovirus	+	?	S
Adenovirus		+	T
Adeno-associated virus (AAV)	+	?	S
Herpesvirus	±	+	?
Vaccina virus	±	+	T
Polio virus	±	+	T
Avian pox virus	±	+	T
Nonviral			
Ligand-DNA conjugates	–	+	T
Adenovirus-ligand -DNA conjugates	–	+	T
Lipofection	±	+	T
Direct injection of DNA	–	+	T
CaPO4 precipitation	±	–	S
Ballistic transfer	+	+	T

+, Major application; ±, some application; –, little or no application; ?, questionable

Methods of Gene Delivery

The transduction of an appropriate target cell represents the first critical step in gene therapy. Consequently, the development of methods of gene transfer has been a major focus of research. Table 1 summarizes methods for delivering genes into mammalian cells that are currently used in clinical gene therapy protocols.

The common feature of these methods is the efficient delivery of genes into cells. In the case of retroviral vectors, the transferred DNA sequences are stably integrated into the chromosome of the target cells. Therefore, these vectors are mainly considered for ex vivo gene therapy. Ex vivo gene therapy involves excision of the target tissue from the body, transduction of the cells in vitro, and subsequent reintroduction of the modified cells into the patient. All other methods result primarily in the introduction of DNA sequences into the nucleus in an unintegrated form, resulting in high, but transient gene expression. Therefore, these techniques are predominantly considered for in vivo gene therapies, in which genetic material is directly transferred into cells and tissues of patients. Numerous variations are in use in the approved clinical protocols. Most studies utilize autologous tumor cells, which necessitates the propagation of patient's own tumor tissue ex vivo; however, because of convenience and better standardization, others use an allogenic tumor cell line for gene transfer and vaccination. Since an autologous melanoma cell line cannot be established in all cases, a third group of clinical studies is currently being performed using autologous or allogeneic fibroblasts as targets for gene transfer; these gene-modified cells are admixed with freshly obtained tumor cells for vaccination (reviewed in [21, 40]. According to a recent Recombinant RNA Advisory Committee (RAC) meeting report (September 1995), almost 65% of the gene therapy trials are aimed at treating cancer. Two thirds of the protocols utilize murine retroviral vectors, whereas a subset of investigators (17%) use adenoviral vectors or liposomes (10%) for gene delivery. The injection of naked DNA for gene delivery, the use of other viral vectors such as adeno-associated viruses, or ballistic gene transfer techniques are currently not commonly in practice [6, 25, 43].

At the Departments of Dermatology and Medical Virology in Zurich, we have produced a retroviral system to transfer genetic material into melanoma cells. For this approach, it is essential that the retrovirus can enter the cells through the appropriate viral receptor on the target cell. Therefore, we had to produce packaging cell lines capable of generating viruses with the ability to infect human cells. In addition, replication of the target cells is necessary for proviral integration to occur. Thus successful gene transfer depends on the ability to induce proliferation of the melanoma cells after the contact with infectious supernatants. Interestingly, one melanoma cell line that was transduced retrovirally with human B7.2 completely lost HLA class I expression. Neither interferon (INF)-α nor INF-γ were capable of inducing any class I expression in the cell line; we therefore concluded that insertion of the retrovirus did affect the essential promoter regions for the class I HLA complex expression in this cell line. The example clearly shows that essential cellular functions have to carefully be controlled after gene transfer with integrating viruses such as retroviruses. Furthermore, the generation of T cell lymphoma after retroviral gene transfer has been described [12].

Additionally, adenovirus vectors are of great interest because of their potential for in vivo gene delivery (reviewed in [9]). Adenoviruses are capable of efficiently infecting nondividing cells and expressing large amounts of gene products. Furthermore, the virus particle is relatively stable and can be purified and concentrated. Most of the adenovirus vectors currently in use carry deletions in the E1A–E1B and E3 regions of the viral genome. Expression of inserted sequences is usually promoted either by the E1A promoter, the major late promoter (MLP) and associated leader sequences, the E3 promoter, or exogeneously added promoter sequences.

Most nonviral methods of gene transfer rely on normal mechanisms used by mammalian cells for the uptake and intracellular transport of macromolecules (reviewed in [29]). Various methods of nonviral gene therapy have been proposed. Some approaches are aimed at developing "artifical viruses" that attempt to mimic the process of viral infection using synthetic materials. Others apply the theory and methods of advanced, particulate drug delivery to deliver DNA to selected somatic targets. DNA complexes containing lipid, protein, peptide, or polymorphic carriers are employed as well as ligands capable of targeting the DNA complex to cell surface receptors on the target cell and ligands for directing the intracellular trafficking of DNA to the nucleus. Nonviral systems have been used to deliver genes to lung, liver, endothelium, epithelium, and tumor cells and have been shown to be safe in more than 15 clinical trials (reviewed in [29]).

State of the Art

Adhesion Molecules and Allogenization

Although melanoma cells usually present various specific HLA class I-associated antigens, such as tyrosinase or MAGE, the presentation of the antigenic peptide by the HLA molecule is not sufficient to activate "naive" T cells and to generate a systemic antitumor immune response. It is speculated that melanoma cells might induce tolerance rather than activation of T cells by presenting antigens without the essential costimulatory signals [2, 3]. These costimulatory signals can be provided by the adhesion molecules B7.1 (CD80) or B7.2 (CD86), two molecules capable of delivering costimulatory signals to T cells via their ligand, CD28 [2, 3, 17–19, 23]. In recent years, the molecular basis of antigen recognition by T cells has been unraveled. Several pathways that control T cell activation and functional specialization, such as the CD28–B7 and the CD40–CD40 ligand, have been identified. Consequently, it is now possible to delineate various strategies for intervention with the immune system, to design protective vaccines, or to induce an effective response to tumor antigens [28].

The immunogenicity of tumor cells is increased if the cells are transfected with human B-7.1 [11]. Expression of the costimulatory ligand B7 on melanoma cells has been shown to induce the rejection of a murine melanoma in vivo [47]. In addition, treatment of mice bearing an 8-day established melanoma by intraperitoneal injection of $B7^+$ tumor cells resulted in complete tumor regression and cure [30]. In human melanomas, B7.1 expression was immunohistologically detected only in regressing lesions [8]. Consequently, gene therapy protocols have been initiated for the treatment of melanoma using melanoma cells genetically engineered to express B7.1 [16].

At Zurich, we have used a retroviral system to transduce $B7.1^+$ [11] and $B7.2^+$ into melanoma cells. After selection, more than 90% of the melanoma cells expressed the transgene. They were used to characterize the immune response of allogenic peripheral blood mononuclear cells (PBMC) after coincubation of irradiated tumor cells to mimic the in vivo situation during vaccination therapy. We were able to confirm results by Sule-Suso and coworkers [45] that $B7^+$ melanoma cells induce an increased proliferation of autologous PBMC as early as after 2 days which continued for up to 5 days. T cell proliferation was accompanied by the upregulated transcription of IL-2 and IFN-γ. However, in our system in Zurich, we found that $B7.2^+$ gene-modified melanoma cells induced IL-4 in addition to IL-2 and IFN-γ secretion. IL-4 secretion was critically dependent on IL-10 secretion, which furthermore caused a dramatic downregulatory effect on IL-2 and IFN-γ regulation, as demonstrated by IL-10-neutralizing antibodies.

IL-10 is not only secreted by T-helper (Th)-2-type T lymphocytes; the analysis of the cytokine spectrum displayed by melanoma cells also revealed that melanoma cells transcribe and secrete significant amounts of IL-10 [3, 5, 33]. IL-10 is a cytokine with a variety of effects, including inhibition of monocytic major histocompatibility complex (MHC) class II-dependent antigen presentation and inhibition of T cell proliferation [3, 10, 26]. In addition, it protects target cells from tumor- and allospecific cytotoxic T cells and downregulates HLA class I expression [32]. The presence of IL-10 can also explain findings by Viret et al. [49] that B7 costimulation did not correct the defect of IL-2 secretion exhibited by many melanoma-reactive T cell clones in response to in vitro antigen presentation by melanoma cells transfected with B7.1. We conclude that the transduction of B7.1 into tumor cells is not sufficient to establish an efficient T cell response due to tumor cell-induced inhibitory factors such as IL-10. Future gene therapy protocols using $B7.1^+$ transduced tumor cells or tumor cells modified by other transgenes as vaccines have to consider strategies to antagonize IL-10.

Antitumor response can be augmented by immunomodulation using gene transfer of cytokines or costimulatory molecules such as B7 as outlined above. In addition, "allogenization" of tumor cells is known to cause tumor rejection in mouse models [27].

Several methods are being explored, including nongenetic approaches such as infection of tumor cells with viruses (e.g., Newcastle disease, vesicular stomatitis; reviewed in [35]) and the introduction of foreign, allogeneic HLA molecules via gene transduction in order to augment antitumor immune responses and to improve clinical outcome. Nabel and coworkers inserted the rare human HLA-B7 gene into melanoma metastases by direct injection of a liposomal DNA mixture, which was associated with partial responses of injected lesions [36].

Suicide Genes

Cytokine gene transfer (see "Cytokines and Cytokine Gene Transfer in Cancer Treatment," this volume) and introduction of molecules such as B7 all aim at an increased immunogenicity and the modulation of the antitumor immune response. However, several other nonimmunologic gene therapy approaches are being worked on, including the use of suicide genes, gene replacement and antisense approaches, and tumor-specific gene targeting.

Suicide genes currently being explored are viral or bacterial enzymes which are not expressed by mammalian cells. Genes encoding these enzymes are introduced into the appropriate vector system to be used for administration as infectious virus particles, as naked DNA, or as liposomal DNA mixture, depending on the target tissue and strategy. This approach is often called virally directed enzyme prodrug therapy (VDEPT), since the enzymes commonly used – herpes simplex virus (HSV) tyrosine kinase (TK) and cytosine deaminase (CD) – convert nontoxic prodrugs such as gancyclovir or Ara-M and 5-fluorocysteine, respectively, into highly toxic metabolites. Current experiments have injected virus vectors containing the genetic information coding for the enzyme directly into the tumor, and the prodrug has been administered systemically. Infected cells locally produce the enzyme, which only locally converts the prodrug. No systemic effects were observed; however, a considerable "bystander" killing effect of uninfected cells due to the diffusion of the toxic metabolites was noted. The bystander effect has the advantage that not all target cells need to be infected to be killed. Calculations range between 70% and 10% of infected cells required to eradicate the injected tumor. Destruction of tumor cells always also leads to an immunologic antitumor response, probably via antigen-presenting cells invading the necrotic and inflamed area [39]. Apart from using the VDEPT strategy, others are exploring the direct expression and targeting of toxins such as ricin A or other bacterial exotoxins. Future gene therapy will probably look into combining locally delivered VDEPT systems with tissue-specific gene regulatory elements [34, 48] and genetically modified tumor cells as vaccines. The main problem of the "suicide" approach continues to be gene delivery to distant organ sites and micrometastases which cannot be injected directly. Nevertheless, several clinical protocols are in progress using retroviral vectors containing the TK gene in order to treat advanced brain tumors via direct stereotactic administration of the gene construct and subsequent systemic application of the appropriate prodrug [6, 21].

Antisense Approaches and Gene Replacement

The identification of an underlying genetic defect made gene therapy an attractive treatment option for a wide variety of diseases, including cancer. Oligonucleotide-mediated modulation of gene expression was established a decade ago, and three applications are currently being explored: (1) "classical" antisense RNA/DNA approaches, (2) use of triplex-forming DNA (anti-gene oligonucleotides), (3) and catalytic RNA (ribozymes).

Gene therapy of cancer using such an approach requires an exact understanding of the genetic and epigenetic events in order to create a rational and effective treatment strategy. Most of the work in the literature has therefore been done dealing with protooncogenes and tumor suppressor genes. The strategy employed involves suppressing or modulating an activated oncogene or replacing a mutated/inactivated tumor suppressor gene with a wild-type/normal one. Both strategies aim at the restoration of normal control of cell growth and differentiation by suppressing the malignant phenotype. Currently, antisense DNA oligonucleotides are most commonly used in vitro, both in animal models and in clinical pilot trials (reviewed in [42, 50, 51]). They have been shown to be effective in various tumor cell lines by inhibiting mostly protooncogenes/oncogenes such as c-*abl*, c-*fos*, c-*fes*, c-*fms*, c-*kit*, c-*myb*, c-*myc*, c-*raf*, c-*src*, and *ras*. The exact mechanism of action of oligonucleotide antisense is not clear at present, and different possibilities are being discussed, including the following: (a) binding of target mRNA and subsequent translation arrest, (b) induction of RNase H cleavage to inhibit translation, (c) interference with transcription, (d) inactivation of splicing sites, and (e) blockage of RNA transport [42, 50, 51]. The main problem for the application of antisense oligonucleotides in vitro and in vivo is the rapid degradation by nucleases, which can only partly be slowed down by phosphorothioate modification of certain oligonucleotides. Further limitations of a broad clinical application are the preferred accumulation in the liver and kidneys, the low cellular uptake, and the lack of delivery specificity. Nevertheless, approximally ten clinical gene therapy trials using an antisense oligonucleotide approach for cancer treatment are currently being performed (see "Cytokines and Cytokine Gene Transfer in Cancer Treatment," this volume). Two studies are aimed at inhibiting the action of growth factors (insulin-like growth factor-1, IGF-1; transforming growth factor-b2, TGF-2) in glioblastoma, and four trials are evaluating the efficacy of antisense directed against the protoonocogenes c-*myc*, c-*fos*, K-*ras*, and *erbB2*; in addition, at least five clinical protocols trying to replace or to inhibit the action of the tumor suppressor gene p53 have been approved.

Antisense RNA, which specifically inhibits gene expression, can be introduced and delivered by routinely used eukaryotic expression vectors, preventing rapid degradation; triplex DNA, which has the advantage over other strategies that it blocks gene expression at the transcriptional rather than the translational level and therefore requires only very few molecules to be therapeutically effective, and ribozymes are still not used in clinical protocols for cancer therapy, and several drawbacks need to be resolved prior to clinical application. However, several in vitro studies and animal models seem promising for the future. All approachs used to date have their own strengths and weaknesses, but the field is still very new and more basic research and development is necessary.

Tissue-Specific Gene Delivery

There is an increasing requirement for efficient and accurate delivery of therapeutic genes to the appropriate target genes. This is particularly important when a therapeutic gene needs to be targeted directly to the (tumor) cell, which is the case for toxins, prodrug-activating enzymes, and oligonucleotide-based strategies. For a significant clinical, therapeutic success, a diffusely growing tumor cell population needs to be reached accurately and with high efficiency in order to eradicate the tumor.

Specificity for gene targeting depends on multiple factors. Target cell surface recognition is one major factor for specific targeting which is being utilized by various viral vector systems (Table 1). For many viruses in use for gene therapy purposes, specific cell surface receptors have been characterized for cell entry. Furthermore, viral infectivity can be regulated and specifically directed by packaging cell lines that naturally display certain envelope proteins with the desired tropism. Furthermore, the unique or restricted expression of certain cell surface molecules can be used to target these cells via virus–ligand conjugates, as has been done for the asialoglycoprotein receptor on hepatocytes. Similarly, the genetic information to be targeted can be complexed with ligands or antibodies recognizing epithelial growth factor (EGF), insulin, or transferrin receptors, which subsequently mediate internalization of the complex (reviewed in [34]). This possibility has several disadvantages, but might nevertheless be feasible in selected approaches. The same is true for the application of liposomes and other molecular conjugates used as carriers.

Targeting of gene expression is also possible at the genetic level by placing the therapeutic gene under the control of a regulatory element which itself depends on tissue-restricted positive or/and negative *trans*-acting transcription factors. Correctly regulated expression may require so-called promoter regions, enhancer elements all located in the noncoding regions, and as the coexpression of (tissue-specific) transcription factors. As well as restricting gene expression, cellular gene-regulatory elements are not inactivated by methylation, which would allow long-term expression, in contrast to viral promoters (reviewed in [34]). At least eight tissue-specific promoters have so far been genetically characterized and are far advanced for gene therapeutic applications in mouse models, which include the *creatine kinase promoter* for treatment of muscle diseases, the *Ig heavy chain promoter/enhancer* for targeting B cell lymphoma, the *promoter of the von Willebrand's factor gene* restricting gene expression to endothelial cells opening ways to target the tumor vasculature as well as providing a tool for the systemic delivery of missing soluble factors, mediators, or hormones, the *myelin basic protein promoter* to target brain tumors, the *carcinoma embryonic antigen (CEA) promoter* to specifically reach gastrointestinal tumor cells, the *albumin* and *a-fetoprotein promoter* are being explored to treat cells of the hepatocyte-lineage, and the *tyrosinase promoter* has been used to deliver therapeutic genes to melanoma cells [48]. Unfortunately, promoter strength of cellular gene-regulatory elements are often weak, and improvements in the efficacy of a vector often compromise its accuracy, and vice versa. Therefore, targeted expression of therapeutic genes will need more time to overcome all the limitations before clinical application will be an effective and successful addition to the therapeutic armamentarium.

Other Vector Systems

In addition to viral gene transfer systems, a number of groups are working on alternative vaccination approaches, including administration of vaccines via the mucosal and oral route. In this context, natural and synthetic polymers are particularly new vaccine delivery systems which are of great interest, since the polymeric delivery systems function as a platform to facilitate direct uptake into the gastrointestinal tract by phagocytic cells (microfold or M cells) and are capable of prolonging antigen presentation and stimulation by Peyer's patches. However, a number of problems need to be solved before effective vaccination strategies can work (reviewed in [44]). Furthermore, alternative approaches for gene therapy strategies exploit the fact that certain bacteria and viruses have high specificity for gastrointestinal epithelial cells. In particular, colonization of Peyer's patches would allow direct access to the underlying lymphatic follicles. Vectors which have been studied include *Salmonella typhi*, *S. typhimurium*, *Yersinia*, and Camille-Guérin bacillus (BCG). In addition, recombinant and attentuated avirulent strains of *Salmonella*, *Shigella*, *Listeria monocytogenes*, and BCG have been shown in several models to be safe and effective [38, 44, 45]. However, oral administration in order to induce systemic immunity is still in its infancy and must overcome a number of obstacles, such as safety of the proposed vector, preexisting immunity to the vector, and development of the appropriate formulations, in order to preserve the viability and immunogenicity of the vector.

Conclusion

Human malignant melanoma in the advanced stage leaves no hope of cure, since conventional therapies, including radiation and chemotherapy, do not alter the course of the disease. Identification of molecules and peptides recognized by cytotoxic T cells, in conjunction with a restricting HLA class I molecule and subsequent target cell killing as well as the emergence of somatic gene therapy as a new form of treatment, has fostered cautious optimism for a more effective melanoma treatment. However, as the first 5 years of somatic gene therapy have shown, the road towards making a significant clinical impact, particularly in cancer therapy, might still be a long one. Gene therapy has already come under harsh criticism [20] because the public's expectations could not be reach immediately and therefore more basic work was called for. Nevertheless, gene therapy is still a very new discipline and success cannot be measured easily [7]. In addition to a number of clinical gene therapy trials involving immunomodulatory approaches, a great deal of effort is being invested in the improvement of delivery systems, including the design of new viral vectors [24] designed to be safer and more efficient. As outlined above, various models are currently being tested in preclinical models and will enter the clinical scene in the next few years. Furthermore, combination approaches combining different gene therapeutic strategies will be evaluated in the near future. Recently, two preliminary abstracts reported on mouse cancer models which were treated with local cell killing via a suicide gene plus virus-mediated coexpression of IL-2 or granulocyte-macrophage colony-stimulating factor (GM-CSF), leading to increased tumor destruction and induction of systemic antitumor immunity (reviewed in [51]). The principal reason for combination gene therapy is the need to increase the effectiveness of any single method that is currently not sufficiently effective to meet therapeutic objectives. Other strategies may be based on advanced tumor immunologic understanding, including T cell activation, antigen presentation, and identification of more tumor antigens. In this context, the physiological role of dendritic cells as potent antigen-presenting cells in inducing systemic tumor immunity should be recognized and appreciated (reviewed in [22]). Based on this, autologous dendritic cells can be transduced with known tumor antigens such as the tyrosinase gene, leading to an appropriate intracellular proteolysis and subsequent presentation of peptides in the context of HLA molecules capable of activating T cell proliferation, as recently described [1].

Taken together, gene therapy is already a highly heterogeneous mixture of various treatment approaches based on precise molecular understanding. However, gene therapy is still in its infancy because in most cases, including malignant melanoma, technical improvements (e.g., delivery systems) are needed as a more advanced knowledge of molecular cascades underlying tumorigenesis, progression, and metastasis formation develops.

Summary

With the initiation of clinical gene therapy trials in 1990, a new era of cancer treatment began. Malignant melanoma has been a major target of such trials, because it is thought to be a tumor which is highly susceptible to immunologic modulation. At present, only very few results of clinical trials are available; however, it has become clear that vector systems and specific gene-targeting delivery systems need substantial improvement if they are to make a significant clinical impact. This chapter describes the recent developments in the gene therapy field, paying special attention to malignant melanoma. Furthermore, a short overview is provided of further genetic approaches used to modify melanoma cell behavior which are currently being worked on and which may appear in the clinic in the near future.

Acknowlegdement. D.S. is a Heisenberg Fellow of the Deutsche Forschungsgemeinschaft (DFG). Work in the laboratory (D.S.) was generously supported by the DFG, the Deutsche Krebshilfe - Dr. Mildred Scheel-Stiftung, and the Sandoz-Stiftung. The continuous support and encouragement of Prof. Beate M. Henz is highly appreciated.

References

1. Alijagic S, Möller P, Jurgovsky K, Czarnetzki BM, Schadendorf D (1995) Transfection of dendritic cells generated from peripheral blood with human tyrosinase induced specific T-cell activation. Eur J Immunol 25:3100–3107
2. Becker JC, Brabletz T, Czerny C, Termeer C, Bröcker EB (1993) Tumor escape mechanisms from immunosurveillance: induction of unresponsiveness in a specific MHC-restricted CD4+ human T cell clone by the autologous MHC class II+ melanoma. Int Immunol 5:1501–1508
3. Becker JC, Czerny C, Bröcker EB (1994) Maintenance of clonal anergy by endogenously produced IL-10. Int Immunol 6:1605–1612
4. Bystryn JC (1989) Immunosurveillance and melanoma. J Invest Dermatol 92:S318–320
5. Chen Q, Daniel V, Maher DW, Hersey P (1994) Production of IL-10 by melanoma cells: examination of its role in immunosuppression mediated by melanoma. Int J Cancer 56:755–760
6. Culver KW (1995) The June 1995 RAC meeting. Gene Ther Newslett 12:1–2
7. Culver KW (1996) Measuring success in clinical gene therapy research. Mol Med Today 6:234–236

8. Denfeld RW, Dietrich A, Wuttig C, Tanczos E, Weiss JM, Vanscheidt W, Schöpf E, Simon JC (1995) In situ expression of B7 and CD28 receptor families in human malignant melanoma: relevance for T-cell-mediated anti-tumor immunity. Int J Cancer 62:259–265
9. Descamps V, Duffour M-T, Mathieu MC, Fernandez N, Cordier L, Abina MA, Kremer E, Perricaudet M, Haddada H (1996) Strategies for cancer gene therapy using adenoviral vectors. J Mol Med 74:183–189
10. deWaal Malefyt R, Yssel H, de Vries JE (1993) Direct effects of IL-10 on subsets of human CD4+ T cell clones and resting T cells. Specific inhibition of IL-2 production and proliferation. J Immunol 150:4754–4765
11. Döhring C, Angman L, Spagnoli G, Lanzavecchia A (1994) T-helper- and accessory-cell-independent cytotoxic responses to human tumor cells transfected with a B7 retroviral vector. Int J Cancer 57:754–759
12. Donahue RE, Kessler SW, Bodine D, McDonagh K, Dunbar C, Goodman S, Agrcola B, Byrne E, Raffeld M, Moen R, Bacher J, Zsebo KM, Nienhuis AW (1992) Helper virus induced T cell lymphoma in nonhuman primates after retroviral mediated gene transfer. J Exp Med 176:1125–1135
13. Dummer R, Welters H, Keilholz U, Tilgen W, Burg G (1990) Interleukin 2: immunologischer Hintergrund und Anwendung in der Tumortherapie. Hautarzt 41:53–55
14. Dummer R, Schafer E, Eilles C, Borner W, Burg G (1991) Lymphokine-activated killer-cell traffic in metastatic melanoma. Lancet 338:456–457
15. Dummer R, Becker JC, Eilles C, Schafer E, Borner W, Burg G (1993) T cells migrate to tumour sites after extracorporeal interleukin 2 stimulation and reinfusion in a patient with metastatic melanoma. Br J Dermatol 128:399–403
16. Fenton RT, Sznol M, Luster DG, Taub DD, Longo DL (1995) A phase I trial of B7-transfected parental lethally irradiated allogeneic melanoma cell lines to induce cell-mediated immunity against tumor-associated antigen presented by HLA-A2 or HLA-A1 in patients with stage IV melanoma NCI protocol T93-0161 BRMP protocol 9401. Hum Gene Ther 6:87–106
17. Freeman GJ, Gray GS, Gimmi CD, Lombard DB, Zhou LJ, White M, Fingeroth JD, Gribben JG, Nadler LM (1991) Structure, expression, and T cell costimulatory activity of the murine homologue of the human B lymphocyte activation antigen B7. J Exp Med 174:625–631
18. Freeman GJ, Gribben JG, Boussiotis VA, Ng JW, Restivo VJ, Lombard LA, Gray GS, Nadler LM (1993) Cloning of B7-2: a CTLA-4 counter-receptor that costimulates human T cell proliferation. Science 262:909–911
19. Freeman GJ, Boussiotis VA, Anumanthan A, Bernstein GM, Ke XY, Rennert PD, Gray GS, Gribben JG, Nadler LM (1995) B7-1 and B7-2 do not deliver identical costimulatory signals, since B7-2 but not B7-1 preferentially costimulates the initial production of IL-4. Immunity 2:523–532
20. Friedmann T (1996) Human gene therapy – an immature genie, but certainly out of the bottle. Nature Med 2:144–147
21. Gilboa E, Lyerly HK (1994) Specific active immunotherapy of cancer using genetically modified tumor vaccines. Biol Ther Cancer Updates 4 (6):1–16
22. Grabbe S, Beissert S, Schwarz T, Granstein RD (1995) Dendritic cells as initiators of tumor immune responses: a possible strategy for immunotherapy? Immunol Today 16:117–121
23. Guinan EC, Gribben JG, Boussiotis VA, Freeman GJ, Nadler LM (1994) Pivotal role of the B7:CD28 pathway in transplantation tolerance and tumor immunity. Blood 84:3261–3282
24. Günzburg WH, Salmons B (1995) Virus vector design in gene therapy. Mol Med Today1:410–417
25. Hengge UR, Chan EF, Foster RA, Walker PS, Vogel JC (1995) Cytokine gene expression in epidermis with biological effects following injection of naked DNA. Nature Genet 10:161–166
26. Howard M, O' Garra A (1992) Biological properties of interleukin 10. Immunol Today 13: 198–200
27. Itaya T, Yamagiwa S, Okada F (1987) Xenogenization of a mouse lung carcinoma (3LL) by transfection with an allogeneic class I major histocompatibility complex gene (H-2L^d). Cancer Res 47:3136–3141
28. Lanzavecchia A (1993) Identifying strategies for immune intervention. Science 260:937–944

29. Ledley FD (1995) Nonviral gene therapy: the promise of genes as pharmaceutical products. Human Gene Ther 6:1129–1144
30. Li Y, McGowan P, Hellstrom I, Hellstrom KE, Chen L (1994) Costimulation of tumor-reactive CD4+ and CD8+ T34S lymphocytes by B7, a natural ligand for CD28, can be used to treat established mouse melanoma. J Immunol 153:421–428
31. Maeurer MJ, Storkus WJ, Kirkwood JM, Lotze MT (1996) New treatment options for patients with melanoma: review of melanoma-derived T-cell epitope-based peptide vaccines. Melanoma Res 6:11–24
32. Matsuda M, Salazar F, Petersson M, Masucci G, Hansson J, Pisa P, Zhang QJ, Masucci MG, Kiessling R (1994) Interleukin 10 pretreatment protects target cells from tumor- and allo-specific cytotoxic T cells and downregulates HLA class I expression. J Exp Med 180:2371–2376
33. Mattei S, Colombo MP, Melani C, Silvani A, Parmiani G, Herlyn M (1994) Expression of cytokine/growth factors and their receptors in human melanoma and melanocytes. Int J Cancer 56:853–857
34. Miller N, Vile R (1995) Targeted vectors for gene therapy. FASEB J 9:190–199
35. Mitchell MS (1996) Immunotherapy of melanoma. J Invest Dermatol Symp Proc 1:215–218
36. Nabel GJ, Nabel EG, Yang ZY, Fox BA, Plautz GE, Gao X, Huang I, Shu S, Gordon D, Chang AE (1993) Direct gene transfer with DNA liposome complexes in melanoma: expression, biologic activity, and lack of toxicity in humans. Proc Natl Acad Sci USA 90:11307–11311
37. Old LJ (1981) Cancer immunology: the search for specificity – GHA Clowes Memorial Lecture. Cancer Res 41:365
38. Pan Z-K, Ikonomidis G, Pardoll D, Paterson Y (1995) Regression of established tumors in mice mediated by the oral admnistration of a recombinant Listeria monocytogenes vaccine. Cancer Res 55:4776–4779
39. Pardoll DM, Beckerleg AM (1995) Exposing the immunology of naked DNA vaccines. Immunity 3:165–169
40. Parmiani G, Colombo MP (1995) Somatic gene therapy of human melanoma: preclinical studies and early clinical trials. Melanoma Res 5:295–301
41. Pockaj BA, Sherry RM, Wei JP, Yannelli JR, Carter CS, Leitman SF, Carasquillo JA, Steinberg SM, Rosenberg SA, Yang JC (1994) Localization of 111indium-labeled tumor infiltrating lymphocytes to tumor in patients receiving adoptive immunotherapy. Augmentation with cyclophosphamide and correlation with response. Cancer 73:1731–1737
42. Scanlon KJ, Ohta Y, Ishida H, Kijima H, Ohkawa T, Kaminski A, Tsai J, Horng G, Kashani-Sabet M (1995) Oligonucleotide-mediated modulation of mammalian gene expression. FASEB J 9:1288–1296
43. Schadendorf D (1997) Cytokines, autologous cell immunostimulatory and gene therapy for cancer treatment. In: Bos JD (ed) Skin immune system, 2nd edn. (in press)
44. Shalaby WSW (1995) Development of oral vaccines to stimulate mucosal and systemic immunity: barriers and novel strategies. Clin Immunol Immunopathol 74:127–134
45. Sizemore DR, Branstrom AA, Sadoff JC (1995) Attenuated Shigella as a DNA vehicle for DNA-mediated immunization. Science 270:299–302
46. Sule-Suso J, Arienti F, Melani C, Colombo MP, Parmiani G (1995) A B7-1-transfected human melanoma line stimulates proliferation and cytotoxicity of autologous and allogeneic lymphocytes. Eur J Immunol 2737–2742
47. Townsend SE, Allison JP (1993) Tumor rejection after direct costimulation of CD8+ T cells by B7-transfected melanoma cells. Science 259:368–370
48. Vile RG, Hart IR (1993) Use of tissue-specific expression of the herpes simplex virus thymidine kinase gene to inhibit growth of established murine melanomas following direct intratumoral injection of DNA. Cancer Res 53:3860 –3864
49. Viret C, Gervois N, Guilloux Y, Le Drean E, Diez E, Jotereau F (1995) T cell activation by antigens on human melanoma cells – co-stimulation by B7-1 is neither sufficient nor necessary to stimulate IL-2 secretion by melanoma-specific T cell clones in vitro. Int Immunol 7:1535–1543
50. Wagner RW (1994) Gene inhibition using antisense oligodeoxynucleotides. Nature 372:333–335
51. Zhang WW (1996) Antisense oncogene and tumor suppressor gene therapy of cancer. J Mol Med 74:191–204

Topical Immunotherapy of Malignant Melanoma

K. Zepter and A. Häffner

Introduction

Topical immunotherapy, the local application of biological response modifiers to lesional sites, has been a stable element within the ever-changing history of "immune-based" treatment approaches to human malignancies. Since the beginning of this comparatively new modality of disease management, reports of nonsystemically administered immunologically active agents made the news, rarely completely appreciated as "genuine" form of therapy, but nevertheless indisputably with their own indications and advantages.

Understandably, it was the dermatologists who took an early interest in the potential of local immunotherapy, as they were confronted with an exceptional situation of diseases often located within easy reach for epidermal, intra- or subcutaneous, and peri- or intralesional routes of drug administration.

With the era of understanding the skin as an immunologically active organ of crucial importance and its cellular components, mainly keratinocytes and dendritic cells, as particularly apt and specialized parts of our self-protecting machinery, topical, immune-based treatment options gained renewed attention as adjuvant – or even alternative – therapeutic pathways.

Although in a very comprehensive form of pharmacological perception, the vast majority of dermatological treatment schemes could be considered as "biologically immune modifications" with corticosteroids, e.g., suppressing leukocyte activities in a nonspecific manner, in the following chapter we will focus on nonsteroidal immune modifiers in the topical treatment of melanoma and non-melanoma skin cancer.

As for cutaneous malignancies, there is an array of reasons to opt for topical immunotherapy as an alternative treatment modality, provided that solitary, reachable, and sensitive tumors and lesions are to be dealt with.

In contrast to systemic application, in which – due to mostly unknown functional interactions – dosage and application intervals of immunologically active agents are determined solely on an empirical basis, the amount of intralesionally administered substance closely correlates with tissue levels achieved. However, for maximum performance, peak levels of active cytokines have to be sustained over sufficiently long periods of time, presenting pharmacokinetic problems still not entirely solved.

Whereas the elimination of bioactive immunotherapeutics given intraveneously has been extensively analyzed, few data exist regarding metabolic kinetics in infiltrated tissue. Koyama and Ishihara report 1% of initial levels for interferon (IFN)-α and about 10% for IFN-β after 24 h [1]. For other agents, such as dinitrochlorobenzene (DNCB) or IL-2, no valid data regarding intralesional concentration or pharmocokinetics have been published so far.

Nevertheless, regardless of the substance used, serum levels in topical treatment schemes routinely are low, thus reducing – although not completely eliminating – the risk of systemic side effects. Whereas almost all immunotherapy regimens using intravenous or intramuscular routes of application suffer from the offset of their beneficiary effects by sometimes severe and life-threatening adverse reactions, apart from intraventricular administration of IFN, no severe side effects in topical treatment schemes have been reported.

Local immunotherapy, therefore, offers itself as a feasible therapeutic alternative in those patients in which the general state of health, concurrent diseases, or failure of prior treatment regimens prohibits further attempts with systemic or surgical interventions. Furthermore, substantiated by several case reports, tumor regression could be achieved by intralesional application of cytokines in patients that failed to respond to systemic treatment modalities.

Moreover, production of antibodies to exogenous cytokines – best analyzed for IFN in systemic immunotherapies – which obviously presents a serious obstacle to immunotherapeutic efforts, is rarely observed after intralesional injection; of 1480 topically treated patients, only 0.2% developed neutralizing antibodies to IFN-α [2], whereas Steis et al. [3] report humoral responses with of up to 61% in patients receiving the same substance by i.v. or i.m. administration.

Recent studies by Balemans and Matijssen [4] added a further dimension to the potential of local immunotherapy; these authors were able to demonstrate that repeated intratumoral and perilymphatic administration of relatively low doses of polyethyleneglycol (PEG)-modified IL-2 in guinea pig hepatocarcinoma results in significant local tumor growth inhibition, a delay in development of regional lymph node metastases, and occasionally cure of tumor. In the latter animals, specific immunity against the syngeneic tumor developed, which could be transferred to naive animals by spleen cells. In a subsequent clinical study, patients with local and regional recurrences of head and neck squamous cell carcinoma (HNSCC) were treated with intratumoral injections of PEG IL-2, resulting in one complete response and stable disease in six patients. Although due to the small number of patients analyzed statistically valid conclusions are not extractable from these studies, topical immunotherapy might be of benefit for selected patient groups and certainly justifies further investigation.

State of the Art

The focus of the following sections is to review and discuss current knowledge about the major locally applied immunotherapeutics and to follow the historic evolution from early attempts using heat-inactivated bacteria to modern chemically modified recombinant cytokines.

Topical Application of Camille-Guérin Bacillus

Almost a quarter of a century ago, Nathanson reported [5] regression of an intradermally situated malignant melanoma after intralesional injection of *Mycobacterium bovis* strain Camille-Guérin bacillus (BCG). Several years later, he conducted a prospective study on 59 patients with metastatic melanoma predominantly localized in the skin, in which patients were randomly assigned to treatment with BCG given either intralesionally or by multiple puncture vaccination at a non-tumor-bearing site in the skin. Interestingly, a strong correlation between clinical symptoms of mycobacterial infection – experienced by half the patients with intralesional application, but only a few of those vaccinated at the distant site – and response rates regarding tumor regression was observed, reaching 45 % in the former compared to 9 % in the latter group [6].

In the early 1970s, intralesional injections of BCG were part of the therapeutic standard in the treatment of cutaneous melanoma lesions [7–9]. The effect of BCG was perceived as a nonspecific lymphocytic stimulus, substantiated by the fact that T cells of therapy responders displayed a marked increase in photohemagglutinin (PHA) mitogenicity assays [10], and systemic antitumoral activity leading to clearance of pulmonary metastases or other distant sites often followed cutaneous BCG injection [11, 12].

However, injection of live bacteria caused several fatal outcomes, preceded by high fevers, major clotting defects, hypotension, and anuria, suggesting that the mechanism was hypersensitivity to BCG [13] and prompting the development of attenuated vaccines, such as methanol extraction residues of BCG (MER). Of 22 patients with cutaneous melanoma metastases, intralesional injections of MER led to complete disappearance of all injected lesions in eight cases. The local reaction consisted of erythema and pustule formation followed by ulceration and tumor necrosis. Side effects included fever, chills, headache, and malaise in the majority of patients; nausea, vomiting, cyanosis, and hypotension occurred infrequently, but hypersensitivity reactions were not observed [14].

Numerous studies cover the utilization of native or fractionated BCG in patients with multiple dermal metastases over a period of more than 15 years [15–19]. Its remarkable success rate in this selective group of patients is exemplified by a case report published in 1981 [20] concerning a patient who, following wide surgical resection of a 1.3-mm-thick primary melanoma with satellite lesions, developed more than 50 dermal metastases. The patient was rendered free of disease over a 2-year period of intralesional injection of BCG, suggesting that aggressive intralesional immunotherapy may complement surgical resection in achieving successful palliation of patients with multiple primary melanomas. Corroborating these findings, a pooled analysis conducted by Tan et al. in 1993 [21] revealed beneficiary effects of intralesional BCG solely in stage III melanoma, primarily in patients with intracutaneous nonvisceral metastases, with complete responses averaging 19 %, partial responses 26 %, and extended survival in 3 % of patients.

Nevertheless, recurrent reports of fatal incidences after BCG vaccination – the most recent dating from 1991 [22–28] – in a period of nontoxic and promising new immunotherapeutics, vastly diminished the importance of intralesionally applied BCG; however, we may see another comeback.

Duda et al. recently genetically engineered BCG to actively express and secrete the cytokine IL-2. This recombinant BCG (rBCG 3A) has been tested as an intratumoral injection and a vaccine therapy in conjunction with irradiated tumor cells against melanoma in the murine B16 melanoma model. Tumor burdens were significantly smaller in the treatment groups with intratumoral and vaccine administration of therapy, and immunization with rBCG 3A and WT BCG 14 days before a B16 challenge resulted in an approximately 45 % smaller tumor burden when compared with controls [29].

Dinitrochlorobenzene-Induced Contact Dermatitis – The "Bystander" Effect

Perception of the intimate relationship between immunologic incompetence and an increased susceptibility to malignancies preceded various approaches to stimulate host defense mechanisms. Vaccinations (using bacterial antigens such as BCG) were performed to reactivate lymphocyte activities in a nonspecific manner, in the hope of "rebalancing" their self-protecting potential. Similarly, the rationale behind sensitization with dinitrochlorobenzene (DNCB) circumvents the obviously failing specific immunosurveillance prinicples in neoplastic development.

The use of DNCB is based on its capacity to elicit a vigorous toxic–allergic reaction, leading to significant inflammation at the chemically exposed site.

Rather than immunologically mediated via a distinct antigen recognition process, tumor cells are eradicated as "innocent bystanders" during necrosis occurring secondary to non-(tumor)-specific allergic and toxic contact dermatitis.

Evidently, critical determinants of tumor regression achievable with this kind of treatment are size, site, and depth of the projected lesions in relationship to their cutaneous surface. Bowen's disease, for example, which consists in superficially spreading squamous cell carcinomas, has been shown to respond particularly well to topical immunotherapy using DNCB as the sensitizing agent. In appropriate concentrations, the substance leads to selective destruction of neoplastic tissue in sensitized patients with neither clinical signs of cytotoxicity on adjacent normal skin nor systemic side effects [30].

A first approach using DNCB as a local immunostimulatory agent in a patient with acrolentiginous melanoma was reported by Malek-Mansour in 1973 [31]. Later, sporadic use of the sensitizer in addition to surgical intervention or – for orthopedic or age-related reasons – sometimes replacing surgery is described in several case reports during the following years [32].

In 1978, a prospective clinical study was conducted comparing 18 patients with multiple recurrences of malignant melanoma without evident distant spread. Patients were randomly assigned to treatment with either intralesional BCG or intralesional DNCB, and in the course of several treatment cycles, both agents were able to destroy approximately 90% of the injected intradermal nodules. As expected, intradermal tumors were more easily obliterated than subcutaneous lesions, and local control of satellites with elimination of all clinically evident tumor sites was achieved only in those patients who had intradermal without subcutaneous disease, regardless of whether BCG or DNCB had been administered. Although the clinical course in the two groups proved to be essentially the same, a profound difference in systemic toxicity was observed, making DNCB preferable to the bacterial mitogenic product [17].

Ten years later, another group of patients with malignant melanoma metastatic to the skin, subcutaneous tissue, or lymph nodes was treated with intralesionally applied DNCB. During the 20-month follow-up period, complete and partial remissions occurred in three out of 16 patients and one patient displayed stabilization of the disease. However, in the remaining 12, not even transient improvement was observed [33].

Because of its limited use in thick lesions, probably nonspecific mode of action, and minor contribution to enhanced survival, lesional application of DNCB has been more or less abandoned, although it may still be useful in selected cases, i.e., in very superficial tumors.

Interferons (IFN)

The IFN, a heterogenous group of proteins, owe their name to the phenomenon of "viral interference" first described in 1955 by Isaacs and Lindenmann [34]. Viral interference refers to the neosynthesis of a soluble protein by virus-infected cells that inhibits viral infection in cells previously incubated with this factor.

IFN are divided into three classes, IFN-α, IFN-β, and IFN-γ. Classification is based on criteria such as antigenicity, typical producers, typical inducers, and biochemical characteristics.

Natural IFN-α comprises a mixture of more than 15 proteins with a relative molecular mass of approximately 19 kDA that binds to the IFN type I receptor; IFN-β is a single molecule with a relative molecular mass of 24 kDa that also interacts with the type I receptor; and IFN-γ is a 45-kDa dimer that corresponds to the IFN type II receptor.

Interesting features of IFN in clinical oncology are their influence on cellular differentiation, their antiproliferative and tumoricidal properties, and their broad immunostimulatory function, affecting natural killer (NK) cell as well as macrophage activity and the expression of major histocompatibility complex (MHC) molecules, respectively.

Following their detection in the mid-1950s, IFN research and clinical use has been hampered for a long time by the limited availability of these substances. The situation did not improve until partially purified, nonrecombinant leukocyte IFN became available for clinical use in the late 1970s.

Consequently, first reports on the topical and systemic use of IFN in the treatment of malignant melanoma date back to that time.

In 1981, Ikic et al. [35] report the intralesional treatment of two patients with metastasizing melanoma. Using 2×10^6 IU natural IFN-α intralesionally seven times a week for 8 weeks and 10^6 IU intramuscularly three times a week, they achieved a complete response in one patient and a partial remission in the other.

Data have since become available from animal experiments demonstrating statistically significant growth-suppressive effects of IFN-β in melanomas (AM-1 and SK-14) transplanted on nude mice, resulting in complete regression of the tumors in three of eight mice carrying SK-14 [36]. Experiments conducted at a later point in the same system using recombinant IFN-α yielded response rates equal to those of human lymphoblastoid IFN-β (HLBI) [37].

Larger series of patients treated by intralesional application of IFN-α were reported by Flodgren et al. [38] (n=20) and Hill et al. [39] (n=32) in 1983. Applying $4–12\times10^6$ IU natural IFN-α two to five times a week, they observed a complete response in five out of 20 and three out of 32 patients, respectively. One out of 20 and three out of 32 patients showed partial responses.

Ishihara et al. [40] achieved partial responses to intralesional treatment with IFN-α in two out of six melanoma patients by injecting natural IFN-β; a complete response was observed in seven out of 41 patients, and 18 patients in this series showed a partial response.

With the exception of a series published by Slater et al. in 1984 [41], in which treatment with $3–6\times10^6$ IU IFN-α/m^2 on 5 days per week led to a complete response in five out of six patients, reported response rates for intralesional treatment with IFN-α range between 20 % and 30 %; the corresponding ratio for topical treatment with IFN-β was higher than 50 % on average.

Interestingly, von Wussow et al. [42], in a study published in 1988, observed not only complete or partial local responses in 23 out of 51 patients, but also a complete or partial systemic response in 18 % of all patients.

With regard to IFN-γ, clinial trials to date have found little evidence for an antitumor activity in the treatment of melanoma, and it has also failed to show significant additive effects in combination with IFN-α. Of 201 patients included in studies involving IFN-γ, only 5 % showed partial responses and 2 % achieved complete remission [42–51]. IFN-γ may, however, play a role in combined treatment strategies such as hyperthermic limb perfusion.

The local application of IFN has several advantages compared to systemic treatment modalities; first, in contrast to systemic treatment there is a direct dose–response correlation, and sufficiently high local concentrations to allow them to unfold their tumoricidal action can be produced; second, whereas systemic application of IFN induces flu-like symptoms and other more severe side effects in almost all patients treated, local application is generally less toxic and systemic IFN levels are low.

Major drawbacks of local IFN treatment are its limited use in disseminated disease and the fact that no controlled prospective randomized trials are available documenting a benefit for overall patient survival. In addition, IFN therapy is impeded by the as yet unpredictable phenomenon of IFN resistance and the formation of potentially blocking IFN antibodies.

Taken together, local IFN therapy, especially with IFN-β, provides a valuable additional treatment option in a setting in which surgical, radiotherapeutic, or chemotherapeutic strategies have failed, e.g., in the palliative treatment of large or widespread metastases in the face or extremities.

Tumor Necrosis Factor-α and Its Use in Combined Treatment Schemes

Tumor necrosis factor (TNF)-α, an extremely potent peptide cytokine, serves as an endogenous mediator of inflammatory, immune, and host defense mechanisms. It originally became known by virtue of two of its functions: (1) induction of cachexia when released in a systemically relevant dose and (2) induction of tissue necrosis when acting locally.

Mainly produced by monocytes and macrophages, it is synthesized as a prohormone of 233 amino acids and later by cleavage of 76 residues processed to the secreted, biologically active form.

While initial studies demonstrated promising cytotoxic effects in experimental cancers in animals, the use of TNF-α in clinical oncology is limited by its toxicity [52, 53]. Moreover, the results obtained in the treatment of metastatic melanoma have been disappointing so far. Feldman et al. [54] report treatment failure in 21 patients with metastasizing melanoma when using TNF-α, and the observed side effects were severe.

However TNF-α may play an important role in regional treatment regimens in which systemic side effects can be avoided. In this respect, the hyperthermic limb perfusion, in particular, using a cocktail of TNF-α, IFN-γ, and melphalan proved to be of substantial benefit in patients with disseminated in-transit metastasis of melanomas of the extremities. The complete remission rate induced by this kind of treatment is as high as 91% in malignant melanoma, as reported by Lienard et al. [55]. In irresectable soft tissue sarcoma, the respective limb can be saved from amputation in 87.5 % of cases. Regional application of high doses of TNF-α and IFN-γ in combination with a chemotherapeutic agent follows a strategy of dual targeting, which means a selective impact on the intratumoral vessels by TNF-α and on the tumor cells by chemotherapy. This approach appears to be the treatment of choice for locally advanced tumours of the limbs.

Interleukin-2

IL-2, a naturally occuring cytokine synthesized and secreted by activated T lymphocytes, exerts a pleiotropic effect on all other cellular components of the immune system, forming an immunomodulation geared towards increased cytotoxic activity.

Originally detected in the supernatant of lectin-activated T lymphocytes, it was thought to be a growth factor and mitogen for these cells, but in fact was soon found to exceed T cell-proliferative responses. Enhancing the differentiation and maturation of activated B cells and increasing both the cytotoxic activity of NK cells and the cytolytic potential of monocytes, its antineoplastic activity was first reported in 1985 by Rosenberg et al., who were able to demonstrate suppression of tumor growth and metastatic ability by concurrent administration of IL-2 and IL-2-activated lymphocytes (LAK) cells [56].

In the following years, adoptive immunotherapy with in vitro IL-2-activated, autologous peripheral or tumor-infiltrating lymphocytes and concomitant systemic application of high doses of IL-2 became an established form of therapy for metastatic malignant melanoma, achieving response rates of up to 25% evident as complete and partial tumor remissions [57].

Corroborating these clinical findings on a histological basis, changing cytokine milieus in lesional infiltrates of nontreated malignant melanoma were observed by Bröcker et al. [58], revealing an extensive loss of IL-2-expressing lymphocytes in infiltrated metastatic nodules, paralleled by decreased IL-2 receptors present in the tumor cell population.

When a few years later monotherapy with systemically administered IL-2 was found to be equally effective, adoptive immunotherapy with LAK or tumor-infiltrating lymphocytes was relinquished and the initial high-dose approach was changed – due to severe toxicity – to low or moderate dosages of $2–10\times10^6$ IU/m^2 per day, starting in 1986.

However, even in considerably reduced concentrations, systemically administered IL-2 coincides in a high percentage of cases with severe toxic reactions, including fever, chill, and nausea, a capillary leak syndrome with hypertension, renal toxicity, or edema, prompting early therapeutic attempts with intralesional injection.

In a pilot study by Gutwald et al. [59], two patients suffering from multiple cutaneous metastases of melanoma were treated with peritumoral injections of a total of 31×10^6 and 39×10^6 IU recombinant IL-2, respectively, in increasing concentrations in one metastasis in each patient. Histologically, almost complete necrosis of the tumor was induced, and in comparison with the control specimen, the T cell-rich infiltrate increased intratumorally and, in particular, peritumorally. While the ratio of T-helper to suppressor T cells remained unchanged, the proportions of NK cells, monocytes/macrophages, and IL-2 receptor-bearing cells increased in treated metastases. Apart from local erythema and swelling, no clinical side effects or laboratory changes were registered in this study [59].

In our hands, intralesional IL-2 as a single agent was successfully used in a patient with recurrent regional metastatic melanoma of the face: four cycles of intracutaneous injections of 9×10^6 IU four times a week at monthly intervals resulted in a complete remission of all regional satellites with a relapse-free survival of now over 12 months (Häffner and Zepter, unpublished communication).

Similarly, Kirkwood et al. [60, 61] consider the regional delivery of cytokines such as IL-2 as a very appropriate and as the least toxic approach, and an ongoing multicenter study includes intralesionally applied IL-2 in dosages of 10×10^6 IU/m^2 per day in combination with several cytostatic agents and IFN-α_{2a} [62].

To overcome the problem of relatively rapid IL-2 turnover in the infiltrated tissue – made responsible for the often short-lived remissions observed – conjugates of IL-2 with PEG have been generated and have provided promising results in topical application schemes.

In a syngeneic tumor model, repeated intratumoral and perilymphatic PEG-modified recombinant human IL-2 caused significant growth inhibition of both the primary tumor and the regional lymph node metastases at lower doses and with less frequent administration than rIL-2. The best schedule for PEG IL-2 was three injections a week for 5 weeks, resulting in cure in four out of 17 and five out of five (*p*.01) animals at the two most efficient dose levels tested. Subsequent experiments indicated that the intratumoral, and not the perilymphatic injection route was essential for the obtained antitumor effect, leading to specific immunity against the syngeneic tumor that was even transferable to naive mice by spleen cells [63, 64].

A initial clinical study performed on 19 patients with local and regional recurrences of head and neck cancer who received intratumoral injections of 200000 U PEG IL-2 three times weekly in courses of 4 weeks resulted in one complete response (6%; duration, 91 weeks) and stable disease in six patients (duration, 8 to 57 weeks), with local edema at the site of injection as the only side effect recorded [65].

In animal experiments, other combinations, such as microwave hyperthermia and local injection of IL-2 [66] or vaccination of melanoma-bearing mice with transfected BCG genetically engineered to actively express and secrete IL-2 [29], have been tested and shown to cause a significant reduction in tumor burden without clinical signs of cytokine-related systemic cytotoxicity. Usage of tissue-specific promoters, in the case of melanoma represented by the 5'-flanking region of the tyrosinase gene, might evolve as an additional molecular genetic approach to further potentiate local IL-2 efficacy without increased systemic injury [67].

In conclusion, topical IL-2, either delivered by genetically engineered cellular sources or as a modified conjugate with an extended half-life and low systemic cytotoxicity, may well continue to be a valuable asset in the repertoire of immunologically active agents for the treatment of recurrent primary or cutaneous metastatic malignant melanoma.

Discussion: Future Perspectives

Far from being able to cover the complete spectrum, the previous sections of this chapter show the range of attempts that researchers and physicians worldwide have made to develop immune-based topical treatment strategies for metastasizing melanoma.

Starting with nonspecific T cell-activating measures using bacterial antigens and contact sensitizers and extending to more refined treatment methods employing recombinant cytokines, highly sophisticated combination schemes (e.g., in hyperthermic limb perfusion) with scientifically proven and clinically significant benefits for patients have been developed. However, as our own experience shows, local therapy of otherwise untreatable melanoma metastases with something as simple as the intratumoral injection of IL-2 can be of substantial help in the palliative care of melanoma patients. In spite of all these accomplishments, it is obvious that a multitude of questions concerning basic tumor immunology remain to be solved. However, especially observations made in the local application of biological response modifiers may enable us to dissect the intricate network of tumor–host interactions that determines to a large degree the patient's fate. In contrast to the systemic administration of cytokines, local application of these signaling molecules generates a more defined and more physiological environment for their activity. The local and the systemic response we are going to observe is therefore more likely to illustrate the physiological tumor–host relationship. An additional step further towards a clearer definition of the microenvironment generated is being made using DNA vectors for tissue-specific expression of cytokine genes, and we await the results of these experiments with great interest.

Summary

For more than two decades, topical immunotherapy has been part of the treatment repertoire in metastasizing melanoma. However, especially in the current era of understanding the skin as an immunologically active organ, topical immune-based strategies have received renewed attention as additional therapeutical pathways. Starting from early attempts using bacterial extracts, topical immunotherapy now includes the local application of chemically modified recombinant cytokines or even genetically engineered vector constructs.

This chapter reviews current knowledge about the major locally applied immunotherapeutics, traces the development of these agents, and discusses future perspectives for the local immunotherapy of malignant melanoma.

References

1. Koyama Y (1983) Pharmacokinetics and clinical trials of HuIFN-b in malignant tumors. In: Kishida T (ed) Interferons. Kyoto, pp 185–195
2. Spiegel RJ, Spicehandler JR, Jacobs SL, Oden EM (1986) Low incidence of serum neutralizing factors in patients receiving recombinant alfa-2b interferon (Intron A). Am J Med 80:223–228
3. Steis RG, Smith JWd, Urba WJ, Clark JW, Itri LM, Evans LM, Schoenberger C, Longo DL (1988) Resistance to recombinant interferon alfa-2a in hairy-cell leukemia associated with neutralizing anti-interferon antibodies. N Engl J Med 318:1409–1413
4. Balemans LT, Mattijssen V, Steerenberg PA, Van Driel BE, De Mulder PH, Den Otter W (1993) Locoregional therapy with polyethylene-glycol-modified interleukin-2 of an intradermally growing hepatocellular carcinoma in the guinea pig induces T-cell-mediated antitumor activity. Cancer Immunol Immunother 37:7–14
5. Nathanson L (1972) Regression of intradermal malignant melanoma after intralesional injection of Mycobacterium bovis strain BCG. Cancer Chemother Rep 56:659–665
6. Nathanson L, Schoenfeld D, Regelson W, Colsky J, Mittelman A (1979) Prospective comparison of intralesional and multipuncture BCG in recurrent intradermal melanoma. Cancer 43:1630–1635
7. Bornstein RS, Mastrangelo MJ, Sulit H, Chee D, Yarbro JW, Prehn LM, Prehn RT (1973) Immunotherapy of melanoma with intralesional BCG. Natl Cancer Inst Monogr 39:213–220

8. Pinsky CM, Hirshaut Y, Oettgen HF (1973) Treatment of malignant melanoma by intratumoral injection of BCG. Natl Cancer Inst Monogr 39:225–228
9. Mastrangelo MJ, Kim YH, Bornstein RS, Chee DO, Sulit HL, Yarbro JW, Prehn RT (1974) Clinical and histologic correlation of melanoma regression after intralesional BCG therapy: a case report. J Natl Cancer Inst 52:19–24
10. Lieberman R, Wybran J, Epstein W (1975) The immunologic and histopathologic changes of BCG-mediated tumor regression in patients with malignant melanoma. Cancer 35:756–777
11. Mastrangelo MJ, Bellet RE, Berkelhammer J, Clark WH Jr (1975) Regression of pulmonary metastatic disease associated with intralesional BCG therapy of intracutaneous melanoma metastases. Cancer 36:1305–1308
12. Sopkova B, Kolar V (1976) Intralesional BCG application in malignant melanoma. Neoplasma 23:421–426
13. McKhann CF, Hendrickson CG, Spitler LE, Gunnarsson A, Banerjee D, Nelson WR (1975) Immunotherapy of melanoma with BCG: two fatalities following intralesional injection. Cancer 35:514–520
14. Krown SE, Hilal EY, Pinsky CM, Hirshaut Y, Wanebo HJ, Hansen JA, Huvos AG, Oettgen HF (1978) Intralesional injection of the methanol extraction residue of Bacillus Calmette-Guerin (MER) into cutaneous metastases of malignant melanoma. Cancer 42:2648–2660
15. Rosenberg SA, Rapp HJ (1976) Intralesional immunotherapy of melanoma with BCG. Med Clin North Am 60:419–430
16. El-Domeiri AA, Nika B, Hsia WC, Crispen R, Sabet TY, Gupta TK (1977) Effectiveness of systemic BCG therapy in advanced melanoma. Arch Surg 112:257–259
17. Cohen MH, Jessup JM, Felix EL, Weese JL, Herberman RB (1978) Intralesional treatment of recurrent metastatic cutaneous malignant melanoma: a randomized prospective study of intralesional Bacillus Calmette-Guerin versus intralesional dinitrochlorobenzene. Cancer 41:2456–2463
18. Lokich JJ, Garnick MB, Legg M (1979) Intralesional immune therapy: methanol extraction residue of BCG or purified protein derivative. Oncology 36:236–241
19. Bartal A, Cohen Y, Mekori T, Haasz R, Robinson E (1979) The effect of methanol extraction residue of BCG on the cellular immune response in patients with malignant melanoma. Med Pediatr Oncol 6:1–10
20. Unger SW, Wanebo HJ, Cooper PH (1981) Multiple cutaneous malignant melanomas with features of primary melanoma. Ann Surg 193:245–250
21. Tan JK, Ho VC (1993) Pooled analysis of the efficacy of bacille Calmette-Guerin (BCG) immunotherapy in malignant melanoma. J Dermatol Surg Oncol 19:985–990
22. Robinson JC (1977) Risks of BCG intralesional therapy: an experience with melanoma. J Surg Oncol 9:587–593
23. Felix EL, Jessup JM, Cohen MH (1978) Severe complications of intralesional BCG therapy in an unsensitized patient. Case report and clinical implications. Arch Surg 113:893–896
24. Voith MA, Lichtenfeld KM, Schimpff SC, Wiernik PH (1979) Systemic complications of MER immunotherapy of cancer: pulmonary granulomatosis and rash. Cancer 43:500–504
25. de la Monte SM, Hutchins GM (1986) Fatal disseminated bacillus Calmette-Guerin infection and arrested growth of cutaneous malignant melanoma following intralesional immunotherapy. Am J Dermatopathol 8:331–335
26. Hatzitheofilou C, Obenchain DF, Porter DD, Morton DL (1982) Granulomas in melanoma patients treated with BCG immunotherapy. Cancer 49:55–60
27. Shea CR, Imber MJ, Cropley TG, Cosimi AB, Sober AJ (1989) Granulomatous eruption after BCG vaccine immunotherapy for malignant melanoma. J Am Acad Dermatol 21:1119–1122
28. Cohen MH, Elin RJ, Cohen BJ (1991) Hypotension and disseminated intravascular coagulation following intralesional bacillus Calmette-Guerin therapy for locally metastatic melanoma. Cancer Immunol Immunother 32:315–324
29. Duda RB, Yang H, Dooley DD, Abu-Jawdeh G (1995) Recombinant BCG therapy suppresses melanoma tumor growth. Ann Surg Oncol 2:542–549
30. Raaf JH, Krown SE, Pinsky CM, Cunningham-Rundles W, Safai B, Oettgen HF (1976) Treatment of Bowen's disease with topical dinitrochlorobenzene and 5-fluorouracil. Cancer 37: 1633–1642

31. Malek-Mansour S (1973) Remission of melanoma with D.N.C.B. treatment. Lancet 2:503–504
32. Sigg C, Schnyder UW (1990) Successful immunotherapy by dinitrochlorobenzene in a case of recurrent acrolentiginous melanoma. Dermatologica 181(3):250–251
33. Budzanowska E, Pawlicki M (1988) An attempt at topical DNCB immunomodulation in advanced malignant melanoma. Tumori 74:519–522
34. Isaacs A, Lindenmann J (1957) Virus interference 1. The Interferon. Proc R Soc B 147:258
35. Ikic D, Brnobic A, Lipozencic J, Malecek J, Smerdel S, Delimar N, Soos E (1981) Topical application of human leukocyte interferon in stasis ulcers and deep burns. Int J Clin Pharmacol Ther Toxicol 19:450–452
36. Kohno M, Ida N, Nagao S, Tanaka N, Sekiguchi F, Uenishi N, Kajita A, Ogawa H (1982) Effects of human fibroblast interferon on human tumors transplanted into nude mice: sensitivity of human tumors to interferon. Gann 73:945–951
37. Hashizume S (1985) Antitumor effects of recombinant human leukocyte interferon (rIFN-alpha A) on human malignomas transplanted into nude mice (in Japanese). Gan To Kagaku Ryoho 12:284–288
38. Flodgren P, Borgstrom S, Jonsson PE, Lindstrom C, Sjogren HO (1983) Metastatic malignant melanoma: regression induced by combined treatment with interferon [HuIFN-alpha(Le)] and cimetidine. Int J Cancer 32:657–665
39. Hill NO, Pardue A, Khan A, Hill RW, Aleman C, Hilario R, Hill JM, Osther K (1983) Interferon and cimetidine for malignant melanoma (letter). N Engl J Med 308:286
40. Ishihara K (1983) Clinical studies of human fibroblast interferon in malignant tumors of the skin – with special reference to local administration. J Jap Soc Cancer Ther 18:41–53
41. Slater D, Krown S, Pinsky C (1984) Human leukocyte (a) interferon and cimetidine in malignant melanoma. Proc Am Soc Clin Oncol 3:54
42. von Wussow P, Block B, Hartmann F, Deicher H (1988) Intralesional interferon-alpha therapy in advanced malignant melanoma. Cancer 61:1071–1074
43. Foon KA, Sherwin SA, Abrams PG, Stevenson HC, Holmes P, Maluish AE, Oldham RK, Herberman RB (1985) A phase I trial of recombinant gamma interferon in patients with cancer. Cancer Immunol Immunother 20:193–197
44. Trautman T, Kirkwood J, Ernstoff M (1985) Phase I trial of recombinant interferon g (IFN g) by 2 or 24 hour infusion in 30 melanoma patients. Proc Am Soc Clin Oncol 4:232
45. Creagan ET, Ahmann DL, Long HJ, Frytak S, Sherwin SA, Chang MN (1987) Phase II study of recombinant interferon-gamma in patients with disseminated malignant melanoma. Cancer Treat Rep 71:843–844
46. Haase KD, Lange OF, Scheef W (1987) Interferon-gamma treatment of metastasized malignant melanoma. Anticancer Res 7:335–336
47. Wagstaff J, Smith D, Nelmes P, Loynds P, Crowther D (1987) A phase I study of recombinant interferon gamma administered by s.c. injection three times per week in patients with solid tumours. Cancer Immunol Immunother 25:54–58
48. Ernstoff MS, Trautman T, Davis CA, Reich SD, Witman P, Balser J, Rudnick S, Kirkwood JM (1987) A randomized phase I/II study of continuous versus intermittent intravenous interferon gamma in patients with metastatic melanoma. J Clin Oncol 5:1804–1810
49. Perez R, Lipton A, Harvey HA, Simmonds MA, Romano PJ, Imboden SL, Giudice G, Downing MR, Alton NK (1988) A phase I trial of recombinant human gamma interferon (IFN-gamma 4A) in patients with advanced malignancy. J Biol Response Mod 7:309–317
50. Landthaler M, Braun-Falco O (1989) Adjuvant therapy of high-risk malignant melanoma patients with gamma interferon. J Am Acad Dermatol 20:687–688
51. Mahrle G, Schulze HJ (1990) Recombinant interferon-gamma (rIFN-gamma) in dermatology. J Invest Dermatol 95:132S–137S
52. Taguchi T (1988) Phase I study of recombinant human tumor necrosis factor (rHu-TNF:PT-050). Cancer Detect Prev 12:561–572
53. Watanabe N, Niitsu Y, Neda H, Yamauchi N, Maeda M, Kuriyama H, Sone H (1988) Anti-tumor effect of human recombinant TNF (in Japanese). Gan To Kagaku Ryoho 15:780–787
54. Feldman E, Creagan E, Schaid D, Ahmann D (1992) Phase II trial of recombinant tumor necrosis factor in disseminated melanoma. Am J Clin Oncol 15:256–269

55. Lienard D, Eggermont AM, Schraffordt Koops H, Kroon BB, Rosenkaimer F, Autier P, Lejeune FJ (1994) Isolated perfusion of the limb with high-dose tumour necrosis factor-alpha (TNF-alpha), interferon-gamma (IFN-gamma) and melphalan for melanoma stage III. Results of a multi-centre pilot study. Melanoma Res 4:21–26
56. Barba D, Saris SC, Holder C, Rosenberg SA, Oldfield EH (1989) Intratumoral LAK cell and interleukin-2 therapy of human gliomas. J Neurosurg 70:175–182
57. Adler A, Stein JA, Kedar E, Naor D, Weiss DW (1984) Intralesional injection of interleukin-2-expanded autologous lymphocytes in melanoma and breast cancer patients: a pilot study. J Biol Response Mod 3:491–500
58. Brocker EB, Zwadlo G, Holzmann B, Macher E, Sorg C (1988) Inflammatory cell infiltrates in human melanoma at different stages of tumor progression. Int J Cancer 41:562–567
59. Gutwald J, Groth W, Mahrle G (1994) Peritumoral administered IL-2-induced tumor regression in melanoma. Pilot study (in German). Hautarzt 45:536–540
60. Kirkwood JM, Ernstoff MS (1990) Role of interferons in the therapy of melanoma. J Invest Dermatol 95:180S–184S
61. Lopez-Hänninen E, Fischer M, Mohr H, Dallmann I, Hadam M et al (1990) Low dose subcutaneous recombinant IL-2 in advanced human malignancies: a phase II outpatient study. Mol Biother 2:18–26
62. Atzpodien J, Kirchner H Sequential combined chemo-immunotherapy of metastatic malignant melanoma using interferon-alpha 2a, IL-2, BCNU, DTIC, cisplatin and tamoxifen (in preparation)
63. Mattijssen V, Balemans LT, Steerenberg PA, De Mulder PH (1992) Polyethylene-glycol-modified interleukin-2 is superior to interleukin-2 in locoregional immunotherapy of established guinea-pig tumors. Int J Cancer 51:812–817
64. Balemans LT, Steerenberg PA, Koppenhagen FJ, Kremer BH, De Mulder PH, Claessen AM, Scheper RJ, Den Otter W (1994) PEG-IL-2 therapy of advanced cancer in the guinea pig. Impact of the primary tumor and beneficial effect of cyclophosphamide. Int J Cancer 58:871–876
65. Mattijssen V, De Mulder PH, De Graeff A, Hupperets PS, Joosten F, Ruiter DJ, Bier H, Palmer PA, Van den Broek P (1994) Intratumoral PEG-interleukin-2 therapy in patients with locoregionally recurrent head and neck squamous-cell carcinoma. Ann Oncol 5:957–960
66. Nakayama J, Urabe A, Toyofuku K, Taniguchi S, Hori Y (1994) Suppression of murine melanoma growth with a combination of microwave hyperthermia and local injection of interleukin 2. Br J Dermatol 130:717–724
67. Vile RG, Hart IR (1994) Targeting of cytokine gene expression to malignant melanoma cells using tissue specific promoter sequences. Ann Oncol 5:59–65

Vaccination with Dendritic Cells – A Specific Immunomodulatory Approach for the Treatment of Malignant Melanoma

D. Schadendorf, S. Grabbe, and F. O. Nestle

Introduction

Malignant melanoma is a tumor with worldwide rising incidence. Typical features are aggressive biological behavior and resistance to most of the currently known therapies. During the last few years, intensive research on the immunology of malignant melanoma has identified cytotoxic T lymphocytes (CTL) as important effector cells in antimelanoma-specific immune responses. CTL attack melanoma cells in a major histocompatibility complex (MHC)-restricted and tumor antigen-specific manner. Some of these tumor antigens have been recently identified. Based on the exact knowledge of the antigen fragments (peptides) which are associated with certain MHC molecules, peptide vaccination seems to be a promising approach for treatment of malignant melanoma. The current problem is that vaccination strategies to induce a sufficiently peptide-specific immune response in a host which is probably already immunosuppressed are not available. Dendritic cells (DC) are of hematopoietic origin and are present in trace amounts at body sites of antigen entry, such as the skin, gut, and lung as well as professional lymphoid organs. They have been called "nature's adjuvant", since they are specialized in the induction and amplification of primary immune responses. Several in vitro and in vivo models have demonstrated the extraordinary capacity of DC to induce tumor antigen-specific immune responses. This has also opened up the possibility of evaluating the powerful antigen-presenting capacity of dendritic cells to induce an antitumor-specific immune response in initial clinical pilot studies.

State of the Art

Phenotype and Function of Dendritic Cells

Cells that are located in the T cell-dependent region of the lymph node and that form a characteristic pattern with cytoplasmic membrane processes using classic silver impregnation techniques have long been known as interdigitating DC. However, it was only after Steinman et al. demonstrated an accessory role for a putative in vitro DC analogue that immunological research began to focus on these cells. DC were subsequently shown [58, 62] to belong to a family of potent antigen-presenting cells (APC) which are located at the zones of foreign antigen entry into the human body. These interface regions include the skin, gut, and lung and the T cell-dependent area of primary lymphoid organs such as the lymph node or the spleen [57]. Because of their strategic location, DC have been proposed to subserve the role of a sentinel cell that is able to induce an adaptive immune response after contact with "dangerous" microbes, tumor cells or tissue injury [38]. The DC is able to transform a peripheral danger signal into a message which can be read by the effector lymphocytes circulating in the professional lymphoid organs. In other words, after contact with foreign antigens, DC bind and process the antigen, move to the adjacent lymph nodes, and present the respective antigenic peptide in the context of MHC class II molecules to naive T lymphocytes, which bear the appropriate T cell receptor.

Four major qualities characterize a DC as an outstanding APC: (1) a cell surface which is specialized for antigen presentation, (2) a highly evolved antigen-capturing and -processing machinery, (3) unique migratory functions, and (4) potent induction of primary MHC class I and II immune responses in vitro and in vivo.

Cell Surface Specialized for Antigen Presentation

A T cell is dependent on three major signals to be activated by an APC: (1) the presentation of the relevant peptide in the groove of an MHC molecule (signal 1), (2) a so-called costimulatory signal (signal 2), and (3) an adhesion signal for efficient T cell clustering. While monocytes have only low levels of MHC class II molecules on their surface, DC express high levels of MHC class II, including HLA-DP and HLA-DQ [32]. DC also express high levels of adhesion molecules, such as intercellular adhesion molecule (ICAM)-1 (CD54), lymphocyte function-associated antigen (LFA)-3 (CD58), and the β_1-integrin (CD29) for effective T cell clustering [18]. Presentation of an antigen (e.g., a tumor antigen) in the absence of a costimulatory signal can lead to unresponsiveness of the T cell which can be long-lasting [12]. Several surface molecules have been shown to be involved in costimulation. The B7 family of surface molecules is among the most important costimulatory molecules [30]. In contrast to monocytes, DC have been shown to express constitutively high levels of this costimulatory molecule [40, 60].

Highly Evolved Antigen-Capturing and -Processing Machinery

DC are not very active in Fcg receptor (FcgR)-mediated phagocytosis, which is consistent with the missing expression of FcgR type I and III [57]. Instead, they have been demonstrated to use two different mechanisms of antigen capture [53]. The first is a high level of constitutive fluid-phase uptake via macropinocytosis. It has been calculated that the DC is able to take up in 1 h a fluid volume that is close to its own volume. The second mechanism of capture is mediated via the mannose receptor in humans [53] and a receptor called DEC-205 in the mouse [29]. There is also a higher level of invariant chain and MHC class II biosynthesis in freshly isolated DC than in other APC [47] and abundant presence of specialized processing compartments for antigen presentation, so-called MHC [42].

Unique Migratory Functions

A prerequisite of an effective immune response is carrying antigen (e.g., tumor antigen) from the periphery into primary lymphoid organs. DC have repeatedly been shown in vitro and in vivo to be the only cell type of the immune system to fulfil this criterium [3, 34]. The factors that stimulate and direct the movement of DC are not clear yet, although certain cytokines or adhesion molecules have been implicated in this process.

Potent Induction of Primary Immune Responses

To raise an effective immune response against a neoantigen or self-antigen (e.g., a tumor antigen), an APC must be able to activate quiescent, naive T cells. Once sensitized, T lymphoblasts readily react to antigenic stimuli. DC have been shown to be the most potent cell for induction of primary immune responses in vitro and in vivo [57, 59]. DC are effective in the induction of a primary T cell response to protein antigens [28], CTL responses to viruses [31], and induction of primary antitumor immune responses (see below).

All the above-mentioned features would make DC an ideal candidate for the generation of a primary immune response in a vaccination setting, e.g., for the induction of antitumor immunity. Unfortunately, one major problem has been the generation of sufficient DC for immunotherapy. Recently, several groups developed techniques to expand sufficient numbers of DC from precursors present in human cord blood, bone marrow, and peripheral blood [9, 49, 52]. This has opened the new possiblility not only of studying DC physiology, but also of using these cells for vaccination in human diseases in which the target of vaccination is well defined (e.g., tumor antigens in melanoma; see below).

Role of Dendritic Cells in Tumor Immunology

Number and Morphology of Dendritic Cells Within Tumors

In a traditional approach to evaluate the role of dendritic APC in tumor immunity, several investigators determined the number and morphology of DC within tumors or in their vicinity. Clinical studies revealed altered numbers and morphology of Langerhans cells (LC) in the vicinity of epithelial malignancies and suggest a correlation between the number of tumor-infiltrating APC and clinical prognosis [5, 50]. Interestingly, most, if not all agents with a known carcinogenic effect on cutaneous tissue also affect the morphology and function of epidermal LC [51]. In rats, tumor-infiltrating DC express high levels of MHC class I and II, CD45, CD11a, and ICAM-1, but relatively low amounts of B7-1. Moreover, a subpopulation of these cells also expressed the CD8 molecule [11]. A series of investigations performed by Halliday et al. [25] indicates that LC migrate into cutaneous neoplasms, possibly due to chemotactic effects of a tumor-derived cytokine. However, no correlation between LC number within cutaneous tumors and type or degree of tumor immunity was found in this tumor system [24]. To address the role of epidermal APC in tumor immunity, initial studies showed that during the latent period of ultraviolet (UV) carcinogenesis, the number of identifiable epidermal LC decreased early in the course of chronic UV irradiation carcinogenesis, correlating with a decrease in antigen-presenting activity after sensitization in the UV-irradiated skin [1]. Thus morphological data favor a role for DC in tumor immunity, but provide no direct evidence for a role of DC in tumor immunosurveillance.

Presentation of Tumor Antigens by Murine Dendritic Epidermal Langerhans Cells and Splenic Dendritic Cells

About 10 years ago, experimental evidence for the capacity of dendritic APC to present tumor-associated antigen (TAA) came from the finding that splenic APC can bind tumor antigens in tumor-bearing mice [55] and that DC are indeed capable of presenting tumor antigens for the generation of specific tumor immunity. In this regard, Knight et al. [33] found that normal splenic DC induce immunity against a methylcholanthrene-induced tumor and that i.v. administration of DC also led to regression of established tumors [33]. Shimizu and coworkers later showed that splenic adherent cells were able to present tumor antigens for induction of tumor immunity in vivo. These authors found that APC remain functional in tumor-bearing mice despite the apparent downregulation of tumor immunity during late stages of tumor progression, but other investigators found both impaired and increased APC activity in tumor-bearing animals [55, 63, 65]. Recently, Nestle and coworkers demonstrated for the first time in humans that tumor-associated DC are deficient in costimulatory molecules and impaired as APC. This has been shown to be mediated by paracrine secretion of interleukin (IL)-10 by the tumor cells and is one possible mechanism to escape immune surveillance [41]. Grabbe et al. [20] addressed the question of whether epidermal LC are able to present TAA in both unprimed and primed systems in vivo. When injected into naive syngeneic mice, TAA-pulsed LC were found to be potently capable of inducing protective tumor immunity, provided that they were incubated in granulocyte-macrophage colony-stimulating factor (GM-CSF) prior to TAA pulse [20]. Likewise, LC were also readily able to present TAA in primed, tumor-immune mice for elicitation of TAA-specific delayed-type hypersensitivity [20]. Finally, Flamand et al. [17] showed that DC induce a protective humoral immune response against a murine plasmacytoma, and Cohen et al. [13] demonstrated that LC induce tumor-specific CTL responses in vitro, further supporting the concept that DC are capable of presenting tumor antigen to primed tumor-specific T cells.

Moreover, LC presentation of TAA was found to be greatly affected by various cytokines. For example, IL-1α, interferon (IFN)-γ, IL-10, and – in certain situations – also tumor necrosis factor (TNF)-α were able to downregulate tumor antigen presentation by epidermal LC, whereas GM-CSF stimulated this capacity [6, 21–23, 61]. Interestingly, the effects of cytokines on the presentation of TAA by LC differed significantly when investigated in unprimed or in primed systems, suggesting that the mechanisms that regulate sensitization of an individual against TAA (activation of naive T cells) differ from those during the actual tumor rejection process (activation of sensitized T cells). Other investigators addressed the question of how cytokines regulate tumor immunity by local application of cytokines at tumor sites or by transfection of cytokine genes into tumor cells. Cytokine-induced tumor rejection may also be mediated via APC. For example, it was hypothesized that the antitumor effects of IL-4 (after local injection or transfection of tumor cells) are mediated via recruitment of APC [8]. Indirect evidence suggests that also in the case of IL-2- or IFN-γ-transfected tumor cells, the generation of tumor immunity is mediated by host APC [4]. In an important study, Dranoff et al. [15] transfected several tumor lines with a whole panel of cytokine genes and assessed their effects on both tumorigenicity and induction of tumor immunity. In this system, specific immunity against the wild-type tumor was observed after cotransfection of tumor cells with IL-2 and GM-CSF or after sublethal X-irradiation of tumor cells transfected with GM-CSF alone. These data indicate that, for in vivo induction of tumor immunity, at least two conditions have to be fulfilled: (1) in vivo tumor cell destruction (generated by IL-2 transfection or X-irradiation) and (2) stimulation of APC function in situ (induced by GM-CSF transfection). In another approach, GM-CSF was administered in vivo using biodegradable microspheres mixed with tumor cells, which again led to induction of tumor-specific immunity [19]. It is likely that this effect of GM-CSF is due to its stimulatory activity on the capacity of dendritic cells to present antigen. Finally, the successful generation of tumor immunity by transfection of costimulatory molecules may also involve APC. By comparing tumor immunity induced by B7-transfected, MHC class I^+ and B7-transfected, MHC class I^- tumor cells, Huang et al. [26] demonstrated that bone marrow-derived APC, and not the transfected tumor cells themselves are the relevant APC for MHC class I-restricted tumor immunity.

Presentation of Tumor Antigens by Ex Vivo-Generated Murine Dendritic Cells

For many years, the question of whether DC are involved in tumor immunity remained academic, since no method was available to generate or isolate sufficient numbers of DC required for tumor immunotherapy. In recent years, however, this situation has changed dramatically, mostly by the finding that large numbers of functionally active DC can be obtained by culture of bone marrow or peripheral blood cells in the presence of GM-CSF and/or other cytokines, such as IL-4, TNF, and stem cell factor (SCF) ligand (for a review, see [45]). Thus a number of studies recently addressed the question of whether these ex vivo-generated DC are also capable of presenting TAA [10, 39, 43, 46, 64]. An excellent study by Mayordomo et al. [39] revealed that DC generated by culture of murine bone marrow in the presence of GM-CSF and IL-4 were indeed potently able to immunize naive mice against subsequent tumor growth as well as to induce regression of already established tumors in syngeneic mice. Moreover, several studies recently demonstrated that tumor immunity induced by DC is not restricted to the "exogenous" MHC class II pathway, but that TAA-pulsed DC also induce CTL-dependent tumor immune responses, mediated by the "endogenous" MHC class I pathway [13, 43, 46, 64].

Melanoma-Associated Tumor Antigens Defined by Cytolytic T Lymphocytes

In order to use DC for vaccination approaches in the therapy of melanoma patients, a number of limitations need to be overcome. The molecular identification and characterization of melanoma-associated tumor antigens is crucial to be able to stimulate a specific antimelanoma immune response. However, the extensive search for tumor-specific melanoma-associated antigens in the last two decades using serological reagents and monoclonal antibodies turned out not to be sucessful in most instances, since antigens detected were not tumor specific. In recent years, it has become increasingly clear that T lymphocytes may play a critical role in antitumor immune responses and surveillance [16]. It is believed that regressions of primary tumors or metastases are caused by the host's immune response to melanoma-associated antigens, which is supported by the following three observations: (1) the magnitude of lymphocytic tumor

Table 1. Melanoma-associated antigens recognized by cytolytic T lymphocytes (CTL)

Target antigen	Restricting HLA molecule	Peptides recognized	Tissue distribution
MAGE-1	HLA-A1 HLA-Cq16	EADPTGJSY SAYGEPRKL	Antigens detected in melanoma and other cancers, but not in normal cells except testis.
MAGE-3	HLA-A1 HLA-A2 HLA-B44	EVDPIGHLY FLWGPRALV MEVDPIGHLY	
BAGE	HLA-Cw16	AARAVFLAL	
GAGE	HLA-Cw6		
pMel-34/Tyrosinase	HLA-A2 HLA-A24, -B44 and HLA-class II HLA-A1	YMNGTMSQV MLLAVLYCL KCDICTDEY	Differenttiation antigens expressed exclusively in melanocytic cells
TRP-1/gp75 TRP-2	HLA-A31 HLA-A31	MSLQRQFLR LLGPGTPYR	
pMel-17/gp100	HLA-A2 HLA-A24 HLA-A3	VLYRYGSFSV KTWGQYWQV YLEPGPVTA LLDGTATLRL VYFFLPDHL ALLAVGATK	
Melan-A/MART-1	HLA-A2	ILTVILGVL AAGIGILTVL GIGILTVL GILTVILGV ALMDKSLHV	
PRAME	HLA-A24	LYVDSLFFL	
N-Acetylglucos aminyl-Transferase V	HLA-A2	VLPDVFIRC	Located in intron sequence expressed in various cell types
p15	HLA-A24	AYGLDFYIL	
β-catenin	HLA-A24	SYLDSGIH*F*	*mutated* genes generating unique T cell epitopes
SR-2	HLA-A3	KIFSEVT*L*K	
MUM-1	HLA-B44	EEKL*I*VVLF	
CDK4	HLA-A2.1	ACDPHSGHFV	

infiltration is an important prognostic parameter [56], (2) tumor-infiltrating lymphocytes can be isolated from regressing melanoma lesions which showed T cell receptor oligoclonality [35, 54], and finally (3) T lymphocytes derived from melanoma lesions or the peripheral blood are capable of mediating impressive tumor regressions in vivo [48].

Since 1991, pioneering work by Boon and coworkers has led to the identification of several tumor antigens presented by MHC class I molecules required for tumor-specific cytolysis by CTL. The availability and further characterization in recent years of such tumor-specific T cell clones led to the identification of several tumor antigens. Both the *genetic approach*, as done by Boon and coworkers (reviewed in [7]) by transfection of cDNA libraries of tumor cells in HLA-matched recipient cells and subsequent analysis by specific CTL clones, and the *peptide elution approach,* based on the elution of HLA-bound peptides by acid treatment and subsequent analysis by mass spectrometry [14], were successful in identifying melanoma-associated antigens. Subsequently, these tumor antigens in human melanoma were shown to fall into three different classes (Table 1), including melanosomal differentiation antigens (e.g., tyrosinase, gp100, tyrosinase-related protein, TRP-1, MelanA/melanoma antigen recognized by T cells, MART-1), mutated antigens (CDK4, β-catenin), and silent antigens which are not expressed in normal cells but on malignant cells (MAGE, BAGE, GAGE) (reviewed in [36]). Fragments of these antigens are presented as peptides by distinct MHC molecules, to be recognized by either MHC class I-restricted $CD8^+$ T cells or MHC class II-restricted $CD4^+$ T cells. Therapeutic strategies based on these new findings were designed using these antigens in an appropriate form for antimelanoma vaccination.

Dendritic Cell Vaccination for Melanoma Patients

Several clinical phase I trials have been initiated or are being planed that utilize selected peptides for immunization. A preliminary report using MAGE peptides for vaccination with some clinical responses have recently been published [37]. In experimental settings, additional approaches are under investigation, including the injection of naked DNA encoding genetic information for a tumor antigen under the gene-regulatory control of a strong eukaryotic promoter (e.g., cytomegalovirus-derived) into muscle. Subsequent expression of this protein leads to a systemic T and B lymphocyte activation with antibody production and CTL generation. In addition, immunization protocols are being developed, including the optimization of adjuvants, vaccination schedules, and routes.

DC are well characterized, highly potent APC that are specialized in the induction and amplification of primary immune responses. From animal tumor models it is known that tumor immunotherapy with DC is both possible and highly effective and that DC are capable of inducing both CD4- and CD8-mediated tumor immunity. It is as yet far too early to predict whether DC vaccination is successful in tumor treatment in the clinical situation. Only one report on the IV infusion of in vitro-generated DC in lymphoma patients has been published, with three out of four showing some clinical responsiveness [27]. Currently protocols for the vaccination of patients with metastatic melanoma using autologous dendritic cells as stimulators and HLA-restricted melanoma peptides as antigens are ongoing, including a cooperative study between Münster, Zurich, and Berlin. In contrast to the published report by Hsu and coworkers, this clinical pilot study utilizes a mixture of peptides (see Table 1) for pulsing depending on the HLA type of the patient and a weekly immunization schedule. Initial clinical and immunological results can be expected in the summer of 1997. Intense investigations are underway to define the conditions that optimize the efficacy of this therapeutic approach, including the transfection of DC with cytokine genes in order to improve the immunostimulatory potential or intrinsic functions of DC as well as the transfection of known melanoma-associated tumor antigens into DC. Recently, the transfection of the tyrosinase gene into in vitro-generated DC led to the appropriate intracellular proteolysis and presentation of antigenic peptides at the cell surface to stimulate a specific T cell response [2]. Although transfection efficacy of DC needs to be improved, transfection with tumor antigens, in particular, allows immunization independent of the HLA type of the patient, in contrast to the restricted use of peptide vaccinations. A further advantage of a DC-based vaccine is the fact that it is independent of (autologous) tumor cells, thus allowing the immunization of melanoma patients with high-risk primary tumors or after lymph node dissection where it is usually difficult to obtain sufficient numbers of autologous tumor cells to grow and prepare tumor cell-based vaccines. Since it is believed that most of the indirect tumor immunological vaccination strategies, including naked DNA and cytokine gene transfer into tumor cells, are dependent on DC [44], direct use as shown in the present chapter should be the most powerful and effective strategy to modulate the host's immune response in favor of the patient and against melanoma. Whether this approach is powerful enough to cure melanoma patients awaits further in vitro and in vivo studies.

Summary

Human melanoma is the main cause of death in patients with skin cancer. Melanoma cells are characterized by a high resistance to any kind of treatment in vitro and in vivo. The underlying mechanisms have not been well studied and are not known. However, several well-known clinical observations, such as regression phenomena of primary tumors and metastases as well as the development of metastases after more than 10 years of latency, have suggested a strong immunological modulation of the natural course of the disease. Human melanoma is now the prototype of an immunogenic tumor in which several tumor antigens are molecularly well defined. Nevertheless, the options based on these new findings to alter the course of the disease, e.g., to prolong the time to first metastases and overall survival time by new therapeutic approaches, have not yet led to any cure or any major therapeutic breakthrough. Fast advances in our immunological understanding and the increasing number of precisely characterized melanoma antigens may open up the way for effective immunological vaccination protocols.

Acknowlegdement. This work was generously supported by grants to D.S. from the Deutsche Forschungsgemeinschaft (DFG), Deutsche Krebshilfe/Dr. Mildred Scheel-Stiftung, and the Sandoz-Stiftung für therapeutische Forschung. Furthermore, grants from the Cancer League Zürich and the Swiss Cancer League to F.O.N. are gratefully acknowledged.

References

1. Alcalay J, Kripke ML (1991) Antigen-presenting activity of draining lymph node cells from mice painted with a contact allergen during ultraviolet carcinogenesis. J Immunol 146: 1717–1721
2. Alijagic S, Möller P, Artuc M, Jurgovsky K, Czarnetzki BM, Schadendorf D (1995) Dendritic cells generated from peripheral blood transfected with human tyrosinase induce specific T cell activation. Eur J Immunol 25:3100–3107
3. Austyn JM, Kupiec-Weglinski JW, Hankins DF, Morris PJ (1988) Migration pattern of dendritic cells in the mouse. Homing to T cell-dependent areas of the spleen, and binding within marginal zone. J Exp Med 167:646–651
4. Bannerji R, Arroyo CD, Cordon-Cardo C, Gilboa E (1994) The role of IL-2 secreted from genetically modified tumor cells in the establishment of antitumor immunity. J Immunol 152:2324–2332

5. Becker Y (1993) Anticancer activity of dendritic cells. Symposium proceedings of the 4th international conference of anticancer research. Crete. In Vivo 7:185–313
6. Beissert S, Hosoi J, Grabbe S, Asahina A, Granstein RD (1995) IL-10 inhibits tumor antigen presentation by epidermal antigen-presenting cells. J Immunol 154:1280–1286
7. Boon T, Gajewski TF, Coulie PG (1995) From defined human tumor antigens to effective immunization. Immunol Today 16:334–336
8. Bosco M, Giovarelli M, Forni M et al (1990) Low doses of IL-4 injected perilymphatically in tumor-bearing mice inhibit the growth of poorly and apparently nonimmunogenic tumors and induce a tumor-specific immune memory. J Immunol 145:3136–3143
9. Caux C, Dezutter-Dambuyant C, Schmitt D, Banchereau J (1992) GM-CSF and TNF- cooperate in the generation of dendritic Langerhans cells. Nature 360:258–261
10. Celluzzi C, Mayordomo JI, Storkus WJ, Lotze MT, Falo LD (1996) Peptide-pulsed dendritic cells induce antigen-specific, CTL-mediated protective tumor immunity. J Exp Med 183:283–287
11. Chaux P, Hammann A, Martin F, Martin M (1993) Surface phenotype and functions of tumor-infiltrating dendritic cells: CD8 expression by a cell subpopulation. Eur J Immunol 23:2517–2525
12. Chen L, Linsley PS, Hellstrøm KE (1993) Costimulation of T cells for tumor immunity. Immunol Today 14:483–486
13. Cohen PJ, Cohen PA, Rosenberg SA, Katz SI, Mule JJ (1994) Murine epidermal Langerhans cells and splenic dendritic cells present tumor-associated antigens to primed T cells. Eur J Immunol 24:315–319
14. Cox AL, Skipper J, Chen Y, Henderson RA, Darrow TL, Shabanowitz, Engelhard VH, Hunt DF, Slingluff CL (1994) Identification of a peptide recognized by five melanoma-specific human cytotoxic T-cell lines. Science 264:716–719
15. Dranoff G, Jaffee E, Lazenby A et al (1993) Vaccination with irradiated tumor cells engineered to secrete murine granulocyte-macrophage colony-stimulating factor stimulates potent, specific, and long-lasting anti-tumor immunity. Proc Natl Acad Sci USA 90:3539–3543
16. Ferrone S (1994) Melanoma, immune surveillance, and immuntherapy. J Clin Invest 93: 1352–1352
17. Flamand V, Sornasse T, Thielemans K et al (1994) Murine dendritic cells pulsed in vitro with tumor antigen induce tumor resistance in vivo. Eur J Immunol 24:605–610
18. Freudenthal PS, Steinman RM (1990) The distinct surface of human blood dendritic cells, as observed after an improved isolation method. Proc Natl Acad Sci USA 87:7698–7702
19. Golumbek PT, Azhari R, Jaffee EM et al (1993) Controlled release, biodegradable cytokine depots: a new approach in cancer vaccine design. Cancer Res 53:5841–5844
20. Grabbe S, Bruvers S, Gallo RL, Knisely TL, Nazareno R, Granstein RD (1991) Tumor antigen presentation by murine epidermal cells. J Immunol 146:3656–3661
21. Grabbe S, Bruvers S, Granstein RD (1992) Effects of immunomodulatory cytokines on the presentation of tumor-associated antigens by epidermal Langerhans cells. J Invest Dermatol 99:66s–68s
22. Grabbe S, Bruvers S, Lindgren AM, Hosoi J, Tan KC, Granstein RD (1992) Tumor antigen presentation by epidermal antigen-presenting cells in the mouse: modulation by granulocyte-macrophage colony stimulating factor, tumor necrosis factor a, and ultraviolet radiation. J Leukoc Biol 52:209–217
23. Grabbe S, Beissert S, Schwarz T, Granstein RD (1995) Dendritic cells as initiators of tumor immune responses – a possible strategy for tumor immunotherapy? Immunol Today 16: 117–121
24. Halliday GM, Reeve VE, Barnetson RSC (1991) Langerhans cell migration into ultraviolet light-induced squamous skin tumors is unrelated to anti-tumor immunity. J Invest Dermatol 97:830–834
25. Halliday GM, Lucas AD, Barnetson RSC (1992) Control of Langerhans' cell density by a skin tumour-derived cytokine. Immunology 77:13–18
26. Huang AY, Golumbek P, Ahmadzadeh M, Jaffee E, Pardoll D, Levitsky H (1994) Role of bone marrow-derived cells in presenting MHC class I-restricted tumor antigens. Science 264: 961–965

27. Hsu FJ, Benike C, Fagnoni F, Liles TM, Czerweinski D, Taidi B, Engleman EG, Levy R (1996) Vaccination of patients with B-cell lymphoma using autologous antigen-pulsed dendritic cells. Nat Med 2:52–58
28. Inaba K, Metlay JP, Crowley MT, Steinman RM (1990) Dendritic cells pulsed with protein antigens in vitro can prime antigen-specific, MHC-restricted T cells in situ. J Exp Med 172:631–640
29. Jiang W, Swiggard WJ, Heufler C, Peng M, Mirza A, Steinman RM, Nussenzweig MC (1995) The receptor DEC-205 expressed by dendritic cells and thymic epithelial cells is involved in antigen processing. Nature 375:151–155
30. June CH, Bluestone JA, Nadler LM, Thompson CB (1994) The B7 and CD28 receptor family. Immunol Today 15:321–331
31. Kast WM, Boog CJP, Roep OB, Voordouw AC, Melief CJM (1988) Failure of success in the restoration of virus-specific cytotoxic T lymphocyte response defects of dendritic cells. J Immunol 140:3186–3193
32. Klareskog L, Malmnäs-Tjerlund UM, Forsum U, Peterson PA (1977) Epidermal Langerhans cells express Ia antigens. Nature 268:248
33. Knight SC, Hunt R, Dore C, Medawar PB (1985) Influence of dendritic cells on tumor growth. Proc Natl Acad Sci USA 82:4495–4497
34. Larsen CP, Steinman RM, Witmer-Pack M, Hankins DF, Morris PJ, Austyn JM (1990) Migration and maturation of Langerhans cells in skin transplants and explants. J Exp Med 172:1483–1493
35. Mackensen A, Carcelain G, Viel S, Raynal M-C, Michalaki H, Triebel F, Bosq J, Hercend T (1994) Direct evidence to support the immunosurveillance concept in a human regressive melanoma. J Clin Invest 93:1391–1402
36. Maeurer MJ, Storkus WJ, Kirkwood JM, Lotze MT (1996) New treatment options for patients with melanoma: review of melanoma-derived T-cell epitope-based peptide vaccines. Melanoma Res 6:11–24
37. Marchand M, Weynants P, Rankin E, Arienti F, Belli F, Parmiani G, Cascinelli N, Bourland A, Vanwijck R, Humblet Y, Canon JL, Laurent C, Naeyaert JM, Plagne R, Deraemaeker R, Knuth A, Jäger E, Brasseur F, Herman J, Coulie PG, Boon T (1995) Tumor regression responses in melanoma patients vaccinated with a peptide encoded by gene MAGE-3. Int J Cancer 63: 883–885
38. Matzinger P (1994) Tolerance, danger, and the extended family. Annu Rev Immunol 12: 991–1045
39. Mayordomo JI, Zorina T, Storkus WJ, Zitvogel L, Celluzzi C, Falo LD, Melief CJ, Ildstad ST, Kast WM, Deleo AB, Lotze MT (1995) Bone marrow-derived dendritic cells pulsed with synthetic tumor peptides elicit protective and therapeutic antitumor immunity. Nature Med 1:1297–1302
40. Nestle FO, Zheng XG, Thompson CB, Turka LA, Nickoloff BJ (1993) Characterization of dermal dendritic cells obtained from normal human skin reveals phenotypic and functionally distinctive subsets (published erratum appears in J Immunol 1994; 152:376). J Immunol 151:6535–6545
41. Nestle FO, Burg G, Fäh J, Wrone-Smith T, Nickoloff BJ (1997) Human basal cell carcinoma associated dendritic cells are deficient in T cell co-stimulatory molecules and are impaired as antigen-presenting cells. Am J Pathol (in press)
42. Nijman HW, Kleijmer MJ, Ossevoort MA, Oorschot VMJ, Vierboom MPM, van der Keur M, Kenemans P, Kast WM, Geuze HJ, Melief CJM (1995) Antigen capture and major histocompatiblity class II compartments of freshly isolated and cultured human blood dendritic cells. J Immunol 182:163–174
43. Paglia P, Chiodoni C, Rodolfo M, Colombo MP (1996) Murine dendritic cells loaded in vitro with soluble protein prime cytotoxic T lymphocytes against tumor antigen in vivo. J Exp Med 183:317–322
44. Pardoll DM, Beckerleg AM (1995) Exposing the immunology of naked DNA vaccines. Immunity 3:165–169
45. Peters JH, Gieseler R, Thiele B, Steinbach F (1996) Dendritic cells: from ontogenetic orphans to myelomonocytic descendants. Immunol Today 17:273–278

46. Porgador A, Snyder D, Gilboa E (1996) Induction of antitumor immunity using bone marrow-generated dendritic cells. J Immunol 156:2918–2926
47. Pure E, Inaba K, Crowley MT, Tardelli L, Witmer-Pack MD, Ruberti G, Fathman G, Steinman RM (1990) Antigen processing by epidermal Langerhans cells corrlates with the level of biosynthesis of major histocompatibility complex class II molecules and expression of invariant chain. J Exp Med 172:1459–1469
48. Robbins PF, El-Gamil M, Kawakami Y, Rosenberg SA (1994) Recognition of tyrosinase by tumor-infiltrating lymphocytes from a patient responding to immunotherapy. Cancer Res 54:3124–3126
49. Romani N, Gruner S, Kämpgen E, Lenz A, Trockenbacher B, Konwalinka G, Fritsch PO, Steinman RM, Schuler G (1994) Proliferating dendritic cell progenitors in human blood. J Exp Med 180:83–93
50. Romerdahl CA, Okamoto H, Kripke ML (1989) Immune surveillance against cutaneous malignancies in experimental animals. Immunol Ser 46:749–767
51. Ruby JC, Halliday GM, Muller HK (1989) Differential effects of benzo[a]pyrene and dimethylbenz[a]-anthracene on Langerhans cell distribution and contact sensitization in murine epidermis. J Invest Dermatol 92:150–155
52. Sallusto F, Lanzavecchia A (1994) Efficient presentation of soluble antigen by cultured human dendritic cells is maintained by granulocyte/macrophage colony-stimulating factor plus interleukin-4 and downregulated by tumor necrosis factor-alpha. J Exp Med 179:1109–1118
53. Sallusto F, Cella M, Danieli C, Lanzavechia A (1995) Dendritic cells use macropinocytosis and the mannnose receptor to concentrate macromolecules in the major histocompatibility complex class II compartment: downregulation by cytokines and bacterial products. J Exp Med 182:389–400
54. Sensi M, Traversari C, Radrizzani M., Salvi S, Maccalli C, Mortarini R, Rivoltini L, Farina C, Nicolini G, Wölfel T, Brichard V, Boon T, Bordignon C, Anichini A, Parmiani G (1995) Cytotoxic T-lymphocyte clones from different patients display limited T-cell-receptor variable region usage in HLA-A2-restricted recognition of the melanoma antigen Melan A/MART-1. Proc Natl Acad Sci USA 92:5674–5678
55. Shimizu J, Suda T, Yoshioka T, Kosugi A, Fujiwara H, Hamaoka T (1989) Induction of tumor-specific in vivo protective immunity by immunization with tumor antigen-pulsed antigen-presenting cells. J Immunol 142:1053–1059
56. Soong SJ (1992) A computerized mathematical model and scoring system predicting outcome in patients with localized melanoma. In: Balch CM, Houghton AN, Milton GW, Sober AJ, Soong SJ (eds) Cutaneous melanoma. Lippincott, Philadelphia, pp 200–214
57. Steinman RM (1991) The dendritic cell system and its role in immunogenicity. Annu Rev Immunol 9:271–296
58. Steinman RM, Witmer MD (1978) Lymphoid dendritic cells are potent stimulators of the primary mixed leukocyte reaction. Proc Natl Acad Sci USA 75:5132–5136
59. Steinman RM, Gutchinov B, Witmer MD, Nussenzweig MC (1983) Dendritic cells are the principal stimulators of the primary mixed leucocyte reaction in mice. J Exp Med 157:613–627
60. Symington FW, Brady W, Linsely PS (1993) Expression and function of B7 on human epidermal Langerhans cells. J Immunol 150:1286–1295
61. Tan KC, Hosoi J, Grabbe S, Asahina A, Granstein RD (1994) Epidermal cell presentation of tumor-associated antigens for induction of tolerance. J Immunol 153:760–767
62. Veerman AJP (1974) On the interdigitating cells in the thymus-dependent area of the rat spleen: a relation between the mononuclear phagocyte system and T-lymphocytes. Cell Tissue Res 148:247–257
63. Yamashita U (1987) Dysfunction of Ia-positive antigen-presenting cells in tumor-bearing mice. Jpn J Cancer Res 78:261–269
64. Zitvogel L, Mayordomo JI, Tjandrawan T, Deleo AB, Clarke ML, Lotze MT, Storkus WJ (1996) Therapy of murine tumors with tumor peptide-pulsed dendritic cells: dependence on T cells, B7 costimulation, and T helper cell 1-associated cytokines. J Exp Med 183:87–97
65. Zou J, Shimizu J, Ikegame K et al (1992) Tumor-bearing mice exhibit a progressive increase in tumor antigen-presenting cell function and a reciprocal decrease in tumor antigen-responsive CD4+ T cell activity. J Immunol 148:648–655

Subject Index

A

Abortions, spontaneous 149
Acantholysis 217
Acitretin 329
Acyclovir 354
Adenovirus vectors 377
Adhesion molecules (ICAM-1) 91, 133, 135, 321
- intercellular 255
Adjuvant interferon therapy 296
Adjuvant melanoma therapy 357
Adjuvant therapy 163
β_2-Adrenoreceptor 132
Adrenocorticoids 131
Adverse 315
- events 73
- reactions 342
- type-1 leprosy reactions 316
AIDS 298
Allergen 273
Allergic contact dermatitis 55
Allergic rhinitis 243
Allergies 11
Allograft 105
Alopecia areata 35
Altered peptide ligands 9
Amyopathic DM 231
ANCA 267, 269
Angina tonsillaris 266
Angiogenesis 109, 257
Angiotensin-converting enzyme inhibitors 230
Anti-CD3 monoclonal antibody 278
Anti-CD4 monoclonal antibodies 233
Anti-inflammatory agent 67
Anti-inflammatory strategies 26
Anti-mouse antibodies 327
Anti-Tac (Fv)-PE38 81
Antibodies 256, 388
- neutralizing 297
Anticardiolipin antibodies 63
Anticytokine 62
Antigen presentation 400
Antigen-presenting cells (APC) 23, 137, 182, 196, 399
- professional (APC) 2, 254
Antiherpetic medications 353
Antimalarials 219
Antimaterial drugs 228
Antiphospholipid antibody 150
Antiphospholipid syndrome 148
Antiproliferative activity 72
Antisense 380
Antitumor immune responses 181, 189
Antiviral compounds 293
AP2 97
APC 4, 137, 184, 400
Apoptosis 91, 95, 136, 174, 343
Arthritis 72
Arthus reaction 263
Atopic allergic 11
Atopic dermatitis 35, 36, 93, 243
Atopic eczema 55, 104
Autoantibodies 63, 217
Autogenous vaccines 294
Autoimmune disease 7, 297
- reactions 254
- thrombocytopenic purpura 147
- thyroiditis 297
Autoimmunity 2
Azathioprine 218, 268, 287
AZT 352

B

B cell epitopes 223
B cell lymphomas 321
B lymphocytes 23
B7 (CD80/86) 2, 5, 104, 235, 378
$B7^+$ 378
B-7.1 378, 401
Bacillus Calmette-Guérin (BCG) 294, 314
Ballistic transfer 188
Basal cell carcinoma 163, 337
Basophils 139
BCG 358, 388
BCG vaccination 316
Bee venom phospholipase A2 136
Benign cutaneous PAN 232
Benign epidermoid cyst 341
bFGF 208

Biochemotherapy 174
Blisters 217
- subepidermal 221
Blueberry muffin rash 152
BNF-1 oncogene 256
Bone marrow transplantation (BMT) 327
- autologous 327
- patient 154
Borrelia 25, 230
BP180 221, 222
- antigen 222
Brain metastases 370
Bronchial asthma 243
Bullous pemphigoid 148, 150, 220
Bullous SLE 228
Bystander effect 379

C
Cachetin 169
Calcineurin 31
Calcium channel blocker 230
Calmette-Guérin 314
Camille-Guérin bacillus (BCG) 388
cAMP-phosphodiesterase 248
Captopril 220
Carcinoembryonic antigen 196
Cardiovascular disease 297
CD3 256
CD4 152, 256
- T cells 341
$CD4^+$ lymphocytes 307
CD8+ 181
- T lymphocytes 152
CD18-deficient polygenic mice 256
CD28 5, 235
CD30 174
CD40 171, 175
CD40L 175
Cell growth 342
Central tolerance 175
Cervical carcinoma 299
Cervical intraepithelial neoplasia (CIN) 294
Chemotaxis 63, 106
Chemotherapy 351
Childhood DM 231
CHS 108
Churg-Strauss granuloma 265, 267
Cimetidine 294, 298
CIN 300
CLA 23
- antigen 22
Clinical phase II studies 73
Clinical phase III studies 74
Clinical protocols 375
Clofazimine 288, 315
Colchicine 222, 268
Coley's toxins 169
Collagen 106, 133
Collagenase 92, 133
Combination therapy 329
Complement factors 267
Complement receptor 3 140
Condyloma 300
Condylomata 164
Connective tissue diseases 35
Connective tissue mast cells 136
Contact hypersensitivity (CHS) 103, 273
Contact sensitivity 273
Conventional treatment 312, 314
Corticosteroids 8, 131, 218, 220, 221, 227, 232, 258, 267, 284
Corynebacterium parvum 358
Costimulatory molecules 175, 400
Costimulatory pathway blockade 175, 235
Costimulatory signals 2, 182, 184, 378
Creutzfeldt-Jacob disease 154
Cromoglycate 285
Cryoglobulinemia 267
Cryosurgery 337
Cryotherapy 293, 295, 349
CTCL 120, 164
CTL (see also cytotoxic T lymphocyte) 182, 399, 404
CTL induction 189
CTLA-4 5
CTLA4Ig 236
Cutaneous B cell lymphomas (CBCL) 321
- immune system 21
- lymphomas 321
- necrotizing vasculitis 263
- necrotizing venulitis 263
- panarteritis nodosa 266
- T cell lymphomas (CTCL) 83, 93, 119, 321
Cyclin D1 256
Cyclo-oxygenase 133
Cyclophilin 31
Cyclophosphamide 218, 222, 230, 268, 288
Cyclosporine 219, 222, 236, 286
Cyclosporine A 29, 244, 254, 268, 284, 326
Cytokines 64, 132, 134, 207, 275, 321, 379
- gene transfer 375, 406
- induced immune modulation 236
- inducer (imiquimod) 294
- inhibitors 236
- receptors 91, 103
- synthesis inhibitory factor 277
Cytotoxic drugs 227
- T cells (CTL) 375
- T lymphocyte (see also CTL) 182
- T-cell responses (CTL) 195

D
D-penicillamine 220, 230
DAB 389 IL-2 83, 328
DAB 486 IL-2 327
DAB 486 α-melanocyte-stimulating hormone 80
DAB 486 interleukin (IL)-2 fusion toxin 80
Danger 24
Dapsone 219, 220, 221, 228, 268, 288, 315
Decoy IL-1 receptor 135
Dehydroorotate dehydrogenase 75
Delayed-type hypersensitivity (DTH) 104, 274
Delayed-type hypersensitivity reactions 47
Dendritic antigen-presenting cells 253
Dendritic cells 5, 23, 90, 104, 137, 254, 274, 330, 399
Dendritic epidermal T cells 275
Dermatitis herpetiformis 223
Dermatitis, palisaded neutrophilic and granulomatous 265
Dermatomyositis 150, 227, 231, 265
- juvenile 148
Desmocollin-1 220
Desmoglein-1 219
Desmoglein-3 217
Dihydrofolate reductase 59
Dinitrochlorobenzene (DNCB) 294, 387, 390
Diphteria toxin 80
Diphtheria toxin A 327
DNA photoproducts 96
- repair enzymes 96
- vaccination 315
- vaccines 195
DNCB 294, 390
Dosage 35
Dose response 392
Drug addict 296
DTIC 162
Dynamic component 22

E
E6 299
E7 299
E-selectin 135
Edema 140
Eicosanoid 134
ELAM 255
ELAM-1 104
Elastase 133
Electrosurgery 293
Endonucleases 132
Endothelial cells 22, 91, 104, 140
Endothelin-1 133
Endotoxic shock 172
Endotoxin 208
Eosinophil 139
Epidermal growth factor (EGF) 94
- receptor 343
Epidermal Langerhans cells 89
Epidermodysplasia verruciformis (EV) 294
Epidermolysis bullosa acquisita 148, 151, 220
Epitope-specific immunostimulatory therapy 294
Epitopes 203
Erysipelas 264
Erythema elevatum et diutinum 264
Erythema gyratum repens 264, 265
Etretinate 220, 329
Exotoxins 79
Extracellular matrix proteins 106

F
Facilitator 200
Fas 95, 96, 171
- antigen 343
- ligand 95, 343
FcεRI 23
Fc receptor 152
Fever 108
Fibroblasts 22, 90
Fibrosis 106
FK-506 43, 287
FK-506-binding proteins, FK-BP 53
Flaky skin mutant mice 256
Flow cytometric dot plot analysis 61
5-fluorouracil 293
Folliculitis 264
Fumagillin 353
Fusion protein 256
Fusion toxins 81, 327

G
Gancyclovir 354
Gastrointestinal symptom 74
Gene targeting 381
Gene therapy 175, 236, 383
- ex vivo 376
Gene-specific repair 97
Giant cell (temporal) arteritis 59, 269
γ-globulin 232
- intravenous 219
- therapy 232
Glucocorticoid 268
- receptor 131
- response elements 131
- therapy in AD, systemic 244
Glucocorticosteroid 131, 244
GM-CSF 5, 31, 132, 137, 139, 182, 351, 402
GMDP 209
Gold 219
gp100 (pmel17) 4, 181, 197, 198

gp75 4
Graft rejection 72
Graft-versus-host-disease (GVHD) 119, 147
Granulocyte-macrophage colony-stimulating factor (GM-CSF) 197
Granulocyte-monocyte colony-stimulating factor (GM-CSF) 351
Granulocytes 91
GVHD 154

H
H2 receptor antagonist 298
Hair loss, reversible 74
Hairy cell leukemia-associated PAN 233
Hapten-specific tolerance 104, 108
Haptens 273, 275
Heat-shock proteins 131
Henoch-Schönlein purpura 264, 267
Heparin 268
Heparin therapy, concurrent 297
Hepatitis B 266
Hepatitis C (cryo-globulinemic vasculitis) 264, 266
Hepatitis C virus 154
Hepatotoxicity 66
HHV-8 348
High-affinity IgE receptor (FceRI) 55
High-dose pulse steroid therapy 286
High-dose UVA1 therapy 89
Histocompatibility complex (MHC) class I 195
History of attacks or psychosis 297
HIV 154, 196, 307
HIV-positive individual 295, 296
HLA 181, 323
- alleles 254
- class II 93
HLA-B27 transgenic rats 256
Hodgkin's disease 174
HPV 293, 300
HPV infections
- latent 293
- subclinical 293
- vulva, persistent subclinical 299
HPV-16 viral capsid proteins L1 and L2 299
Human immunodeficiency virus (HIV) 102
Human Leishmaniasis, forms of 312
Human papillomaviruses (HPV) 293
Human T lymphotropic virus (HTLV)-1-associated adult T cell leukemia 82
Human-chorionic gonadotropin 353
Hypereosinophilia 139
Hypergammaglobulinemia 267
Hypersensitivity angiitis 263
Hypertrophic DLE 228

I
ICAM-1 93, 104, 133, 135, 341
IFN (Interferon) 132, 315
- antibodies 323
- contraindications 297
- intralesional injection 295
- parenterally in the form of intramuscular or subcutaneous injections 295
- therapy, intralesional 295
- topically as a gel 295
- treatment, continuous 296
- treatment, cyclic 296
IFN-α 161, 166, 323, 329
- BCC 163
- condylomata 164
- CTCL 164
- intralesional 391
- melanoma adjuvant therapy 163
- melanoma advanced 161
- melanoma palliative therapy 162
- SCC 164
- therapy 161
IFN-α_{2a} 342
IFN-α_{2b} 339
IFN-β 324, 387, 391
IFN-γ 91, 103, 165, 313, 314, 315, 317, 324, 340, 931
- production 324
- receptor 328
Ig synthesis 63
IgA 223
- deficiency 154
IgE 108, 136, 147, 243
IgE-recpeptor, high-affinity 55
IgG 136, 147
- polyclonal 152
IL-1β 276
IL-1 62, 93, 101, 132, 153, 276, 321, 328
- receptor 94
- receptor antagonist (IL-1ra) 62, 101, 153
IL-2 6, 132, 162, 182, 308, 314, 315, 317, 325, 359, 365, 388, 393
- PE 81
- receptor 81, 233, 256, 325
- soluble 325
- toxin 233
IL-3 132
IL-4 132, 322
IL-5 132, 139, 322
IL-6 91, 132, 208
IL-7 93, 188, 321
- receptor 328
IL-8 132, 328
- receptor 54
IL-10 10, 91, 92, 96, 103, 134, 182, 275, 277, 378, 402

IL-11 132
IL-12 104, 132, 188, 275, 314, 317, 329
IL-13 132
IL-1RI 94
IL-1RII 94
Imidazaquinolinamines 301
Imidazoquinolinamine derivative 298
Imiquimod 298
Immune intervention 1
- response 399
- system 258
Immunisation
- low zone 315
- schedule 190
Immunobullous diseases 35
Immunocompetent 301
Immunocompromised patient 295
Immunocytes 253
Immunodeficient 301
Immunofluorescence 217
- direct 217
Immunogenicity 2, 379
Immunoglobulin 268
Immunoglobulin therapy, intravenous 353
Immunologic microenvironment 22
Immunological activation 253
Immunological tolerance 223
Immunomodulation 25
Immunomodulator 298
Immunophillins 53
Immunosuppression 227, 297
Immunosuppressive strategies 26
Immunosuppressive treatment 284
Immunotherapy 387
- intralesionally 387
- intravenously 387
- local 387
- nonsystemically 387
- topical 387
Immunotherapeutic vaccination 316
Immunotoxins 79, 233
- therapy 175
Increased eosinophil survival 139
Indomethacin 268
Inducible protein (IP)-10 324
Infected tissue
- destruction of 293
- excision of 293
Inflammation 23
Inflammatory activation 253
- dendritic epidermal cells (IDEC) 23, 54
- edema 140
- skin diseases 59
Influenza A 195
Inhibitory κBα (IκBα) 133
Innocent bystanders 390
Inosine pranobex 294, 299
Integration 204
Intercellular adhesion molecule 255
Interferon (IFN) 245, 255, 294, 295, 322, 337, 359, 391
- intralesional 337
Interferon-α 268, 322, 349
Interferon-β 323
Interferon-γ 313, 324
Interleukin (see also IL)-1 91, 92
- (see also IL)-2 2, 30, 256, 325
Internal ribosomal entry sites (IRES) 199
Intraepidermal blisters 218
Intratumoral 388
IRES (see Internal ribosomal entry sites) 199
Irritation 273
Isotretinoin 329

J
Juvenile rheumatoid arthritis 150

K
Kaposi's sarcoma (KS) 166, 347
- African 347
- AIDS-associated 347
- epidemiological forms 347
- iatrogenic 347
Kawasaki disease 269
Kawasaki syndrome 148, 149
KC 33, 35
55-kD TNF receptor 172
75-kD TNF receptor 172
Keratinocytes 22, 90, 103, 134, 207, 253, 258, 275, 294, 321
Ki-1/CD30 anaplastic large cell lymphoma (ALCL) 174

L
L-tryptophan 229
LAK cell 325
Laminin-5 222
Langerhans cells (LC) 23, 54, 90, 104, 137, 274, 294, 401
Laser surgery 293
Leflunomide 8, 71
Leishmaniasis 311
Leishmanization 314
Leprosy 311
Leukocyte cyclic adenosine monophosphate (cAMP) phosphodiesterase (PDE) 248
Leukocytoclastic vasculitis 263
Leukocytosis 108
Leukotrienes 139
Levamisole 294
(LFA)-1 93
Lichen planus 35

Lipid A partial structure analogues 211
Lipocortin 132, 134
Lipopolysaccharide 169
Liposomal formulation 352
Lipotropic CTCL 324
5-lipoxygenase (5-LO) metabolites 64
Listeria monocytogenes 172
Livedo racemosa 266
- reticularis 266
- vasculitis 267
Local hypothermia 329
Long-term toxicity 66
Low zone immunisation 315
LT-α 170
LT-β 170
- receptor 170
Lupus erythematosus (hypergammaglobulinemic vasculitis) 29, 126, 227, 228, 264, 265
- systemic 148
Lupus nephritis 229
Lymph nodes 5
Lymphocyte activation, two-signal model of 2
Lymphocyte function-associated antigen (LFA)-1 255
Lymphocytes 23, 136
Lymphokine-activated killer (LAK) cells 353
Lymphoma 321

M
Macrolide 43, 53
Macrophage 137
- activating factor 324
- inflammatory protein 276
- migration inhibitory factor 135
MAGE 182, 197, 375
MAGE-1 4
Major histocompatibility complex (MHC) 2, 324
- class II alleles 294
Malignant melanoma 181
Malignant skin tumor 25
Malignant tumors 24
MART-1 (see Melanoma antigen recognized by T cells) 197, 375
Mast cells 91
MDP(Lys)GDP 211
MDP-LYS-L18 209
MDT (see also multidrug therapy) 315, 318
Melan A/MART-1 4, 371
Melanocortin (MC) receptors 107
Melanocyte lineage specific proteins 371
Melanocyte-stimulating hormone (MSH) 107
Melanoma 4, 103, 161, 181, 190, 202, 382, 387, 399
Melanoma antigen recognized by T cells (see MART) 197
Melanoma-associated antigen 404
Methotrexate 59, 218, 233, 254, 268
MHC 4, 7, 23
- antagonist peptides 234
- class II 137
- linkage 173
Migration inhibitory factor 132
Minocycline 289
MIP 308
MIP-1α 132
Miscellaneous 328
Mohs' micrographic surgery 340
Monoclonal antibodes (mAb) 79, 327
Monocytes 137
Mononeuritis multiplex 266
Morphea 229
MSH (α-MSH) 92, 109
MTP-PE 209
MTX
- mode of action of 65
- polyglutamates 66
Mucosal mast cells 136
Multidrug therapy (MDT) 315
Muramyl peptides 208
- derivatives 209
MY7 (CD13) 328
Myobacterium bovis 388
Mycobacterium ϖ vaccine 316, 318
Mycosis fungoides (MF) 323
Myocytes 196

N
Nail psoriasis 59
Natural killer (NK) 322
Necrosis 392
Negative feedback mechanism 25
Neoadjuvant therapy 362
Neuropeptides 91, 92, 107
Neutral endopeptidase 132
Neutrophilic skin disease 283
Neutrophils 140
NF-κB 31, 62, 133, 173
NF-AT 134
NF-ATp 53
Niacinamide 220, 221, 223
Nitric oxide synthase 135
NK cells 393
NK-1 receptors 133
Non-Hodgkin's lymphoma 82
Non-melanoma skin cancer 337
Non-self 24
Nonviral methods of gene transfer 377
Nuclear Factor-κB (see also NF-κB) 133
Nuclear transcription factors 176

O
Oligonucleotides 380
Omenn's syndrome 246

Oncogenes 380
Oral tolerization 235
Oxidative mechanism 97

P
Palpable purpura 263
Panarteritis nodosa 263
- classic 265
- microscopic 265
Pansclerotic morphea 230
Papillomavirus 293
Paraneoplastic DM 231
Parvovirus B19 infection, chronic 233
PDGF 208
PEG IL-2 394
Pemphigus 217
- erythematosus 219
- foliaceus 148
- vulgaris 122, 148, 151
Penicillin 230, 267
Penicillin G 230
Pentostatin 329
Peptide 3, 9, 234, 301, 405
Perforin-deficient mice 202
Perfusion 361
Peripheral tolerance 174
Peritumoral infiltrate 341
Phospholipase A2 133
Photocarcinogenesis 89
Photochemotherapy 89, 329
- extracorporeal 119, 329
Photoimmunology 89
- therapeutic 97
Photopheresis, extracorporeal 95, 219, 222
Phototherapy 89
Pityriasis lichenoides et varioliformis 59
Pityriasis rubra pilaris 59
PLA_2 134
Plasmapheresis 219, 268
Plasminogen activator 133
- inhibitor 132
Plasmocytoma 264
PMN accumulation 63
Podophyllin 293
Podophyllotoxin 293
Polyangiitis, microscopic 232
Polyarteritis nodosa 59, 227, 232
Polyclonal IgG 152
Polymyositis 150
Polyvinyl chloride 229
Prostaglandin E2 92, 248
Pregnancy 222, 297
Primary immune defects 243
Primary immune response 24
Prohormone convertase 107
Prolylhydroxylase inhibitors 230
Promoter 381, 405
Proopiomelanocortin 92
Proopiomelanocortin (POMC) 107
Prostanoids 91
Protooncogenes 380
Pruritus 299, 326
Pseudomonas exotoxin 81
Psoralen 120
Psoriasis 34, 35, 47, 55, 59, 71, 85, 89, 102, 297
- severe 59
PUVA 27, 89, 121
Pyoderma gangraenosum 35, 148, 151, 283

R
Radiotherapy 337, 349
RANTES 132, 138
Rapamycin 8, 54
Rash/allergic reaction 73
Receptors for hormones and cytokines 132
Recombinant BCG 389
Recombinant IFN (rIFN)-α_{2a}, given cyclically 296
Reiter's disease 59
Renal dysfunction 297
Renal transplant recipients 294
13-*cis*-Retinoic acid 329, 330
Reticuloendothelial system 152
Retinoids 228, 294, 298, 329, 353
Retroviral system 377
Retroviral vector 190
Rheumatoid arthritis (rheumatoid vasculitis) 29, 47, 59, 71, 103, 148, 150, 264, 265
- juvenile 150
Ribonucleases 132
Ribozymes 380
Rifampicin 315
rIFN-α treatment, cyclic 297
rIFN-α_{2a} treatment, continuous 297
Risk factors 66
Rotamases 31

S
SALT 23
SCF 132
SCID
- mice 257
- human skin chimeric animal model 257
Scl-70 229
Scleroderma 91, 125, 229
Secretory leukocyte inhibitory protein 132
Self 24
Self-Nonself discrimination 1
Sensitization 273
Serum IgE levels 245
Severe general disease 297
Sexually transmitted disease 348

Sézary syndrome 83, 95, 323, 329
Sialyl Lewis antigen 255
Side effects 65, 141, 297, 323, 326, 388
- of CsA 33
Sigma ligands 213
Silica 229
Singlet oxygen 95
Skin
- homing T cells 22
- immune response 25
- immune system 23
- infection 25
Soluble mediators 91
Somatostatin 136
Spanish rapseed oil 229
Spontaneous abortions 149
Squamous cell carcinoma 164, 337
- of the anus 299
- of the outer genitalia 299
- of the skin 299
- of the upper respiratory tract 299
Static component 22
Streptococcal 255
Streptomyces tsukubaensis 53
Subacute cutaneous LE 227
Superantigen 154, 255
Suppression of the immune response 7
Suppressor factors 101
Surgery 337
Sweet syndrome 264
Systemic (large vessel) vasculitis 264
Systemic sclerosis 227

T
T cell 134, 136
- epitopes 223
- nactivation 184
- proliferation 74
- receptor (TCR) 1
- subsets 11
T cell lymphoma 321
- cutaneous 82, 83
T helper cells 134
T lymphocytes 91, 152, 253, 404
T-101 327
T-helper (Th)1-type cytokine networks 258
Tac antigen 325
Tacrolimus (FK-506) 53
Takayasu's arteritis 59, 269
TCR 6, 22, 30
- vaccination 235
Teenage girl 299, 300
Tetracycline 220, 221, 223, 267
TGF-α 208
TGF-β 231
Th1 11, 25, 91, 104, 235, 243, 255, 311
- cells 311
- cytokines 311
- profile 322
- type cells 134
Th1/Th2 dichotomy 25
Th2 11, 25, 94, 235, 243, 278, 311
- cells 311
- cytokine pattern 322
- cytokine profile 322
- type cells 134
Th3 11
Therapy regimen 296
Thrombocytes, low levels of 297
Thrombocytopenic purpura 297
Thymine dimers 96
Thymopentin 328
Thymopoietin 247, 328
TNF 236, 328
- receptor 94
TNF-α 31, 132, 153, 169, 208, 308, 351, 392
- gene polymorphism 173
- inhibitors 172
TNFR 170
Tolerance 72, 273
Topical immunotherapy 387
Topical treatment 324
Total cumulative dose 67
Toxicity 328
Transforming growth factor (TGF)-β 105, 106
Transcription factor activator Protein-1 133
Transcription factors 133
Transduction 376
Transfection 405
- of cytokine genes 402
Transformation 326
Transgenic mouse 104
Treponema 25
Trichloroacetic acid 293
Triplex-forming DNA 380
Tumor
- antigens 181, 401, 402, 403, 405
- associated antigen 402
- Buschke-Löwenstein 295
- cell vaccines 185, 190
- cells, terminal differentiation of 343
- immunity 188, 189, 402, 403
- immunology 3
- infiltrating APC 401
- large 295
- necrosis factor (TNF) 150, 343
- necrosis factor (TNF)-α 102, 392
- regression 343
- rejection 184, 188
- specific antigens 3
Type-2 leprosy 315

Tyrosinase 4, 181, 371, 375
Tyrosine kinase (TK) 75, 379

U
Ultraviolet (UV) light 101
Urticarial vasculitis 264
UV irradiation 401
UV-treated skin 274
UVA 27, 89
UVA1 therapy, high-dose 89
UVB 27, 89
- 311-nm 89

V
Vβ genes 254
Vaccination 184, 189, 293, 316, 330, 399
- CTL epitope 301
- immunotherapeutic 316
- population-based 299
- therapy 330
Vaccines 299
- DNA 301
- live virus expression vector-based 301
- prophylactic 299, 301
- subunit 301
- synthetic peptide-based 301
- therapeutic 299
Vascular cell adhesion molecule 255
Vascular permeability 140
Vasculitis 59
- leukocytoclastic 263
- systemic 149
Vasculitis allergica 263
Vasocortin 132
VDEPT 379
Vector 198
Vector system 375
Vestibulitis 295
Vinblastine 351
Vincristine 351
Viral-persistence phase 300
Virus-like particles (VLP) 300
Vitamin A 298
Vitamin A acid, local 295
Vitiligo 370
VLP 301
Vulvodynia 295

W
Warts 293
- calcitrant anogenital 295
- facial flat 295
- genital 295
Wegener's granulomatosis 264
Weight loss 74
Winiwarter Bürger disease 269
Wound healing 107, 308

X
X-linked hyper-IgM syndrome 171